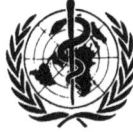

WORLD HEALTH ORGANIZATION

INTERNATIONAL AGENCY FOR RESEARCH ON CANCER

IARC MONOGRAPHS

ON THE

EVALUATION OF CARCINOGENIC

RISKS TO HUMANS

*Occupational Exposures in Insecticide Application,
and Some Pesticides*

VOLUME 53

This publication represents the views and expert opinions
of an IARC Working Group on the
Evaluation of Carcinogenic Risks to Humans,
which met in Lyon,

16-23 October 1990

1991

IARC MONOGRAPHS

In 1969, the International Agency for Research on Cancer (IARC) initiated a programme on the evaluation of the carcinogenic risk of chemicals to humans involving the production of critically evaluated monographs on individual chemicals. In 1980 and 1986, the programme was expanded to include the evaluation of the carcinogenic risk associated with exposures to complex mixtures and other agents.

The objective of the programme is to elaborate and publish in the form of monographs critical reviews of data on carcinogenicity for agents to which humans are known to be exposed, and on specific exposure situations; to evaluate these data in terms of human risk with the help of international working groups of experts in chemical carcinogenesis and related fields; and to indicate where additional research efforts are needed.

This project is supported by PHS Grant No. 2UO1CA33193-09 awarded by the US National Cancer Institute, Department of Health and Human Services. Additional support has been provided since 1986 by the Commission of the European Communities.

ISBN 92 832 1253-3

ISSN 0250-9555

Distributed for the International Agency for Research on Cancer
by the Secretariat of the World Health Organization

PRINTED IN THE UK

CONTENTS

CONTENTS

NOTE TO THE READER

The term 'carcinogenic risk' in the *IARC Monographs* series is taken to mean the probability that exposure to an agent will lead to cancer in humans.

Inclusion of an agent in the *Monographs* does not imply that it is a carcinogen, only that the published data have been examined. Equally, the fact that an agent has not yet been evaluated in a monograph does not mean that it is not carcinogenic.

The evaluations of carcinogenic risk are made by international working groups of independent scientists and are qualitative in nature. No recommendation is given for regulation or legislation.

Anyone who is aware of published data that may alter the evaluation of the carcinogenic risk of an agent to humans is encouraged to make this information available to the Unit of Carcinogen Identification and Evaluation, International Agency for Research on Cancer, 150 cours Albert Thomas, 69372 Lyon Cedex 08, France, in order that the agent may be considered for re-evaluation by a future Working Group.

Although every effort is made to prepare the monographs as accurately as possible, mistakes may occur. Readers are requested to communicate any errors to the Unit of Carcinogen Identification and Evaluation, so that corrections can be reported in future volumes.

IARC WORKING GROUP ON THE EVALUATION
OF CARCINOGENIC RISKS TO HUMANS:
OCCUPATIONAL EXPOSURES IN INSECTICIDE APPLICATION, AND SOME PESTICIDES

Lyon, 16-23 October 1990

LIST OF PARTICIPANTS

Members[1]

U.G. Ahlborg, Unit of Toxicology, National Institute of Environmental Medicine, Karolinska Institute, Box 60208, 10401 Stockholm, Sweden

N.O. Bianchi, Multidisciplinary Institute of Cellular Biology, CC 403, 1900 La Plata, Argentina

E. Bingham, Department of Environmental Health, Kettering Laboratory, University of Cincinnati Medical Center, 3223 Eden Avenue, Cincinnati, OH 45267, USA (*Chairperson*)

A. Blair, Occupational Studies Section, Environmental Epidemiology Branch, National Cancer Institute, Executive Plaza North, Room 418, Bethesda, MD 20892, USA

J.R. Bucher, National Toxicology Program, National Institute of Environmental Health Sciences, PO Box 12233, Research Triangle Park, NC 27709, USA

L. Dencker, Institute of Toxicology, Biomedical Center, Uppsala University, Box 594, 75123 Uppsala, Sweden

R. Greenhalgh, Xenos Laboratories Inc., 2319 St-Laurent Blvd, Unit 100, Ottawa, Ontario, Canada K1G 4K6

J. Jeyaratnam, Department of Community, Occupational and Family Medicine, National University of Singapore, Lower Kent Ridge Road, Singapore 0511, Republic of Singapore

W.M.F. Jongen, Agrotechnical Research Institute, Haagsteeg 6, Mailbox 17, 6700 AA Wageningen, The Netherlands

---

[1]Unable to attend, M.S. Rao, Department of Pathology, Northwestern University Medical School, Ward Memorial Building, 303 East Chicago Avenue, Chicago, IL 60611, USA

M. Lotti, Institute of Occupational Medicine, University of Padua, via Facciolati 71, 35127 Padua, Italy

E. Lynge, Danish Cancer Registry, Institute of Cancer Epidemiology, Rosenvaengets Hovedvej 5, Box 839, 2100 Copenhagen Ø, Denmark

D.R. Mattison, Graduate School of Public Health, University of Pittsburgh, Room 111, Parran Hall, 130 DeSoto Street, Pittsburgh, PA 15261, USA

N.E. Pearce, Department of Medicine, Wellington School of Medicine, University of Otago, PO Box 7343, Wellington South, New Zealand

B. Priestly, Department of Clinical and Experimental Pharmacology, University of Adelaide, Box 498 GPO, Adelaide, SA 5001, Australia

J.P. Seiler, Department of Medicine, Intercantonal Control Point for Drugs, Erlachstrasse 8, 3000 Bern 9, Switzerland

M. Sorsa, Department of Industrial Hygiene and Toxicology, Institute of Occupational Health, Topeliuksenkatu 41 a A, 00250 Helsinki, Finland

T. Shirai, Department of Pathology, Nagoya City University Medical School, 1 Kawasumi, Mizuho-cho, Mizuho-ku, Nagoya 467, Japan

H.D. Tandon, B7/8 Safdarjung Enclave, New Delhi 110029, India

V.S. Turusov, Cancer Research Centre, USSR Academy of Medical Sciences, Karshirskoye Shosse 24, 115478 Moscow, USSR (*Vice-Chairperson*)

P. Vineis, Unit of Cancer Epidemiology, Department of Biomedical Science and Human Oncology, via Santena 7, 10126 Turin, Italy

M. Wassermann, Department of Occupational Health, The Hebrew University, Hadassah Medical School, PO Box 1172, 91010 Jerusalem, Israel

M.D. Waters, Genetic Toxicology Division (MD-68), Environmental Protection Agency, Health Effects Research Laboratory, Research Triangle Park, NC 27711, USA

Representative and observers[1]

Representative of ILSI Risk Science Institute

S. Olin, International Life Sciences Institute Risk Science Institute, 1126 Sixteenth Street NW, Washington DC 20036, USA

Commission of the European Communities

C. Griffiths, DG XI/A/2, Commission of the European Communities, Breydel 6th Floor/234, 200 rue de la Loi, 1049 Brussels, Belgium

J. Osman, Health and Safety Executive, Magdalen House, Room 236, Stanley Precinct, Bootle, L20 39Z Merseyside, United Kingdom

---

[1]Unable to attend, S.M. Sieber, Division of Cancer Etiology, National Cancer Institute, Building 31, Room 11A03, Bethesda, MD 20892, USA

US Environmental Protection Agency

R. Engler, US Environmental Protection Agency (H7509C), 401 M Street SW, Washington DC 20460, USA

International Group of National Associations of Manufacturers of Agrochemical Products

G.R. Gardiner, International Group of National Associations of Manufacturers of Agrochemical Products, 79a avenue Albert Lancaster, 1180 Brussels, Belgium

A. Pelfrène, International Registration and Regulatory Affairs, Agchem Division, Pennwalt France SA, 1 rue des Frères Lumière, 78370 Plaisir, France

European Chemical Industry, Ecology and Toxicology Centre

J. Ishmael, Imperial Chemical Industries Plc, Central Toxicology Laboratory, Alderley Park, Macclesfield, Cheshire SK10 4TJ, United Kingdom

US National Agricultural Chemicals Association

J.F. McCarthy, Scientific & Regulatory Affairs, National Agricultural Chemicals Association, 7249 Wapello Drive, Rockville, MD 20855, USA

National Veterinary School of Lyon

G. Keck, National Veterinary School of Lyon, Route de Sain Bel, Marcy l'Etoile, 69260 Charbonnières les Bains, France

Secretariat

International Programme on Chemical Safety/World Health Organization

R. Plestina, Division of Environmental Health, International Programme on Chemical Safety, World Health Organization, 1211 Geneva 27, Switzerland

IARC

P. Boffetta, Unit of Analytical Epidemiology
J.R.P. Cabral, Unit of Mechanisms of Carcinogenesis
E. Cardis, Unit of Biostatistics Research and Informatics
M. Friesen, Unit of Environmental Carcinogenesis and Host Factors
M.-J. Ghess, Unit of Carcinogen Identification and Evaluation
E. Heseltine, Lajarthe, St Léon-sur-Vézère, France
M. Kogevinas, Unit of Analytical Epidemiology
V. Krutovskikh, Unit of Mechanisms of Carcinogenesis

M. Marselos, Unit of Carcinogen Identification and Evaluation[1]
D. McGregor, Unit of Carcinogen Identification and Evaluation
D. Mietton, Unit of Carcinogen Identification and Evaluation
G. Nordberg, Unit of Carcinogen Identification and Evaluation[2]
I. O'Neill, Unit of Environmental Carcinogenesis and Host Factors
C. Partensky, Unit of Carcinogen Identification and Evaluation
I. Peterschmitt, Unit of Carcinogen Identification and Evaluation, Geneva
D. Shuker, Unit of Environmental Carcinogenesis and Host Factors
L. Shuker, Unit of Carcinogen Identification and Evaluation
S. Swierenga, Unit of Carcinogen Identification and Evaluation[3]
L. Tomatis, Director
H. Vainio, Chief, Unit of Carcinogen Identification and Evaluation
J. Wilbourn, Unit of Carcinogen Identification and Evaluation
H. Yamasaki, Unit of Mechanisms of Carcinogenesis

Secretarial assistance

J. Cazeaux
M. Lézère
M. Mainaud
S. Reynaud
S. Ruiz

---

[1]Present address: Department of Pharmacology, Medical School, University of Ioannina, 45110 Ioannina, Greece
[2]Present address: Department of Environmental Medicine, University of Umeå, 901 87 Umeå, Sweden
[3]Present address: Health and Welfare Canada, Drugs Directorate, Tunney's Pasture, Ottawa, Ontario, Canada K1A OL2

PREAMBLE

IARC MONOGRAPHS PROGRAMME ON THE EVALUATION
OF CARCINOGENIC RISKS TO HUMANS[1]

PREAMBLE

1. BACKGROUND

In 1969, the International Agency for Research on Cancer (IARC) initiated a programme to evaluate the carcinogenic risk of chemicals to humans and to produce monographs on individual chemicals. The *Monographs* programme has since been expanded to include consideration of exposures to complex mixtures of chemicals (which occur, for example, in some occupations and as a result of human habits) and of exposures to other agents, such as radiation and viruses. With Supplement 6 (IARC, 1987a), the title of the series was modified from *IARC Monographs on the Evaluation of the Carcinogenic Risk of Chemicals to Humans* to *IARC Monographs on the Evaluation of Carcinogenic Risks to Humans*, in order to reflect the widened scope of the programme.

The criteria established in 1971 to evaluate carcinogenic risk to humans were adopted by the working groups whose deliberations resulted in the first 16 volumes of the *IARC Monographs* series. Those criteria were subsequently re-evaluated by working groups which met in 1977 (IARC, 1977), 1978 (IARC, 1978), 1979 (IARC, 1979), 1982 (IARC, 1982) and 1983 (IARC, 1983). The present preamble was prepared by two working groups which met in September 1986 and January 1987, prior to the preparation of Supplement 7 (IARC, 1987b) to the *Monographs* and was modified by a working group which met in November 1988 (IARC, 1988).

2. OBJECTIVE AND SCOPE

The objective of the programme is to prepare, with the help of international working groups of experts, and to publish in the form of monographs, critical reviews and evaluations of evidence on the carcinogenicity of a wide range of human exposures. The *Monographs* may also indicate where additional research efforts are needed.

The *Monographs* represent the first step in carcinogenic risk assessment, which involves examination of all relevant information in order to assess the strength of the available

[1]This project is supported by PHS Grant No. 2 UO1 CA33193-09 awarded by the US National Cancer Institute, Department of Health and Human Services, and with a subcontract to ILSI Risk Science Institute. Since 1986, this programme has also been supported by the Commission of the European Communities.

evidence that certain exposures could alter the incidence of cancer in humans. The second step is quantitative risk estimation, which is not usually attempted in the *Monographs*. Detailed, quantitative evaluations of epidemiological data may be made in the *Monographs*, but without extrapolation beyond the range of the data available. Quantitative extrapolation from experimental data to the human situation is not undertaken.

The term 'carcinogen' is used in these monographs to denote an agent or mixture that is capable of increasing the incidence of malignant neoplasms; the induction of benign neoplasms may in some circumstances (see p. 22) contribute to the judgement that the exposure is carcinogenic. The terms 'neoplasm' and 'tumour' are used interchangeably.

Some epidemiological and experimental studies indicate that different agents may act at different stages in the carcinogenic process, probably by fundamentally different mechanisms. In the present state of knowledge, the aim of the *Monographs* is to evaluate evidence of carcinogenicity at any stage in the carcinogenic process independently of the underlying mechanism involved. There is as yet insufficient information to implement classification according to mechanisms of action (IARC, 1983).

The monographs may assist national and international authorities in making risk assessments and in formulating decisions concerning any necessary preventive measures. The evaluations of IARC working groups are scientific, qualitative judgements about the degree of evidence for carcinogenicity provided by the available data on an agent. These evaluations represent only one part of the body of information on which regulatory measures may be based. Other components of regulatory decisions may vary from one situation to another and from country to country, responding to different socioeconomic and national priorities. *Therefore, no recommendation is given with regard to regulation or legislation, which are the responsibility of individual governments and/or other international organizations.*

The *IARC Monographs* are recognized as an authoritative source of information on the carcinogenicity of chemicals and complex exposures. A users' survey, made in 1988, indicated that the *Monographs* are consulted by various agencies in 57 countries. Each volume is generally printed in 4000 copies for distribution to governments, regulatory bodies and interested scientists. The *Monographs* are also available *via* the Distribution and Sales Service of the World Health Organization.

3. SELECTION OF TOPICS FOR MONOGRAPHS

Topics are selected on the basis of two main criteria: (a) that they concern agents and complex exposures for which there is evidence of human exposure, and (b) that there is some evidence or suspicion of carcinogenicity. The term agent is used to include individual chemical compounds, groups of chemical compounds, physical agents (such as radiation) and biological factors (such as viruses) and mixtures of agents such as occur in occupational exposures and as a result of personal and cultural habits (like smoking and dietary practices). Chemical analogues and compounds with biological or physical characteristics similar to those of suspected carcinogens may also be considered, even in the absence of data on carcinogenicity.

The scientific literature is surveyed for published data relevant to an assessment of carcinogenicity; the IARC surveys of chemicals being tested for carcinogenicity (IARC, 1973-1990) and directories of on-going research in cancer epidemiology

(IARC, 1976-1989/90) often indicate those exposures that may be scheduled for future meetings. An ad-hoc working group convened by IARC in 1984 gave recommendations as to which chemicals and exposures to complex mixtures should be evaluated in the *IARC Monographs* series (IARC, 1984, 1989).

As significant new data on subjects on which monographs have already been prepared become available, re-evaluations are made at subsequent meetings, and revised monographs are published.

4. DATA FOR MONOGRAPHS

The *Monographs* do not necessarily cite all the literature concerning the subject of an evaluation. Only those data considered by the Working Group to be relevant to making the evaluation are included.

With regard to biological and epidemiological data, only reports that have been published or accepted for publication in the openly available scientific literature are reviewed by the working groups. In certain instances, government agency reports that have undergone peer review and are widely available are considered. Exceptions may be made on an ad-hoc basis to include unpublished reports that are in their final form and publicly available, if their inclusion is considered pertinent to making a final evaluation (see pp. 25 *et seq.*). In the sections on chemical and physical properties, on analysis, on production and use and on occurrence, unpublished sources of information may be used.

5. THE WORKING GROUP

Reviews and evaluations are formulated by a working group of experts. The tasks of this group are five-fold: (i) to ascertain that all appropriate data have been collected; (ii) to select the data relevant for the evaluation on the basis of scientific merit; (iii) to prepare accurate summaries of the data to enable the reader to follow the reasoning of the Working Group; (iv) to evaluate the results of experimental and epidemiological studies; and (v) to make an overall evaluation of the carcinogenicity of the exposure to humans.

Working Group participants who contributed to the considerations and evaluations within a particular volume are listed, with their addresses, at the beginning of each publication. Each participant who is a member of a working group serves as an individual scientist and not as a representative of any organization, government or industry. In addition, representatives from national and international agencies and industrial associations may be invited as observers.

6. WORKING PROCEDURES

Approximately one year in advance of a meeting of a working group, the topics of the monographs are announced and participants are selected by IARC staff in consultation with other experts. Subsequently, relevant biological and epidemiological data are collected by IARC from recognized sources of information on carcinogenesis, including data storage and retrieval systems such as CHEMICAL ABSTRACTS, MEDLINE and TOXLINE— including EMIC and ETIC for data on genetic and related effects and teratogenicity, respectively.

The major collection of data and the preparation of first drafts of the sections on chemical and physical properties, on analysis, on production and use and on occurrence are carried out under a separate contract funded by the US National Cancer Institute. Efforts are made to supplement this information with data from other national and international sources. Representatives from industrial associations may assist in the preparation of sections on production and use.

Information on production and trade is obtained from governmental and trade publications and, in some cases, by direct contact with industries. Separate production data on some agents may not be available because their publication could disclose confidential information. Information on uses is usually obtained from published sources but is often complemented by direct contact with manufacturers.

Six months before the meeting, reference material is sent to experts, or is used by IARC staff, to prepare sections for the first drafts of monographs. The complete first drafts are compiled by IARC staff and sent, prior to the meeting, to all participants of the Working Group for review.

The Working Group meets in Lyon for seven to eight days to discuss and finalize the texts of the monographs and to formulate the evaluations. After the meeting, the master copy of each monograph is verified by consulting the original literature, edited and prepared for publication. The aim is to publish monographs within nine months of the Working Group meeting.

The available studies are summarized by the Working Group, with particular regard to the qualitative aspects discussed below. In general, numerical findings are indicated as they appear in the original report; units are converted when necessary for easier comparison. The Working Group may conduct additional analyses of the published data and use them in their assessment of the evidence and may include them in their summary of a study; the results of such supplementary analyses are given in square brackets. Any comments are also made in square brackets; however, these are kept to a minimum, being restricted to those instances in which it is felt that an important aspect of a study, directly impinging on its interpretation, should be brought to the attention of the reader.

7. EXPOSURE DATA

Sections that indicate the extent of past and present human exposure, the sources of exposure, the persons most likely to be exposed and the factors that contribute to exposure to the agent, mixture or exposure circumstance are included at the beginning of each monograph.

Most monographs on individual chemicals or complex mixtures include sections on chemical and physical data, on analysis, on production and use and on occurrence. In monographs on, for example, physical agents, biological factors, occupational exposures and cultural habits, other sections may be included, such as: historical perspectives, description of an industry or habit, exposures in the work place or chemistry of the complex mixture.

The Chemical Abstracts Services Registry Number, the latest Chemical Abstracts Primary Name and the IUPAC Systematic Name are recorded. Other synonyms are given, but the list is not necessarily comprehensive.

Information on chemical and physical properties and, in particular, data relevant to identification, occurrence and biological activity are included. A description of technical products includes trades names, relevant specifications and available information on composition and impurities. Some of the trade names given may be those of mixtures in which the agent being evaluated is only one of the ingredients.

The purpose of the section on analysis is to give the reader an overview of current methods cited in the literature, with emphasis on those widely used for regulatory purposes. No critical evaluation or recommendation of any of the methods is meant or implied. Methods for monitoring human exposure are also given, when available. The IARC publishes a series of volumes, *Environmental Carcinogens: Methods of Analysis and Exposure Measurement (IARC, 1978-1988)*, that describe validated methods for analysing a wide variety of agents and mixtures.

The dates of first synthesis and of first commercial production of a chemical or mixture are provided; for agents which do not occur naturally, this information may allow a reasonable estimate to be made of the date before which no human exposure to the agent could have occurred. The dates of first reported occurrence of an exposure are also provided. In addition, methods of synthesis used in past and present commercial production and different methods of production which may give rise to different impurities are described.

Data on production, foreign trade and uses are obtained for representative regions, which usually include Europe, Japan and the USA. It should not, however, be inferred that those areas or nations are necessarily the sole or major sources or users of the agent being evaluated.

Some identified uses may not be current or major applications, and the coverage is not necessarily comprehensive. In the case of drugs, mention of their therapeutic uses does not necessarily represent current practice nor does it imply judgement as to their clinical efficacy.

Information on the occurrence of an agent or mixture in the environment is obtained from data derived from the monitoring and surveillance of levels in occupational environments, air, water, soil, foods and animal and human tissues. When available, data on the generation, persistence and bioaccumulation of the agent are also included. In the case of mixtures, industries, occupations or processes, information is given about all agents present. For processes, industries and occupations, a historical description is also given, noting variations in chemical composition, physical properties or levels of occupational exposure with time.

Statements concerning regulations and guidelines (e.g., pesticide registrations, maximal levels permitted in foods, occupational exposure limits) are included for some countries as indications of potential exposures, but they may not reflect the most recent situation, since such limits are continuously reviewed and modified. The absence of information on regulatory status for a country should not be taken to imply that that country does not have regulations with regard to the exposure.

8. STUDIES OF CANCER IN HUMANS

(a) Types of studies considered

Three types of epidemiological studies of cancer contribute to the assessment of carcinogenicity in humans—cohort studies, case-control studies and correlation studies.

Rarely, results from randomized trials may be available. Case reports of cancer in humans may also be reviewed.

Cohort and case-control studies relate individual exposures under study to the occurrence of cancer in individuals and provide an estimate of relative risk (ratio of incidence in those exposed to incidence in those not exposed) as the main measure of association.

In correlation studies, the units of investigation are usually whole populations (e.g., in particular geographical areas or at particular times), and cancer frequency is related to a summary measure of the exposure of the population to the agent, mixture or exposure circumstance under study. Because individual exposure is not documented, however, a causal relationship is less easy to infer from correlation studies than from cohort and case-control studies. Case reports generally arise from a suspicion, based on clinical experience, that the concurrence of two events—that is, a particular exposure and occurrence of a cancer—has happened rather more frequently than would be expected by chance. Case reports usually lack complete ascertainment of cases in any population, definition or enumeration of the population at risk and estimation of the expected number of cases in the absence of exposure. The uncertainties surrounding interpretation of case reports and correlation studies make them inadequate, except in rare instances, to form the sole basis for inferring a causal relationship. When taken together with case-control and cohort studies, however, relevant case reports or correlation studies may add materially to the judgement that a causal relationship is present.

Epidemiological studies of benign neoplasms and presumed preneoplastic lesions are also reviewed by working groups. They may, in some instances, strengthen inferences drawn from studies of cancer itself.

(b) Quality of studies considered

The monographs are not intended to summarize all published studies. Those that are judged to be inadequate or irrelevant to the evaluation are generally omitted. They may be mentioned briefly, particularly when the information is considered to be a useful supplement to that in other reports or when they provide the only data available. Their inclusion does not imply acceptance of the adequacy of the study design or of the analysis and interpretation of the results, and limitations are clearly outlined in square brackets at the end of the study description.

It is necessary to take into account the possible roles of bias, confounding and chance in the interpretation of epidemiological studies. By 'bias' is meant the operation of factors in study design or execution that lead erroneously to a stronger or weaker association than in fact exists between disease and an agent, mixture or exposure circumstance. By 'confounding' is meant a situation in which the relationship with disease is made to appear stronger or to appear weaker than it truly is as a result of an association between the apparent causal factor and another factor that is associated with either an increase or decrease in the incidence of the disease. In evaluating the extent to which these factors have been minimized in an individual study, working groups consider a number of aspects of design and analysis as described in the report of the study. Most of these considerations apply equally to case-control, cohort and correlation studies. Lack of clarity of any of these aspects in the reporting of a study can decrease its credibility and its consequent weighting in the final evaluation of the exposure.

Firstly, the study population, disease (or diseases) and exposure should have been well defined by the authors. Cases in the study population should have been identified in a way that was independent of the exposure of interest, and exposure should have been assessed in a way that was not related to disease status.

Secondly, the authors should have taken account in the study design and analysis of other variables that can influence the risk of disease and may have been related to the exposure of interest. Potential confounding by such variables should have been dealt with either in the design of the study, such as by matching, or in the analysis, by statistical adjustment. In cohort studies, comparisons with local rates of disease may be more appropriate than those with national rates. Internal comparisons of disease frequency among individuals at different levels of exposure should also have been made in the study.

Thirdly, the authors should have reported the basic data on which the conclusions are founded, even if sophisticated statistical analyses were employed. At the very least, they should have given the numbers of exposed and unexposed cases and controls in a case-control study and the numbers of cases observed and expected in a cohort study. Further tabulations by time since exposure began and other temporal factors are also important. In a cohort study, data on all cancer sites and all causes of death should have been given, to avoid the possibility of reporting bias. In a case-control study, the effects of investigated factors other than the exposure of interest should have been reported.

Finally, the statistical methods used to obtain estimates of relative risk, absolute cancer rates, confidence intervals and significance tests, and to adjust for confounding should have been clearly stated by the authors. The methods used should preferably have been the generally accepted techniques that have been refined since the mid-1970s. These methods have been reviewed for case-control studies (Breslow & Day, 1980) and for cohort studies (Breslow & Day, 1987).

(c) Quantitative considerations

Detailed analyses of both relative and absolute risks in relation to age at first exposure and to temporal variables, such as time since first exposure, duration of exposure and time since exposure ceased, are reviewed and summarized when available. The analysis of temporal relationships can provide a useful guide in formulating models of carcinogenesis. In particular, such analyses may suggest whether a carcinogen acts early or late in the process of carcinogenesis (IARC, 1983), although such speculative inferences cannot be used to draw firm conclusions concerning the mechanisms of action and hence the shape (linear or otherwise) of the dose-response relationship below the range of observation.

(d) Criteria for causality

After the quality of individual epidemiological studies has been summarized and assessed, a judgement is made concerning the strength of evidence that the agent, mixture or exposure circumstance in question is carcinogenic for humans. In making their judgement, the Working Group considers several criteria for causality. A strong association (i.e., a large relative risk) is more likely to indicate causality than a weak association, although it is recognized that relative risks of small magnitude do not imply lack of causality and may be important if the disease is common. Associations that are replicated in several studies of the same design or using different epidemiological approaches or under different circumstances of exposure are more likely to represent a causal relationship than isolated observations from single studies. If there are inconsistent results among investigations, possible reasons are sought (such as differences in amount of exposure), and results of studies judged to be of high quality are given more weight than those from studies judged to be methodologically less sound. When suspicion of carcinogenicity arises largely from a single study, these data are not combined with those from later studies in any subsequent reassessment of the strength of the evidence.

If the risk of the disease in question increases with the amount of exposure, this is considered to be a strong indication of causality, although absence of a graded response is not necessarily evidence against a causal relationship. Demonstration of a decline in risk after cessation of or reduction in exposure in individuals or in whole populations also supports a causal interpretation of the findings.

Although a carcinogen may act upon more than one target, the specificity of an association (i.e., an increased occurrence of cancer at one anatomical site or of one morphological type) adds plausibility to a causal relationship, particularly when excess cancer occurrence is limited to one morphological type within the same organ.

Although rarely available, results from randomized trials showing different rates among exposed and unexposed individuals provide particularly strong evidence for causality.

When several epidemiological studies show little or no indication of an association between an exposure and cancer, the judgement may be made that, in the aggregate, they show evidence of lack of carcinogenicity. Such a judgement requires first of all that the studies giving rise to it meet, to a sufficient degree, the standards of design and analysis described above. Specifically, the possibility that bias, confounding or misclassification of exposure or outcome could explain the observed results should be considered and excluded with reasonable certainty. In addition, all studies that are judged to be methodologically sound should be consistent with a relative risk of unity for any observed level of exposure and, when considered together, should provide a pooled estimate of relative risk which is at or near unity and has a narrow confidence interval, due to sufficient population size. Moreover, no individual study nor the pooled results of all the studies should show any consistent tendency for relative risk of cancer to increase with increasing level of exposure. It is important to note that evidence of lack of carcinogenicity obtained in this way from several epidemiological studies can apply only to the type(s) of cancer studied and to dose levels and intervals between first exposure and observation of disease that are the same as or less than those observed in all the studies. Experience with human cancer indicates that, in some cases, the period from first exposure to the development of clinical cancer is seldom less than 20 years; latent periods substantially shorter than 30 years cannot provide evidence for lack of carcinogenicity.

9. STUDIES OF CANCER IN EXPERIMENTAL ANIMALS

For several agents (e.g., 4-aminobiphenyl, bis(chloromethyl)ether, diethylstilboestrol, melphalan, 8-methoxypsoralen (methoxsalen) plus ultra-violet radiation, mustard gas and vinyl chloride), evidence of carcinogenicity in experimental animals preceded evidence obtained from epidemiological studies or case reports. Information compiled from the first 41 volumes of the *IARC Monographs* (Wilbourn *et al.*, 1986) shows that, of the 44 agents and mixtures for which there is *sufficient* or *limited evidence* of carcinogenicity to humans (see p. 26), all 37 that have been tested adequately experimentally produce cancer in at least one animal species. Although this association cannot establish that all agents and mixtures that cause cancer in experimental animals also cause cancer in humans, nevertheless, *in the absence of adequate data on humans, it is biologically plausible and prudent to regard agents and mixtures for which there is sufficient evidence (see p. 26) of carcinogenicity in experimental animals as if they presented a carcinogenic risk to humans.*

The nature and extent of impurities or contaminants present in the agent or mixture being evaluated are given when available. Animal strain, sex, numbers per group, age at start of treatment and survival are reported.

Experiments in which the agent or mixture was administered in conjunction with known carcinogens or factors that modify carcinogenic effects are also reported. Experiments on the carcinogenicity of known metabolites and derivatives may be included.

For experimental studies with mixtures, consideration is given to the possibility of changes in the physicochemical properties of the test substance during collection, storage, extraction, concentration and delivery. Either chemical or toxicological interactions of the components of mixtures may result in nonlinear dose-response relationships.

An assessment is made as to the relevance to human exposure of samples tested in experimental systems, which may involve consideration of: (i) physical and chemical characteristics, (ii) constituent substances that indicate the presence of a class of substances, (iii) the results of tests for genetic and related effects, including genetic activity profiles, DNA adduct profiles, oncogene expression and mutation and suppressor gene inactivation.

(a) Qualitative aspects

An assessment of carcinogenicity involves several considerations of qualitative importance, including (i) the experimental conditions under which the test was performed, including route and schedule of exposure, species, strain, sex, age, duration of follow-up; (ii) the consistency of the results, for example, across species and target organ(s); (iii) the spectrum of neoplastic response, from benign tumours to malignant neoplasms; and (iv) the possible role of modifying factors.

As mentioned earlier (p. 15), the monographs are not intended to summarize all published studies. Those studies in experimental animals that are inadequate (e.g., too short a duration, too few animals, poor survival; see below) or are judged irrelevant to the evaluation are generally omitted. Guidelines for adequate long-term carcinogenicity experiments have been outlined (e.g., Montesano *et al.*, 1986).

Considerations of importance to the Working Group in the interpretation and evaluation of a particular study include: (i) how clearly the agent was defined and, in the case of mixtures, how adequately the sample characterization was reported; (ii) whether the dose was adequately monitored, particularly in inhalation experiments; (iii) whether the doses used were appropriate and whether the survival of treated animals was similar to that of controls; (iv) whether there were adequate numbers of animals per group; (v) whether animals of each sex were used; (vi) whether animals were allocated randomly to groups; (vii) whether the duration of observation was adequate; and (viii) whether the data were adequately reported. If available, recent data on the incidence of specific tumours in historical controls, as well as in concurrent controls, should be taken into account in the evaluation of tumour response.

When benign tumours occur together with and originate from the same cell type in an organ or tissue as malignant tumours in a particular study and appear to represent a stage in the progression to malignancy, it may be valid to combine them in assessing tumour incidence (Huff *et al.*, 1989). The occurrence of lesions presumed to be preneoplastic may in certain instances aid in assessing the biological plausibility of any neoplastic response observed.

Of the many agents and mixtures that have been studied extensively, few induced only benign neoplasms. Benign tumours in experimental animals frequently represent a stage in the evolution of a malignant neoplasm, but they may be 'endpoints' that do not readily undergo transition to malignancy. However, if an agent or mixture is found to induce only benign neoplasms, it should be suspected of being a carcinogen and it requires further investigation.

(b) *Quantitative aspects*

The probability that tumours will occur may depend on the species and strain, the dose of the carcinogen and the route and period of exposure. Evidence of an increased incidence of neoplasms with increased level of exposure strengthens the inference of a causal association between the exposure and the development of neoplasms.

The form of the dose-response relationship can vary widely, depending on the particular agent under study and the target organ. Since many chemicals require metabolic activation before being converted into their reactive intermediates, both metabolic and pharmacokinetic aspects are important in determining the dose-response pattern. Saturation of steps such as absorption, activation, inactivation and elimination of the carcinogen may produce nonlinearity in the dose-response relationship, as could saturation of processes such as DNA repair (Hoel *et al.*, 1983; Gart *et al.*, 1986).

(c) *Statistical analysis of long-term experiments in animals*

Factors considered by the Working Group include the adequacy of the information given for each treatment group: (i) the number of animals studied and the number examined histologically, (ii) the number of animals with a given tumour type and (iii) length of survival. The statistical methods used should be clearly stated and should be the generally accepted techniques refined for this purpose (Peto *et al.*, 1980; Gart *et al.*, 1986). When there is no difference in survival between control and treatment groups, the Working Group usually compares the proportions of animals developing each tumour type in each of the groups. Otherwise, consideration is given as to whether or not appropriate adjustments have been made for differences in survival. These adjustments can include: comparisons of the proportions of tumour-bearing animals among the 'effective number' of animals alive at the time the first tumour is discovered, in the case where most differences in survival occur before tumours appear; life-table methods, when tumours are visible or when they may be considered 'fatal' because mortality rapidly follows tumour development; and the

Mantel-Haenszel test or logistic regression, when occult tumours do not affect the animals' risk of dying but are 'incidental' findings at autopsy.

In practice, classifying tumours as fatal or incidental may be difficult. Several survival-adjusted methods have been developed that do not require this distinction (Gart *et al.*, 1986), although they have not been fully evaluated.

10. OTHER RELEVANT DATA

(a) *Absorption, distribution, metabolism and excretion*

Concise information is given on absorption, distribution (including placental transfer) and excretion in both humans and experimental animals. Kinetic factors that may affect the dose-response relationship, such as saturation of uptake, protein binding, metabolic activation, detoxification and DNA repair processes, are mentioned. Studies that indicate the metabolic fate of the agent in humans and in experimental animals are summarized briefly, and comparisons of data from humans and animals are made when possible. Comparative information on the relationship between exposure and the dose that reaches the target site may be of particular importance for extrapolation between species.

(b) *Toxic effects*

Data are given on acute and chronic toxic effects (other than cancer), such as organ toxicity, immunotoxicity, endocrine effects and preneoplastic lesions.

(c) *Reproductive and developmental effects*

Effects on reproduction, teratogenicity, feto- and embryotoxicity are also summarized briefly.

(d) *Genetic and related effects*

Tests of genetic and related effects may indicate possible carcinogenic activity. They can also be used in detecting active metabolites of known carcinogens in human or animal body fluids, in detecting active components in complex mixtures and in the elucidation of possible mechanisms of carcinogenesis.

The adequacy of the reporting of sample characterization is considered and, where necessary, commented upon. Considerations with regard to complex mixtures are similar to those described for animal carcinogenicity tests, described on p. 21. The available data are interpreted critically by phylogenetic group according to the endpoints detected, which may include DNA damage, gene mutation, sister chromatid exchange, micronuclei, chromosomal aberrations, aneuploidy and cell transformation. The concentrations (doses) employed are given and mention is made of whether an exogenous metabolic system was required. These data are given as listings of test systems, data and references; bar graphs (activity profiles) and corresponding summary tables with detailed information on the preparation of the profiles are given in appendices.

Positive results in tests using prokaryotes, lower eukaryotes, plants, insects and cultured mammalian cells suggest that genetic and related effects (and therefore possibly carcinogenic effects) could occur in mammals. Results from such tests may also give information about the types of genetic effect produced and about the involvement of metabolic activation. Some endpoints described are clearly genetic in nature (e.g., gene mutations and chromosomal aberrations), others are to a greater or lesser degree associated with genetic effects (e.g., unscheduled DNA synthesis). In-vitro tests for tumour-promoting activity and for cell transformation may detect changes that are not necessarily the result of genetic alterations but that may have specific relevance to the process of carcinogenesis. A critical appraisal of these tests has been published (Montesano *et al.*, 1986).

Genetic or other activity detected in the systems mentioned above is not always manifest in whole mammals. Positive indications of genetic effects in experimental mammals and in humans are regarded as being of greater relevance than those in other organisms. The demonstration that an agent or mixture can induce gene and chromosomal mutations in whole mammals indicates that it may have the potential for carcinogenic activity, although this activity may not be detectably expressed in any or all species tested. Relative potency in tests for mutagenicity and related effects is not a reliable indicator of carcinogenic potency. Negative results in tests for mutagenicity in selected tissues from animals treated *in vivo* provide less weight, partly because they do not exclude the possibility of an effect in tissues other than those examined. Moreover, negative results in short-term tests with genetic endpoints cannot be considered to provide evidence to rule out carcinogenicity of agents or mixtures that act through other mechanisms. Factors may arise in many tests that could give misleading results; these have been discussed in detail elsewhere (Montesano *et al.*, 1986).

The adequacy of epidemiological studies of reproductive outcomes and genetic and related effects in humans is evaluated by the same criteria as are applied to epidemiological studies of cancer.

(e) Structure-activity considerations

This section describes structure-activity relationships that may be relevant to an evaluation of the carcinogenicity of an agent.

11. SUMMARY OF DATA REPORTED

In this section, the relevant epidemiological and experimental data are summarized. Only reports, other than in abstract form, that meet the criteria outlined on p. 15 are considered for evaluating carcinogenicity. Inadequate studies are generally not summarized: such studies are usually identified by a square-bracketed comment in the text.

(a) Exposures

Human exposure is summarized on the basis of elements such as production, use, occurrence in the environment and determinations in human tissues and body fluids. Quantitative data are given when available.

(b) Carcinogenicity in humans

Results of epidemiological studies that are considered to be pertinent to an assessment of human carcinogenicity are summarized. When relevant, case reports and correlation studies are also considered.

(c) Carcinogenicity in experimental animals

Data relevant to the evaluation of carcinogenicity in animals are summarized. For each animal species and route of administration, it is stated whether an increased incidence of neoplasms was observed, and the tumour sites are indicated. If the agent or mixture produced tumours after prenatal exposure or in single-dose experiments, this is also indicated. Dose-response and other quantitative data may be given when available. Negative findings are also summarized.

(d) Other relevant data

Data on biological effects in humans of particular relevance are summarized. These may include kinetic and metabolic considerations and evidence of DNA binding, persistence of DNA lesions or genetic damage in exposed humans.

Toxicological information and data on kinetics and metabolism in experimental animals are given when considered relevant. The results of tests for genetic and related effects are summarized for whole mammals, cultured mammalian cells and nonmammalian systems.

When available, comparisons of such data for humans and for animals, and particularly animals that have developed cancer, are described.

Structure-activity correlations are mentioned when relevant.

12. EVALUATION

Evaluations of the strength of the evidence for carcinogenicity arising from human and experimental animal data are made, using standard terms.

It is recognized that the criteria for these evaluations, described below, cannot encompass all of the factors that may be relevant to an evaluation of carcinogenicity. In considering all of the relevant data, the Working Group may assign the agent, mixture or exposure circumstance to a higher or lower category than a strict interpretation of these criteria would indicate.

(a) Degrees of evidence for carcinogenicity in humans and in experimental animals and supporting evidence

It should be noted that these categories refer only to the strength of the evidence that an exposure is carcinogenic and not to the extent of its carcinogenic activity (potency) nor to the mechanisms involved. A classification may change as new information becomes available.

An evaluation of degree of evidence, whether for a single substance or a mixture, is limited to the materials tested, and these are chemically and physically defined. When the materials evaluated are considered by the Working Group to be sufficiently closely related, they may be grouped for the purpose of a single evaluation of degree of evidence.

(i) Carcinogenicity data in humans

The applicability of an evaluation of the carcinogenicity of a mixture, process, occupation or industry on the basis of evidence from epidemiological studies depends on the variability over time and place of the mixtures, processes, occupations and industries. The Working Group seeks to identify the specific exposure, process or activity which is considered most likely to be responsible for any excess risk. The evaluation is focused as narrowly as the available data on exposure and other aspects permit.

The evidence relevant to carcinogenicity from studies in humans is classified into one of the following categories:

Sufficient evidence of carcinogenicity: The Working Group considers that a causal relationship has been established between exposure to the agent, mixture or exposure circumstance and human cancer. That is, a positive relationship has been observed between the exposure and cancer in studies in which chance, bias and confounding could be ruled out with reasonable confidence.

Limited evidence of carcinogenicity: A positive association has been observed between exposure to the agent, mixture or exposure circumstance and cancer for which a causal interpretation is considered by the Working Group to be credible, but chance, bias or confounding could not be ruled out with reasonable confidence.

Inadequate evidence of carcinogenicity: The available studies are of insufficient quality, consistency or statistical power to permit a conclusion regarding the presence or absence of a causal association.

Evidence suggesting lack of carcinogenicity: There are several adequate studies covering the full range of levels of exposure that human beings are known to encounter, which are mutually consistent in not showing a positive association between exposure to the agent, mixture or exposure circumstance and any studied cancer at any observed level of exposure. A conclusion of 'evidence suggesting lack of carcinogenicity' is inevitably limited to the cancer sites, conditions and levels of exposure and length of observation covered by the available studies. In addition, the possibility of a very small risk at the levels of exposure studied can never be excluded.

In some instances, the above categories may be used to classify the degree of evidence for carcinogenicity for specific organs or tissues.

(ii) *Carcinogenicity in experimental animals*

The evidence relevant to carcinogenicity in experimental animals is classified into one of the following categories:

Sufficient evidence of carcinogenicity: The Working Group considers that a causal relationship has been established between the agent or mixture and an increased incidence of malignant neoplasms or of an appropriate combination of benign and malignant neoplasms (as described on p. 22) in (a) two or more species of animals or (b) in two or more independent studies in one species carried out at different times or in different laboratories or under different protocols.

Exceptionally, a single study in one species might be considered to provide sufficient evidence of carcinogenicity when malignant neoplasms occur to an unusual degree with regard to incidence, site, type of tumour or age at onset.

In the absence of adequate data on humans, it is biologically plausible and prudent to regard agents and mixtures for which there is *sufficient evidence* of carcinogenicity in experimental animals as if they presented a carcinogenic risk to humans.

Limited evidence of carcinogenicity: The data suggest a carcinogenic effect but are limited for making a definitive evaluation because, e.g., (a) the evidence of carcinogenicity is restricted to a single experiment; or (b) there are unresolved questions regarding the adequacy of the design, conduct or interpretation of the study; or (c) the agent or mixture increases the incidence only of benign neoplasms or lesions of uncertain neoplastic potential, or of certain neoplasms which may occur spontaneously in high incidences in certain strains.

Inadequate evidence of carcinogenicity: The studies cannot be interpreted as showing either the presence or absence of a carcinogenic effect because of major qualitative or quantitative limitations.

Evidence suggesting lack of carcinogenicity: Adequate studies involving at least two species are available which show that, within the limits of the tests used, the agent or mixture is not carcinogenic. A conclusion of evidence suggesting lack of carcinogenicity is inevitably limited to the species, tumour sites and levels of exposure studied.

(iii) *Supporting evidence of carcinogenicity*

Other evidence judged to be relevant to an evaluation of carcinogenicity and of sufficient importance to affect the overall evaluation is then described. This may include data on tumour pathology, genetic and related effects, structure-activity relationships, metabolism and pharmacokinetics, physicochemical parameters, chemical composition and possible mechanisms of action. For complex exposures, including occupational and industrial exposures, the potential contribution of carcinogens known to be present is considered by the Working Group in its overall evaluation of human carcinogenicity. The Working Group also determines to what extent the materials tested in experimental systems are relevant to those to which humans are exposed. The available experimental evidence may also help to specify more precisely a causal factor.

(b) *Overall evaluation*

Finally, the body of evidence is considered as a whole, in order to reach an overall evaluation of the carcinogenicity to humans of an agent, mixture or circumstance of exposure.

An evaluation may be made for a group of chemical compounds that have been evaluated by the Working Group. In addition, when supporting data indicate that other, related compounds for which there is no direct evidence of capacity to induce cancer in animals or in humans may also be carcinogenic, a statement describing the rationale for this conclusion is added to the evaluation narrative; an additional evaluation may be made for this broader group of compounds if the strength of the evidence warrants it.

The agent, mixture or exposure circumstance is described according to the wording of one of the following categories, and the designated group is given. The categorization of an agent, mixture or exposure circumstance is a matter of scientific judgement, reflecting the strength of the evidence derived from studies in humans and in experimental animals and from other relevant data.

Group 1—The agent (mixture) is carcinogenic to humans.
The exposure circumstance entails exposures that are carcinogenic to humans.

This category is used only when there is *sufficient evidence* of carcinogenicity in humans.

Group 2

This category includes agents, mixtures and exposure circumstances for which, at one extreme, the degree of evidence of carcinogenicity in humans is almost sufficient, as well as those for which, at the other extreme, there are no human data but for which there is experimental evidence of carcinogenicity. Agents, mixtures and exposure circumstances are assigned to either 2A (probably carcinogenic) or 2B (possibly carcinogenic) on the basis of epidemiological, experimental and other relevant data.

Group 2A—The agent (mixture) is probably carcinogenic to humans.
The exposure circumstance entails exposures that are probably carcinogenic to humans.

This category is used when there is *limited evidence* of carcinogenicity in humans and *sufficient evidence* of carcinogenicity in experimental animals. Exceptionally, an agent, mixture or exposure circumstance may be classified in this category solely on the basis of *limited evidence* of carcinogenicity in humans or of *sufficient evidence* of carcinogenicity in experimental animals strengthened by supporting evidence from other relevant data.

Group 2B—The agent (mixture) is possibly carcinogenic to humans.
The exposure circumstance entails exposures that are possibly carcinogenic to humans.

This category is generally used for agents, mixtures and exposure circumstances for which there is *limited evidence* of carcinogenicity in humans in the absence of *sufficient evidence* of carcinogenicity in experimental animals. It may also be used when there is *inadequate evidence* of carcinogenicity in humans or when human data are nonexistent but there is *sufficient evidence* of carcinogenicity in experimental animals. In some instances, an agent, mixture or exposure circumstance for which there is *inadequate evidence* of or no data on carcinogenicity in humans but *limited evidence* of carcinogenicity in experimental animals together with supporting evidence from other relevant data may be placed in this group.

Group 3—The agent (mixture, exposure circumstance) is not classifiable as to its carcinogenicity to humans.

Agents, mixtures and exposure circumstances are placed in this category when they do not fall into any other group.

Group 4—The agent (mixture, exposure circumstance) is probably not carcinogenic to humans.

This category is used for agents, mixtures and exposure circumstances for which there is *evidence suggesting lack of carcinogenicity* in humans together with *evidence suggesting lack of carcinogenicity* in experimental animals. In some instances, agents, mixtures or exposure circumstances for which there is *inadequate evidence* of or no data on carcinogenicity in humans but *evidence suggesting lack of carcinogenicity* in experimental animals, consistently and strongly supported by a broad range of other relevant data, may be classified in this group.

References

Breslow, N.E. & Day, N.E. (1980) *Statistical Methods in Cancer Research*, Vol. 1, *The Analysis of Case-control Studies* (IARC Scientific Publications No. 32), Lyon, IARC

Breslow, N.E. & Day, N.E. (1987) *Statistical Methods in Cancer Research*, Vol. 2, *The Design and Analysis of Cohort Studies* (IARC Scientific Publications No. 82), Lyon, IARC

Gart, J.J., Krewski, D., Lee, P.N., Tarone, R.E. & Wahrendorf, J. (1986) *Statistical Methods in Cancer Research*, Vol. 3, *The Design and Analysis of Long-term Animal Experiments* (IARC Scientific Publications No. 79), Lyon, IARC

Hoel, D.G., Kaplan, N.L. & Anderson, M.W. (1983) Implication of nonlinear kinetics on risk estimation in carcinogenesis. *Science*, *219*, 1032-1037

Huff, J.E., Eustis, S.L. & Haseman, J.K. (1989) Occurrence and relevance of chemically induced benign neoplasms in long-term carcinogenicity studies. *Cancer Metastasis Rev.*, *8*, 1-21

IARC (1973-1990) *Information Bulletin on the Survey of Chemicals Being Tested for Carcinogenicity/Directory of Agents Being Tested for Carcinogenicity*, Numbers 1-14, Lyon

Number 1 (1973)	52 pages
Number 2 (1973)	77 pages
Number 3 (1974)	67 pages
Number 4 (1974)	97 pages
Number 5 (1975)	88 pages
Number 6 (1976)	360 pages
Number 7 (1978)	460 pages
Number 8 (1979)	604 pages
Number 9 (1981)	294 pages
Number 10 (1983)	326 pages
Number 11 (1984)	370 pages
Number 12 (1986)	385 pages
Number 13 (1988)	404 pages
Number 14 (1990)	369 pages

IARC (1976-1989/90)

Directory of On-going Research in Cancer Epidemiology 1976. Edited by C.S. Muir & G. Wagner, Lyon

Directory of On-going Research in Cancer Epidemiology 1977 (IARC Scientific Publications No. 17). Edited by C.S. Muir & G. Wagner, Lyon

Directory of On-going Research in Cancer Epidemiology 1978 (IARC Scientific Publications No. 26). Edited by C.S. Muir & G. Wagner, Lyon

Directory of On-going Research in Cancer Epidemiology 1979 (IARC Scientific Publications No. 28). Edited by C.S. Muir & G. Wagner, Lyon

Directory of On-going Research in Cancer Epidemiology 1980 (IARC Scientific Publications No. 35). Edited by C.S. Muir & G. Wagner, Lyon

Directory of On-going Research in Cancer Epidemiology 1981 (IARC Scientific Publications No. 38). Edited by C.S. Muir & G. Wagner, Lyon

Directory of On-going Research in Cancer Epidemiology 1982 (IARC Scientific Publications No. 46). Edited by C.S. Muir & G. Wagner, Lyon

Directory of On-going Research in Cancer Epidemiology 1983 (IARC Scientific Publications No. 50). Edited by C.S. Muir & G. Wagner, Lyon

Directory of On-going Research in Cancer Epidemiology 1984 (IARC Scientific Publications No. 62). Edited by C.S. Muir & G. Wagner, Lyon

Directory of On-going Research in Cancer Epidemiology 1985 (IARC Scientific Publications No. 69). Edited by C.S. Muir & G. Wagner, Lyon

Directory of On-going Research in Cancer Epidemiology 1986 (IARC Scientific Publications No. 80). Edited by C.S. Muir & G. Wagner, Lyon

Directory of On-going Research in Cancer Epidemiology 1987 (IARC Scientific Publications No. 86). Edited by D.M. Parkin & J. Wahrendorf, Lyon

Directory of On-going Research in Cancer Epidemiology 1988 (IARC Scientific Publications No. 93). Edited by M. Coleman & J. Wahrendorf, Lyon

Directory of On-going Research in Cancer Epidemiology 1989/90 (IARC Scientific Publications No. 101). Edited by M. Coleman & J. Wahrendorf, Lyon

IARC (1977) *IARC Monographs Programme on the Evaluation of the Carcinogenic Risk of Chemicals to Humans. Preamble* (IARC intern. tech. Rep. No. 77/002), Lyon

IARC (1978) *Chemicals with* Sufficient Evidence *of Carcinogenicity in Experimental Animals*—IARC Monographs *Volumes 1-17* (IARC intern. tech. Rep. No. 78/003), Lyon

IARC (1978-1988) *Environmental Carcinogens. Methods of Analysis and Exposure Measurement*:

> Vol. 1. *Analysis of Volatile Nitrosamines in Food* (IARC Scientific Publications No. 18). Edited by R. Preussmann, M. Castegnaro, E.A. Walker & A.E. Wasserman (1978)

> Vol. 2. *Methods for the Measurement of Vinyl Chloride in Poly(vinyl chloride), Air, Water and Foodstuffs* (IARC Scientific Publications No. 22). Edited by D.C.M. Squirrell & W. Thain (1978)

> Vol. 3. *Analysis of Polycyclic Aromatic Hydrocarbons in Environmental Samples* (IARC Scientific Publications No. 29). Edited by M. Castegnaro, P. Bogovski, H. Kunte & E.A. Walker (1979)

> Vol. 4. *Some Aromatic Amines and Azo Dyes in the General and Industrial Environment* (IARC Scientific Publications No. 40). Edited by L. Fishbein, M. Castegnaro, I.K. O'Neill & H. Bartsch (1981)

> Vol. 5. *Some Mycotoxins* (IARC Scientific Publications No. 44). Edited by L. Stoloff, M. Castegnaro, P. Scott, I.K. O'Neill & H. Bartsch (1983)

> Vol. 6. N-*Nitroso Compounds* (IARC Scientific Publications No. 45). Edited by R. Preussmann, I.K. O'Neill, G. Eisenbrand, B. Spiegelhalder & H. Bartsch (1983)

> Vol. 7. *Some Volatile Halogenated Hydrocarbons* (IARC Scientific Publications No. 68). Edited by L. Fishbein & I.K. O'Neill (1985)

> Vol. 8. *Some Metals: As, Be, Cd, Cr, Ni, Pb, Se, Zn* (IARC Scientific Publications No. 71). Edited by I.K. O'Neill, P. Schuller & L. Fishbein (1986)

> Vol. 9. *Passive Smoking* (IARC Scientific Publications No. 81). Edited by I.K. O'Neill, K.D. Brunnemann, B. Dodet & D. Hoffmann (1987)

> Vol. 10. *Benzene and Alkylated Benzenes* (IARC Scientific Publications No. 85). Edited by L. Fishbein & I.K. O'Neill (1988)

IARC (1979) *Criteria to Select Chemicals for* IARC Monographs (IARC intern. tech. Rep. No. 79/003), Lyon

IARC (1982) *IARC Monographs on the Evaluation of the Carcinogenic Risk of Chemicals to Humans, Supplement 4, Chemicals, Industrial Processes and Industries Associated with Cancer in Humans* (IARC Monographs, *Volumes 1 to 29*), Lyon

IARC (1983) *Approaches to Classifying Chemical Carcinogens According to Mechanism of Action* (IARC intern. tech. Rep. No. 83/001), Lyon

IARC (1984) *Chemicals and Exposures to Complex Mixtures Recommended for Evaluation in* IARC Monographs *and Chemicals and Complex Mixtures Recommended for Long-term Carcinogenicity Testing* (IARC intern. tech. Rep. No. 84/002), Lyon

IARC (1987a) *IARC Monographs on the Evaluation of Carcinogenic Risks to Humans*, Supplement 6, *Genetic and Related Effects: An Updating of Selected* IARC Monographs *from Volumes 1 to 42*, Lyon

IARC (1987b) *IARC Monographs on the Evaluation of Carcinogenic Risks to Humans*, Supplement 7, *Overall Evaluations of Carcinogenicity: An Updating of* IARC Monographs *Volumes 1 to 42*, Lyon

IARC (1988) *Report of an IARC Working Group to Review the Approaches and Processes Used to Evaluate the Carcinogenicity of Mixtures and Groups of Chemicals* (IARC intern. tech. Rep. No. 88/002), Lyon

IARC (1989) *Chemicals, Groups of Chemicals, Mixtures and Exposure Circumstances to be Evaluated in Future IARC Monographs, Report of an ad hoc Working Group* (IARC intern. tech. Rep. No. 89/004), Lyon

Montesano, R., Bartsch, H., Vainio, H., Wilbourn, J. & Yamasaki, H., eds (1986) *Long-term and Short-term Assays for Carcinogenesis—A Critical Appraisal* (IARC Scientific Publications No. 83), Lyon, IARC

Peto, R., Pike, M.C., Day, N.E., Gray, R.G., Lee, P.N., Parish, S., Peto, J., Richards, S. & Wahrendorf, J. (1980) Guidelines for simple, sensitive significance tests for carcinogenic effects in long-term animal experiments. In: *IARC Monographs on the Evaluation of the Carcinogenic Risk of Chemicals to Humans*, Supplement 2, *Long-term and Short-term Screening Assays for Carcinogens: A Critical Appraisal*, Lyon, pp. 311-426

Wilbourn, J., Haroun, L., Heseltine, E., Kaldor, J., Partensky, C. & Vainio, H. (1986) Response of experimental animals to human carcinogens: an analysis based upon the IARC Monographs Programme. *Carcinogenesis*, 7, 1853-1863

GENERAL REMARKS

In this fifty-third volume of *IARC Monographs*, the carcinogenic risks to humans from exposure to eight individual insecticides, four fungicides and five herbicides, as well as from occupational exposure in spraying and application of insecticides are reviewed. Eight of the pesticides considered were evaluated previously in the *IARC Monographs* programme; those compounds were re-evaluated in this volume owing to the availability of new data on carcinogenicity in exposed populations and/or in experimental animals. Pesticides and related occupational exposures that were evaluated by previous IARC working groups are listed in Table 1.

Table 1. Pesticides and related occupational exposures that have been evaluated previously in the *IARC Monographs*

Compound	Year	Degree[a] of evidence for carcinogenicity		Overall evaluation of carcinogenicity to humans
		Human	Animal	
Insecticides				
Agents and groups of agents				
Aldrin	1987	I	L	3
Aramite®	1974	ND	S	2B
Arsenic and arsenic compounds	1987	S	L	1[b]
Carbaryl	1976	ND	I	3
Chlordane/heptachlor[c]	1987	I	L	3
Chlordecone	1979	ND	S	2B
Chlordimeform	1983	ND	I	3
Chlorobenzilate	1983	ND	L	3
DDT	1987	I	S	2B
Dichlorvos[c]	1987	ND	I	3
Dicofol	1983	ND	L	3
Dieldrin	1987	I	L	3
Endrin	1974	ND	I	3
Hexachlorocyclohexanes (HCH)	1987	I		2B
Technical-grade HCH			S	
α-HCH			S	
β-HCH			L	
γ-HCH (Lindane)			L	
Malathion	1983	ND	I	3
Methoxychlor	1979	ND	I	3

Table 1 (contd)

Compound	Year	Degree[a] of evidence for carcinogenicity		Overall evaluation of carcinogenicity to humans
		Human	Animal	
Insecticides (contd)				
Agents and groups of agents (contd)				
Methyl parathion	1987	ND	ESL	3
Mirex	1979	ND	S	2B
Parathion	1983	ND	I	3
Piperonyl butoxide	1983	ND	I	3
Tetrachlorvinphos	1983	ND	L	3
Trichlorfon	1983	ND	I	3
Zectran[d]	1976	ND	I	3
Mixtures				
Terpene polychlorinates (Strobane®)	1974	ND	L	3
Toxaphene (polychlorinated camphenes)	1979	ND	S	2B
Fungicides				
Captan	1983	ND	L	3
Chlorophenols	1987	L		2B
Pentachlorophenol[c]			I	
2,4,5-Trichlorophenol[e]			I	
2,4,6-Trichlorophenol[e]			S	
Chlorothalonil	1983	ND	L	3
Copper 8-hydroxyquinoline	1977	ND	I	3
Ferbam	1976	ND	I	3
Hexachlorobenzene	1987	I	S	2B
Maneb	1976	ND	I	3
ortho-Phenylphenol	1983	ND	I	3
Quintozene (Pentachloronitrobenzene)	1974	ND	L	3
Sodium *ortho*-phenylphenate	1987	ND	S	2B
Thiram[c]	1976	ND	I	3
Zineb	1976	ND	I	3
Ziram[c]	1976	ND	I	3
Herbicides				
Amitrole	1987	I	S	2B
Chlorophenoxy herbicides	1987	L		2B
2,4-D			I	
2,4,5-T			I	
MCPA			ND	
Chloropropham	1976	ND	I	3
Diallate	1983	ND	L	3
Fluometuron	1983	ND	I	3

Table 1 (contd)

Compound	Year	Degree[a] of evidence for carcinogenicity		Overall evaluation of carcinogenicity to humans
		Human	Animal	
Herbicides (contd)				
Monuron	1976	ND	L	3
Nitrofen (technical-grade)	1983	ND	S	2B
Propham	1976	ND	I	3
Sulfallate	1983	ND	S	2B
Other				
1,2-Dibromo-3-chloropropane[f]	1987	I	S	2B
Dimethylcarbamoyl chloride[g]	1987	I	S	2A
Ethylene dibromide[h]	1987	I	S	2A
Naphthylthiourea (ANTU)[i]	1987	I	I	3
Sodium diethyldithiocarbamate[h]	1976	ND	I	3

[a]I, inadequate evidence; S, sufficient evidence; L, limited evidence; ND, no data; ESL, evidence suggesting lack of carcinogenicity
[b]This evaluation applies to the group of chemicals as a whole and not necessarily to all individual chemicals within the group.
[c]Previous evaluation
[d]And molluscicide
[e]Primarily used as chemical intermediate
[f]Soil fumigant/nematicide
[g]Pesticide intermediate
[h]Soil fumigant
[i]Rodenticide

About 1500 chemicals are registered for use in thousands of pesticide formulations; however, fewer than 50 pesticides account for about 75% of those used (Salem & Olajos, 1988).

Crops are affected by different pests and by competition from weeds, with large variations between climatic and agricultural regions. Several insects and other arthropods, fungi, molluscs and bacteria attack crops, resulting in quantitative and qualitative crop losses. The introduction of new plant species and cultivars in plantation and cash crop farming of monocultures can lead to increased problems. The crop losses caused by pests are great in developed as well as developing countries. In North America, Europe and Japan, losses are estimated to be in the range 10-30%, but in developing parts of the world they are substantially higher: Crop losses due to pests and plant diseases of the order of 40% are common in these areas, and losses of as much as 75% have been reported (WHO/UNEP, 1990).

During the last four decades, chemical control of pests and weeds has been dramatically expanded worldwide to minimize such losses. A study by Smith and Gratz (1984) showed that the greatest demand for pesticides in urban vector control was for insecticides. Pesticides are used worldwide, albeit in varying degrees, depending on dominating crops, stage of development, climatic conditions and prevalence of pests. The general development of agropesticide use has been summarized (WHO/UNEP, 1990); this shows the diversified and increasing use of pesticides in agriculture in five stages, from very low to very high. The stages coincide to a certain extent with the general economic development of countries; however, in an individual country, different agricultural stages may occur at the same time in different farming regions. Some countries may also be at different stages for different variables (agropesticide use level, product range, development of local pesticide industry, distribution structure, regulatory infrastructure, area under control and general level of agricultural development).

Worldwide consumption of pesticides in 1985 was estimated at about 3 million tonnes. According to available data, 20% (equivalent to 600 000 tonnes annually) of the whole market is exported to and used in developing countries (WHO/UNEP, 1990). The major applications of pesticides in 1985 were herbicides (46%), insecticides (31%) and fungicides (18.4%) (Anon., 1985). Estimates of world pesticide sales in 1985 are shown in Table 2.

Table 2. Pesticide market value, 1985, by area and product; million US$[a]

Area	Herbicides	Insecticides	Fungicides	Others	Total
USA	3100	1090	330	330	4850
Western Europe	1475	850	1100	400	3825
East Asia	775	1300	785	90	2950
Latin America	485	655	250	60	1450
Eastern Europe	625	450	230	95	1400
Rest of the world	615	655	105	50	1425
World total	7075	5000	2800	1025	15 900
% of total	44.5	31.4	17.6	6.4	

[a]From Wood Mackenzie Agrochemical Service, personal communication, cited in WHO/UNEP (1990)

Overall pesticide use in agriculture, in terms of amounts applied per hectare, has been very much greater in Japan, Europe and the USA (about 75%) than in the rest of the world, although China is also a major user. The fastest growing market, however, is Africa, with a sales increase of 182% between 1980 and 1984. Other rapidly expanding markets are Central and South America (32%), Asia (28%) and the Middle East (26%). Although herbicide sales have been greater than those of insecticides and fungicides in developed countries and some developing countries and are increasing rapidly, this pattern is not being repeated in other developing countries, where by far the greatest proportion of pesticides used are still insecticides. The 15 most widely used pesticides in seven Asian countries (Bangladesh, India, Nepal, Pakistan, Philippines, Republic of Korea and Thailand) are as follows: carbaryl (insecticide), malathion (insecticide), methyl parathion (insecticide), diazinon (insecticide), monocrotophos (insecticide), endosulfan (insecticide), carbofuran (insecticide), mancozeb (fungicide), paraquat (herbicide), aluminium phosphide (insecticide), methyl oxydemeton (insecticide), phosphamidon (insecticide), 2,4-D [(2,4-dichlorophenoxy)acetic acid] (herbicide), 2-sec-butylphenyl methylcarbamate (insecticide) and zinc phosphide (insecticide) (WHO/UNEP, 1990).

Another factor of importance for assessing the potential public health impact of pesticides is the seasonality of their use. Each pest is of importance only during a limited part of the growing season, and human exposures are therefore likely to be limited to the same seasons, when pesticide use occurs. For example, in some parts of West Africa, herbicides and fungicides tend to be used early in the growing season, whereas insecticides are used at a later stage (WHO/UNEP, 1990).

The future use of pesticides depends on several factors. The need for pest control using the available products is important. Other factors are marketing regulations, environmental concerns and the availability of alternative methods. About 25% of all pesticides is presently used in developing countries, mainly on cash crops. Depending on the stage of development of a country, the type and amounts of pesticides will change from a low level of organochlorines on a few crops to a wide range and higher total dosage of insecticides, fungicides and herbicides on a large variety of crops. The present trend is that many crops are submitted to pesticide treatment as soon as land-use is intensified. Public health programmes for control of vector-borne diseases are the other important pesticide application, and the amounts used may currently, in some developing countries, far exceed the amounts used for the control of agricultural pests and diseases (WHO/UNEP, 1990).

Reliable global estimates of morbidity and mortality due to acute exposures to pesticides are not available. In some countries, however, when data are available, they indicate that the problem varies greatly from place to place. For instance, a comparison of mortality due to pesticides in the USA for 1973 and 1974 with the rates of the previous years indicates a decline in pesticide-related fatalities from 152 to 52 between 1956 and 1974. An average of 35 pesticide-related deaths per annum was recorded throughout the 1970s; the majority of these deaths involved either gross safety violations or incompetence. The numbers of deaths due to occupational exposure to pesticides were reported as five in 1973 and seven in 1974 (Hayes & Vaugh, 1977).

In Sri Lanka, on the contrary, yearly pesticide-related deaths in 1975-80 were about 1000 out of 13 000 hospital admissions; of these deaths, about 10-15% were related to occupational exposures. Similar findings were obtained in Indonesia, Malaysia and Thailand (Jeyaratnam et al., 1982, 1987). Educational and safety programmes have been developed by international organizations, such as WHO, UNEP and FAO, to prevent acute poisoning.

The monograph on **occupational exposures in spraying and application of insecticides** specifically covers studies of workers exposed during the use of insecticides; the few studies on workers exposed during the manufacture of insecticides were not included in the monograph. Many epidemiological studies of cancer refer to 'agricultural workers' or to exposures to pesticides generally rather than to insecticides specifically, and these studies were also not evaluated. Surprisingly few epidemiological studies are available on occupational exposures in spraying and application of insecticides, given that many of these compounds have been in common use since 1950. For several chemicals considered in this volume, the available epidemiological studies concerned populations with multiple exposures to different pesticides, and the information often did not allow the Working Group to disentangle their separate effects. Groups recorded as exposed to insecticides specifically may be exposed to one or a number of the insecticides considered in this volume, to other specified insecticides or, as is more usually the case, to unspecified insecticides. All such studies were taken into account in evaluating the carcinogenic risk of occupational exposure in the spraying and application of insecticides.

Of the insecticides reviewed in this volume, **aldicarb** is used only for agricultural purposes; **dichlorvos** is used to protect stored grain, in veterinary medicine and in the control of insects in houses and other buildings; **chlordane** and **heptachlor** are also used for insect control (notably termites) in buildings. The synthetic pyrethroids, **permethrin**, **deltamethrin** and **fenvalerate**, are used in agriculture as well as in houses and gardens and for the protection of stored products. **DDT** has been used in crop protection but has also been used extensively for the control of insect-borne diseases.

Captafol is a non-systemic, protective and curative fungicide that has been used on plants and for seed treatment; it has also been used as a wood preservative. **Ziram** and **thiram** are both foliar fungicides; thiram is also used in seed treatment, and both are used as curing agents in the rubber industry. **Pentachlorophenol** is used principally as a wood preservative; it is used to protect against wood-boring insects and as a herbicide. Pentachlorophenol is also a widespread environmental pollutant; residues are found in all media and in humans. The US National Human Monitoring Program for Pesticides found in a three-year study with the collaboration of the US Public Health Service that pentachlorophenol occurred in 85% of urine samples from the general population of the USA (Kutz *et al.*, 1978).

Of the herbicides, **monuron** is used for total weed control in non-crop areas; **trifluralin** is a selective herbicide used for pre-emergence control of grasses and broad-leafed weeds; and **picloram** and the triazines, **atrazine** and **simazine**, are used in crop and non-crop areas against broad-leafed weeds and/or grasses. Simazine is also used as an aquatic herbicide and algicide.

Some pesticides reviewed in this volume, e.g., chlordane, DDT, captafol, aldicarb, monuron, trifluralin, picloram and pentachlorophenol, now have restricted use in some countries. Use of the organochlorine insecticides DDT and chlordane in agriculture reached a maximum in the 1960s but has declined since, and they have been banned in several countries. There continues, however, to be widespread general exposure to persistent organochlorine pesticides in developing countries. These compounds are known to bioaccumulate in the environment and in food chains. Exposure of humans to pesticide residues in food has been reported in only two 'market basket' surveys from North America; the lack of such data from developing countries makes it difficult to estimate exposure or potential exposure and bioaccumulation for these regions.

Several quantitative and qualitative difficulties are encountered in evaluating the precise exposures of people working with pesticides:

(i) Workers involved in the production of pesticides are exposed both to technical products, which generally contain about 95% pure material, as well as to formulated products, which contain from 10 to 50% of the active ingredient.

(ii) Formulations contain 'inert' non-pesticidal ingredients, some of which are known carcinogens and mutagens, although efforts have been made to remove them (US

Environmental Protection Agency, 1987, 1989). Such substances are added to pesticide products as solvents, emulsifiers and aerosol propellants and may, at some dose, have toxicological effects; however, the toxicity of these chemicals has generally not been tested.

(iii) Public health and agricultural use of pesticides involves handling formulated products, mixing them for spraying, spraying, eventually disposing of excess material and cleaning spray equipment. Formulations are generally prepared for application by the applicators themselves, and technical products and application patterns differ in various parts of the world. Workers in developing countries may have high occupational exposures to pesticides owing to inadequate working conditions (lack of protective clothing, unsafe pesticide spraying and storage practices) or to deficient sociocultural conditions (illiteracy, bad housing, inefficient garbage disposal and sewage systems, etc.). Residues in food and water are another potential source of exposure. In this case, the levels of pesticides involved are several orders of magnitude lower than those associated with production and application.

(iv) Nitroso derivatives of pesticides may occur as impurities in technical products; these include N-nitrosodi-n-propylamine in trifluralin and N-nitrosodiethylamine and N-nitrosodiisopropylamine in picloram. In both situations, the amount of nitrosamines permissible in technical material has been regulated. Where possible, the Working Group took note of the likely effect of these and other impurities when evaluating the reported studies. Since the interaction of nitrite with chemicals is considered to be a general phenomenon, however, not specifically related to the use of pesticides, and has been dealt with in other *IARC Monographs*, such studies are not included in the evaluations in these monographs.

Biologically active impurities are known to arise from synthesis, formulation and storage of pesticides. Regulatory bodies require the specification of technical material in order to identify impurities present at levels higher than 0.1-1% (WHO, 1985). Furthermore, in some cases, data on toxicity are required for impurities present at levels higher than 1%.

Impurities may also be formed owing to interaction with coformulants and to storage under inappropriate conditions (WHO, 1986), but little information is available. There are indications that the resulting impurities might be much more acutely toxic than the original compound (WHO/UNEP, 1990), but the Working Group was not aware of any study showing increased long-term toxicity due to contamination. Dioxins and other impurities found in technical products, such as pentachlorophenol and 2,4,5-T, have been discussed in detail elsewhere (IARC, 1977).

For several of the chemicals that are considered in this volume, occupational cohorts were studied but no information was available on smoking habits. Since smoking is a well-known cause of several cancers, including those of the lung, larynx, oesophagus and bladder, the possibility must be entertained that any association found between occupational exposure and tobacco-related cancer sites is due in fact to smoking. In making such an evaluation, the following points are usually considered:

(i) The occurrence of only *one* tobacco-related cancer in association with the exposure under consideration makes tobacco use an unlikely explanation; in particular, the incidence of or mortality from non-neoplastic diseases related to tobacco should be taken into consideration.

(ii) When exposure-response patterns are observed, it is unlikely that tobacco use is an explanation, because use of tobacco rarely parallels an exposure pattern (Siemiatycki *et al.*, 1988).

(iii) Comparison between crude and smoking-adjusted odds ratios for lung cancer across different occupations showed no systematic difference between the two (Blair *et al.*, 1985). Analysis of smoking habits among occupational categories in large populations also suggests that differences are not likely to exert a strong confounding effect (Brackbill *et al.*, 1988; Stellman *et al.*, 1988; Levin *et al.*, 1990).

(iv) Since the relative risks for cancers caused by tobacco are known quite precisely, it is possible to calculate the magnitude of a smoking differential that must occur in order to explain differences in many observed cancer rates. It can be shown arithmetically that in order to distort risk estimates appreciably, the distribution of smoking habits in an occupational cohort must be quite different from that of the comparison population.

(v) Tobacco use complicates evaluation of tobacco-related cancers among farmers, since data from around the world indicate that they have a lower prevalence of smoking than the general population. This is especially relevant for the monograph on occupational exposures in spraying and application of insecticides. Farmers in several countries, however, have increased risks for soft-tissue sarcomas and for cancers of the lymphohaematopoietic system, brain, prostate, stomach and lip (Pearce & Reif, 1990).

In general, the published studies on carcinogenicity and toxicity in experimental systems were carried out using pesticidally active material (nonetheless, sometimes of unspecified purity) rather than using a formulated product; human exposure, in contrast, is often to a number of formulated products. Extrapolation from experimental data based on pure compounds to the human situation in which technical products are used is therefore not straightforward.

In several studies of the carcinogenicity of DDT in mice (see pp. 202 *et seq.*), an inverse relationship was observed between the incidence of liver neoplasia and lymphoma; more specifically, increases in the incidence of liver tumours appeared to be related to decreases in that of lymphoma. In some studies, this phenomenon may be explained by a reduction in survival due to toxicity or other factors in high-dose groups—those groups that have often shown increased incidences of liver tumours; however, this explanation does not apply to all cases in which the phenomenon has been observed. The Working Group reported the incidence of lymphomas in those studies in which it differed in treated groups from that in controls. It was the position of the Working Group that the observation of decreases in the incidences of certain tumours is generally not relevant to an evaluation of carcinogenicity as defined by the IARC: 'an increase in the incidence of malignant neoplasms; the induction of benign neoplasms may in some circumstances contribute to the judgement that (an) exposure is carcinogenic'.

Pesticides hold a somewhat unique position among man-made chemicals. Because of their high biological activities, numerous studies have been performed on their toxicology. Unfortunately, for a number of reasons, such data have rarely been published and therefore cannot be evaluated here, even though they are summarized in other WHO publications. Mention is made whenever information was derived from such publications.

WHO (1985) has established specifications for many pesticides used in public health. These include a description of the material and its ingredients, its chemical and physical properties and methods for determining those properties. Specifications have been set for both technical-grade products and common formulations. FAO (1987) has similar specifications for plant protection products. These also include specifications for the technical material and common formulations.

Codex maximum residue limits are applied to pesticide residues present in raw agricultural products treated with a pesticide according to good agricultural practice. They are usually at the parts per million level. For commodities entering international trade, maximum residue limits are applicable at the point of entry into a country. In addition, each country has its own national maximum residue limits or tolerances, which may differ from that of the Codex Alimentarius (FAO, 1978; Codex Committee on Pesticide Residues, 1990).

References

Anon. (1985) A look at world pesticide markets. *Farm Chemicals*, September, pp. 26, 29, 30, 32, 34

Blair, A., Hoar, S.K. & Walrath, J. (1985) Comparison of crude and smoking-adjusted standardized mortality ratios. *J. occup. Med.*, *27*, 881-884

Brackbill, R., Frazier, T. & Shilling, S. (1988) Smoking characteristics of US workers, 1978-1980. *Am. J. ind. Med.*, *13*, 5-41

Codex Committee on Pesticide Residues (1990) *Guide to Codex Maximum Limits for Pesticide Residues*, Part 2 (CAC/PR 2—1990; CCPR Pesticide Classification No. 120), The Hague

FAO (1978) *Pesticide Residues in Foods—Report 1977*, Rome

FAO (1987) *Manual on the Development and Use of FAO Specifications for Plant Protection Products* (FAO Plant Production and Protection Paper 85), 3rd rev. ed., Rome

Hayes, W.J., Jr & Vaughn, W.K. (1977) Mortality from pesticides in the United States in 1973 and 1974. *Toxicol. appl. Pharmacol.*, *42*, 235-252

IARC (1977) *IARC Monographs on the Evaluation of the Carcinogenic Risk of Chemicals to Man*, Vol. 15, *Some Fumigants, the Herbicides 2,4-D and 2,4,5-T, Chlorinated Dibenzodioxins and Miscellaneous Industrial Chemicals*, Lyon, pp. 41-102

Jeyaratnam, J., de Alwis Seneviratne, R.S. & Copplestone, J.F. (1982) Survey of pesticide poisoining in Sri Lanka. *Bull. World Health Organ.*, *60*, 615-619

Jeyaratnam, J., Lun, K.C. & Phoon, W.O. (1987) Survey of acute pesticide poisoning among agricultural workers in four Asian countries. *Bull. World Health Organ.*, *65*, 521-527

Kutz, F.W., Murphy, R.S. & Strassman, S.C. (1978) *Survey of Pesticide Residues and Their Metabolites in Urine from the General Population*. In: Rao, K.R., ed., *Pentachlorophenol*, New York, Plenum

Levin, L.I., Silverman, D.T., Hartge, P., Fears, T.R. & Hoover, R.N. (1990) Smoking patterns by occupation and duration of employment. *Am. J. ind. Med.*, *17*, 711-725

Pearce, N. & Reif, J.S. (1990) Epidemiologic studies of cancer in agricultural workers. *Am. J. ind. Med.*, *18*, 133-148

Salem, H. & Olajos, E.J. (1988) Review of pesticides: chemistry, uses and toxicology. *Toxicol. ind. Health*, *4*, 291-321

Siemiatycki, J., Wacholder, S., Dewar, R., Cardis, E., Greenwood, C. & Richardson, L. (1988) Degree of confounding bias related to smoking, ethnic group and socioeconomic status in estimates of the associations between occupation and cancer. *J. occup. Med.*, *30*, 617-625

Smith, A. & Gratz, N.G. (1984) *Urban Vector and Rodent Control Services* (VBC/84.4), Geneva, WHO

Stellman, S.D., Boffetta, P. & Garfinkel, L. (1988) Smoking habits of 800,000 American men and women in relation to their occupations. *Am. J. ind. Med.*, *13*, 43-58

US Environmental Protection Agency (1987) Inert ingredients in pesticide products; policy statement. *Fed. Reg.*, *52*, 13305-13309

US Environmental Protection Agency (1989) Inert ingredients in pesticide products; policy statement; revision and modification of lists. *Fed. Reg.*, *54*, 48314-48316

WHO (1985) *Specifications for Pesticides Used in Public Health*, 6th ed., Geneva

WHO (1986) *Organophosphorus Insecticides: A General Introduction* (Environmental Health Criteria 63), Geneva

WHO/UNEP (1990) *Public Health Impact of Pesticides Used in Agriculture*, Geneva

INSECTICIDES

OCCUPATIONAL EXPOSURES IN SPRAYING
AND APPLICATION OF INSECTICIDES[1]

1. Exposure Data

The public health impact of pesticides, including insecticides, used in agriculture has recently been reviewed (WHO/UNEP, 1990). The overview presented in sections 1.1 and 1.2.1 of this monograph makes extensive reference to that document.

1.1 Historical perspectives

The use of inorganic chemicals to control insects possibly dates back to classical Greece and Rome. Homer mentioned the fumigant value of burning sulfur; Pliny the Elder advocated the insecticidal use of arsenic and referred to the use of soda and olive oil for treating legume seeds. The Chinese were employing moderate amounts of arsenicals as insecticides by the sixteenth century, and, not long afterwards, nicotine was used, in the form of tobacco extracts. By the nineteenth century, both pyrethrum (a natural insecticide obtained by extraction of chrysanthemum flowers) and soap were being used for insect control, as was a combined wash of tobacco, sulfur and lime to combat insects and fungi.

The middle of the nineteenth century marked the first systematic scientific studies into the use of chemicals for crop protection. Work on arsenic compounds led to the introduction in 1867 of Paris green, an impure copper arsenite, used in the USA to check the spread of the Colorado beetle; by 1900, its use was so widespread that probably the first insecticide legislation in the world was enacted to control its use.

In the years between the two World Wars, both the number and the complexity of chemicals for crop protection increased. Tar oils, which include anthracene, creosote and naphtha, were used to control eggs of aphids on dormant trees. During the Second World War, the insecticidal potential of DDT was discovered in Switzerland and insecticidal organophosphorus compounds were developed in Germany. In 1945, the first soil-active carbamate herbicides were discovered by researchers in the United Kingdom, and the organochlorine insecticide chlordane was introduced in the USA and in Germany. Shortly afterwards, the insecticidal carbamates were developed in Switzerland.

During the 1970s and 1980s, many new insecticides were introduced. Typically, these are based on a new understanding of biological and biochemical mechanisms of pest control and

---

[1]Insecticidal use of arsenicals is not included in this monograph. The carcinogenic activity of arsenic and arsenic compounds was evaluated by previous IARC working groups (IARC, 1980, 1987).

are often effective at lower doses than the older ones. A new, important group of insecticides is the synthetic light-stable pyrethroids, which were developed from naturally occurring pyrethrins. Increasing knowledge of host–pest interactions has led to a new approach to the design of insecticides and new formulations and ways of application.

1.2 Use and exposure

1.2.1 *Trends in worldwide use of insecticides*

A wide range of insecticides, fungicides, molluscicides, bactericides and herbicides, including fumigants, are used, mainly in developed countries but also (and increasingly so) in developing countries. Organochlorine insecticides are still used in the latter but are being replaced gradually by organophosphorus, carbamate and pyrethroid insecticides. Another important use for insecticides is in the control of ectoparasites.

The pests responsible for the greatest losses are locusts, but effective, inexpensive insecticides to control the massive locust infestations that plague some parts of the world have yet to be developed. The crop on which most insecticides are used is cotton.

The most common formulations are emulsifiable concentrates and ultra-low volume concentrates. In urban areas, organochlorine insecticides are now little used; they have been replaced by pyrethrins, pyrethroids and organophosphorus insecticides, such as chlorpyrifos, dichlorvos, fenitrothion, fenthion, malathion and temephos. The worldwide requirements for pesticides in urban public health programmes worldwide are substantial, the annual cost being over US $ 100 million. In 1980, about 50 000 tonnes of pesticides were used in public health programmes in developing countries. It was estimated that such programmes account for about 10% of total pesticide use, the remainder being used mainly in agriculture.

Insecticides are used on a number of crops of different relative importance for world agricultural production (Table 1). Herbicides are used mainly on corn and soya beans, insecticides mainly on cotton and horticultural crops and fungicides mainly on horticultural crops and wheat. Worldwide use of insecticides in 1985 was approximately 29% in Japan and the Far East, 23% in the USA, 12% in western Europe, and 36% in the rest of the world; the corresponding values for herbicides were: 10, 46, 21 and 22%, respectively.

Table 1. The insecticide market by crop in 1985 (million US $ in 1984)[a]

Crop	USA	Western Europe	Japan & Far East	Rest of world	Total
Maize	262	70	28	96	456
Cotton	206	24	149	590	969
Wheat	16	34	23	35	108
Sorghum	20	6	6	24	56
Rice	24	7	498	104	633
Other grains	7	22	5	12	46
Soya beans	30	4	27	67	128
Tobacco	33	8	31	38	108
Peanuts (Groundnuts)	22	1	19	23	65
Sugar beets	8	59	6	24	97
Sugar cane	6	—	9	27	42

Table 1 (contd)

Crop	USA	Western Europe	Japan & Far East	Rest of world	Total
Coffee	—	—	5	39	44
Cocoa	—	—	13	25	38
Tea	—	—	38	19	57
Rubber	—	—	11	8	19
Other field crops	22	43	45	60	170
Alfalfa	18	8	2	4	32
Other hay and forage	2	3	2	6	13
Pasture and rangeland	6	2	2	9	19
Fruit, vegetables and horticultural crops	299	213	329	327	1168
Total	981 (23%)	504 (12%)	1248 (29%)	[1537] (36%)	4268 (100%)

[a]From WHO/UNEP (1990)

1.2.2 *Application principles and techniques*

Methods of application of pesticides, including insecticides, have been reviewed (Haskell, 1985). The aim of insecticide application is to distribute a small amount of active ingredient to the appropriate insect with minimal contamination of non-target organisms. The diversity of possible targets—e.g., insects, plants, soil, walls of dwellings— necessitates a variety of application techniques, which can be summarized in five groups:

- (i)   release or propulsion through the air to the target either
  - in the solid state as dusts or granules, or
  - in the liquid state as sprays;
- (ii) application directly to or injection into the plant;
- (iii) injection into the soil;
- (iv) release into irrigation water; or
- (v)   release into the air with diffusion to the target (fumigation).

Hazards due to drift and inhalation of particles less than 30 μm in diameter have resulted in a decline in the use of dusts, except for treating seeds and small seedlings at the time of transplanting, for which specialized equipment is available. Seed treatment is ideal for protecting young plants with minimal quantities of toxicant, but as phytotoxicity can be a problem the use of granules accurately placed alongside seeds at sowing has increased. Equipment is also available for spot treatment of individual plants, and granules are often broadcast, sometimes by hand; but this requires a higher dose than other application techniques (Matthews, 1985).

Special equipment is needed to meter granules, so the majority of pesticides are applied as sprays. The volume of spray liquid applied varies with the size of target and on whether discrete droplets or a complete film of spray is to be distributed on the target. While 50 to more than 1000 litres/ha may be applied to field crops, bushes and trees, as little as 5 litres/ha of pesticides may be applied using newer ultra-low volume spray techniques (Matthews, 1985).

Less than 0.1% of the applied dose may reach insect pests in a field crop treated with a foliar spray, whereas up to 30% of an applied herbicide penetrated experimental plants sprayed in a greenhouse (Matthews, 1985). The low efficiency of sprays has been due largely to the wide range of droplet sizes emitted by traditional spraying equipment; control of droplet size is designed to suit the intended target and the method of application (Table 2).

Table 2. Optimal droplet sizes[a]

Target	Droplet size (μm)
Flying insects	10-50
Insects on foliage	30-50
Foliage	40-100
Soil (and avoidance of drift)	250-500
Aerial applications	> 500

[a]Adapted from Matthews (1985)

The five basic classes of ground application equipment include hydraulic sprayers, air sprayers, foggers and aerosol generators, power dusters and hand-held equipment (Anon., 1981). In hydraulic sprayers, the pesticide is delivered under pressure by a pump to one or more nozzles. The type of nozzle regulates droplet size and spray pattern. Hydraulic sprayers are of four basic types:

(i)   *Multiple-purpose sprayers* provide versatility for a variety of problems. Spray pressure is adjustable; tank size ranges from 190 to 750 litres; sprayers are skid- or wheel-mounted and powered by auxiliary engines or a power take-off; spray is dispensed through a hand-gun or field boom.

(ii)   *Small general-purpose sprayers* are useful for small jobs, for instance in green-houses, large gardens and golf courses. Tank size ranges up to 100 litres; power is provided by a small engine that furnishes a wide range of pressures (50-500 psi [3.5-35.2 kg/cm^2]); spray is dispensed through a hand-gun or short boom, and the sprayers are usually mounted on a hand-operated cart or attached to a garden tractor.

(iii)   *Low-pressure, low-volume sprayers* are commonly used on crops. They can be mounted directly on equipment or are equipped with wheels; tank size ranges up to 950 litres; power is usually provided by a power take-off, but may be supplied by an auxiliary engine; operating pressure is up to 100 psi [7.0 kg/cm^2] and spray is dispensed through a field boom.

(iv)   *High-pressure, high-volume sprayers* are used by fruit growers and truck farmers in order to obtain good penetration and coverage in tall growing trees and dense crop growths. These sprayers are essentially the same as multiple purpose sprayers except that larger engines provide up to 1000 psi [70.3 kg/cm^2] and tank size ranges up to 2300 litres (Anon., 1981).

Air sprayers (also known as ultra-low-volume, concentrate blower, airblast and airmist sprayers) are used for spraying orchards, large shade trees and field crops. Pesticides are applied in concentrated form, using relatively small volumes of water, in contrast to hydraulic sprayers. A low-volume pump delivers the liquid spray under low pressure to the fan, where it is discharged into an air stream in small droplets by a group of nozzles or shear plates. Pump pressures range from 50 to 400 psi [3.5-28.1 kg/cm^2], and fans deliver 5000-25 000 ft^3/mn [2.4-11.8 m^3/s] or air velocities of 100-150 mile/h [160-240 km/h] (Anon., 1981; Joyce, 1985).

Foggers or aerosol generators are designed primarily for control of mosquitoes and flies in large buildings, parks, resorts and communities. These machines disperse fine particles of pesticides into the air, as fogs or mists, where they remain for a considerable time. Fogs and aerosols are produced by either thermal or mechanical methods or a combination. Aerosol equipment is not practical for application of most agricultural pesticides because of its tendency to create drifts (Anon., 1981).

Power dusters are run by engine or power take-offs. Like airblast sprayers, dusters also utilize air streams from a centrifugal fan to carry the pesticide to the target area. They may have single or multiple outlets. Dusters may be impractical for application of some pesticides because of drift hazard (Anon., 1981).

Hand-held equipment is designed primarily for application of pesticides in small areas; this type of equipment includes hand-pump atomizers, aerosol dispensers, compressed air sprayers, knapsack sprayers and dusters. The *hand-pump atomizer* has a hand-operated pump to force an air stream over the tip of a siphon tube; pesticide is sucked from the tube and atomized in the air stream. These sprayers were commonly used to control flying insects in houses but have been almost completely replaced by aerosol dispensers. *Aerosol dispensers* are probably the most common type of applicator for household pest sprays. The pesticide and a propellant, usually freon, are forced, under pressure, through an atomizing nozzle. *Compressed air sprayers* are designed to hold 4-12 litres in the tank. A hand pump is used to pressurize the tank and deliver the pesticide, under pressure, to the nozzle. Spray patterns and droplet size can be regulated by nozzle type. Solutions, emulsions and suspensions of pesticides can be used at pressures of 30-50 psi (2.2-3.5 kg/cm^2]. *Knapsack hand sprayers* are carried on the back and usually have a capacity of 20 litres; a hand-operated piston or diaphragm pump provides the pressure (30-100 psi [2.2-7.0 kg/cm^2]) to expel the pesticide. *Duster hand sprayers* range from small self-contained units to those mounted on wheelbarrows. Air velocity for dispensing the dust is created by a plunger, hand crank or belt attached to a fan or blower (Anon., 1981).

The subject of aerial spray equipment and accessories is complex; however, many aspects of aerial application are similar to ground application. For example, sprayers are basically constructed of the same components. Several classes of aircraft may be used for the application of pesticides, including high-wing monoplanes, low-wing monoplanes, biplanes, multi-engine aircraft (used extensively in forest and rangeland application) and helicopters. Helicopters have some advantages over fixed-wing aircraft: operation at slower speeds; increased safety; improved accuracy of swath, coverage and placement of chemical; and operation without airport facilities. Pesticides are generally released at greater heights than from conventional sprayers (Anon., 1981).

Application equipment can be constructed for dispersing dry or liquid pesticides. Dry chemicals are dispensed from fixed-wing aircraft primarily by ram-air spreaders and spinners. In a ram-air spreader, dry materials are metered from a hopper into the propeller slip stream. The fact that ram-air systems cannot spread materials in a wide swath led to the development of spinners, which consist of spinning vanes mounted under the hopper that throw material outward in a uniform pattern. The use of spreaders and blowers can nearly double the swath width. In helicopters, two types of dispenser are used: a blower driven by the engine forces dry material from two side tanks and out of short booms, but the material may be spread using spinners instead of the boom; or a single hopper can be suspended on a cable and dry material is dispensed using spinners (Anon., 1981).

Two types of liquid spray systems exist for fixed- and rotary-wing aircraft: the pressure type, in which the spray is applied under specific pressures; and the gravity-feed type, in which the flow of spray solution from the tank dispersion unit relies on gravity. Swath widths of 12-18 m, in the application range of 1.5 to 15 litres/ha, are normal when material is released 1.5-2.5 m above the ground. Booms for fixed- and rotary-wing aircraft, although mounted differently, are basically the same in construction. Boom pipes are round or aerodynamic in cross section. In a fixed-wing aircraft, they are mounted on the trailing edge of the wing and are usually three-quarters the wing length. Atomizers have a nozzle and a variety of spinning screen cages, discs and wire brushes; they are usually driven by fans or electric motors. Atomizers produce droplets of more uniform size and are useful in low-volume spraying, such as for grasshopper and mosquito control (Anon., 1981).

The present trend in pesticide use is to apply highly concentrated material at low rates: ultra-low-volume rates for mosquito control are as low as 0.15 litres/ha. The use of such formulations requires the use of special equipment and application procedures, as the systems must deliver fine droplets to be effective. This can be accomplished by using spinning or flat fan nozzles that discharge 0.15 litres/ha at 40-55 psi [2.8-3.9 kg/cm^2]. For helicopter operations, a single spinning nozzle may provide adequate output at very low rates such as required for mosquito control. Because the ultra-low-volume systems produce fine droplets, the location of the nozzles is important (Anon., 1981).

1.2.3 Occupational exposures

Occupational exposures may occur during the manufacture and processing of insecticides as well as during their use. In addition, pesticide residues on plants or fruits may cause significant exposure of farm workers picking or handling the products. Among the more specific occupations with potential exposure are: manufacturers (production workers), formulators, vendors, transporters, mixers, loaders, applicators/operators (farmers or professionals) and pickers and growers.

The relative importance of the routes of occupational exposure is usually in the following order: dermal exposure > respiratory exposure > oral exposure. The occupational groups can have long-term exposure of this type, but very few reports of any effects are available, and further studies are needed to describe better the conditions of chronic exposure that do occur. It is relatively easy to identify people in occupations where exposure to pesticides is common and/or heavier than in the general population, but documentation or measurements of exposure to specific pesticides are seldom available. Furthermore, even if monitoring data or other documentation of exposure are available, it is difficult to evaluate risks associated with specific pesticides because most applicators have contact with a variety of pesticides and because variation in work practices can greatly affect the delivered dose.

Different levels of exposure are encountered depending on the type of application equipment used (Table 3). Furthermore, considerable differences in exposure have been found among the different jobs; most frequently, mixer-loaders have been found to receive the highest exposures, as they work with large quantities of concentrated materials.

Table 3. Estimated exposure of applicators using different application equipment[a]

Type of equipment	Average exposure[b] (range)	No. of observations
Airblast	790 (109-2826)	283
Hand-held hydraulic sprayguns	340 (0.8-2175)	12
Knapsack sprayers	320 (20-11 518)	20
Portable mistblowers	150 (19-546)	6
Hydraulic ground boom sprayers	210 (0.03-3460)	15

[a]From Dover (1985)
[b]Micrograms active ingredient per 100 cm² surface area per hour

Selected studies in which occupational exposures in spraying and application of insecticides have actually been measured are presented in Table 4.

Table 4. Occupational exposures in spraying and application of insecticides

Chemical	Population	Levels[a]	Reference
Indoor application			
Malathion	Spraymen treating interior household surfaces for mosquito control in Pakistan	330 mg (average daily dermal exposure)	Baker et al. (1978)
Chlorpyrifos	Applicators treating 20 single-family housing units with a paint-on application method (application time per unit was 1.3 h) in Omaha, NE, USA	2.1 μg/cm²/h (D) 0.01 μg/l/h (R)	Gold et al. (1981)
	Applicators treating 20 single-family housing units with a spray application method (application time per unit was 0.81 h) in Omaha, NE, USA	4.1 μg/cm²/h (D) 0.07 μg/l/h (R)	
Dichlorvos	Commercial pest control applicators treating 20 single-family houses with hand sprayers in NE, USA	Total estimated exposure: 28 μg/kg bw/h (D) 0.4 μg/kg bw/h (R)	Gold & Holcslaw (1985)
Pirimiphosmethyl	Applicators spraying tomato plants in greenhouses in Hungary	424.8 mg/h (D)[b] 44.3 mg/h (D)[c] 165 μg/h (R)[b] 39 μg/h (R)[c]	Adamis et al. (1985)
Dimethoate	Applicators spraying tomato plants in greenhouses in Hungary	346.0 mg/h (D)[b] 10.5 mg/h (D)[c] 59 μg/h (R)[b] 1 μg/h (R)[c]	Adamis et al. (1985)

Table 4 (contd)

Chemical	Population	Levels[a]	Reference
Indoor application (contd)			
Permethrin	Applicators spraying tomato plants in greenhouses in Hungary	3.9 mg/h (D)[c] 4 μg/h (D)[c]	Adamis *et al.* (1985)
Fenoxycarb	Two technicians treating 20 houses in Omaha, NE, USA, for cockroach infestation	Total exposure: 21.2 mg/h (D) 1.6 mg/h (R)	Ogg & Gold (1988)
Fluvalinate	Tractor driver using boom sprayer to treat ornamental plants at commercial greenhouse in Cortez, FL, USA	265 μg/h (estimated mean total body accumulation rate excluding hands)	Stamper *et al.* (1989)
	Tractor driver using span sprayer to treat ornamental plants at commercial greenhouse in Cortez, FL, USA	3 μg/h (estimated mean total body accumulation rate excluding hands)	
Chlorpyrifos	Tractor driver using boom sprayer to treat ornamental plants at commercial greenhouse in Cortez, FL, USA	3958 μg/h (estimated mean total body accumulation rate excluding hands)	Stamper *et al.* (1989)
	Tractor driver using span sprayer to treat ornamental plants at commercial greenhouse in Cortez, FL, USA	203 μg/h (estimated mean total body accumulation rate excluding hands)	
Lawn, turf and forest application			
Chlorthion	Workers treating pasture land for mosquitoes with aerosol generator in CA, USA		Culver *et al.* (1956)
	14 runs over 2.58 h	9-15 mg (total skin exposure)[d]	
	14 runs over 2.12 h	1-5 mg (total skin exposure)[e]	
Malathion	Workers treating pasture land for mosquitoes with aerosol generator in CA, USA		Culver *et al.* (1956)
	23 runs over 5.23 h	32-86 mg (total skin exposure)[d]	
	23 runs over 5.07 h	6-14 mg (total skin exposure)[e]	
Fenthion	Mosquito control workers using power sprayers (treatment site not stated)	Mean potential exposure: 3.6 mg/h (D) < 16 μg/h (R)	Wolfe *et al.* (1974)
	Mosquito control workers using hand pressure sprayer (treatment site not stated)	Mean potential exposure: 3.6 mg/h (D) < 21 μg/h (R)	

Table 4 (contd)

Chemical	Population	Levels[a]	Reference
Lawn, turf and forest application (contd)			
Fenthion (contd)	Mosquito control workers using hand granular dispersal (treatment site not stated)	Mean potential exposure: 12.3 mg/h (D) 88 μg/h (R)	
Carbaryl 80WP[f]	Two applicators spraying trees (9 times) in NE, USA	Mean total: 128.4 mg/h (D) 0.1 mg/h (R)	Leavitt et al. (1982)
	Five applicators spraying trees (once for 25 min) in NE, USA	Total exposure: 59.4 mg/h (D) 0.1 mg/h (R)	
Carbaryl	Five workers using low-pressure garden pump sprayers on a telescoping pole to treat tree boles in Placerville, CA, USA	Mean total body exposure: 62.7 mg	Haverty et al. (1983)
	Five workers using high-pressure sprayers to treat tree boles in Placerville, CA, USA	Mean total body exposure: 1.5 mg	
Diazinon	Three sprayers treating lawns (with compressed air sprayers) to duplicate around-the-house use in WA, USA	Mean potential exposure, hands: 5.5 mg/h (D) Mean potential exposure: 1.9 μg/h (R)	Davis et al. (1983)
	Three sprayers treating shrubs (with compressed air sprayers) to duplicate around-the-house use in WA, USA	Mean potential exposure, hands: 6.8 mg/h (D) Mean potential exposure: 2.9 μg/h (R)	
	Three sprayers treating lawns (with hose-end sprayers) to duplicate around-the-house use in WA, USA	Mean potential exposure, hands: 25.0 mg/h (D) Mean potential exposure: 7.4 μg/h (R)	
Diazinon	Professional lawn workers using spray guns or rotary spreaders (total work time: 300-400 min) in IN, USA	13-23 ng/m^3 (R) 3.9-130.2 μg/100 cm^2 (D, wrist areas) 30-592 μg/100 cm^2 (D, thigh areas)	Freeborg et al. (1985)
Trichlorfon	Professional lawn workers using spray guns (total work time: 456 min) in IN, USA	2 ng/m^3 (R) ND-0.35 μg/100 cm^2 (D, wrist areas)	Freeborg et al. (1985)
Chlorpyrifos	Six lawn sprayers monitored for 1 h in MI, USA	Mean calculated exposure: 135 mg/day (D) 22 μg/day (R)	Copley (1987)

Table 4 (contd)

Chemical	Population	Levels[a]	Reference
Agricultural application			
Dimethoate	Eight spraymen using a knapsack spray-er for treatment of crops in Sudan	Total calculated exposure: 175.8 μg/cm^2/day to 8.3 mg/cm^2/day (D); 5.1–19.9 μg/day (R)	Copplestone et al. (1976)
Pyrethroid formulation	Seven applicators spraying cotton in the Ivory Coast	Total exposure: 2.8–42.2 mg/h (D); < 100–200 μg/m^3 (R)	Prinsen & Van Sittert (1980)
Carbaryl	Applicator treating apples with a hand-gun hose-nozzle sprayer in WA, USA	Mean total exposure: 19.6 mg/h (D)	Maitlen et al. (1982)
	Applicators treating peas or potatoes with tractor-mounted boom sprayer in WA, USA	Total exposure: 1.6 mg/h (D) (wettable powder); 2.8 mg/h (D) (liquid suspension)	
Parathion	Spray-rig drivers treating citrus trees using an airblast sprayer (from an open tractor) in CA, USA	Mean exposure: 0.33 μg/cm^2/h (D)	Carman et al. (1982)
	Spray-rig drivers treating citrus trees using an airblast sprayer (from a cab unit with both side-windows open) in CA, USA	Mean exposure: 0.48 μg/cm^2/h (D)	
	Spray rig drivers treating citrus trees using an airblast sprayer (from a cab unit with windows closed) in CA, USA	Mean exposure: 0.01 μg/cm^2/h (D)	
	Spray rig drivers treating citrus trees using an oscillating boom sprayer (from an open tractor) in CA, USA	Mean exposure: 4.8 μg/cm^2/h (D)	
	Spray rig drivers treating citrus trees using an oscillating boom sprayer (from a cab unit with both side windows open) in CA, USA	Mean exposure: 2.4 μg/cm^2/h (D)	
	Spray rig drivers treating citrus trees using an oscillating boom sprayer (from a cab unit with windows closed) in CA, USA	Mean exposure: 0.03 μg/cm^2/h (D)	
Dimethoate	Spray rig drivers treating citrus trees using an airblast sprayer (from an open tractor) in CA, USA	Mean exposure: 2.5 μg/cm^2/h (D)	Carman et al. (1982)
	Spray rig drivers treating citrus trees using an airblast sprayer (from a cab unit with both side windows open) in CA, USA	Mean exposure: 1.5 μg/cm^2/h (D)	
	Spray rig drivers treating citrus trees using an airblast sprayer (from a cab unit with windows closed) in CA, USA	Mean exposure: < 0.01 μg/cm^2/h (D)	

Table 4 (contd)

Chemical	Population	Levels[a]	Reference
Agricultural application (contd)			
Chlorobenzilate	Four applicators using airblast sprayers pulled by canopied tractors treating citrus groves in FL, USA	[32.7] mg/h (estimated mean total body exposure)	Nigg & Stamper (1983)
	Two pesticide mixer-loaders at a citrus grove in FL, USA	[8.3] mg/h (estimated mean total body exposure)	
Cypermethrin	Applicators treating crops in the United Republic of Tanzania, the Ivory Coast and Paraguay using an Electrodyn[g] sprayer	3.0–26.9 mg/h (D) (total contamination)	Dover (1985)
	Applicators treating crops in the Republic of Tanzania and the Ivory Coast using a spinning disc sprayer	17.8–369.9 mg/h (D) (total contamination)	
	Applicators treating crops in Paraguay using a knapsack sprayer	29.5 mg/h (D) (total contamination)	
Carbaryl	Applicators treating tall vegetables (maize) in home gardens for 15 min (clothing worn afforded six increasing levels of protection) in PA, USA	0.5–9.9 mg (dust) 0.2–7.7 mg (wettable powder) 0.2–11 mg (aqueous suspension)[h]	Kurtz & Bode (1985)
	Applicators treating low vegetables (green beans) in home gardens for 15 min (clothing worn afforded six increasing levels of protection) in PA, USA	0.5–10.2 mg (dust)[h] 0.2–5.4 mg (wettable powder)[h] 0.2–6.8 mg (aqueous suspension)[h]	
Imidan	Applicators treating fruit trees for 14 h with airblast sprayers (tractors not equipped with spray cabs) in NY, USA	Total exposure: 56.3 μg/cm^2 (D)	Spittler & Bourke (1985)
	Applicators treating fruit trees for 31.3 h with airblast sprayers (tractors equipped with spray cabs) in NY, USA	Total exposure: 40.3 μg/cm^2 (D)	
Terbufos	Eleven Canadian farmers using planter-mounted granular applicators for crop treatment while planting maize	Mean estimated exposure: 72.4 μg/h (D); 11.3 μg/h (R)	Devine et al. (1986)
Azinphosmethyl	Orchard sprayers in Ontario, Canada	5.2 mg (D) (mean exposure)	Franklin et al. (1986)
	Orchard sprayers in Nova Scotia, Canada	4.3 mg (D) (mean exposure excluding hands) 5.6 mg (D) (mean exposure including hands)	

Table 4 (contd)

Chemical	Population	Levels[a]	Reference
Agricultural application (contd)			
Malathion	Seven mixers for treatment of citrus in CA, USA	762 μg[i] 2161 μg[j]	Fenske (1987)
Aerial application			
Carbaryl	Applicators treating maize from a helicopter with a boom sprayer in WA, USA	Total exposure: 7.4 mg/h (D) (wettable powder); 3.4 mg/h (D) (water-based flowable); 26.5 mg/h (D) (liquid suspension)	Maitlen et al. (1982)
Chlordimeform	200 workers including mixers, loaders, applicators, flaggers and cleaners in CA, USA	90 μg/l urine with levels highest in mixer-loaders and lowest in pilots and flaggers	Maddy et al. (1986)
Cypermethrin	Pilots using ultra-low-volume spray to treat commercial cotton on farms in MS, USA	0.66 mg/8 h (actual exposure) 1.07 mg/8 h (potential exposure)[k]	Nye (1986)
	Mixer-loaders for ultra-low-volume application to treat commercial cotton on farms in MS, USA	2.43 mg/8 h (actual exposure) 10.5 mg/8 h (potential exposure)[k]	

[a]Abbreviations: bw, body weight; (D), dermal; (R), respiratory
[b]Applicator moved forward and passed through area sprayed
[c]Applicator moved backward
[d]Jeep driver; also did the formulating
[e]During the insecticide application, this man walked behind and along the upwind side of the equipment in order to regulate the machinery and help clock the speed of the jeep; he also did the formulating
[f]80% wettable powder
[g]Glass bottle with built-in nozzle instead of spray tank
[h]Mean estimated exposures to unprotected body areas
[i]Estimated head exposure using fluorescent tracer technique
[j]Estimated head exposure using patch technique
[k]Actual exposure estimates represent the uncovered areas of the head and hands of the workers; potential exposure estimates represent the sum of the residues from the overalls plus the cotton gloves and nylon socks worn by the workers.

In a study of the exposure of agricultural workers to carbaryl, Maitlen et al. (1982) found that the mixer-loader operation was not inherently different for ground, aerial or hand-gun applications. Factors that affected the hourly dermal exposure of mixer-loaders included: the formulation used; the use of gloves; and the method (scooping or pouring) of removing powdered insecticide from its container prior to mixing. Powdered formulations resulted in higher total hourly dermal exposures (43.3 mg/h with gloves; 107 mg/h without gloves) than liquid formulations (3.0 mg/h with gloves; 40 mg/h without gloves). An average of 76% of the total exposure of all mixer-loaders was on the hands. The techniques of scooping and pouring powdered formulations from the container without wearing gloves resulted in total average hourly dermal exposures of 176 and 38 mg/h, respectively.

Dermal exposure to malathion was monitored for mosquito control spray teams treating interior household surfaces in Pakistan. Exposure was found to vary with job category: spraymen experienced the highest exposure to the forehead (mean, 39.3 $\mu g/cm^2$) and chest (mean, 13.6 $\mu g/cm^2$), while mixers had the highest exposure to the arms (mean, 49.6 $\mu g/cm^2$). Supervisors had the lowest exposures to the arms (mean, 2.9 $\mu g/cm^2$). During this study, the authors observed improper work practices which increased dermal exposure to malathion. Spraymen's clothes were wet at the end of the working day, smelled strongly of pesticide, and were worn for several days without washing. Both spraymen and mixers had extensive skin contact with the pesticide while filling and pressurizing the spray tanks. Some mixers mixed the malathion suspension with their hands. Many spray cans leaked pesticide onto the arms, hands and chests of the spraymen. When spray nozzles became clogged, the spraymen sometimes blew through them to unclog them (Baker *et al.*, 1978).

Nye (1986) found that during aerial application of cypermethrin, pilots were exposed primarily *via* contact with the aircraft when entering and leaving, as well as from the cockpit ventilation system. Dermal exposure was predominantly *via* the hands and to a lesser degree, the trunk. For mixer-loaders, exposure was more uniform, but the trunk, gloves and forearms contained most of the cypermethrin residues. Pilots were, on average, exposed to ten times less cypermethrin than mixer-loaders. The author noted that mixer-loaders worked principally with the formulation concentrate, while the pilots were exposed principally to diluted spray.

1.2.4 *Exposure monitoring*

Human exposure can either be measured directly or inferred. Examples of methods for direct measurement are collection of pesticides in breathing-zone air or on pads or clothing worn by workers. These techniques provide a direct, calculable measure of human exposure under actual conditions. Most often, however, direct measurement is not possible; for example, in retrospective studies, exposures may only be inferred from the available information. Coupling biochemical measures with traditional exposure evaluation procedures used in epidemiological studies of cancer offers the best opportunity for improving the assessment of historical pesticide exposures (Moseman & Oswald, 1980; Blair *et al.*, 1989).

Exposure to pesticides has usually been estimated by monitoring the ambient environment. In some cases, exposure by inhalation has been measured using personal sampler pumps with absorbent filters approximating the breathing zone of the worker (Franklin, 1989). A new technique for estimating exposure by inhalation is to measure the level of the chemical in exhaled breath (Morgan *et al.*, 1989). Exposure by dermal contact is estimated by placing absorbent patches on the worker's body or clothing or by solvent extraction of clothing worn during application. Exposure estimates obtained from ambient monitoring (personal samplers, patches, clothing, tracers) indicate the amount of pesticide that impinges on the surface of the body (contact exposure) and not the absorbed dose (Franklin, 1989).

A number of definitions have been developed for the biological monitoring of exposures in general and for that of insecticides in particular (Foa *et al.*, 1987; Clarkson *et al.*, 1988; Wang *et al.*, 1989). In this monograph, the term 'biological monitoring' is used to cover all those procedures for assessing dose and the biochemical and physiological effects (possibly reversible) in human biological specimens after exposure to insecticides. Industrial hygiene practices and clinical diagnostic procedures are not included in this discussion. Within the limits of this definition, it is obvious that the identification of risks and of groups of subjects at risk is crucial.

Biochemical effects of organophosphorus pesticides can be assessed by measuring the inhibition of certain blood enzymes, as their inhibition usually mirrors that of the corresponding enzyme within the nervous system which represents the molecular target of the organophosphate. Thus, measurement of acetylcholinesterase in red blood cells is widely used to assess cholinergic effects, whereas inhibition of neuropathy target esterase in lymphocytes might be used to assess the delayed neurotoxic effects of some organo-phosphate insecticides (Hayes *et al.*, 1980; Ames *et al.*, 1989; Lotti, 1989; WHO/UNEP, 1990).

Insecticides can be measured in biological samples by the usual analytical techniques (see the monographs on individual insecticides) or by biological methods. A number of reports are available in which insecticides and/or their metabolites have been measured in body fluids after occupational exposures (Coye *et al.*, 1986; Maroni, 1986; Wang *et al.*, 1989). Examples include the measurement of dialkylphosphates in urine after exposure to organophosphorus insecticides (Coye *et al.*, 1986), of *para*-nitrophenol after exposure to parathion and methylparathion (Wolfe *et al.*, 1970) and of 1-naphthol after exposure to carbaryl (Comer *et al.*, 1975) (e.g., see Coye *et al.*, 1986). Although these procedures are used for quantitative assessments of dose, interpretation of the results is hampered in the absence of pharmacokinetic data in man. Such data are also essential when extrapolating data on toxicity across species.

A somewhat different approach to biological monitoring is the measurement of adducts to proteins (Shugart *et al.*, 1989). Adducts to haemoglobin have been detected with several pesticides (Sabbioni & Neumann, 1990). The advantages of such measurements include the possibility of assessing dose closer to the target, of assessing individual capacity to form electrophiles and of extrapolating data on toxicity more easily across species. When the mechanism of action of a pesticide is understood, more specific markers can be used.

2. Studies of Cancer in Humans

Epidemiological studies on cancer risk following exposure to insecticides can be divided into three types: (a) those referring to specific insecticides with or without mention of insecticides in general; (b) those mentioning only insecticides in general; and (c) those referring to populations exposed to 'pesticides' or 'pesticides/herbicides'. Studies under (a) were considered both in the specific monographs and in the present one. Studies under (b) are reviewed only in the present monograph. As for category (c), in a few cases, the Working Group included studies of populations exposed to 'pesticides' because they provide special information relevant to the evaluation of insecticides.

2.1 Descriptive and ecological studies

2.1.1 *Mortality statistics*

In Central Luzon in the Philippines, the use of organophosphate and organochlorine insecticides increased after adoption of modern rice varieties in the late 1960s. Insecticides were applied by backpack sprayer, usually by men. Protective clothing was not worn. Mortality was studied in three rural municipalities, with a population of 96 000 in 1980 and where more than 80% of the heads of households in typical villages were employed primarily in rice farming. The study covered two periods: 1961-71, with low use of insecticides, and 1972-84, with high use. For men aged 15-54 years, the mean age-standardized mortality rate per 100 000 for cancer (all sites except brain) increased from 21.1 to 25.9. Mortality from leukaemia among men increased from 0.6 to 3.6 per 100 000. Seven of the 11 leukaemia cases recorded since 1961 occurred in 1979-84. The leukaemia rates for women in the same periods were 0.6 and 0.7 per 100 000, respectively (Loevinsohn, 1987).

2.1.2 *Proportionate mortality studies*

Several studies have been undertaken on the basis of death certificates from Wisconsin, USA (Blair & Watts, 1980; Blair & White, 1981; Cantor, 1982; Cantor & Blair, 1984; Saftlas *et al.*, 1987). In the most recent of these, a study population was selected of 35 972 white men, 18 years and older, who resided in 69 of the 70 Wisconsin counties and died in 1968-76 and whose occupation on the death certificate was farm owner, tenant or labourer. Proportionate mortality ratio (PMR) and proportionate cancer mortality ratio (PCMR) values were calculated using mortality of white, non-farming Wisconsin men for comparison. Data from the agricultural censuses in 1949, 1964 and 1969 and from the population census in 1960 were used for constructing indicators of exposures in agriculture in each county. The PMR for all cancers was significantly lower than expected (5634 observed; PMR, 0.92 [95% confidence interval (CI), 0.90-0.94]). This deficit was due in particular to tobacco-related cancers. When the data were analysed after excluding smoking-related causes of death, statistically significant excess risks were found for cancers of the stomach (PCMR, 1.1 [95% CI, 1.0-1.2]), prostate (PCMR, 1.1 [1.1-1.2]) and eye (PCMR, 3.4 [2.2-5.2]) and for all lymphopoietic cancers (PCMR, 1.1 [1.0-1.2]). Analysis by agricultural exposure level revealed a statistically significant excess risk for cancers of other lymphatic tissue (two-thirds were multiple myelomas) in counties with heavy use of insecticides (28 observed; PCMR, 1.6 [1.0-2.2]). The risk was also increased in counties with heavy use of herbicides and fertilizers and a high proportion of maize production.

2.1.3 *Case-control studies with ecological information on exposure*

Several case-control studies employed similar methods to evaluate cancer risks and potential exposure to agricultural insecticides in the USA (Blair & Thomas, 1979; Burmeister *et al.*, 1982, 1983; Cantor & Blair, 1984). Deceased cases were ascertained from death certificates, and controls were deceased residents from the same state, matched to the cases by date of birth, date of death, race, sex and county of residence. Usual occupation as a farmer was determined from the death certificate. Potential exposure of farmers to insecticides was classified on the basis of their county of residence and insecticide use patterns for that county. Thus, these studies employed both ecological and individual assessments.

Blair and Thomas (1979) found mortality from leukaemia to be elevated among farmers in Nebraska, but the risks were similar among farmers in counties using less insecticides (odds ratio, 1.2; 95% CI, 0.94-1.6) and in counties using more insecticides (odds ratio, 1.3; 1.0-1.7). Similar findings were obtained in Iowa, where the risks for leukaemia among farmers did not appear to be higher among those residing in counties where insecticides were used heavily than in counties where they were used to a lesser extent (Burmeister *et al.*, 1982).

In Iowa, the odds ratio for death due to multiple myeloma for farmers born after 1890 residing in counties in the upper tercile of insecticide use was 2.0 ($p \leq 0.05$) (Burmeister *et al.*, 1983). Cantor and Blair (1984) evaluated risks for multiple myeloma in association with ecological assessments of exposure to insecticides in Wisconsin. Using nonfarmers residing in counties where insecticide use was low as unexposed controls, the odds ratios were 0.9 (95% CI, 0.7-1.3) for nonfarmers residing in counties with high insecticide use, 1.2 (0.9-1.7) for farmers residing in counties with low insecticide use and 1.9 (1.1-3.5) for farmers living in counties with high insecticide use. [These results are based on the same data as those of Saftlas *et al.* (1987).]

Proportionate mortality studies and case-control studies with ecological information on exposure are summarized in Table 5.

2.2 Cohort studies

Mortality rates were studied for a cohort of male pesticide applicators in the USA whose exposures included fumigants, carbamates, chlorinated hydrocarbons and organophosphates (Wang & MacMahon, 1979). The cohort was formed of employees from three nationwide pest control companies during the approximately 10 years for which centralized personnel records had been maintained. From a total of 44 083, records were selected for men who had been employed for at least three months between 1 January 1967 and 30 June 1976 by two of the companies and between 1 January 1968 and 30 June 1976 by the other and whose name, social security number, date of birth and dates of employment had been recorded. Examination of a sample of records for 4000 men who had been excluded showed that information was missing for 18%. Individual follow-up was not attempted. In the most recent analysis (MacMahon *et al.*, 1988), the cohort (16 124 men) was linked to Social Security Administration files in 1977 and 1981 and to the National Death Index for 1979-84. A total of 1082 deaths were thus identified, and death certificates were obtained for 994 (92%). The 88 deaths from unknown cause were allocated to causes of death according to the distribution of the deaths of known cause. National mortality rates for US white men were used for comparison, because the majority of the subjects were known to be white. The standardized mortality ratio (SMR) for deaths from all causes was 0.98 (90% CI, 0.93-1.03), and the SMR for all cancers was 1.1 (90% CI, 1.0-1.2]. Analysis by cause of death showed a statistically significant excess risk of lung cancer (SMR, 1.4; 90% CI, 1.1-1.6), which was present throughout the study period; the risk did not increase with duration of employment,

Table 5. Summary of findings for cancers at selected sites from descriptive and ecological studies on use of insecticides in the USA

Reference	Location	Cancer site	Relative risk	95% CI	Comments
Saftlas et al. (1987)	Wisconsin	Other lymphatic tissue	1.6	[1.0-2.2]	Farmers in high-use areas
Blair & Thomas (1979)	Nebraska	Leukaemia	1.3	1.0-1.7	Farmers in high-use areas
Burmeister et al. (1982)	Iowa	Leukaemia	1.3	0.9-1.9	Farmers in high-use areas (born (1890-1900)
			1.1	0.8-1.7	Farmers in high-use areas (born after 1900)
			1.4	1.1-1.8	Farmers in low-use areas (born 1890-1900)
			1.5	1.2-2.0	Farmers in low-use areas (born after 1900)
Burmeister et al. (1983)	Iowa	Multiple myeloma	2.0[a]	NA	Farmers in high-use areas (born (1890-1900)
			2.0[a]	NA	Farmers in high-use areas (born after 1900)
			1.4	NA	Farmers in low-use areas (born 1890-1900)
			1.2	NA	Farmers in low-use areas (born after 1900)
Cantor & Blair (1984)	Wisconsin	Multiple myeloma	1.9	1.1-3.5	Farmers in high-use counties
			1.2	0.9-1.7	Farmers in low-use counties
			0.9	0.7-1.3	Nonfarmers in high-use counties
			1.0	Reference	Nonfarmers in low-use counties

[a]$p \leq 0.05$

the SMRs being 1.4 for 0-4 years of employment, 1.1 for 5-9 years and 0.75 for 10 years or more. The SMRs were 1.3 (90% CI, 0.65-2.2) for skin cancer, 1.2 (0.50-2.5) for cancer of the bladder and 1.0 (0.67-1.4) for lymphatic and haematopoietic cancers. [The Working Group noted that exposure to arsenic was not mentioned but may have occurred.]

A national programme in the USA to monitor the health status of people occupationally exposed to pesticides enlisted 2620 volunteers in 13 states between 1971 and 1973. An effort was made to recontact these subjects in 1977-78, and 70% were successfully traced; 62 deaths were identified, and the cause of death was known for 59. Mortality data were analysed for the 1995 white men, using mortality rates for US white men for comparison. The SMR for neoplastic diseases was 0.39 (10 observed [95% CI, 0.2-0.7]) (Morgan et al., 1980). [The Working Group noted that the study was based on volunteers and that follow-up was incomplete.]

A cohort study of licensed pest control workers in Florida was undertaken (Blair et al., 1983). The authors stated that pest control workers apply a variety of pesticides, including chlorinated hydrocarbons, carbamates, organophosphates, phenoxyacetic acids, phthalimides, coumarins, arsenical insecticides and fungicides. The 4411 workers were identified from licence applications submitted by pest control firms in 1965-66. For each worker, full name, social security number, address, date of birth, primary duty in 1965-66, specific years licensed, and individual and firm certification categories were retrieved from the files. The cohort was followed up until 1 January 1977, and 96% were successfully traced. Death certificates were obtained for 389 of the 428 deceased subjects. Mortality rates for the US national population were used for comparison. The SMR for overall mortality among white male workers was 1.0 (378 observed, 367.5 expected [95% CI, 0.9-1.1]). An excess risk was found for lung cancer (34 observed, 25.1 expected; SMR, 1.4 [0.9-1.9]). Mortality from brain cancer was also elevated (5 observed, 2.5 expected; SMR, 2.0 [0.6-4.7]). The SMRs were [1.3 (0.2-4.8)] for skin cancer, [1.6 (0.3-4.6)] for cancer of the bladder, [2.7 (0.6-8.0)] for laryngeal cancer and [1.3 (0.4-3.4)] for leukaemia. The excess lung cancer risk increased by length of licensure; the SMRs were 1.0 [0.6-1.7] for < 10 years, 1.6 [0.8-2.8] for 10-19 years and 2.9 [1.2-5.6] for > 20 years; this pattern did not change when mortality rates for Florida were used for comparison. The lung cancer mortality was highest for workers employed by firms licensed for controlling rodents and general household pests, but it was elevated in other licensing categories also. [The Working Group noted that potential contact with arsenical insecticides complicates interpretation.]

A proportionate mortality analysis indicated an excess risk for neoplasms of the lymphatic and haematopoietic system and for cancers of the pancreas, lung and prostate among various subgroups of deceased members of the American Federation of Grain Millers' life insurance plan (Alavanja et al., 1987). Following this observation, a cohort study (which included these deaths) was published (Alavanja et al., 1990). Since 1955, which was the year the insurance plan started, 40 247 current or former members had been enrolled. A total of 22 938 white men with complete enrolment records were included in the study. Information on general pesticide use in the grain mills was obtained from interviews with senior employees and managers, from a survey among current union members and from various other sources, but could not be linked to individuals. In the analysis, the cohort was subdivided into workers in flour mills, workers in other grain industries, and workers in unidentified grain companies. In general, a wider variety of pesticides appeared to be used at the flour mills than at the other facilities. The pesticides most frequently cited as being used in all the flour mills included carbon tetrachloride, ethylene dibromide, malathion, methyl bromide, phosphine and pyrethrum. In a questionnaire survey in 1985-86, 31% of the flour millers reported that they applied pesticides, whereas this proportion was 16% among the other grain millers. The cohort was followed through to 1985. A total of 3668 deaths were identified, and death certificates were found for 3460 (94%). Mortality rates for US white men were used for comparison. The total of 3668 deaths was compared to an expected number of 4125.6 (SMR, 0.89; 95% CI, 0.86-0.92). The SMRs for all causes were 0.85 [0.8-0.9] for flour mills, 1.04 [1.0-1.1] for other grain industries and 0.58 [0.5-0.7] for unidentified grain companies. The SMRs for lung cancer were 0.78 [0.7-0.9] for flour mill workers and 1.1 [0.9-1.4] for workers in other grain industries. Workers in flour mills had slightly elevated risks of developing non-Hodgkin's lymphoma (SMR, 1.5 [0.9-2.3], based on 21 deaths), pancreatic cancer (SMR, 1.3 [0.9-1.9]; 33 deaths) and leukaemia (SMR, 1.4 [0.9-2.0]; 25 deaths); mortality from these causes was not increased among the other grain mill workers. The risk for non-Hodgkin's lymphoma among the flour mill workers increased by time elapsed since first employment, from an SMR of 0.64 for < 5 years, 0.49 for 5-9 years, 1.3 for 10-19 years and 2.3 (95% CI, 1.2-4.0) for > 20 years. A similar pattern was seen for pancreatic cancer (0.87 for < 5 years; 0.30 for 5-9 years; 1.2 for 10-19 years; and 1.9 (1.1-3.0) for ≥ 20 years). No trend by elapsed time was seen for leukaemia. Similar observations were made in a case-control study undertaken within the cohort. A survey showed that the flour mill workers did not differ from the other grain millers in educational level or in smoking habits, but they had a slightly higher consumption of alcohol. The risk for non-Hodgkin's lymphoma is not known to be associated with alcohol consumption, and the excess risk among the flour millers was therefore hypothesized to be associated with use of pesticides in flour mills. The risk for pancreatic cancer could be due to excessive alcohol consumption, but it was noted that mortality from cirrhosis of the liver was not elevated. [The Working Group noted that this cohort is unlikely to have been exposed to arsenic.]

Cancer incidence was studied in a cohort of 25 945 male farmers licensed for use of pesticides in 1970-74 in the Piedmont region of Italy. The pesticides were mainly in toxicological classes I and II according to Italian law. The cohort was matched to the Piedmont Hospital Discharge File for the period 1976-83, and 631 cancer cases were found. The number of person-years accumulated by the cohort members in 1976-83 was estimated. Cancer incidence rates for non-licensed men were used for comparison, estimated by subtracting cases and person-years for licensed men from those of the total population. The total of 631 cancer cases observed in the licensed group was compared with 877.8 expected cases. The standardized incidence ratios (SIR) were 0.7 (95% CI, 0.6-0.8) for all cancers, 1.4 (1.0-1.8) for malignant neoplasms of the skin, 1.4 (1.0-1.9) for malignant lymphoma, 1.0 (0.6-1.4) for malignancies of the nervous system and 1.1 (0.8-1.5) for leukaemia and multiple myeloma. Other cancer sites were not included in the analysis. The risk for malignant lymphomas was higher in residents of villages with a high proportion of arable land (SIR, 1.8; 95% CI, 1.2-2.5) (Corrao et al., 1989).

A study of 316 pesticide-exposed workers in Neubrandenburg in eastern Germany indicated an excess risk for lung cancer (Barthel, 1976). A subsequent study was therefore undertaken of 1658 men who had worked as agricultural plant protection workers or plant protection agronomists for at least five years in the 14 districts of the eastern part of Germany (excluding Berlin) during 1948-72 (Barthel, 1981a,b). About 70% of the potential study population was identified and included in the study. Respiratory protective equipment was rarely used. Before 1960, the pesticides included the insecticides calcium arsenate (banned since 1955), DDT, hexachlorocyclohexanes, methyl parathion and toxaphene, the fungicide cupral and the herbicides 4,6-dinitro-*ortho*-cresol, (2,4-dichlorophenoxy)acetic acid (2,4-D) and 4-chloro-2-methylphenoxyacetic acid (MCPA). A variety of pesticides was gradually introduced after 1960, of which zineb, maneb, simazine and chloral hydrate were used to a large extent. The cohort was followed up for cancer incidence and mortality through to 1978, and 169 malignant neoplasms were observed. Tumour incidence rates for the eastern part of Germany in 1973 were used to calculate expected numbers of tumour cases for the years 1970-78. Fifty bronchial carcinomas were observed in this period, where 27.5 cases were expected (SIR, 1.8 [95% CI, 1.4-2.4]). The lung cancer risk increased with length of exposure: SIR for < 10 years, 1.2 [0.5-2.5]; 10-19 years, 1.7 [1.1-2.4]; and > 19 years, 3.0 [1.7-4.7]. There was, however, no difference for workers first exposed in 1948-60 (SIR, 1.8 [1.3-2.5]) or those first exposed in 1961-72 (SIR, 1.7 [0.5-3.9]). A questionnaire survey among 163 randomly selected pesticide workers and an equivalent number of population controls showed no difference in smoking habits.

Cancer incidence was studied in a cohort of 20 245 licensed pesticide applicators in Sweden (Wiklund *et al.*, 1986, 1987, 1989). Since 1965, a licence has been mandatory for using the most acutely toxic pesticides. The workers in the study had been issued a licence between 1965 and 1976 and were followed up for cancer incidence to 31 December 1982. A survey on a random sample of 268 workers showed that 15% had used insecticides in the 1950s, 34% in the 1960s and 46% in the 1970s. During the 1950s and 1960s, DDT was the insecticide used most frequently, and in the 1970s, fenitrothion; 72% of the workers had been exposed to phenoxyacetic acid herbicides, and exposure to other herbicides and fungicides was also reported. Cancer incidence rates for the Swedish population were used for comparison. A total of 558 cancer cases were observed in the cohort (SIR, 0.86; 95% CI, 0.79-0.93). Excess risks were observed for lip cancer (14 observed; 1.8; 0.96-2.9), testicular cancer (18 observed; 1.6; 0.92-2.5) and Hodgkin's disease (11 observed; 1.2; 0.60-2.2) but not for lung cancer (38 observed, 0.50; 0.35-0.68), non-Hodgkin's lymphoma (21 observed; 1.0; 0.63-1.5) or cancer at any other site. The SIR for testicular cancer increased with time since licensure (0-4 years, 0.94; 5-9 years, 1.4; ≥ 10 years, 2.5; based on four, six and eight cases, respectively). The SIR for lung cancer increased with years since first employment from 0.31 (0-4 years) to 0.49 (5-9 years) to 0.56 (≥ 10 years). The authors provided data showing that smoking was less prevalent among pesticide applicators than among other occupational categories in Sweden, strongly suggesting that the observed deficit of lung cancer was due to lower cigarette consumption. A follow-up from date of licensure until 31 December 1984 indicated no excess risk for soft-tissue sarcomas (seven cases observed; SIR, 0.9; 95% CI, 0.4-1.9) (Wiklund *et al.*, 1988).

Cohort studies are summarized in Table 6.

Table 6. Summary of findings in cohort studies on spraying and application of insecticides

Reference	Location	Occupation	Cancer site	SMR	95% CI	Comments
MacMahon et al. (1988)	USA	Pest control workers	Lung	1.4	1.1–1.6	No trend for lung cancer with duration of employment; 90% confidence interval
			Skin	1.3	0.65–2.2	
			Bladder	1.2	0.50–2.5	
			Lymphatic & haematopoietic	1.0	0.67–1.4	
Blair et al. (1983)	USA	Licensed pest control workers	Larynx	[2.7]	[0.6–8.0]	Trend for lung cancer with duration of licensure
			Lung	1.4	[0.9–1.9]	
			Skin	[1.3]	[0.2–4.8]	
			Bladder	[1.6]	[0.3–4.6]	
			Leukaemia	[1.3]	[0.4–3.4]	
			Brain	2.0	[0.6–4.7]	
Alavanja et al. (1990)	USA	Flour millers	Lung	0.78	[0.7–0.9]	Trend for lymphomas and pancreas with time since first employment
			Leukaemia	1.4	[0.9–2.0]	
			Non-Hodgkin's lymphoma	1.5	[0.9–2.3]	
			Pancreas	1.3	[0.9–1.9]	
Corrao et al. (1989)	Italy	Farmers licensed for use of pesticides (Tox. class I + II)	Skin	1.4	1.0–1.8	SIR
			Lymphomas	1.4	1.0–1.9	
			Haematopoietic	1.1	0.8–1.5	
			Nervous system	1.0	0.6–1.4	
Barthel (1981a,b)	Germany	Plant protection workers and agronomists	Lung	1.8	[1.4–2.4]	SIR; trend with length of exposure
Wiklund et al. (1989)	Sweden	Licensed pesticide applicators	Lung	0.50	0.35–0.68	SIR; trend for testicular and lung cancer with time
			Non-Hodgkin's lymphoma	1.0	0.63–1.5	
			Hodgkin's disease	1.2	0.60–2.2	
			Lip	1.8	0.96–2.9	
			Testis	1.6	0.92–2.5	

2.3 Case-control interview studies

2.3.1 *Lymphatic and haematopoietic systems and soft-tissue sarcoma*

Hoar *et al*. (1986) conducted a population-based case-control study of white male residents of Kansas, USA, 21 years or older. Information was collected on 139 histo-logically confirmed cases of soft-tissue sarcoma and 132 of Hodgkin's disease diagnosed in 1976-82 and on a random sample of 172 cases of non-Hodgkin's lymphoma diagnosed in 1979-81. Three population controls were matched to each case on age and vital status: living controls up to 64 years of age were selected by random digit dialling; older subjects were selected from Medicare files; and deceased controls were selected from state mortality files, after excluding index neoplasms, a malignancy at an ill-defined site, homicide and suicide. After exclusions, a total of 1005 controls were selected. Patients and controls, or their next of kin, were interviewed by telephone about farming practices. Interviews were obtained for 96% of patients and 94% of controls. Information on herbicide and insecticide use provided by a sample of farmers among enrolled subjects was validated by interviewing their pesticide suppliers. A small excess of non-Hodgkin's lymphoma (odds ratio, 1.5; 95% CI, 0.9-2.4) was found among patients reporting use of any insecticides. Odds ratios by year of first use of insecticides among farmers were 1.7 for use prior to 1946, 1.5 for 1946-55, 0.7 for 1956-65 and 1.5 for 1966 or later. No association was observed with number of hectares treated. Adjustment for days per year of herbicide use reduced the odds ratio for insecticide use to 1.1 (95% CI, 0.6-2.2). Risks for non-Hodgkin's lymphoma increased slightly, however, with days per year of insecticide use, even after adjusting for exposure to herbicides (odds ratio, 1.2 (95% CI, 0.5-2.8) for one to two days of insecticide use; and 1.4 (0.6-3.1) for more than two days of insecticide use). A further analysis of these data was undertaken by Hoar Zahm *et al*. (1988). A small excess risk for soft-tissue sarcoma was seen among farmers using insecticides on animals (odds ratio, 1.6; 95% CI, 0.9-2.5) but not among those using insecticides on crops (0.8; 0.4-1.6). Relative risks for use on animals rose with time since first use to 4.9 (0.6-64.1) among farmers who first used them in 1945 or earlier. Potentially greater exposure might be expected during treatment of animals because higher concentrations are sprayed in confined spaces, such as barns. Excess risks were associated with most of the major classes of insecticides. No association was observed between the risk for Hodgkin's disease and use of insecticides.

In a study of similar design to the study in Kansas, all non-Hodgkin's lymphomas occurring among white men 21 years or older between 1983 and 1986 in 66 counties in eastern Nebraska were ascertained through local hospitals (Hoar Zahm *et al*., 1990). Population-based controls were frequency matched to cases on race, age and vital status. A total of 227 cases of non-Hodgkin's lymphoma and 831 controls were selected. Telephone interviews were conducted to obtain detailed information on specific agricultural chemicals used, and responses were obtained from 201 cases (91%) and 725 controls (87%). There was little evidence of an association between non-Hodgkin's lymphoma among farmers and use of insecticides overall (odds ratio, 1.1; 95% CI, 0.7-1.6); but non-Hodgkin's lymphoma was associated with use of organophosphorus insecticides (odds ratio, 2.4, adjusted for use of 2,4-D). Risks rose with days per year of use of organophosphorus compounds (odds ratios,

1.7 for 1-5 days/year, 1.8 for 6-20 days/year and 3.1 for 21 or more days/year). [Numbers of exposed subjects and confidence intervals were not provided.]

A population-based case-control study was conducted in Washington State (USA) to investigate the relationship between soft-tissue sarcoma and non-Hodgkin's lymphoma and past exposure to phenoxyacetic acid herbicides and chlorinated phenols (Woods *et al.*, 1987). Between 1981 and 1984, 206 soft-tissue sarcomas and 746 non-Hodgkin's lymphomas were diagnosed in men aged 20-79 years. Of these cases, 13% were excluded due to physicians' refusal; 91% of the remaining patients (or their proxies) were interviewed and information was derived about pesticide exposures. Of the remaining 163 soft-tissue sarcoma cases, 33 were excluded on the basis of a pathology review, and two were excluded for other reasons, leaving 128 soft-tissue sarcoma cases to be included in the analysis. Of the remaining 586 non-Hodgkin's lymphoma cases, 10 were excluded for various reasons, leaving 576 cases to be included in the analysis. Controls for living cases were selected by random-digit telephone dialling (for those aged 20-64 years) and from Health Case Financing Administration files (for those aged 65-79 years); deceased controls were obtained from death certificates and matched on five-year age group. Interviews were obtained for 694 of the 910 controls (76%). Odds ratios for potential exposure to chlordane were 1.6 (95% CI, 0.7-3.8) for non-Hodgkin's lymphoma and 0.96 (0.2-4.8) for soft-tissue sarcoma. Potential exposure to DDT yielded odds ratios of 1.8 (1.0-3.2) for non-Hodgkin's lymphoma and 1.1 (0.4-3.2) for soft-tissue sarcoma. Adjustment for exposure to some other pesticides did not substantially change these risk estimates. Another evaluation of the data from this study restricted analyses to farmers (Woods & Polissar, 1989). The relative risks for non-Hodgkin's lymphoma among farmers potentially exposed were 1.6 (0.5-5.1) for chlordane and 1.7 (0.9-3.3) for DDT.

A population-based, multicentre case-control study of multiple myeloma in people under 80 years of age was carried out between 1977 and 1981 in four US areas covered by cancer registries (Morris *et al.*, 1986). Interviews were obtained with 698 cases (89% of eligible subjects) and 1683 controls (83%); 32% of case interviews and 1% of those for controls were with next-of-kin. Controls were obtained by household sampling in one area and by random digit dialling in the remaining three areas; they were matched to cases on age, sex and race. Self-reported exposures to chemicals were grouped into 20 categories, some of which were further subdivided. The odds ratio for exposure to pesticides was 2.6 (95% CI, 1.5-4.6); an odds ratio of similar magnitude was obtained when reports from surrogate respondents were excluded (2.9; 1.5-5.5). The numbers of cases and controls who reported exposure to various classes of insecticides were two cases and five controls for organophosphorus compounds [odds ratio, 1.0; 0.2-5.1], nine cases and eight controls for organochlorines [2.8; 1.1-7.0] and three cases and five controls for arsenicals [1.5; 0.4-6.2]. [Subjects exposed to other pesticides were excluded when calculating these odds ratios.]

A case-control study on multiple myeloma was conducted within a prospective study of 1.2 million American Cancer Society volunteers who in 1982 filled in a self-administered questionnaire on diseases and several cancer risk factors, including occupation and exposure to pesticides and herbicides. They were followed for mortality up to 1984 or 1986, and 282 deceased subjects with mention of multiple myeloma on their death certificate were identified. Prevalent cases of multiple myeloma and subjects with related symptoms identified at the time of entry into the cohort were excluded, leaving 128 incident cases, who were matched on sex, age, residence and race to four randomly selected controls. A logistic regression analysis adjusting for potential confounders was presented. The odds ratio for occupation as a farmer was 2.7 (95% CI, 1.3-5.7; based on 16 cases and 28 controls exposed); the odds ratio for exposure to pesticides and herbicides was 1.6 (0.7-3.7; 12 cases and 25 controls). When these variables were combined, nonfarmers exposed to pesticides and herbicides experienced no excess risk (crude odds ratio, 1.0; 95% CI, 0.3-3.1), whereas exposed farmers had an elevated risk (crude odds ratio, 4.3; 95% CI, 1.7-10.9), which was greater than that of unexposed farmers (crude odds ratio, 1.7; 95% CI, 0.8-4.0) (Boffetta *et al.*, 1989).

A population-based case-control study of leukaemia among white men aged 30 years or older in Iowa (1981-83) and in Minnesota (1980-82) covered a total of 669 eligible cases (Brown *et al.*, 1990). Living controls were selected by random digit dialling (< 65 years) and from Medicare records (> 65 years); deceased controls were selected from death certificates. Interviews were completed with 86% of the cases or close relatives and with 77-79% of the controls; the study thus included 578 cases and 1245 controls. A standardized questionnaire was used to obtain detailed information on residential history, drinking-water source, nonfarm occupational history, smoking and alcohol use, use of unpasteurized dairy products, medical conditions, family history of cancer and farm activities, including information on 24 animal insecticides and 34 crop insecticides. Relative risks were calculated by comparison to subjects who were nonfarmers, adjusting for age, vital status, state of residence, tobacco use, family history of lymphopoietic cancer, high-risk occupations and high-risk exposures. The risk for leukaemia overall was not significantly associated with reported use of any insecticide (odds ratio, 1.1; 95% CI, 0.9-1.3) among farmers. An excess risk was observed for chronic lymphocytic leukaemia (1.3; 1.0-1.8), but not for other histological types: acute nonlymphocytic leukaemia, 1.0 (0.7-1.6), chronic myelogenous, 1.0 (0.5-1.8) and acute lymphocytic, 0.8 (0.2-2.5). The risk for leukaemia tended to be greater with use of insecticides on animals than on crops. Significant excesses occurred with use on animals of natural insecticides (odds ratio, 1.5; 95% CI, 1.0-2.2) and organophosphates (1.5; 1.0-2.1). Time since first use of insecticides also influenced risk: after a 20-year latency, significant excesses of leukaemia were noted with use on animals of several insecticides, including DDT (1.4; 1.0-2.0), dichlorvos (2.4; 1.1-5.4), famphur (11.6; 1.2-107.0), nicotine (2.0; 1.2-3.4) and pyrethrins (3.8; 1.0-14.8). Nonsignificant odds ratios of 2.0 or more were observed with use of carbaryl (3.0; 0.7-3.1), coumaphos (2.3; 0.6-8.8), methoxychlor (2.1; 0.7-6.6) and toxaphene (2.6; 0.8-8.8). The relative risk for leukaemia associated with frequent use on animals (> 10 days/year) was statistically significant for dichlorvos (3.8; 1.0-14.8) and malathion (3.2; 1.0-10.0); the risk increased with frequency of use of DDT on animals, from 0.6 (0.3-1.4) for 1-4 days per year to 1.1 (0.4-2.7) for 5-9 days per year, to 2.1 (1.1-3.9) for 10 or more days per year. These estimates for agricultural exposures were not mutually adjusted.

Patients with chronic lymphatic leukaemia diagnosed in five hospitals in the middle and south-east of Sweden between 1964 and 1984 who were still alive after 1981 were compared with population controls living in the catchment areas of the hospitals (Flodin *et al.*, 1988). Subjects over 80 years or mentally disabled were excluded, leaving 111 cases (response rate,

91%) and 431 controls (response rate, 83%; replacements were sought for the 17% who did not respond). Information on exposure to ionizing radiation, DDT, solvents and engine exhausts as well as a history of previous diseases, smoking and occupation were collected using a self-administered questionnaire. Results of a stratified analysis based on a confounder score including age, sex, exposure to fresh wood, solvents, engine exhausts, DDT and horses and employment as farmer were presented. Exposure to DDT was reported by six cases and four controls; the odds ratio was 6.0 (95% CI, 1.5-23.0). [The Working Group noted the limitation of inclusion of prevalent cases because of the potential influence on recall of exposure.]

A study on Hodgkin's disease and non-Hodgkin's B-cell lymphomas was conducted in one of the areas included in the study described above. The same criteria were applied for selection of cases, and the same controls were used. There were 54 cases of Hodgkin's disease and 106 of non-Hodgkin's lymphoma (overall response rate, 97%) and 275 controls. Logistic regression analysis was carried out including sex, age, farming, exposure to fresh wood and all exposures that gave a crude odds ratio greater than 2.0. Exposure to DDT was reported by three patients with Hodgkin's disease, none with non-Hodgkin's lymphoma and three controls. The odds ratio for Hodgkin's disease was 7.5 (90% CI, 0.8-70.0) (Persson et al., 1989). [The limitation of the study by Flodin et al. (1988) noted above also applies to this study.]

A case-control study on malignant lymphomas in northern Sweden considered primarily exposure to phenoxyacetic acid herbicides and chlorophenols (Hardell et al., 1981). Cases were all men aged 25-85 years with histologically verified malignant lymphoma admitted to the control hospital in the area in 1974-78. A total of 60 cases of Hodgkin's disease and 109 of non-Hodgkin's lymphoma were matched to 338 population controls (responses available from 335) by age, sex, place of residence, vital status and year of death for deceased cases and controls. Information from self-administered questionnaires was supplemented by telephone interviews when the data were incomplete. A total of 22 cases and 26 controls reported exposure to DDT [odds ratio, 1.8; 95% CI, 1.0-3.2]. Seven cases and 11 controls reported exposure to DDT and not to phenoxyacetic acid herbicides [odds ratio, 1.6; 95% CI, 0.6-4.1]. Information on use of DDT was not presented separately for patients with Hodgkin's disease and those with non-Hodgkin's lymphoma.

Four case-control studies in Sweden assessed the risk of soft-tissue sarcoma alone, primarily in association with exposure to phenoxyacetic acid herbicides and chlorophenols (Hardell & Sandström, 1979; Eriksson et al., 1981; Hardell & Eriksson, 1988; Eriksson et al., 1990). Exposure was assessed by methods similar to those described above, using questionnaires mailed to subjects or next-of-kin. For subgroups of the subjects, information was supplemented with telephone interviews.

A case-control study in northern Sweden included 52 male cases of histologically reviewed soft-tissue sarcoma (100% response) and 206 population controls (99% response), matched for age, sex, place of residence and year of death for deceased cases and controls (Hardell & Sandström, 1979). Four cases and 14 controls reported exposure to DDT (crude odds ratio, 1.2 [95% CI, 0.4-3.7]).

A population-based case-control study in southern Sweden included 110 cases of histologically verified soft-tissue sarcoma and 219 controls (responses obtained from all but one), matched for age, place of residence and year of death for dead cases and controls (Eriksson *et al.*, 1981). Seven cases and 11 controls reported exposure to DDT [crude odds ratio, 1.3; 95% CI, 0.5-3.4].

A population-based case-control study in northern Sweden included 54 male cases of soft-tissue sarcoma (responses obtained from all but one) (Hardell & Eriksson, 1988). Two control groups were used: one was population-based, with 311 subjects (94% response) matched for age and place of residence, and the second consisted of 179 cases of malignant disease (94% response) diagnosed in the same period as the cases. Six cases, 19 population-based controls and eight cancer controls reported exposure to DDT [crude odds ratio, 1.9; 95% CI, 0.7-5.0 (population controls); 2.7; 0.9-7.8 (cancer controls)]. Crude odds ratios for exposure to DDT without exposure to phenoxyacetic acid herbicides were [0.6 (0.1-5.0)] for population controls and [1.2 (0.1-11.6)] for cancer controls.

All male patients diagnosed with histologically confirmed soft-tissue sarcoma between 1978 and 1986 were identified from a regional cancer registry in central Sweden. Interviews were completed with 218 (92%) of the cases identified. One control per case was drawn from the National Population Registry matched on age, sex, vital status and county of residence; 212 controls (89%) of those selected were interviewed. Twelve controls who were contacted could not complete the questionnaire and were replaced by the next person on the population register. Subjects or next-of-kin completed a 12-page questionnaire regarding exposures of interest; these data were supplemented by telephone interviews for subjects employed in agriculture, forestry, horticulture, carpentry and sawmills. The odds ratios for soft-tissue sarcoma were 0.61 (95% CI, 0.34-1.1) for potential exposure to DDT and 0.52 (0.19-1.4) for potential exposure to pesticides other than DDT or mercury seed dressings (Eriksson *et al.*, 1990).

2.3.2 *Other cancers*

A proportionate analysis of occupational mortality in Washington State, USA, identified a 30% increased risk for respiratory cancer among orchardists (Milham, 1983), and a case-control study was undertaken on mortality from respiratory cancer in Washington State in 1968-80 (Wicklund *et al.*, 1988). Death certificates were selected that contained the occupational codes for orchardists, orchard labourers and brush pickers, and farm owners and tenants. Cases were men who had died from respiratory cancer, and potential controls were men who had died from other causes, matched by county of residence, year of death, age at death and occupational code. An attempt was made to contact surviving next-of-kin or other informants. Interviews were obtained for 87.1, 79.6 and 60.5%, respectively, of the three occupational groups. On the basis of the information obtained, orchardists were limited to men who had been involved in orchard work for at least 10 years or 25% of their working history or had been associated with at least one orchard of five or more acres [> 2 ha]. Information on occupational exposures and smoking was obtained from a structured questionnaire. If the informant was unable to recall whether a specific pesticide had been sprayed by the deceased but was able to recall the precise year of his orchard work, a 'presumed' history of spraying a particular pesticide was obtained. Lead arsenate was used by orchardists before 1945 and was replaced by DDT subsequently; thus, if a deceased man had worked prior to 1945, he was presumed to have a positive history of lead arsenate spraying, and if he had worked after 1945 he was presumed to have a positive history of DDT spraying. Information was obtained for all but 7% of the 155 cases and 4.9% of the 155 matched controls. A total of 89 cases and 89 controls were assumed to have had exposure to DDT. When men exposed to DDT but not to lead arsenate were considered, there were 33 cases and 29 controls, and the odds ratio (adjusted for smoking) was 0.91 (95% CI, 0.40-2.1). [The Working Group noted that the unexposed group included men for whom details on exposure to DDT were not available, which may have biased the odds ratio towards the null.]

Two case-control studies in Sweden examined the risks for colon cancer (Hardell, 1981) and nasal and nasopharyngeal cancer (Hardell et al., 1982), primarily in relation to exposure to phenoxyacetic acid herbicides and chlorophenols. The same control group, consisting of 541 people, was used in these two studies and in two previous studies conducted by the same group (Hardell & Sandström, 1979 [see above]; Hardell et al., 1981). There were 154 cases of colon cancer and 71 cases of nasal and nasopharyngeal cancer. Odds ratios for exposure to DDT, without controlling for other agricultural exposures, were [0.8; 0.4-1.7] for colon cancer and [1.2; 95% CI, 0.5-2.9] for nasal and nasopharyngeal cancer. In the study of colon cancer, exposure to DDT was also analysed after excluding subjects who had been exposed to phenoxyacetic acids and chlorophenols; the odds ratio was [0.5; 0.2-1.6].

Men aged 25-80 who had been diagnosed with liver cancer between 1974 and 1981 and reported to the Department of Oncology, Umeå, Sweden, were included in another case-control study (Hardell et al., 1984). Microscope slides were reviewed for the 166 assembled cases, and 103 cases of primary liver cancer were retained for the study; 206 population-based controls were matched to cases on age and residence. Information on exposure was obtained as in previous studies (see Hardell & Sandström, 1979); responses were obtained for 102 cases and 200 controls. The analysis was restricted to the 98 cases of hepatocellular or cholangiocellular carcinoma. Odds ratios for exposure to DDT, without controlling for other agricultural exposures, were [0.4; 95% CI, 0.1-1.1] for exposure to DDT in farming and [1.3; 0.4-4.0] for exposure to DDT in forestry.

A total of 240 cases of brain glioma were collected from two hospitals in Milan, Italy, between 1983 and 1984. Patients with non-glioma brain tumours (465) and patients with non-neoplastic neurological diseases (277) recruited from the same hospitals and matched for age and sex to the cases formed two series of controls [response rates not given]. Subjects were asked about their occupational history as well as their use of fertilizers, herbicides and insecticides or fungicides. Exposure of farmers to insecticides or fungicides gave an odds ratio of 2.0 (95% CI, 1.2-3.2) using all controls and of 2.1 (1.3-3.6) using only cancer controls (Musicco et al., 1988).

2.3.3 Childhood cancer

A case-control study of brain tumours in Baltimore, MD, USA, included all cases under 20 years of age diagnosed in 1965-75, and two groups of controls—one selected from birth certificates of the state and one from children with other malignancies. Controls were matched individually to cases on sex, race and date of birth; cancer controls were also matched on date of diagnosis. Interviews were conducted with 84 of 127 (66%) identified cases; interviews with controls yielded 73 matched pairs with population controls and 78 matched pairs with cancer controls. Parents were interviewed with respect to environmental exposures, including insect exterminations in the household, as well as child and family characteristics. A matched-pair analysis was conducted. Insect extermination was more common in houses of cases with respect to population controls (odds ratio, 2.3 [95% CI, 0.9-6.6]) but not to cancer controls (1.2 [0.5-2.8]) (Gold *et al.*, 1979).

The results of the case-control studies are summarized by site in Tables 7-9.

3. Other Relevant Data in Humans

3.1 Toxic effects

The toxicology of insecticides in humans has been reviewed (Hayes, 1982).

[The Working Group noted that useful information on chronic illness resulting from human exposure to insecticides is limited (WHO, 1990). The reasons include variable exposure to insecticides, the large number of compounds used (also in combination), the presence of many confounding factors, and the lack of sensitive, specific endpoints for different types of toxicity. Consequently, it seems unlikely that broad surveys in which exposure is not characterized will be adequate to identify the effects of insecticides. Several reports infer that insecticides have chronic effects, but because of constraints such as those described above and often because of the lack of an appropriate epidemiological design, the results cannot be interpreted. Well-designed studies of occupational exposures, combined with appropriate biomonitoring procedures, are perhaps the only way of collecting information on this issue.]

Some of the studies that purport to show an association between adverse health effects and exposure to insecticides are listed below. Disorders of the cardiovascular system (Bezugly & Gorskaya, 1976; Fokina & Bezugly, 1978; Kaskevich, 1980), nervous system (Bezugly *et al.*, 1973); sensory organs, respiratory system (Muminov & Fershtat, 1973; Barthel, 1974; Werner *et al.*, 1978) and reduced lung function (Kolpakov, 1979; Lings, 1982) have been reported following exposure to pesticides (including specified and unspecified insecticides). Skin disorders, including dermatitis (Wassermann *et al.*, 1960; Mirakhmedov & Yusupov, 1973; Takahashi *et al.*, 1975; Nagata *et al.*, 1976a; Tsugane *et al.*, 1978; Yokoyama *et al.*, 1978), headache, nausea (Tsugane *et al.*, 1978; Yokoyama *et al.*, 1978) and blood disorders (Bezugly *et al.*, 1973; Nakajima & Kawabata, 1977) have also been reported.

Abnormal electroencephalograms were observed in some but not all studies on farm workers exposed to organochlorine, organophosphorus and carbamate insecticides (Kontek *et al.*, 1971; Horiguchi, 1973; Horiguchi *et al.*, 1976a,b).

Altered liver enzyme activities have been reported among pesticide workers exposed to organophosphorus pesticides alone or in combination with organochlorine and/or other pesticides (Liska & Tildyova, 1974; Dzhaparov & Karimov, 1978).

Table 7. Case-control studies on malignant lymphomas containing information on insecticide exposure

Reference	Location	Cancer	No. of exposed cases/controls	Relative risk	95% CI	Comments
Hoar et al. (1986)	Kansas, USA	Non-Hodgkin's lymphoma	54/275	1.5	0.9–2.4	Insecticides; not adjusted for herbicide use
			24/99	1.1	0.6–2.2	Adjusted for herbicide use; farmers only
Hoar Zahm et al. (1988)	Kansas, USA	Hodgkin's disease	38/275	0.8	0.5–1.4	Insecticide use
			32/214	0.9	0.5–1.5	Insecticide use on animals
			25/132	1.1	0.6–1.9	Insecticide use on crops Unadjusted for other agricultural exposures
Hoar Zahm et al. (1990)	Nebraska, USA	Non-Hodgkin's lymphoma	104/321	1.1	0.7–1.6	Insecticides; not adjusted for herbicide use
			NA	2.4	NA	Organophosphates; adjusted for 2,4-D use Risks rose with days per year of organophosphate insecticides after adjustment for herbicides
Woods et al. (1987); Woods & Polissar (1989)	Washington, USA	Non-Hodgkin's lymphoma	NA	1.6	0.7–3.8	Chlordane
			NA	1.8	1.0–3.2	DDT
			NA	1.6	0.5–5.1	Chlordane for farmers only
			NA	1.7	0.9–3.3	DDT for farmers only Not adjusted for other agricultural exposures
Persson et al. (1989)	Sweden	Non-Hodgkin's lymphoma	0/3	–	–	DDT exposure
Persson et al. (1989)	Sweden	Hodgkin's disease	3/3	7.5	0.8–70.0	DDT; adjusted for some agricultural exposures; 90% CI
Hardell et al. (1981)	Sweden	Malignant lymphoma	22/26	[1.8]	[1.0–3.2]	DDT; crude risk calculated from data in paper. Not adjusted for other agricultural exposures
			7/11	[1.6]	[0.6–4.1]	Crude risk for DDT, without exposure to phenoxyacetic acid herbicides

NA, not available

Table 8. Case-control studies of soft-tissue sarcomas containing information of insecticide exposure

Reference	Location	No. of exposed case/controls	Relative risk	95% CI	Comments
Hoar Zahm et al. (1988)	Kansas, USA	50/275 46/214 14/132	1.3 1.6 0.8	0.8–2.2 0.9–2.5 0.4–1.6	Insecticide use Insecticide use on animals Insecticide use on crops Not adjusted for other agricultural exposures
Woods et al. (1987)	Washington, USA	NA NA	0.96 1.1	0.2–4.8 0.4–3.2	Chlordane DDT Not adjusted for other exposures
Hardell & Sandström (1979)	Sweden	4/14	1.2	[0.4–3.7]	DDT Crude risk calculated from data in paper; not adjusted for other agricultural exposures
Eriksson et al. (1981)	Sweden	7/11	[1.3]	[0.5–3.4]	DDT Crude risk calculated from data in paper; not adjusted for other agricultural exposures
Hardell & Eriksson (1988)	Sweden	6/19 6/8	[1.9][a] [2.7][b]	[0.7–5.0] [0.9–7.8]	DDT Crude relative risk calculated from data in paper; not adjusted for other agricultural exposures
		1/10 1/3	[0.6][a] [1.2][b]	[0.1–5.0] [0.1–11.6]	Crude risk for exposure to DDT and not phenoxyacetic acid
Eriksson et al. (1990)	Sweden	6/11	0.52	0.19–1.4	Pesticides other than DDT and mercury seed dressings
		22/33	0.61	0.34–1.1	DDT Not adjusted for other agricultural exposures

[a]Population controls
[b]Cancer controls

Table 9. Case-control studies of other cancers containing information on insecticide exposure

Reference	Location	Cancer[a]	No. of cases/ controls	Relative risk	95% CI	Comments
Morris et al. (1986)	USA	Multiple myeloma	28/25 2/5 9/8	2.6 [1.0] [2.8]	1.5–4.6 [0.2–5.1] [1.1–7.0]	Pesticides Organophosphorus Organochlorines
Boffetta et al. (1989)	USA	Multiple myeloma	12/25 4/17 8/20 8/8	1.6 1.0[b] 1.7[b] 4.3[b]	0.7–3.7 0.3–3.1 0.8–4.0 1.7–10.9	Pesticides and herbicides; adjusted for other exposures Exposed nonfarmers Unexposed farmers Exposed farmers
Brown et al. (1990)	Iowa and Minnesota, USA	Leukaemia ALL CLL AML CML	250/588 5/588 122/588 58/588 20/588	1.1 0.8 1.3 1.0 1.0	0.9–1.3 0.2–2.5 1.0–1.8 0.7–1.6 0.5–1.8	Use of any insecticide Adjusted for vital status, age, state, tobacco, family history of lymphopoietic cancer, high-risk occupations, high-risk exposures
Flodin et al. (1988)	Sweden	Chronic lymphatic leukaemia	6/4	6.0	1.5–23.0	DDT; adjusted for other exposures
Wiklund et al. (1988b)	USA	Respiratory	33/29	0.91	0.40–2.1	DDT Both cases and controls were orchard workers
Hardell et al. (1981)	Sweden	Colon	9/40	[0.8]	[0.4–1.7]	DDT Crude risk calculated from data in paper; not adjusted for other agricultural exposures
		Colon	3/21	[0.5]	[0.2–1.6]	DDT Crude risk calculated from data in paper; for exposure to DDT and not phenoxyacetic acids or chlorophenols
Hardell et al. (1982)	Sweden	Nose, nasopharynx	6/40	[1.2]	[0.5–2.9]	DDT Crude risk calculated from data in paper; not adjusted for other agricultural exposures

Table 9 (contd)

Reference	Reference	Cancer	No. of cases/ controls	Relative risk	95% CI	Comments
Hardell et al. (1984)	Sweden	Primary liver	4/20	[0.4]	[0.1–1.1]	DDT Crude risk calculated from data in paper; not adjusted for other agricultural exposures; farmers
		Primary liver	5/8	[1.3]	[0.4–4.0]	DDT Crude risk calculated from data in paper; not adjusted for other agricultural exposures; foresters
Musicco et al. (1988)	Italy	Brain	37/55 37/31	2.0 2.1	1.2–3.2 1.3–3.6	All controls Tumour controls only Insecticides and fungicides
Study of children						
Gold et al. (1979)	USA	Brain	19/10 21/19	2.3[c] 1.2[d]	[0.9–6.6] [0.5–2.8]	Exterminations in house

[a]ALL, acute lymphocytic leukaemia; CLL, chronic lymphocytic leukaemia; AML, acute myeloid leukaemia; CML, chronic myeloid leukaemia
[b]Crude odds ratio
[c]Population controls
[d]Cancer controls

3.2 Reproductive and developmental effects in humans

In an ecological study, all cases of cleft lip or cleft palate occurring among white, liveborn singletons in rural areas in Iowa or Michigan (USA) in 1974-75 were identified, together with a 2% sample of all livebirths, who served as controls. Cases and controls were assigned an exposure score based on the proportion of hectares of land on which insecticides or herbicides were used for pest control, by county. An odds ratio of 2.9 (95% CI, 1.5-5.4) was found in Iowa, indicating that the risk of cleft lip or cleft palate was almost three times higher in children born in counties with a high proportion of cropland treated with insecticides or herbicides, compared to other counties. In Michigan, the odds ratio was 1.7 (95% CI, 1.0-2.8). The study did not distinguish between insecticides and herbicides (Gordon & Shy, 1981). [The Working Group noted that the study has the limitations of ecological analyses.]

A study on a population of 8867 people (2951 men and 5916 women) engaged in floriculture in Colombia and exposed to 127 different types of pesticides has been reported. Information on reproductive outcomes before and after employment in the industry was collected by means of a detailed interview. The odds ratio for spontaneous abortion after employment in floriculture was 2.2 (95% CI, 1.8-2.7) among female workers and 1.8 (1.2-2.8) among wives of male workers. The odds ratios for premature birth were 1.9 (1.6-2.2) and 2.8 (2.0-3.8), respectively. The authors point out difficulties in the interpretation of their findings, particularly in regard to recall bias. They did not analyse fungicides and insecticides separately (Restrepo *et al.*, 1990).

In a study of 12 couples (wife and husband) employed in grape gardens in India and of 15 comparable but unexposed couples, reproductive histories were collected. There were 14 spontaneous abortions (44% of 32 pregnancies) and one stillbirth in the exposed group and three spontaneous abortions (8% of 40 pregnancies) and no stillbirth in the unexposed group. The excess of abortions was significant ($p < 0.05$). The workers were exposed to several pesticides, including DDT, lindane, parathion, dichlorvos and dieldrin (Rita *et al.*, 1987).

3.3 Genetic and related effects

Only those studies that provide information on exposure to insecticides were considered. Nevertheless, interpretation of the observed effects was impeded by two fundamental problems: the lack, in almost all studies, of quantitative information on exposure to insecticides and the multiplicity of exposures. People exposed occupationally to insecticides during spraying and application handle large numbers of pesticide formulations, only a proportion of which may be insecticide formulations. Within these formulations, so-called inert ingredients usually form the bulk of the materials, and many of these are biologically highly reactive substances. Consequently, it is difficult or impossible to attribute effects observed in sprayers and applicators specifically to insecticide formulations or even to any named pesticidal component.

3.3.1 *Cytogenetic studies*

Sixteen agricultural workers who had been exposed predominantly to insecticides (mainly the organophosphorus compounds, demeton, ethyl parathion, trichlorfon and naled) in the USA, with a mean exposure time of 12 years, were compared with 16 controls with a variety of occupations not involving pesticides. Blood samples were taken off-season and mid-season from both groups, and 25 metaphase-arrested lymphocytes from each person were scored on each occasion for chromatid breaks and gaps. The frequency of chromatid breaks in mid-season samples was increased from 0.44 ± 0.22 (SD) in the control group to 1.56 ± 0.29 in the exposed group (Yoder *et al.*, 1973). There was no difference in the occurrence of chromatid gaps either off-season or mid-season or of chromatid breaks in off-season samples. [The Working Group noted that no attempt was made to control for confounding factors such as tobacco smoking, that small numbers of cells were scored from each person and that individual results were not reported.]

The effects of low levels of the insecticide fumigant, ethylene dibromide, upon the frequencies of sister chromatid exchange and chromosomal aberrations were examined among forestry workers in mainland USA (Steenland *et al.*, 1985) and papaya workers in Hawaii (Steenland *et al.*, 1986). Blood samples were taken from 14 forestry workers who sprayed pine trees before and after exposure (8-h time-weighted average, 80 ppb [616 $\mu g/m^3$], with a peak of up to 281 ppb [2164 $\mu g/m^3$]) and compared with those from six unexposed controls. No effect of exposure to ethylene dibromide was observed, although smoking did increase the frequency of sister chromatid exchange. A group of 60 papaya workers exposed to ethylene dibromide at a geometric mean of 88 ppb [678 $\mu g/m^3$] (8-h time-weighted average), but with peak exposures of up to 262 ppb [2017 $\mu g/m^3$], were compared with a control group of 42 workers from a nearby sugar mill. The two groups were matched for age, tobacco, marijuana and coffee use and race. No difference was found in the total frequencies of either chromosomal aberrations or sister chromatid exchange. The frequency of the latter, however, was increased in men who smoked either tobacco or marijuana, and that of chromosomal aberrations showed an increasing trend with age.

Floriculturists (36 men and women) in Argentina involved in spraying various pesticides, including organophophosphates, carbamates and organochlorines, were studied for chromosomal aberrations and sister chromatid exchange. Symptoms of chronic intoxication were observed in 21 workers. The control group consisted of 15 healthy scientists and technicians. A significant difference was seen in sister chromatid exchange frequencies between the symptomatic and non-symptomatic floriculturists as well as between a matched group of controls and sprayers. The frequency of only dicentric and ring type chromosomal aberrations was increased when the whole group of floriculturists and controls was compared (Dulout *et al.*, 1985).

In a study from Hungary, 80 male workers were involved in mixing and spraying pesticides (80 formulations were recorded, including insecticides such as organophosphates, organochlorines, pyrethroids and carbamates). At least 12 weeks' continuous contact with pesticides was recorded during the spraying season. A group of 24 administrative workers and mechanics served as controls. A significant increase in the frequency of chromosomal aberrations was seen in the group of pesticide workers as compared with controls; that of chromosome-type aberrations increased with duration of exposure (Páldy *et al*,. 1987).

Forty producers of potted plants (17 smokers) working in greenhouses in Argentina and exposed to a mixture of organophosphorus, organochlorine, carbamate and some miscellaneous pesticides, were examined for chromosomal aberrations (Dulout *et al.*, 1987). The control group consisted of 32 healthy hospital blood donors (10 smokers) with no known exposure to pesticides. Since some of the control individuals showed toxic symptoms that are seen after chronic exposure to pesticides, a second control group was selected consisting of 12 blood donors (six smokers) with no symptom of exposure. No difference was observed between the control groups with respect to frequency of chromosomal aberrations or between the producers of potted plants and the controls as a whole.

The frequencies of chromosomal aberrations in 15 vineyard workers in India who were exposed to seven insecticides (DDT, lindane, quinalphos, metasystox, parathion, dichlorvos and dieldrin) and two fungicides (dithane M_{45} and copper sulfate) were compared with those in 10 controls of similar age and socioeconomic status, but not exposed to pesticides (Rita et al., 1987). The proportion of metaphase cells with chromatid breaks was significantly increased in the exposed group.

In another Hungarian study, 55 male workers were involved in spraying and applying pesticides in greenhouses, plastic tents and open fields. Among the pesticide formulations, various organophosphates, carbamates and pyrethroids were listed. The control group consisted of 60 male blood donors. A slight increase in the frequency of chromosomal aberrations was recorded among the open-field sprayers; however, the values for closed-space workers were at the control level (Nehéz et al., 1988).

Cotton field workers (pesticide mixers and sprayers) in India were studied for the effects of exposure to pesticides (particularly insecticides) on the frequency of chromosomal aberrations (Rupa et al., 1989a) and of sister chromatid exchange (Rupa et al., 1989b). Peripheral lymphocytes were examined from 50 smokers and compared with those from 20 nonsmokers and 27 smokers, none of whom were occupationally exposed to pesticides. The frequency of chromosomal aberrations was significantly increased in the pesticide-exposed group as compared with either of the control groups. Sister chromatid exchange frequencies showed similar responses to both smoking and pesticides exposure; there was a trend towards an increasing number of sister chromatid exchanges with years of exposure to pesticides.

In a study of chromosomal aberrations, 52 nonsmoking cotton-field workers exposed to pesticides (mainly insecticides) were compared with 25 controls. The insecticides mentioned included malathion, methyl parathion, dimethoate, DDT and fenvalerate. The prevalence of chromosomal aberrations was significantly increased in the group of workers, and there was a positive trend with duration of exposure (Rupa et al., 1989c).

Fumigation of phosphine produced from aluminium or magnesium phosphide pellets is used commonly in the grain industry to control beetles. Of 24 professional fumigant applicators, nine were exposed to phosphine alone (mean level, 2.97 mg/m^3 in grain bin areas; average duration of exposure, over 20 min daily). This group had a five-fold higher frequency of chromosomal deletions than the control subjects, and the frequency of breaks was also significantly increased. Chromosome banding analysis showed that chromosomal rearrangements were six times more frequent in the exposed workers than in the controls. Sister chromatid exchange frequency was not increased. In lymphocytes in vitro, no sister chromatid exchange was induced, but the frequency of chromosomal aberrations was increased in a dose-related manner (Garry et al., 1989).

Carbonell *et al.* (1990) studied 27 agricultural workers in Spain who had used insecticides such as fenvalerate, deltamethrin and methomyl. No sister chromatid exchange was induced.

The results of studies on cytogeneticity are summarized in Table 10.

3.3.2 *Urine mutagenicity studies*

Urine samples were taken from 12 greenhouse owners (11 men and 1 woman) who daily sprayed fungicides and insecticides (dichlorvos, orthene (acephate) and pentac (dienochlor) mentioned) in greenhouses in central New York for 1-40 years. The samples, collected 8 h after spraying, and control samples taken three days later were tested for mutagenicity using *Salmonella typhimurium* (strains TA100 and TA98) both with and without an exogenous metabolic system. No increase in mutagenic activity was detected in urine from seven subjects. Three subjects who had elevated urine mutagenicity had been working with poor protection. Two of the subjects reported smoking during the days of sample collection (Shane *et al.*, 1988).

San *et al.* (1989) and See *et al.* (1990) assayed the urine of nonsmoking orchardists in Canada using chromosomal aberrations in Chinese hamster ovary cells as the endpoint. People were exposed to organophosphates among other pesticides. Chromosome damaging activity was significantly elevated in samples collected during the pesticide spraying season as compared to samples collected during the non-spraying season or to urine samples from nonsmoking controls.

4. Summary of Data Reported and Evaluation

4.1 Exposure data

Chemicals have been used to control insects for centuries but have come into widespread use only within the past century, with the development of a variety of synthetic insecticides. Of the several hundred chemicals that have been applied for insecticidal purposes, fewer than one hundred have been used extensively.

The principal classes of compounds that have been used as insecticides are organochlorine, organophosphorus, carbamate and pyrethroid compounds and various inorganic compounds. Insecticides comprise a higher proportion of the total pesticide usage in developing countries than in developed countries.

Insecticides are applied by aerial spraying and by various ground-based techniques, ranging from hand-held sprayers and dusters to vehicle-mounted hydraulic sprayers, air sprayers, foggers and power dusters.

Occupational exposures occur in the mixing and loading of equipment and in the spraying and application of insecticides. Absorption resulting from dermal exposure is the most important route of uptake for exposed workers.

4.2 Carcinogenicity in humans

4.2.1 *Descriptive and ecological studies*

Several death certificate case-control studies in the USA evaluated cancer risks in association with ecological measures of insecticide exposure. The risk for multiple myeloma

Table 10. Summary of results from cytogenetic biomonitoring studies on pesticide applicators

Job description	Exposure data	Insecticides listed	Number of subjects (exposed/ controls)	Cytogenetic effect[a] CA	SCE	Reference
Crop dusters, formulators, spray rig operators, farmers in Idaho, USA	Mean exposure time, 12 years	Organophosphates (10), organochlorines (5), phenolics (1), carbamates (1)	16/16	+	ND	Yoder et al. (1973)
Floriculturists in Argentina	Chronic intoxication symptoms in 21 individuals, at least 10 years of employment	Organophosphates (5), organochlorines (7), carbamates (5)	36/15	(+)	+	Dulout et al. (1985)
Pesticide mixers and field sprayers in Hungary	0.2–15 years of exposure; long exposure group, 11–15 years	80 different formulations: insecticides (organophosphates, pyrethroids), herbicides, fungicides	80/24	+	ND	Páldy et al. (1987)
Growers of potted plants in Argentina	Haematological tests normal, cholinesterase decreased in only 3/40; employment time, > 10 years	About 40 different formulations: organophosphates (3), organochlorines (3), permethrin, carbamates (5), and other pesticides	40/32	−	ND	Dulout et al. (1987)
Vineyard workers in India	5–15 years of exposure	Various (9) pesticides used throughout the year including 7 insecticides (e.g., DDT, dichlorvos, lindane, parathion)	15/10	+	ND	Rita et al. (1987)
Farmers and greenhouse workers in Hungary	Better protection in greenhouse than in open field; most exposed for 2–10 years	Various formulations of agrochemicals (insecticides: organophosphates (7), carbamates (3), pyrethroids (5); fungicides)	55/60	(+)	ND	Nehéz et al. (1988)
Mixers and sprayers of pesticides in cotton fields in India	Several years of exposure, 8 h/day; 9 months/year; all cotton-field workers were smokers	Insecticides (11) including DDT, BHC, malathion, fenvalerate, cypermethrin	50/47	+	+	Rupa et al. (1989a,b)

Table 10 (contd)

Job description	Exposure data	Insecticides listed	Number of subjects (exposed/controls)	Cytogenetic effect[a] CA	Cytogenetic effect[a] SCE	Reference
Mixers and sprayers of pesticides in cotton fields in India	Several years of exposure, 8 h/day; 9 months/year; all cotton-field workers were non-smokers	Insecticides (11) including: DDT, BHC, malathion, fenvalerate	52/25	+	ND	Rupa et al. (1989c)
Fumigant applicators in grain industry	Daily exposure over 20 min in closed space with phosphine at 0.4-5.8 mg/m^3	Groups exposed to phosphine alone (n = 9) and to phosphine and other pesticides (n = 15)	9/24	+	-	Garry et al. (1989)
Horticultural and flori-cultural workers in Spain	Over 10 years of work in family enterprises	Various pesticides, including insecticides (methomyl, fenvalerate, deltamethrin)	27/28	ND	-	Carbonell et al. (1990)

[a]CA, chromosomal aberration; SCE, sister chromatid exchange; +, statistically significant positive result; (+), suggestive positive result; -, negative result; ND, no data

tended to be greater for farmers residing in counties where insecticides were more heavily used, but that for leukaemia did not.

4.2.2 *Cohort studies*

A cohort of workers from a large pest control company in the USA had an excess lung cancer risk. Similarly, in a cohort of licensed pest control workers from Florida, there was significantly increased mortality from lung cancer, which was particularly high among workers licensed for 20 years or more; a nonsignificant excess risk for brain cancer was also seen. A follow-up of deaths among plant protection workers and agronomists in eastern Germany showed an increased risk of lung cancer which also increased with length of exposure; survey data indicated that the smoking habits of these pesticide workers were similar to those of the general population.

Among farmers licensed for pesticide use in the Piedmont region of Italy, increased risks for skin cancer and malignant lymphomas were reported; lung cancer incidence was not studied.

A cohort of licensed pesticide applicators in Sweden showed excess risks for cancers of the lip and testis, a slight excess risk for Hodgkin's disease, and risks similar to those of the general population for non-Hodgkin's lymphoma and soft-tissue sarcoma. Overall, there was a deficit of lung cancer risk that was probably related to the lower smoking rates of the applicators.

In a study of a large cohort of grain millers in the USA, flour-mill workers had excess risks for non-Hodgkin's lymphoma and pancreatic cancer; the risk for lung cancer was not increased.

4.2.3 *Case-control studies*

The risk for non-Hodgkin's lymphoma rose with frequency of use of organo-phosphorus insecticides among farmers in Nebraska, an association that could not be accounted for by use of phenoxyacetic acid herbicides. In Kansas, the risk increased slightly with frequency of use of insecticides as a group. In a study in Washington State, non-Hodgkin's lymphoma was associated with potential contact with chlordane and DDT. DDT use was also associated with non-Hodgkin's lymphoma in one of two studies in Sweden.

Multiple myeloma was associated with use of pesticides (particularly organochlorine insecticides) in a study in the USA. The risk for multiple myeloma was also elevated among farmers in the USA exposed to unspecified herbicides and pesticides.

The results of six studies in Sweden and the USA on soft-tissue sarcoma in association with exposure to insecticides were inconsistent.

Chronic lymphocytic leukaemia has been associated with use of insecticides in the USA and with use of DDT in Sweden.

The risk for brain cancer was associated with exposure to insecticides and fungicides in farmers in Italy.

Overall, the strongest evidence that exposure to nonarsenical insecticides causes cancer in humans comes from the cohort studies of applicators. Two of these studies showed significant excesses of lung cancer. Two showed rising risks with duration of exposure, whereas the third showed an inverse association. These findings were based on small numbers in the subgroups with the longest exposure, and applicators in some of these studies had potential contact with arsenical insecticides. Some case-control studies of multiple myeloma and other tumours of B-cell origin show small excesses among people exposed to insecticides. In most studies, however, potential confounding by other agricultural exposures had not been fully explored.

4.3 Other relevant data

In a study in India, an excess of spontaneous abortions was reported among couples exposed to several pesticides in grape gardens. In a population in Colombia, where exposure to many different pesticides occurred, increased risks for spontaneous abortion and decreased birth weight were reported.

Several studies on the cytogenetic effects of work with pesticide formulations are described. Only in the case of ethylene dibromide and phosphine was exposure to a single, identified insecticide: No cytogenetic effect was observed with exposure to ethylene dibromide, while a significant excess of chromosomal aberrations was observed among the phosphine fumigators. All other studies were of workers handling not only a mixture of insecticide formulations but also other pesticide formulations. The majority of these studies reported increases in the frequency of chromosomal aberrations and/or sister chromatid exchange among the exposed workers. With the exceptions noted above, in no instance, however, could the involvement of non-insecticides be eliminated.

4.4 Evaluation[1]

There is *limited evidence* that occupational exposures in spraying and application of nonarsenical insecticides[2] entail a carcinogenic risk.

Overall evaluation

Spraying and application of nonarsenical insecticides[2] entail exposures that *are probably carcinogenic to humans (Group 2A).*

5. References

Adamis, Z., Antal, A., Fuezesi, I., Molnár, J., Nagy, L. & Susán, M. (1985) Occupational exposure to organophosphorus insecticides and synthetic pyrethroid. *Int. Arch. occup. environ. Health, 56,* 299-305

Alavanja, M.C.R., Rush, G.A., Stewart, P. & Blair, A. (1987) Proportionate mortality study of workers in the grain industry. *J. natl Cancer Inst., 78,* 247-252

Alavanja, M.C.R., Blair, A. & Masters, M.N. (1990) Cancer mortality in the US flour industry. *J. natl Cancer Inst., 82,* 840-848

---

[1]For definitions of the italicized terms, see Preamble, pp. 26-28.
[2]Arsenic and arsenic compounds are carcinogenic to humans (IARC, 1987). This evaluation applies to the group of chemicals as a whole and not necessarily to all individual chemicals within the group.

Ames, R.G., Brown, S.K., Mengle, D.C., Kahn, E., Stratton, J.W. & Jackson, R.J. (1989) Cholinesterase activity depression among California agricultural pesticide applicators. *Am. J. ind. Med.*, *15*, 143-150

Anon. (1981) *Basic Pesticide Equipment Manual*, Helena, MT, Department of Agriculture

Baker, E.L., Jr, Zack, M., Miles, J.W., Alderman, L., Warren, M., Dobbin, R.D., Miller, S. & Teeters, W.R. (1978) Epidemic malathion poisoning in Pakistan malaria workers. *Lancet*, *i*, 31-34

Barthel, E. (1974) Pulmonary fibroses in persons exposed to pesticides (Ger.). *Z. Erkr. Atmungsorg.*, *141*, 7-17

Barthel, E. (1976) High incidence of lung cancer in persons with chronic occupational exposure to pesticides in agriculture (Ger.). *Z. Erkr. Atm.-Org.*, *146*, 266-274

Barthel, E. (1981a) Increased risk of lung cancer in pesticide-exposed male agricultural workers. *J. Toxicol. environ. Health*, *8*, 1027-1040

Barthel, E. (1981b) Cancer risk in pesticide-exposed agricultural workers (Ger.) *Arch. Geschwulstforsch.*, *51*, 579-585

Bezugly, V.P. & Gorskaya, N.Z. (1976) The role of the complex of organochlorine and organophosphorus pesticides in the development of atherosclerosis (Russ.). *Vrach. Delo.*, *2*, 99-102

Bezugly, V.P., Odintsova, I.L. & Gorskaya, N.S. (1973) Morphological composition of the blood in persons working with a complex of organochlorine and organophosphorus pesticides (Russ.). *Vrach. Delo*, *11*, 134-138

Blair, A. & Thomas, T.L. (1979) Leukemia among Nebraska farmers: a death certificate study. *Am. J. Epidemiol.*, *110*, 264-273

Blair, A. & Watts, D. (1980) Bladder cancer and dairy farming (Letter to the Editor). *J. occup. Med.*, *22*, 576-577

Blair, A. & White, D.W. (1981) Death certificate study of leukemia among farmers from Wisconsin. *J. natl Cancer Inst.*, *66*, 1027-1030

Blair, A., Grauman, D.J., Lubin, J.H. & Fraumeni, J.F., Jr (1983) Lung cancer and other causes of death among licensed pesticide applicators. *J. natl Cancer Inst.*, *71*, 31-37

Blair, A., Hoar Zahm, S., Cantor, K.P. & Stewart, P.A. (1989) Estimating exposure to pesticides in epidemiological studies of cancer. In: Wang, R.G.M., Franklin, C.A., Honeycutt, R.C. & Reinert, J.C., eds, *Biological Monitoring for Pesticide Exposure. Measurement, Estimation, and Risk Reduction* (ACS Symposium Series 382), Washington DC, American Chemical Society, pp. 38-46

Boettiger, L.E. (1979) Epidemiology and aetiology of aplastic anemia. *Haematol. Bluttransfus.*, *24*, 27-37 (116)

Boffetta, P., Stellman, S.D. & Garfinkel, L. (1989) A case-control study of multiple myeloma nested in the American Cancer Society prospective study. *Int. J. Cancer*, *43*, 554-559

Brown, L.M., Blair, A., Gibson, R., Everett, G.D., Cantor, K.P., Schuman, L.M., Burmeister, L.F., Van Lier, S.F. & Dick, F. (1990) Pesticide exposures and other agricultural risk factors for leukemia among men in Iowa and Minnesota. *Cancer Res.*, *50*, 6585-6591

Burmeister, L.F., Van Lier, S.F. & Isacson, P. (1982) Leukemia and farm practices in Iowa. *Am. J. Epidemiol.*, *115*, 720-728

Burmeister, L.F., Everett, G.D., Van Lier, S.F. & Isacson, P. (1983) Selected cancer mortality and farm practices in Iowa. *Am. J. Epidemiol.*, *118*, 72-77

Cantor, K.P. (1982) Farming and mortality from non-Hodgkin's lymphoma: a case-control study. *Int. J. Cancer*, *29*, 239-247

Cantor, K.P. & Blair, A. (1984) Farming and mortality from multiple myeloma: a case-control study with the use of death certificates. *J. natl Cancer Inst.*, 72, 251-255

Carbonell, E., Puig, M., Xamena, N., Creus, A. & Marcos, R. (1990) Sister chromatid exchange in lymphocytes of agricultural workers exposed to pesticides. *Mutagenesis*, 5, 403-405

Carman, G.E., Iwata, Y., Pappas, J.L., O'Neal, J.R. & Gunther, F.A. (1982) Pesticide applicator exposure to insecticides during treatment of citrus trees with oscillating boom and airblast units. *Arch. environ. Contam. Toxicol.*, 11, 651-659

Clarkson, T.W., Friberg, L., Nordberg, G.F. & Sager, P.R., eds (1988) *Biological Monitoring of Toxic Metals*, New York, Plenum

Comer, S.W., Staiff, D.C., Armstrong J.F. & Wolfe, H.R. (1975) Exposure of workers to carbaryl. *Bull environ. Contam. Toxicol.*, 13, 385-391

Copley, K. (1987) Dow studies measure applicator exposure. *Grounds Maint.*, 22, 42, 46

Copplestone, J.F., Fakhri, Z.I., Miles, J.W., Mitchell, C.A., Osman, Y. & Wolfe, H.R. (1976) Exposure to pesticides in agriculture: a survey of spraymen using dimethoate in the Sudan. *Bull. World Health Organ.*, 54, 217-223

Corrao, G., Calleri, M., Carle, F., Russo, R., Bosia, S. & Piccioni, P. (1989) Cancer risk in a cohort of licensed pesticide users. *Scand. J. Work Environ. Health*, 15, 203-209

Coye, M.J., Lowe, J.A. & Maddy, K.J. (1986) Biological monitoring of agricultural workers exposed to pesticides: II. Monitoring of intact pesticides and their metabolites. *J. occup. Med.*, 28, 628-636

Culver, D., Caplan, P. & Batchelor, G.S. (1956) Studies of human exposure during aerosol application of malathion and chlorthion. *Arch. ind. Health*, 13, 37-50

Davis, J.E., Stevens, E.R., Staiff, D.C. & Butler, L.C. (1983) Potential exposure to diazinon during yard applications. *Environ. Monit. Assess.*, 3, 23-28

Devine, J.M., Kinoshita, G.B., Peterson, R.P. & Picard, G.L. (1986) Farm worker exposure to terbufos [phosphorodithioic acid, *S*-(*tert*-butylthio)methyl *O,O*-diethyl ester] during planting operations of corn. *Arch. environ. Contam. Toxicol.*, 15, 113-119

Dover, M.J. (1985) *A Better Mousetrap: Improving Pest Management for Agriculture*, Washington DC, World Resources Institute

Dulout, F.N., Pastori, M.C., Olivero, O.A., Cid, M.G., Loria, D., Matos, E., Sobel, N., de Bujan, E.C. & Albiano, N. (1985) Sister-chromatid exchanges and chromosomal aberrations in a population exposed to pesticides. *Mutat. Res.*, 143, 237-244

Dulout, F.N., Pastori, M.C., Cid, M.G., Matos, E., von Guradze, H.N., Maderna, C.R., Loria, D., Sainz, L., Albiano, N. & Sobel, N. (1987) Cytogenetic analysis in plant breeders. *Mutat. Res.*, 189, 381-386

Dzhaparov, A.K. & Karimov, V.A. (1978) State of metabolites and the activity of carbohydrate metabolizing enzymes in patients with chronic organochlorine and organophosphorus pesticide poisoning (Russ.). *Gig. Tr. prof. Zabol.*, 11, 28-29

Eriksson, M., Hardell, L., Berg, N.O., Möller, T. & Axelson, O. (1981) Soft-tissue sarcomas and exposure to chemical substances: a case-referent study. *Br. J. ind. Med.*, 38, 27-33

Eriksson, M., Hardell, L. & Adami, H.-O. (1990) Exposure to dioxins as a risk factor for soft tissue sarcoma: a population-based case-control study. *J. natl Cancer Inst.*, 82, 486-490

Fenske, R.A. (1987) Assessment of dermal exposure to pesticides: a comparison of the patch technique and the video imaging/fluorescent tracer technique. In: Greenhalgh, R. & Roberts, T.R., eds, *Pesticide Science and Technology* (Proceedings of the 6th International Congress on Pesticides Chemistry), Oxford, Blackwell Scientific Publishers, pp. 579-582

Flodin, U., Fredriksson, M., Persson, B. & Axelson, O. (1988) Chronic lymphatic leukaemia and engine exhausts, fresh wood, and DDT: a case-referent study. *Br. J. ind. Med.*, *45*, 33-38

Foa, V., Emmett, E.A., Maroni, M. & Colombi, A. (1987) *Occupational and Environmental Chemical Hazards, Cellular and Biochemical Indices for Monitoring Toxicity*, Chichester, Ellis Horwood

Fokina, K.V. & Bezugly, V.P. (1978) Role of combinations of organochlorine and organophosphorus pesticides in the development of cerebral atherosclerosis (Russ.). *Vrach. Delo*, *4*, 19-23

Franklin, C.A. (1989) Biological monitoring for pesticide exposure. In: Wang, R.G.M., Franklin, C.A., Honeycutt, R.C. & Reinert, J.C., eds, *Biological Monitoring for Pesticide Exposure. Measurement, Estimation, and Risk Reduction* (ACS Symposium Series 382), Washington DC, American Chemical Society, pp. 2-5

Franklin, C.A., Muir, N.I. & Moody, R.P. (1986) The use of biological monitoring in the estimation of exposure during the application of pesticides. *Toxicol. Lett.*, *33*, 127-136

Freeborg, R.P., Daniel, W.H. & Konopinski, V.J. (1985) Applicator exposure to pesticides applied to turfgrass. In: Honeycutt, R.C., Zweig, G. & Ragsdale, N.N., eds, *Dermal Exposure Related to Pesticide Use: Discussion of Risk Assessment* (ACS Symposium Series 273), Washington DC, American Chemical Society, pp. 287-295

Garry, V.F., Griffith, J., Danzl, T.J., Nelson, R.L., Whorton, E.B., Krueger, L.A. & Cervenka, J. (1989) Human genotoxicity: pesticide applicators and phosphine. *Science*, *246*, 251-255

Gold, R.E. & Holcslaw, T. (1985) Dermal and respiratory exposure of applicators and residents to dichlorvos-treated residences. In: Honeycutt, R.C., Zweig, G. & Ragsdale, N.N., eds, *Dermal Exposure Related to Pesticide Use: Discussion of Risk Assessment* (ACS Symposium Series 273), Washington DC, American Chemical Society, pp. 253-264

Gold, E., Gordis, L., Tonascia, J. & Szklo, M. (1979) Risk factors for brain tumors in children. *Am. J. Epidemiol.*, *109*, 309-319

Gold, R.E., Leavitt, J.R.C. & Ballard, J. (1981) Effect of spray and paint-on applications of a slow-release formulation of chlorpyrifos on German cockroach control and human exposure. *J. Econ. Entomol.*, *74*, 552-554

Gordon, J.E. & Shy, C.M. (1981) Agricultural chemical use and congenital cleft lip and/or palate. *Arch. environ. Health*, *36*, 213-220

Hardell, L. (1981) Relation of soft-tissue sarcoma, malignant lymphoma and colon cancer to phenoxy acids, chlorophenols and other agents. *Scand. J. Work Environ. Health*, *7*, 119-130

Hardell, L. & Eriksson, M. (1988) The association between soft tissue sarcomas and exposure to phenoxyacetic acids. *Cancer*, *62*, 652-656

Hardell, L. & Sandström, A. (1979) Case-control study soft tissue sarcomas and exposure to phenoxyacetic acids or chlorophenols. *Br. J. Cancer*, *39*, 711-717

Hardell, L., Eriksson, M., Lenner, P. & Lundgren, E. (1981) Malignant lymphoma and exposure to chemicals, especially organic solvents, chlorophenols and phenoxy acids: a case-control study. *Br. J. Cancer*, *43*, 169-176

Hardell, L., Johansson, B. & Axelson, O. (1982) Epidemiological study of nasal and nasopharyngeal cancer and their relation to phenoxy acid or chlorophenol exposure. *Am. J. ind. Med.*, *3*, 247-257

Hardell, L., Bengtsson, N.O., Jonsson, U., Eriksson, S. & Larsson, L.G. (1984) Aetiological aspects on primary liver cancer with special regard to alcohol, organic solvents and acute intermittent porphyria—an epidemiological investigation. *Br. J. Cancer*, *50*, 389-397

Haskell, P.T., ed. (1985) *Pesticide Application: Principles and Practice*, Oxford, Clarendon Press

Haverty, M.I., Page, M., Shea, P.J., Hoy, J.B. & Hall, R.W. (1983) Drift and worker exposure resulting from two methods of applying insecticides to pine bark. *Bull. environ. Contam. Toxicol.*, *30*, 223-228

Hayes, W.J., Jr (1982) *Pesticides Studied in Man*, Baltimore, Williams & Wilkins Co.

Hayes, A.L., Wise, R.A. & Weir, F.W. (1980) Assessment of occupational exposure to organophosphates in pest control operators. *Am. ind. Hyg. Assoc. J.*, *41*, 568-575

Hoar, S.K., Blair, A., Holmes, F.F., Boysen, C.D., Robel, R.J., Hoover, R. & Fraumeni, J.F., Jr (1986) Agricultural herbicide use and risk of lymphoma and soft-tissue sarcoma. *J. Am. med. Assoc.*, *256*, 1141-1147

Hoar Zahm, S., Blair, A., Holmes, F.F., Boysen, C.D. & Robel, R.J. (1988) A case-referent study of soft-tissue sarcoma and Hodgkin's disease. Farming and insecticide use. *Scand. J. Work Environ. Health*, *14*, 224-230

Hoar Zahm, S., Weisenburger, D.D., Babbitt, P.A., Saal, R.C., Vaught, J.B., Cantor, K.P. & Blair, A. (1990) A case-control study of non-Hodgkin's lymphoma and the herbicide 2,4-dichlorophenoxyacetic acid (2,4-D) in eastern Nebraska. *Epidemiology*, *1*, 349-356

Horiguchi, Y. (1973) Studies on the influence of organophosphorus pesticides on the central nervous system. Part 2. Effects on the human body (Jpn.). *J. Jpn. Assoc. rural Med.*, *22*, 294-295

Horiguchi, Y., Yanagisawa, T., Ide, H. & Sasaki, K. (1976a) Studies on the effect of organophosphorus pesticides in the human central nervous system (Jpn.). *J. Jpn. Assoc. rural Med.*, *25*, 627-628

Horiguchi, Y., Yanagisawa, T., Sasaki, K., Ide, H., Ueki, S., Abe, E. & Kurosawa, K. (1976b) Neurological studies on the treatment of organophosphorus insecticide intoxication. Part 5. Electroencephalographic study of pesticide applicators (Jpn.). In: [Studies on the Effects of Pesticides on Living Bodies], pp. 68-70

IARC (1980) *IARC Monographs on the Evaluation of the Carcinogenic Risk of Chemicals to Humans*, Vol. 23, *Some Metals and Metallic Compounds*, Lyon, pp. 39-141

IARC (1986) *IARC Monographs on the Evaluation of Carcinogenic Risks to Humans*, Suppl. 6, *Genetic and Related Effects: An Updating of Selected* IARC Monographs *from Volumes 1 to 42*, Lyon, pp. 296-300

IARC (1987) *IARC Monographs on the Evaluation of Carcinogenic Risks to Humans*, Suppl. 7, *Overall Evaluations of Carcinogenicity: An Updating of* IARC Monographs *Volumes 1 to 42*, Lyon, pp. 100-106

Joyce, R.J.V. (1985) Application from the air. In: Haskell, P.T., ed., *Pesticide Application: Principles and Practices*, Oxford, Clarenden Press, pp. 118-152

Kaskevich, L.M. (1980) On the character of pre-clinical changes under the effect of a complex of chloro- and phosphororganic pesticides (Russ.). *Vrach. Delo*, *4*, 105-107

Kolpakov, I.E. (1979) Demonstration of early changes in the respiratory function and gas exchange of workers exposed to pesticides. *Gig. Tr. prof. Zabol.*, *1*, 36-37

Kontek, M., Marcinkowska, B. & Pietraszek, Z. (1971) Electroencephalograms in farmers professionally exposed to pesticides (Pol.). *Med. Prac.*, *22*, 433-440

Korsak, R.J. & Sato, M.M. (1977) Effects of chronic organophosphate pesticide exposure on the central nervous system. *Clin. Toxicol.*, *11*, 83-95

Kurtz, D.A. & Bode, W.M. (1985) Application exposure to the home gardener. In: Honeycutt, R.C., Zweig, G. & Ragsdale, N.N., eds, *Dermal Exposure Related to Pesticide Use: Discussion of Risk Assessment* (ACS Symposium 273), Washington DC, American Chemical Society, pp. 139-162

Leavitt, J.R.C., Gold, R.E., Holcslaw, T. & Tupy, D. (1982) Exposure of professional pesticide applicators to carbaryl. *Arch. environ. Contam. Toxicol.*, *11*, 57-62

Lings, S. (1982) Pesticide lung: a pilot investigation of fruit-growers and farmers during the spraying season. *Br. J. ind. Med.*, *39*, 370-376

Liska, D. & Tildyova, K. (1974) Study of the changes of activity of some enzymes in the blood of pilots and engineers exposed to organophosphorus pesticides (Czech.). *Cesk. Hyg.*, *19*, 289-295

Loevinsohn, M.E. (1987) Insecticide use and increased mortality in rural central Luzon, Philippines. *Lancet, i,* 1359-1362

Lotti, M. (1989) Neuropathy target esterase in blood lymphocytes: monitoring the interaction of organophosphates with a primary target. In: Wang, R.G.M., Franklin, C.A., Honeycutt, R.C. & Reinert, J.C., eds, *Biological Monitoring for Pesticide Exposure. Measurement, Estimation, and Risk Reduction* (ACS Symposium Series 382), Washington DC, American Chemical Society, pp. 117-123

MacMahon, B., Monson, R.R., Wang, H.H. & Zheng, T. (1988) A second follow-up of mortality in a cohort of pesticide applicators. *J. occup. Med.*, *30*, 429-432

Maddy, K.T., Knaak, J.B. & Gibbons, D.B. (1986) Monitoring the urine of pesticide applicators in California for residues of chlordimeform and its metabolites 1982-1985. *Toxicol. Lett.*, *33*, 37-44

Maitlen, J.C., Sell, C.R., McDonough, L.M. & Fertig, S.N. (1982) Workers in the agricultural environment: dermal exposure to carbaryl. In: Plimmer, J.R., ed., *Pesticide Residues and Exposure* (ACS Symposium Series 182), Washington DC, American Chemical Society, pp. 83-103

Marinova, G., Osmakova, D., Dermendzhieva, L.L., Khadzhikolev, I., Chakurova, O. & Kaneva, Y. (1973) Professional injuries—pesticides and their effects on the reproductive function of women working with pesticides (Hung.). *Akush. Ginecol. (Sofia)*, *12*, 138-140

Maroni, M. (1986) Organophosphorus pesticides. In: Alessio, L., Berlin, A., Boni, M. & Roi, R., eds, *Biological Indicators for the Assessment of Human Exposure to Industrial Chemicals*, Luxembourg, Commission of the European Communities, pp. 47-77

Matthews, G.A. (1985) Application from the ground. In: Haskell, P.T., ed., *Pesticide Application: Principles and Practice*, Oxford, Clarendon Press, pp. 95-117

Milham, S., Jr (1983) *Occupational Mortality in Washington State, 1950-1979* (DHHS (NIOSH) Publication No. 83-116), Cincinnati, OH, National Institute for Occupational Safety and Health

Mirakhmedov, U.M. & Yusupov, B.Y. (1973) Clinical aspects of dermatoses caused by poisonous chemicals in agricultural workers (Russ.). *Gig. Tr. prof. Zabol.*, *17*, 48-49

Morgan, D.P., Lin, L.I. & Saikaly, H.H. (1980) Morbidity and mortality in workers occupationally exposed to pesticides. *Arch. environ. Contam. Toxicol.*, *9*, 349-382

Morgan, M.S., Phillips, G.S. & Kirkpatrick, E.M. (1989) Convenient field sampling method for monitoring volatile compounds in exhaled breath. In: Wang, R.G.M., Franklin, C.A., Honeycutt, R.C. & Reinert, J.C., eds, *Biological Monitoring for Pesticide Exposure. Measurement, Estimation, and Risk Reduction* (ACS Symposium Series 382), Washington DC, American Chemical Society, pp. 56-69

Morris, P.D., Koepsell, T.D., Daling, J.R., Taylor, J.W., Lyon, J.L., Swanson, G.M., Child, M. & Weiss, N.S. (1986) Toxic substance exposure and multiple myeloma: a case-control study. *J. natl Cancer Inst.*, *76*, 987-994

Moseman, R.F. & Oswald, E.O. (1980) Development of analytical methodology for assessment of human exposure to pesticides. In: Harvey, J., Jr & Zweig, G., eds, *Pesticide Analytical Methodology* (ACS Symposium Series 136), Washington DC, American Chemical Society, pp. 251-257

Muminov, A.I. & Fershtat, V.N. (1973) The status of the upper respiratory tract in people working with combinations of organophosphorus and organochlorine pesticides (Russ.). *Vestn. Otorinolaringol.*, 35, 96

Musicco, M., Sant, M., Molinari, S., Filippini, G., Gatta, G. & Berrino, F. (1988) A case-control study of brain gliomas and occupational exposure to chemical carcinogens: the risk to farmers. *Am. J. Epidemiol.*, 128, 778-785

Nagata, H., Izumiyama, T., Kamata, K., Takano, S., Saito, M., Suzuki, K., Tajiri, H., Kobayashi, S. & Kurotani, S. (1976) Results of multiphase health examination of pesticide applicators in grape and apple orchards with combined pesticides (Jpn.). *J. Jpn. Assoc. rural Med.*, 25, 196-197

Nakajima, H. & Kawabata, M. (1977) Health examination results from a model rural village in Yamaguchi Prefecture (Jpn.). *J. Jpn. Assoc. rural Med.*, 26, 177

Nehéz, M., Boros, P., Ferke, A., Mohos, J., Palotás, M., Vetró, G., Zimányi, M. & Dési, I. (1988) Cytogenetic examination of people working with agrochemicals in the southern region of Hungary. *Regul. Toxicol. Pharmacol.*, 8, 37-44

Nigg, H.N. & Stamper, J.H. (1983) Exposure of spray applicators and mixer-loaders to chlorobenzilate miticide in Florida citrus groves. *Arch. environ. Contam. Toxicol.*, 12, 477-482

Nye, D.E. (1986) Aerial applicator and mixer-loader exposure to cypermethrin during ULV application to cotton. In: *Proceedings of the Beltwide Cotton Production Research Conferences, Las Vegas, Nevada, January 4-9, 1986*, Memphis, TN, National Cotton Council and The Cotton Foundation, pp. 198-200

Ogg, C.L. & Gold, R.E. (1988) Exposure and field evaluation of fenoxycarb for German cockroach (*Orthoptera*: Blattellidae) control. *J. Econ. Entomol.*, 81, 1408-1413

Páldy, A., Puskás, N., Vincze, K. & Hadházi, M. (1987) Cytogenetic studies on rural populations exposed to pesticides. *Mutat. Res.*, 187, 127-132

Persson, B., Dahlander, A.-M., Fredriksson, M., Brage, H.N., Ohlson, C.-G. & Axelson, O. (1989) Malignant lymphomas and occupational exposures. *Br. J. ind. Med.*, 46, 516-520

Prinsen, G.H. & Van Sittert, N.J. (1980) Exposure and medical monitoring study of a new synthetic pyrethroid after one season of spraying on cotton in Ivory Coast. In: Tordoir, W.F. & van Heemstra-Lequin, E.A.H., eds, *Field Worker Exposure During Pesticide Application* (Studies in Environmental Science No. 7), Amsterdam, Elsevier, pp. 105-120

Restrepo, M., Muñoz, N., Day, N.E., Parra, J.E., de Romero, L. & Nguyen-Dinh, X. (1990) Prevalence of adverse reproductive outcomes in a population occupationally exposed to pesticides in Colombia. *Scand. J. Work Environ. Health*, 16, 232-238

Rita, P., Reddy, P.P. & Vankatram Reddy, S. (1987) Monitoring of workers occupationally exposed to pesticides in grape garden of Andhra Pradesh. *Environ. Res.*, 44, 1-5

Rupa, D.S., Reddy, P.P. & Reddi, O.S. (1989a) Frequencies of chromosomal aberrations in smokers exposed to pesticides in cotton fields. *Mutat. Res.*, 222, 37-41

Rupa, D.S., Reddy, P.P. & Reddi, O.S. (1989b) Analysis of sister-chromatid exchanges, cell kinetics and mitotic index in lymphocytes of smoking pesticide sprayers. *Mutat. Res.*, 223, 253-258

Rupa, D.S., Reddy, P.P. & Reddi, O.S. (1989c) Chromosomal aberrations in peripheral lymphocytes of cotton field workers exposed to pesticides. *Environ. Res.*, 49, 1-6

Sabbioni, G. & Neumann, H.-G. (1990) Biomonitoring of arylamines: hemoglobin adducts of urea and carbamate pesticides. *Carcinogenesis*, 11, 111-115

Saftlas, A.F., Blair, A., Cantor, K.P., Hanrahan, L. & Anderson, H.A. (1987) Cancer and other causes of death among Wisconsin farmers. *Am. J. ind. Med.*, 11, 119-129

San, R.H.C., Rosin, M.P., See, R.H., Dunn, B.P. & Stich, H.F. (1989) Use of urine for monitoring human exposure to genotoxic agents. In: Wang, R.G.M., Franklin, C.A., Honeycutt, R.C. & Reinert, J.C., eds, *Biological Monitoring for Pesticide Exposure. Measurement, Estimation, and Risk Reduction* (ACS Symposium Series 382), Washington DC, American Chemical Society, pp. 98-116

See, R.H., Dunn, B.P. & San, R.H.C. (1990) Clastogenic activity in urine of workers occupationally exposed to pesticides. *Mutat. Res., 241*, 251-259

Shane, B.S., Scarlett-Kranz, J.M., Reid, W.S. & Lisk, D.J. (1988) Mutagenicity of urine from greenhouse workers. *J. Toxicol. environ. Health, 24*, 429-437

Shugart, L.R., Adams, S.M., Jiminez, B.D., Talmage, S.S. & McCarthy, J.F. (1989) Biological markers to study exposure in animals and bioavailability of environmental contaminants. In: Wang, R.G.M., Franklin, C.A., Honeycutt, R.C. & Reinert, J.C., eds, *Biological Monitoring for Pesticide Exposure. Measurement, Estimation, and Risk Reduction* (ACS Symposium Series 382), Washington DC, American Chemical Society, pp. 85-97

Spittler, T.D. & Bourke, J.B. (1985) Potential exposure in the application of pesticides to orchard and field crops. In: Honeycutt, R.C., Zweig, G. & Ragsdale, N.N., eds, *Dermal Exposure Related to Pesticide Use: Discussion of Risk Assessment* (ACS Symposium Series 273), Washington DC, American Chemical Society, pp. 297-310

Stamper, J.H., Nigg, H.N., Mahon, W.D., Nielsen, A.P. & Royer, M.D. (1989) Applicator exposure to fluvalinate, chlorpyrifos, captan, and chlorothalonil in Florida ornamentals. *J. agric. Food Chem., 37*, 240-244

Steenland, K., Carrano, A., Clapp, D., Ratcliffe, J., Ashworth, L. & Meinhardt, T. (1985) Cytogenetic studies in humans after short-term exposure to ethylene dibromide. *J. occup. Med., 27*, 729-732

Steenland, K., Carrano, A., Ratcliffe, J., Clapp, D., Ashworth, L. & Meinhardt, T. (1986) A cytogenetic study of papaya workers exposed to ethylene dibromide. *Mutat. Res., 170*, 151-160

Takahashi, M., Akaboshi, S. & Nishiya, N. (1975) On occupational intoxication caused by pesticides in persons engaging in pesticide application for pest control (Jpn.). *Ind. Med., 17*, 52-53

Tsugane, S., Hirabayashi, H., Tajima, J., Yokoyama, T., Tsugane, Y., Sakurai, K., Nakamura, S., Ide, H. & Asanuma, S. (1978) Actual status of pesticide application and health management of pesticide applicators in vegetable-growing highlands (Jpn.). *J. Jpn. Assoc. rural Med., 27*, 446-447

Wang, H.H. & MacMahon, B. (1979) Mortality of pesticide applicators. *J. occup. Med., 21*, 741-744

Wang, R.G.M., Franklin, C.A., Honeycutt, R.C. & Reinert, J.C., eds (1989) *Biological Monitoring for Pesticide Exposure, Measurement Estimation and Risk Reduction* (ACS Symposium Series 382), Washington DC, American Chemical Society

Wassermann, M., Iliesçu, S., Mandric, G. & Horvath, P. (1960) Toxic hazards during DDT- and BHC-spraying of forests against Lymantria monacha. *Arch. ind. Health, 21*, 503-508

Werner, E., Meyer, P. & Thiele, E. (1978) Examination of the mucous membranes of the upper respiratory tract and of parotid secretion of people working in agriculture after exposure to agrochemicals (Ger.). *Z. ges. Hyg., 24*, 335-337

WHO/UNEP (1990) *Public Health Impact of Pesticides Used in Agriculture*, Geneva

Wicklund, K.G., Daling, J.R., Allard, J. & Weiss, N.S. (1988b) Respiratory cancer among orchardists in Washington State, 1968 to 1980. *J. occup. Med., 30*, 561-564

Wiklund, K., Dich, J. & Holm, L.-E. (1986) Testicular cancer among agricultural workers and licensed pesticide applicators in Sweden (Letter to the Editor). *Scand. J. Work Environ. Health, 12*, 630-631

Wiklund, K., Dich, J. & Holm, L.-E. (1987) Risk of malignant lymphoma in Swedish pesticide appliers. *Br. J. Cancer, 56*, 505-508

Wiklund, K., Dich, J. & Holm, L.-E. (1988) Soft tissue sarcoma risk in Swedish licensed pesticide applicators. *J. occup. Med., 30*, 801-804

Wiklund, K., Dich, J., Holm, L.-E. & Eklund, G. (1989) Risk of cancer in pesticide applicators in Swedish agriculture. *Br. J. ind. Med., 46*, 809-814

Wolfe, H.R., Durham, W.F. & Armstrong, J.F. (1970) Urinary excretion of insecticide metabolites. Excretion of *para*-nitrophenol and DDA as indicators of exposure to parathion. *Arch. environ. Health, 21*, 711-716

Wolfe, H.R., Armstrong, J.F. & Durham, W.F. (1974) Exposure of mosquito control workers to fenthion. *Mosquito News, 34*, 263-267

Woods, J.S. & Polissar, L. (1989) Non-Hodgkin's lymphoma among phenoxy herbicide-exposed farm workers in western Washington State. *Chemosphere, 18*, 401-406

Woods, J.S., Polissar, L., Severson, R.K., Heuser, L.S. & Kulander, B.G. (1987) Soft tissue sarcoma and non-Hodgkin's lymphoma in relation to phenoxyherbicide and chlorinated phenol exposure in western Washington. *J. natl Cancer Inst., 78*, 899-910

Yoder, J., Watson, M. & Benson, W.W. (1973) Lymphocyte chromosome analysis of agricultural workers during extensive occupational exposure to pesticides. *Mutat. Res., 21*, 335-340

Yokoyama, T., Yanagasawa, T., Tsugane, S., Kikuchi, Y. & Taguchi, F. (1978) Status of application of pesticides for vegetables in highland fields and the health status of farmers applying pesticides to the vegetables (Jpn.). *J. Jpn. Assoc. rural Med., 27*, 203

ALDICARB

1. Exposure Data

1.1 Chemical and physical data

1.1.1 *Synonyms, structural and molecular data*

Chem. Abstr. Serv. Reg. No.: 116-06-3

Chem. Abstr. Name: 2-Methyl-2-(methylthio)propanal, *O*-[(methylamino)carbonyl]-oxime

IUPAC Systematic Name: 2-Methyl-2-(methylthio)propionaldehyde *O*-methylcarba-moyloxime

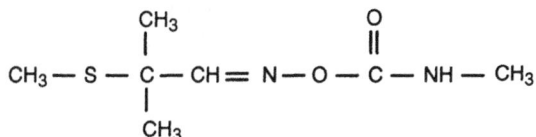

$$CH_3 - S - \underset{\underset{CH_3}{|}}{\overset{\overset{CH_3}{|}}{C}} - CH = N - O - \overset{\overset{O}{\parallel}}{C} - NH - CH_3$$

$C_7H_{14}N_2O_2S$ Mol. wt: 190.30

1.1.2 *Chemical and physical properties*

(a) *Description*: Colourless crystals (Worthing & Walker, 1987)

(b) *Boiling-point*: Decomposes (Rhone-Poulenc Ag Co., 1987)

(c) *Melting-point*: 98-100°C (Worthing & Walker, 1987)

(d) *Spectroscopy data*: Infrared spectroscopy data have been reported (US Environmental Protection Agency, 1976).

(e) *Solubility*: Slightly soluble in water (6 g/l at 20°C); soluble in most organic solvents: at 25°C, acetone, 350 g/kg; dichloromethane, 300 g/kg; benzene, 150 g/kg; xylene, 50 g/kg; practically insoluble in heptane (Worthing & Walker, 1987)

(f) *Volatility*: Vapour pressure, 9.75×10^{-5} mm Hg [1.3×10^{-5} Pa] at 25°C (Worthing & Walker, 1987)

(g) *Stability*: Stable in neutral, acidic and weakly alkaline media; hydrolysed by concentrated alkalis; decomposes above 100°C; rapidly converted by oxidizing agents to the sulfoxide, which is more slowly oxidized to the sulfone (Worthing & Walker, 1987; Royal Society of Chemistry, 1989)

(h) *Conversion factor for airborne concentrations*[1]: mg/m^3 = 7.78 × ppm

---

[1]Calculated from: mg/m^3 = (molecular weight/24.45) × ppm, assuming standard temperature (25°C) and pressure (760 mm Hg [101.3 kPa])

1.1.3 *Trade names, technical products and impurities*

Some common trade names are AI3-27 093, Aldicarb, ENT 27 093, OMS 771, Temik and UC 21149.

Aldicarb is available in the USA as a technical grade product with a purity of 98% (minimum) (Rhone-Poulenc Ag Co., 1987).

It is formulated in the USA and Europe as a granular product with the concentration of active ingredient ranging from 5 to 15%; some formulated products also contain gypsum and dichloromethane (Royal Society of Chemistry, 1986; Rhone-Poulenc Ag Co., 1990a,b; see IARC, 1987a). Aldicarb is also formulated as mixtures with pentachloronitrobenzene (see IARC, 1974, 1987b), 5-ethoxy-3-(trichloromethyl)-1,2,4-thiadiazole and lindane (see IARC, 1987c) (Royal Society of Chemistry, 1986; Rhone-Poulenc Ag Co., 1990c). The granular carrier material is impregnated with aldicarb and a bonding agent which helps prevent dustiness that may be caused by abrasion during shipping; dust is also removed during the manufacturing process to minimize inhalation exposure and hazards of direct handling (Baron & Merriam, 1988).

1.1.4 *Analysis*

Selected methods for the analysis of aldicarb in various matrices are given in Table 1. Several more methods and the environmental fate and transport of aldicarb and its metabolites have been reviewed (Moye & Miles, 1988).

Table 1. Methods for the analysis of aldicarb

Sample matrix	Sample preparation[a]	Assay procedure[a]	Limit of detection	Reference
Water	Filter; inject into reversed-phase HPLC column; separate analytes using gradient elution chromatography; hydrolyse with 0.05 N NaOH; react with *ortho*-phthalaldehyde and 2-mercaptoethanol	HPLC/FL	1.0 μg/l (2.0)[b]	US Environmental Protection Agency (1989a)
Drinking-water	Adsorb on Amberlite XAD-2 resin; elute with acetone	HPLC/UV	1 μg/l	Narang & Eadon (1982)
Crops, animal tissue	Extract with acetone/water (3:1); add peracetic acid to oxidize residues to sulfone; clean-up on activated Florisil column	GC/FPD[c]	0.01–0.05 ppm (mg/kg)	US Food and Drug Administration (1989a)
Milk	Precipitate solids with phosphoric acid and filter; add peracetic acid to oxidize residues to sulfone; extract into chloroform; clean-up on activated Florisil column	GC/FPD[c]	0.001 ppm (mg/l)	US Food and Drug Administration (1989a)
Cotton-seed	Grind sample; extract and oxidize with acetonitrile/peracetic acid solution; clean-up on activated Florisil column	GC/FPD[c]	0.02 ppm (mg/kg)	US Food and Drug Administration (1989a)

Table 1 (contd)

Sample matrix	Sample preparation[a]	Assay procedure[a]	Limit of detection	Reference
Grapes, potatoes	Extract with methanol; clean-up by liquid-liquid partitioning and column chromatography	LC/FL	Not reported	Association of Official Analytical Chemists (1985)
Formulations	Extract and dilute with dichloro-methane; measure absorbance at 5.75 μm and compare with standard	IR	Not reported	Romine (1974); Williams (1984)

[a]Abbreviations: GC/FPD, gas chromatography/flame photometric detection; HPLC/FL, high-performance liquid chromatography/fluorescence detection; HPLC/UV, high-performance liquid chromatography/ultra-violet detection; IR, infrared spectroscopy; LC/FL, liquid chromatography/fluorimetric detection
[b]Estimated limit of detection for aldicarb sulfone and aldicarb sulfoxide
[c]Total residues of aldicarb and its carbamate metabolites are determined as aldicarb sulfone

1.2 Production and use

1.2.1 *Production*

Aldicarb was first prepared by Payne and Weiden (1965) and was first made available as a commercial product in 1970, following its registration in the USA for use on cotton (Romine, 1974).

Aldicarb is synthesized by reacting nitrosyl chloride with isobutylene to obtain 2-chloro-2-methyl-1-nitrosopropane dimer, which is further reacted with methyl mercaptan and sodium hydroxide to obtain 2-methyl-2-(methylthio)propionaldoxime. Aldicarb is obtained by reaction of the oxime with methyl isocyanate (Romine, 1974).

Aldicarb is currently produced in the USA and in France (Meister, 1990). Production in the USA in 1979-81 was estimated at 2000 tonnes per annum (US Environmental Protection Agency, 1987).

1.2.2 *Use*

Aldicarb acts as a systemic insecticide, acaricide and nematicide and is applied to soil under cotton, potatoes, sugar beets, peanuts, soya beans, ornamental plants, sweet potatoes, pecans, citrus (grapefruit, lemons, limes and oranges only), dry beans, sorghum and sugar-cane (Rhone-Poulenc Ag Co., 1989; Meister, 1990). In the USA during 1979-81, annual usage of aldicarb (active ingredient) was estimated as follows (tonnes; %): cotton, 520 (29%); potatoes, 430 (25%); peanuts, 250 (14%); soya beans, 205 (12%); pecans, 180 (10%); ornamental plants (lilies, roses, holly), 45 (3%); sugar beets, 45 (3%); citrus, 34 (2%); sweet potatoes, 22 (< 1%); and tobacco, 6 (< 1%) (Holtorf, 1982). In Finland, 132 kg aldicarb (active ingredient) were sold in 1988 (Hynninen & Blomqvist, 1989). In the USA in 1989, about 1000-1500 tonnes aldicarb are believed to have been used. Aldicarb use is restricted in certain areas in various parts of the world, usually because of its potential to leach to groundwater (IRPTC/UNEP, 1990).

1.3 Occurrence

1.3.1 *Air*

Few studies are available on the stability or migration of aldicarb in air over or near treated fields. Laboratory studies with ^{14}C-labelled aldicarb in various soil types resulted in its loss, which could be explained only on the grounds that aldicarb or its decomposition products had been transferred to the vapour phase. Subsequent experiments showed that transfer of radioactivity to the atmosphere was inversely proportional to the depth of application in the soil (Coppedge *et al.*, 1977). Little aldicarb was released from a clay soil treated with this pesticide and placed in a volatilizer (Supak *et al.*, 1977).

1.3.2 *Water*

Aldicarb has been detected in ground- and drinking-water in 15 states in the USA at levels ranging from traces to 500 μg/kg (WHO, 1991).

It was detected in water in Suffolk County, NY, in August 1979: a monitoring programme for aldicarb in water indicated that 1121 (13.5%) of 8404 wells examined exceeded the State recommended guideline of 7 μg/l. Of the contaminated wells, 52% contained between 8 and 30 μg/l, 32% between 31 and 75 μg/l and 16% contained more than 75 μg/l (Zaki *et al.*, 1982). Following the banning of aldicarb in Suffolk County in 1979, approximately 74% of all wells sampled in the County in 1981 contained no detectable level of aldicarb. Of the 27% of wells (2054 samples) that did, residue levels were 1-10 μg/l in 56%, 11-100 μg/l in 40% and > 100 μg/l in 4% (US Environmental Protection Agency, 1988). Data derived from monitoring of all drinking-water wells in Suffolk County in which contamination had occurred are shown in Table 2.

Table 2. Numbers of wells containing aldicarb residues in Suffolk County, NY, 1980-85[a]

Year	No. of samples	No. of wells containing aldicarb	
		> 8 μg/l	1-7 μg/l
1980	8595	1193	1167
1981	677	190	275
1982	2905	380	265
1983	4659	804	661
1984	3974	670	546
1985	4022	942	688

[a]From US Environmental Protection Agency (1988)

Extensive monitoring studies in the USA have mostly been related to potato and citrus production. Relatively high percentages (5–> 50%) of positive findings occurred in Wisconsin and north-eastern states (New York, Massachusetts, Rhode Island, Connecticut, Maine). There was substantial evidence for leaching to shallow groundwater associated with citrus production in Florida (US Environmental Protection Agency, 1988; WHO, 1991).

1.3.3 *Soil*

Numerous studies have been carried out with aldicarb under field and laboratory conditions to study its translocation, persistence and degradation (WHO, 1991). It has a half-time in soil of approximately 30 days; this can vary depending on microbial populations, soil composition, moisture, temperature and farming practices (Meister, 1990). Its half-time in the root zone varied from one week to over two months. The primary mode of degradation in this zone is oxidative metabolism by microorganisms, although some hydrolysis may occur. Warm soil temperatures, high moisture content and high organic contents may result in more rapid degradation (US Environmental Protection Agency, 1988; WHO, 1991).

Aldicarb is mobile in most types of soil, with adsorption coefficients typically of < 1.0 and often 0.1. Incidents of groundwater contamination have primarily been associated with sandy soils, to which aldicarb residues are poorly bound (US Environmental Protection Agency, 1988).

Aldicarb has been used extensively since 1979-80 to control cotton whitefly in the Sudan, reaching a maximum of nearly 84 000 ha in 1984-85. When uptake and distribution were studied and the maximum uptake recorded two weeks after application of aqueous treatments and four weeks after application of granular formulations, no aldicarb or its sulfoxide or sulfone metabolites were detected in plant tissues or in soil at harvest (El-Zorgani *et al.*, 1988).

1.3.4 *Food*

In a market-basket survey carried out in the USA in 1983-85 on 491 samples of raw agricultural commodities, 76 (72 of white potatoes, two of sweet potatoes, one peach and one collard green) contained aldicarb residues. The mean residue level in potato samples taken in 1984 and 1985 was 200 µg/kg, while that taken in 1983 was 720 µg/kg (US Environmental Protection Agency, 1988).

In 1984-85 to 1988-89 in Canada, aldicarb residues were found in 13 of 30 samples of potatoes, at 0.02-0.78 mg/kg (mean, 0.13 mg/kg). No residue was detected in samples of bananas, oranges, cucumbers or wine (Government of Canada, 1990).

In 1978, national monitoring of potatoes treated at 3 kg/ha active ingredient in the Netherlands found total residues (expressed as the sulfone) in 23 samples, ranging from < 0.03 to 0.38 mg/kg, 100-205 days after broadcast application (mean, 0.11 mg/kg). Monitoring in 1982 of potatoes treated similarly showed residues of < 0.03-0.25 mg/kg (mean, 0.06 mg/kg) (FAO/WHO, 1986).

In a total diet study in 1986-88, 3737 domestic and imported food samples were analysed in the USA. Of these, 3656 (98%) contained no detectable residue. Potatoes (312) were included and residues found in 18% of samples, the highest level being 0.71 mg/kg. No residue was found in 98% of bananas sampled (55); one sample contained 0.12 mg/kg (US Food and Drug Administration, 1989b).

1.4 Regulations and guidelines

Limits for residues of aldicarb in foods in various countries or regions are given in Table 3.

Table 3. National or regional residue limits for aldicarb in foods[a]

Country or region	Residue limit (mg/kg)	Commodities
Australia	0.2	Potatoes, strawberries
	0.05[b]	Cottonseed
	0.02[b]	Cereal grain, sugar-cane
	0.01[b]	Citrus
Austria	0.05[c]	All foodstuffs of vegetable origin
	0.01[c]	All foodstuffs of animal origin
Belgium	0.05[d]	Brussels sprouts, potatoes
	0[e] (0.02)	Other foodstufs of vegetable origin
Brazil	1.0	Potatoes
	0.3	Bananas
	0.2	Citrus fruit
	0.1	Cottonseed, coffee (raw beans)
	0.05	Peanuts
	0.02	Beans, sugar-cane, tomatoes
Canada	0.5[f]	Potatoes
Denmark	0.2[d]	Citrus fruit, potatoes
	0.5[d]	Bananas
	0.05[d]	Onions
Finland	0.2[d]	Citrus fruit
	0.05[d]	Other foodstuffs (except cereal grains)
Germany	0.5[c]	Potatoes
	0.3[c]	Citrus fruit
	0.1[c]	Beans, citrus juices, cottonseed, raw coffee
	0.05[c]	Maize, onions, peanuts, soya beans, sugar beets, strawberries
	0.01[c]	All foodstuffs of animal orign
Hungary	0.05	Sugar beets
	0.01	Sugar
Israel	0.1	Cottonseed
Italy	0.05	Sugar beets
Kenya	0.1	Cottonseed
Mexico	1.0	Cotton, potatoes
	0.6	Citrus fruit (processed), tomatoes (processed)
	0.5	Nuts, sorghum forage
	0.3	Pecans
	0.1	Beans, coffee
	0.05	Peanuts, sorghum grain
	0.02	Soya beans, sugar-cane and sweet potatoes (negligible)
Netherlands	0.5[d]	Bananas, pecan nuts, potatoes
	0.2[d]	Sorghum
	0.1[d]	Beans (dry), coffee beans, cottonseed, sweet potatoes
	0.05[g]	Brussels sprouts, onions, peanuts
	0.01[g]	Meat, milk
	0 (0.02)[h]	Other crops or food

Table 3 (contd)

Country or region	Residue limit (mg/kg)	Commodities
South Africa	1.0[c]	Potatoes
	0.5[c]	Bananas
	0.2[c]	Citrus (except lemons), grapes, tomatoes
	0.1[c]	Cottonseed, sugar-cane
	0.05[c]	Macadamia nuts, mealies (green), pecan nuts
Spain	5.00[c]	Tobacco
	1.00[c]	Beetroot tops
	0.50[c]	Potatoes
	0.30[c]	Bananas
	0.20[c]	Citrus fruit
	0.10[c]	Cottonseed
	0.05[c]	Other plant products
Sweden	0.2[c]	Citrus fruit
	0.05[c]	Potatoes
Switzerland	0.02[f]	Maize
	0.01	Sugar beets
Taiwan	0.5	Fruit vegetables, root vegetables, tropical fruit
	0.2	Citrus fruit
	0.1	Beans (dry)
USA	1[f]	Potatoes, sugar beets (tops)
	0.6	Dried citrus pulp (feed)
	0.5	Peanuts (hulls), pecans, sorghum (fodder), sorghum bran (feed)[i]
	0.3	Bananas, cottonseed hulls (feed), grapefruit, lemons, limes, oranges
	0.2	Sorghum (grain)
	0.1	Beans (dry), coffee beans, cottonseed, sugar-cane (fodder, forage), sweet potatoes, sorghum bran[i]
	0.05	Peanuts, sugar beets
	0.02	Soya beans, sugar-cane
	0.01	Cattle, goats, hogs, horses and sheep (fat, meat and meat by-products)
	0.002	Milk
Yugoslavia	0.05[f]	Sugar beets

[a]From Health and Welfare Canada (1990); US Environmental Protection Agency (1989b,c)

[b]The maximum residue limit has been set at or about the limit of analytical determination.

[c]Sum of aldicarb, aldicarb sulfoxide and aldicarb sulfone (total calculated as aldicarb)

[d]Sum of aldicarb, its sulfoxide and its sulfone

[e]The figure in parentheses is the lower limit for determining residues in the corresponding product according to the standard method of analysis.

[f]Including the metabolites aldicarb sulfoxide and aldicarb sulfone

[g]A pesticide may be used on an eating or drinking ware or raw material without a demonstrable residue remaining; the value listed is considered the highest concentration at which this requirement is deemed to have been met.

[h]Residues shall be absent; the value in parentheses is the highest concentration at which this requirement is still deemed to have been met.

[i]Interim tolerance

The FAO/WHO Joint Meeting on Pesticide Residues evaluated aldicarb at meetings in 1979, 1982, 1985 and 1988 (FAO/WHO, 1980, 1983a, 1986, 1988). In 1982, an acceptable daily intake in food of 0.005 mg/kg bw was established (FAO/WHO, 1983b).

Maximum residue levels have been established by the Codex Alimentarius Commission for aldicarb (sum of aldicarb, its sulfoxide and its sulfone, expressed as aldicarb) in or on the following commodities (in mg/kg): maize forage, 5; sugar beets (leaves or tops), 1; bananas, dry sorghum (straw and fodder), pecans, potatoes, 0.5; citrus fruit, sorghum, 0.2; coffee beans, dry beans, cottonseed, sweet potatoes, 0.1; maize, onion (bulb), peanuts, sugar beets, 0.05; dry soya beans, 0.02; meat, milk, 0.01 (Codex Commission on Pesticide Residues, 1990).

The Office of Drinking Water of the US Environmental Protection Agency established a Health Advisory Level of 10 ppb (μg/l) for residues of aldicarb in drinking-water (US Environmental Protection Agency, 1984), with a proposed revision of 3 ppb (μg/l) (US Environmental Protection Agency, 1991). Aldicarb was included in the 1987 Canadian guidelines for drinking-water quality, with a maximum acceptable concentration of 9 μg/l (Minister of National Health and Welfare, 1987).

The technical product aldicarb has been classified as 'extremely hazardous' by WHO (1990).

2. Studies of Cancer in Humans

No data were available to the Working Group.

3. Studies of Cancer in Experimental Animals

Oral administration

Mouse

Groups of 50 male and 50 female B6C3F$_1$ mice, six weeks old, were fed aldicarb (approximately 99% pure) at 2 or 6 mg/kg of diet for 103 weeks. A control group of 25 males and 25 females was available. Survival at 90 weeks was 21/25 control, 48/50 low-dose and 45/50 high-dose males and 19/25 control, 45/50 low-dose and 44/50 high-dose females. No reduction in body weight was observed in treated animals, and there was no treatment-related increase in tumour incidence at any site. The authors stated that the dietary concentrations of aldicarb used were too low to be considered a maximum tolerated dose (US National Cancer Institute, 1979).

Rat

Groups of 50 male and 50 female Fischer 344/N rats, eight weeks of age, were fed aldicarb (approximately 99% pure) at 2 or 6 mg/kg of diet for 103 weeks. A control group of 25 males and 25 females was available. Survival at 90 weeks was 18/25 control, 44/50 low-dose and 39/50 high-dose males and 24/25 control, 44/50 low-dose and 46/50 high-dose females. No reduction in body weight was observed in treated animals, and there was no treatment-related increase in tumour incidence at any site. The authors stated that the dietary concentrations of aldicarb used were too low to be considered a maximum tolerated dose (US National Cancer Institute, 1979).

4. Other Relevant Data

The toxicity of aldicarb has been reviewed (FAO/WHO, 1980, 1983a; Risher *et al.*, 1987; Baron & Merriam, 1988; WHO, 1991).

4.1 Absorption, distribution, metabolism and excretion

The metabolism of aldicarb is shown in Figure 1 (Risher *et al.*, 1987).

4.1.1 *Humans*

Most carbamate insecticides are readily absorbed from the gastrointestinal tract. They may also be absorbed to varying degrees through the skin (Feldman & Maibach, 1970; Sterling, 1983).

Reports on the toxicity of aldicarb in humans (section 4.2.1) suggest that it enters the human body following skin contact, inhalation and ingestion. It is metabolized to aldicarb sulfoxide and aldicarb sulfone. Aldicarb derivatives (aldicarb, aldicarb sulfoxide and aldicarb sulfone) were found in the tissues of a 20-year-old man run over by a tractor following overexposure for about 2 h without adequate protection. The levels found were 482 µg/l in blood, 187 µg/kg in liver, 683 µg/kg in kidney and 823 µg/kg in skin from the hand. Aldicarb itself was not detected in blood, but aldicarb sulfoxide was present at 108 ppb [µg/l] and aldicarb sulfone at 374 ppb [µg/l], indicating an almost complete two-step oxidation process. The same trend was seen in the liver and kidney, while aldicarb occurred at the highest level in the skin. The total body burden of aldicarb was estimated at 18.2 mg (equivalent to 0.275 mg/kg bw) (Lee & Ransdell, 1984).

4.1.2 *Experimental systems*

Aldicarb is readily absorbed through the gut in rats and cows and through the skin in rats and rabbits. It is rapidly metabolized and excreted within 24 h of exposure, almost all of the toxic and nontoxic metabolites being excreted in urine (Risher *et al.*, 1987). Signs of poisoning were reported to occur only a few minutes after administration of higher doses in rats given aldicarb at up to 0.1 mg/kg bw by intubation (Cambon *et al.*, 1979). In rats administered radiolabelled aldicarb orally, 80% of the label was excreted in the urine within 24 h; less than 0.4% consisted of unchanged aldicarb (Andrawes *et al.*, 1967). Almost complete absorption *via* the gut was observed in cows (Dorough & Ivie, 1968; Dorough *et al.*, 1970).

Analysis of tissue samples taken from rats one to four days following oral administration of radiolabelled aldicarb indicated general distribution and elimination (Andrawes *et al.*, 1967).

The metabolism of aldicarb in rats involves both hydrolysis of the carbamate ester and oxidation of the sulfur to the sulfoxide and sulfone derivatives (Andrawes *et al.*, 1967). While the hydrolysis results in compounds with little or no insecticidal activity or toxicity to other organisms, the sulfoxide and sulfone metabolites are active cholinesterase inhibitors (Bull *et*

Fig. 1. Metabolic pathways of aldicarb in rats (from Risher *et al.*, 1987)

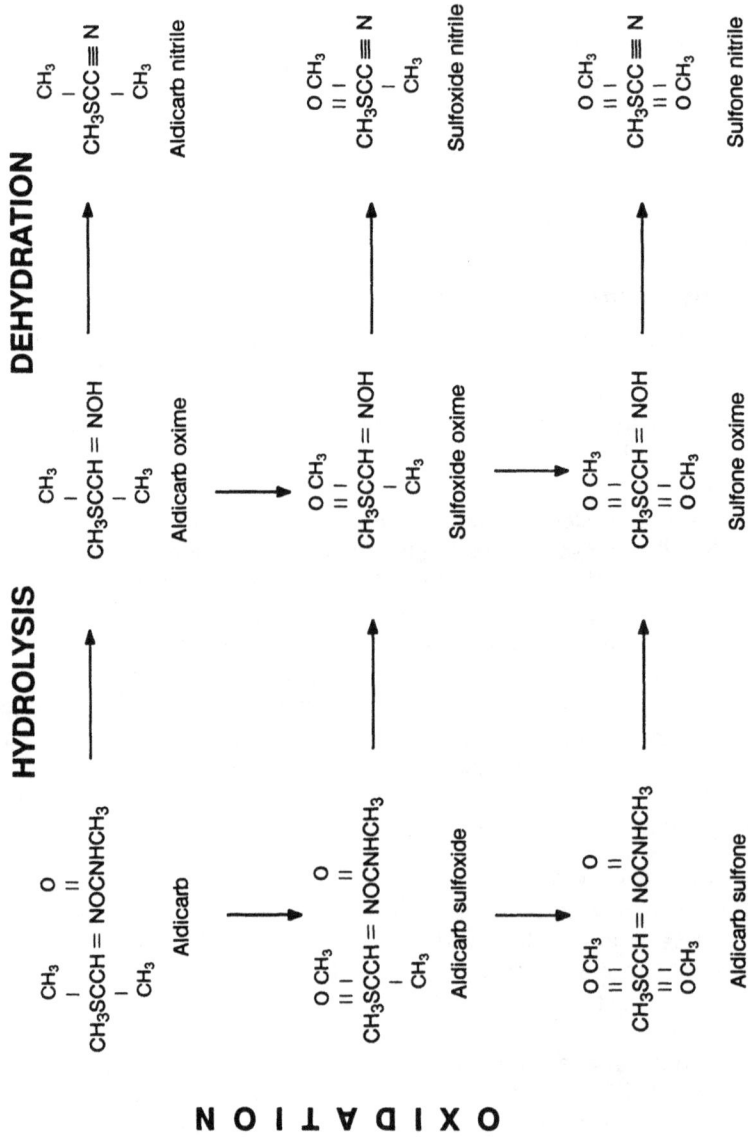

al., 1967; Risher *et al.*, 1987). In rats, the sulfoxide and the oxime sulfoxide constitute the major urinary metabolites, at 40% and 30%, respectively (Knaak *et al.*, 1966).

4.2 Toxic effects

4.2.1 *Humans*

Aldicarb is one of the most toxic pesticides known (Marshall, 1985). Its toxicity is based on a transient inhibition of acetylcholinesterase. Carbamates form unstable complexes with chlolinesterases by carbamoylation of the active sites of the enzymes (Done, 1979; Mortensen, 1986). Unlike the relatively irreversible anticholinesterase activity of the organophosphorus insecticides, the carbamoylation process which produces the esterase inhibition is quickly reversible.

Several reports on the acute and chronic toxicity of aldicarb are summarized in Table 4. In most exposure situations, the clinical symptoms observed were consistent with the known mechanism of action (inhibition of acetylcholinesterase). In some of the studies, the dose has been estimated. Cholinesterase measurements have been of additional use in characterizing dose or extent of exposure.

4.2.2 *Experimental systems*

The acute toxicity of alidcarb is high, with oral LD_{50}s in rats and mice generally below 1 mg/kg bw. Depression of cholinesterase activity has been reported in rats administered aldicarb, its sulfoxide or its sulfone. The relative order of inhibition of cholinesterase was plasma > red blood cells > brain (DePass *et al.*, 1985; studies reported by Risher *et al.*, 1987).

After a review of several studies, Risher *et al.* (1987) concluded there was no effect of subchronic and chronic oral feeding to rats of aldicarb at 0.3 mg/kg bw/day; of aldicarb sulfoxide at 0.3 mg/kg bw/day; of aldicarb sulfone at 2.4 mg/kg bw/day; or of 1:1 aldicarb sulfoxide:sulfone mixture at 0.6 mg/kg bw/day. The latter was tested owing to the observation that residues found in drinking-water are generally present as this mixture.

Suppressed humoral immune response (splenic plaque-forming cell assay) has been reported after exposure of mice to aldicarb in drinking-water for up to 34 days. Suppression on day 34 was significant, however, only at 1 ppb [µg/l] water and was less pronounced and not significant at 10, 100 or 1000 µg/l water (Olson *et al.*, 1987). In a similar study in mice exposed to aldicarb in drinking-water at levels of 0.1-1000 ppb [µg/l] for 34 days, using a variety of immunological endpoints including that used by Olson *et al.*, no significant effect on the immunological system was noted (Thomas *et al.*, 1987). Shirazi *et al.* (1990), however, performed a follow-up experiment using the same assay and aldicarb at 0.01-1000 µg/l in drinking-water but prolonging the study time up to 180 days. After extensive statistical analysis, the authors concluded that there was a stimulatory effect at 30 and 60 days and an inhibitory effect at 90 and 180 days. Dean *et al.* (1990) reported that aldicarb given intraperitoneally to mice at doses of 0.01-100 ng per mouse (0.1 ml of a 0.1, 1, 10, 100 or 1000 ppb solution) decreased the stimulatory function of macrophages without affecting T-lymphocyte function. There was no clear dose-response relationship.

Table 4. Acute and chronic toxicity of aldicarb in human populations

Type of exposure/population studied	No. of cases	Clinical symptom reported[a]	Estimated dose	Other endpoints/comments	Reference
Foreman running mechanical bagging machine for one day	1	+	NR[b]	Decrease in plasma and red blood cell AChE[c]	US Environmental Protection Agency (1975)
California, USA, 1974-76 Acute occupational intoxication as reported by physicians; dermal and inhalation exposure	38	+	NR	Not reported	Peoples et al. (1978)
Florida, USA, 1981 Interview survey of 436 citrus growers	1	+	NR	Intoxication confirmed by unspecified laboratory tests	Griffith & Duncan (1985)
Farm worker exposed ~2 h without adequate protection	1	-	0.275 mg/kg bw	Incapacitation due to intoxication thought to contribute to death in an accident	Lee & Ransdell (1984)
Woman ate leaf of spearmint growing near roses sprayed three weeks previously	1	+	NR	NR	Marshall (1985)
Nebraska, USA, 1977 and 1978 Two incidents of intoxication following ingestion of cucumbers; aldicarb contamination identified in later incident	14	+	(0.025–0.041 mg/kg bw)[d]	No abnormal blood chemistry	Goes et al. (1980)
Vancouver, Canada, 1985 Ingestion of cucumbers contaminated with aldicarb	140	+	0.01–0.03 mg/kg bw	NR	Hirsch et al. (1987)

Table 4 (contd)

Type of exposure/population studied	No. of cases	Clinical symptom reported[a]	Estimated dose	Other endpoints/comments	Reference
Oregon and California, USA **Ingestion of watermelon**					
Oregon, aldicarb residues in 10/16 melons eaten by definite cases	61 definite, 43 suspected 264 reported	+		NR	Green et al. (1987)
California, aldicarb sulfoxide residues in 10/250 melons	690 probable of 1350 reported	+	0.002–0.06 mg/kg bw	NR	Jackson & Goldman (1986); Jackson et al. (1986)
Suffolk County, NY, USA, 1981 Questionnaire survey of 1500 households with well-water aldicarb levels > 7 ppb (μg/l)	641 individuals evaluated from 204 questionnaires	–	NR	Trend in neurological syndromes reported with increasing aldicarb concentration	Sterman & Varma (1983)
Portage County, WI, USA, 1985 37 women from households supplied by well-water screened for aldicarb and 13 from households supplied with municipal water	23 exposed to detectable levels of aldicarb, 27 controls	–	0.3–48 μg/day	Increased number of T8 cells; increased % of total lymphocytes as T8 cells; decreased ratio T4:T8 cells in exposed versus controls	Fiore et al. (1986)

[a]Clinical symptoms reported consistent with inhibition of acetylcholinesterase, +; no such symptom reported, –
[b]NR, none reported and no details given to estimate dose
[c]AChE, acetylcholinesterase
[d]Dose estimated by Jackson & Goldman (1986)

4.3 Reproductive and developmental effects

4.3.1 *Humans*

No data were available to the Working Group.

4.3.2 *Experimental systems*

Few data are available on the reproductive and developmental effects of aldicarb. In two studies described in a review by Risher *et al.* (1987), there was reported to be no evidence of toxicity in the offspring of rats treated with aldicarb in the feed at doses as high as 1 mg/kg bw [near the LD_{50}] throughout pregnancy and lactation, and offspring of rabbits treated with aldicarb by gavage at doses of up to 0.5 mg/kg bw on days 7-27 of gestation were reported to exhibit no developmental toxicity. Rats investigated in a three-generation study in which aldicarb was incorporated into the diet were also reported to exhibit no significant difference in any parameter assessed compared to control animals.

Cambon *et al.* (1979, 1980) evaluated the effects of administering a single dose of aldicarb (0-0.1 mg/kg bw) on gestation day 18 on acetylcholinesterase activity in maternal and fetal tissue of Sprague-Dawley rats. Maternal blood acetylcholinesterase activity was reduced at doses greater than 0.001 mg/kg, and fetal blood acetylcholinesterase activity was reduced at doses of 0.001 mg/kg and above in samples taken > 1 h after dosing. The effect persisted for up to 24 h at doses of 0.01 mg/kg and above. Tissues were stored overnight at 4°C before analysis. Acetylcholinesterase was assayed in maternal and fetal brain homogenates 1 h after administration of 0.1 mg/kg bw aldicarb, and isoenzymes were analysed using polyacrylamide electrophoresis. Both maternal and fetal brain acetyl-cholinesterase levels were decreased by aldicarb; the levels of two of three cholinesterase isozymes were decreased in fetal brain and that of only one of the cholinesterase isozymes was decreased in maternal brain.

4.4 Genetic and related effects (see Table 5 and Appendices 1 and 2)

4.4.1 *Humans*

No data were available to the Working Group.

4.4.2 *Experimental systems*

Aldicarb induced differential toxicity in *Salmonella typhimurium* but not in strains of *Escherichia coli*. Aldicarb was not mutagenic to bacteria, whereas mutations were induced in cultured mammalian cells. Gene mutation, sister chromatid exchange and chromosomal aberrations were induced by aldicarb in cultured human cells. In a single study, no DNA strand breakage was observed in human cells.

In vivo, aldicarb induced chromosomal aberrations in cells of rat bone marrow.

5. Summary of Data Reported and Evaluation

5.1 Exposure data

Aldicarb is a moderately persistent systemic insecticide, acaricide and nematicide formulated as granules. It was first used in 1970 and is applied mainly on cotton and potatoes.

Exposure to aldicarb may occur during its production and application and, at lower levels, *via* contamination of groundwater and consumption of food containing residues.

Table 5. Genetic and related effects of aldicarb

Test system	Result[a] Without exogenous metabolic system	With exogenous metabolic system	Dose[b] LED/HID	Reference
SAD, *Salmonella typhimurium* TA1538/1978, differential toxicity	+	0	1000.0000	Rashid & Mumma (1986)
ERD, *Escherichia coli* WP2, differential toxicity	−	0	2000.0000	Rashid & Mumma (1986)
ERD, *Escherichia coli* K12, differential toxicity	−	0	2000.0000	Rashid & Mumma (1986)
SA0, *Salmonella typhimurium* TA100, reverse mutation	−	−	5000.0000	Dunkel *et al.* (1985)
SA0, *Salmonella typhimurium* TA100 reverse mutation	−	−	5000.0000	Zeiger *et al.* (1988)
SA5, *Salmonella typhimurium* TA1535, reverse mutation	−	−	5000.0000	Dunkel *et al.* (1985)
SA5, *Salmonella typhimurium* TA1535, reverse mutation	−	−	5000.0000	Zeiger *et al.* (1988)
SA7, *Salmonella typhimurium* TA1537, reverse mutation	−	−	5000.0000	Dunkel *et al.* (1985)
SA7, *Salmonella typhimurium* TA1537, reverse mutation	−	−	5000.0000	Zeiger *et al.* (1988)
SA8, *Salmonella typhimurium* TA1538, reverse mutation	−	−	5000.0000	Dunkel *et al.* (1985)
SA9, *Salmonella typhimurium* TA98, reverse mutation	−	−	5000.0000	Dunkel *et al.* (1985)
SA9, *Salmonella typhimurium* TA98, reverse mutation	−	−	5000.0000	Zeiger *et al.* (1988)
SAS, *Salmonella typhimurium* TA97, reverse mutation	−	−	5000.0000	Zeiger *et al.* (1988)
ECW, *Escherichia coli* WP2 *uvr*A, reverse mutation	−	−	5000.0000	Dunkel *et al.* (1985)
G5T, Gene mutation, mouse lymphoma L5178Y cells, *tk* locus	+	0	2600.0000	Caspary *et al.* (1988)
G5T, Gene mutation, mouse lymphoma L5178Y cells, *tk* locus	+	+	1300.0000	Mitchell *et al.* (1988)
G5T, Gene mutation, mouse lymphoma L5178Y cells, *tk* locus	−	+	1000.0000	Myhr & Caspary (1988)
DIH, DNA strand breakage, human skin fibroblasts *in vitro*	−	0	1.9000	Blevins *et al.* (1977)
GIH, Gene mutation, human lymphoblastoid TK6 cells, *tk* locus	+	0	1600.0000	Caspary *et al.* (1988)
SHL, Sister chromatid exchange, human lymphocytes *in vitro*	+	+	0.0000	Debuyst & Van Larebeke (1983; abstract)
SHL, Sister chromatid exchange, human lymphocytes *in vitro*	(+)	+	40.0000	Cid & Matos (1984)
CHL, Chromosomal aberrations, human lymphocytes *in vitro*	(+)	+	350.0000	Cid & Matos (1987)
CBA, Chromosomal aberrations, rat bone-marrow *in vivo*	+	0	0.0012 × 5 i.p.	Sharaf *et al.* (1982)

[a] +, positive; (+), weak positive; −, negative; 0, not tested

[b] In-vitro tests, μg/ml; in-vivo tests, mg/kg bw

5.2 Carcinogenicity in humans

No data were available to the Working Group.

5.3 Carcinogenicity in experimental animals

Aldicarb has not been tested adequately for carcinogenicity in experimental animals.

5.4 Other relevant data

Aldicarb is highly acutely toxic: it is one of the most potent cholinesterase-inhibiting carbamate insecticides.

No data were available on the genetic and related effects of aldicarb in humans.

Aldicarb induced chromosomal aberrations in rat bone-marrow cells *in vivo*. It induced various kinds of chromosomal damage and gene mutation in cultured human cells and induced gene mutation in rodent cells. It did not cause mutation in bacteria.

5.5 Evaluation[1]

No data were available from studies in humans.

There is *inadequate evidence* for the carcinogenicity of aldicarb in experimental animals.

Overall evaluation

Aldicarb *is not classifiable as to its carcinogenicity to humans (Group 3).*

6. References

Andrawes, N.R., Dorough, H.W. & Lindquist, D.A. (1967) Degradation and elimination of Temik in rats. *J. Econ. Entomol.*, *60*, 979-987

Association of Official Analytical Chemists (1985) Changes in methods. *N*-Methylcarbamate insecticide and metabolite residues. Liquid chromatographic method. First action. *J. Assoc. off. anal. Chem.*, *68*, 386-388

Baron, R.L. & Merriam, T.L. (1988) Toxicology of aldicarb. *Rev. environ. Contam. Toxicol.*, *105*, 2-70

Blevins, R.D., Lijinsky, W. & Regan, J.D. (1977) Nitrosated methylcarbamate insecticides: effect on the DNA of human cells. *Mutat. Res.*, *44*, 1-7

Bull, D.L., Lindquist, D.A. & Coppedge, J.R. (1967) Metabolism of 2-methyl-2-(methylthio)-propionaldehyde O-(methylcarbamoyl)oxime (Temik, UC-21149) in insects. *J. agric. Food Chem.*, *15*, 610-616

Cambon, C., Declume, C. & Derache, R. (1979) Effect of the insecticidal carbamate derivatives (carbofuran, pirimicarb, aldicarb) on the activity of acetylcholinesterase in tissues from pregnant rats and fetuses. *Toxicol. appl. Pharmacol.*, *49*, 203-208

---

[1]For definition of the italicized terms, see Preamble, pp. 26-28.

Cambon, C., Declume, C. & Derache, R. (1980) Foetal and maternal rat brain acetylcholinesterase: isoenzymes changes following insecticidal carbamate derivatives poisoning. *Arch. Toxicol.*, *45*, 257-262

Caspary, W.J., Langenbach, R., Penman, B.W., Crespi, C., Myhr, B.C. & Mitchell, A.D. (1988) The mutagenic activity of selected compounds at the TK locus: rodent vs. human cells. *Mutat. Res.*, *196*, 61-81

Cid, M.G. & Matos, E. (1984) Induction of sister-chromatid exchanges in cultured human lymphocytes by aldicarb, a carbamate pesticide. *Mutat. Res.*, *138*, 175-179

Cid, M.G. & Matos, E. (1987) Chromosomal aberrations in cultured human lymphocytes treated with aldicarb, a carbamate pesticide. *Mutat. Res.*, *191*, 99-103

Codex Committee on Pesticide Residues (1990) *Guide to Codex Maximum Limits for Pesticide Residues*, Part 2 (CAC/PR 2—1990; CCPR Pesticide Classification No. 117), The Hague

Coppedge, J.R., Bull, D.L. & Ridgway, R.L. (1977) Movement and persistence of aldicarb in certain soils. *Arch. environ. Contam. Toxicol.*, *5*, 129-141

Dean, T.N., Selvan, R.S., Misra, H.P., Nagarkatti, M. & Nagarkatti, P.S. (1990) Aldicarb treatment inhibits the stimulatory activity of macrophages without affecting the T-cell responses in the syngeneic mixed lymphocyte reaction. *Int. J. Immunopharmacol.*, *12*, 337-348

Debuyst, B. & Van Larebeke, N. (1983) Induction of sister-chromatid exchanges in human lymphocytes by aldicarb, thiofanox and methomyl (Abstract No. 35). *Mutat. Res.*, *113*, 242-243

DePass, L.R., Weaver, E.V. & Mirro, E.J. (1985) Aldicarb sulfoxide/aldicarb sulfone mixture in drinking water of rats: effects on growth and acetylcholinesterase activity. *J. Toxicol. environ. Health*, *16*, 163-172

Done, A.K. (1979) The toxic emergency. The great equalizers? II. Anticholinesterases. *Emerg. Med.*, *11*, 167-175

Dorough, H.W. & Ivie, G.W. (1968) Temik-S^{35} metabolism in a lactating cow. *J. agric. Food Chem.*, *16*, 460-464

Dorough, H.W., Davis, R.B. & Ivie, G.W. (1970) Fate of Temik-carbon-14 lactating cows during a 14-day feeding period. *J. agric. Food Chem.*, *18*, 135-142

Dunkel, V.C., Zeiger, E., Brusick, D., McCoy, E., McGregor, D., Mortelmans, K., Rosenkranz, H.S. & Simmon, V.F. (1985) Reproducibility of microbial mutagenicity assays. II. Testing of carcinogens and noncarcinogens in *Salmonella typhimurium* and *Escherichia coli*. *Environ. Mutagenesis*, *7* (Suppl. 5), 1-248

El-Zorgani, G.A., Bakhiet, T.N. & Eldin, N.S. (1988) Distribution of residues of ^{14}C-aldicarb applied to cotton plants in Gezira, Sudan. *Int. atomic Energy Agency*, *297*, 149-156

FAO/WHO (1980) *Pesticide Residues in Food: 1979 Evaluations. The Monographs* (FAO Plant Production and Protection Paper 20 Sup.), Rome

FAO/WHO (1983a) *Pesticide Residues in Food—1982 Evaluations. The Monographs* (FAO Plant Production and Protection Paper 49), Rome

FAO/WHO (1983b) *Pesticide Residues in Food—1982* (FAO Plant Production and Protection Paper 46), Rome

FAO/WHO (1986) *Pesticide Residues in Food—1985* (FAO Plant Production and Protection Paper 72/1), Rome

FAO/WHO (1988) *Pesticide Residues in Food—1988. Evaluations. Part I. Residues* (FAO Plant Production and Protection Paper 93/1), Rome

Feldman, R.J. & Maibach, H.I. (1970) Pesticide percutaneous penetration in man (Abstract No. 5). *J. invest. Dermatol.*, *54*, 435-436

Fiore, M.C., Anderson, H.A., Hong, R., Golubjatnikov, R., Seiser, J.E., Nordstrom, D., Hanrahan, L. & Belluck, D. (1986) Chronic exposure to aldicarb-contaminated groundwater and human immune function. *Environ. Res.*, *41*, 633-645

Goes, E.A., Savage, E.P., Gibbons, G., Aaronson, M., Ford, S.A. & Wheeler, H.W. (1980) Suspected foodborne carbamate pesticide intoxications associated with ingestion of hydroponic cucumbers. *Am. J. Epidemiol.*, *111*, 254-260

Government of Canada (1990) *Report on National Surveillance Data from 1984/85 to 1988/89*, Ottawa

Green, M.A., Heumann, M.A., Wehr, H.M., Foster, L.R., Williams, L.P., Jr, Polder, J.A., Morgan, C.L., Wagner, S.L., Wanke, L.A. & Witt, J.M. (1987) An outbreak of watermelon-borne pesticide toxicity. *Am. J. public Health*, *77*, 1431-1434

Griffith, J. & Duncan, R.C. (1985) Grower reported pesticide poisoning among Florida citrus fieldworkers. *J. environ. Sci. Health*, *B20*, 61-72

Health and Welfare Canada (1990) *National Pesticide Residue Limits in Foods*, Ottawa, Bureau of Chemical Safety, Food Directorate, Health Protection Branch

Hirsch, G.H., Mori, B.T., Morgan, G.B., Bennett, P.R. & Williams, B.C. (1987) Report of illnesses caused by aldicarb-contaminated cucumbers. *Food Addit. Contam.*, *5*, 155-160

Holtorf, R.C. (1982) *Preliminary Quantitative Usage Analysis of Aldicarb as a Pesticide*, Washington DC, US Environmental Protection Agency, Office of Pesticide Programs

Hynninen, E.-L. & Blomqvist, H. (1989) Sales of pesticides in Finland in 1988 (Fin.). *Kemia Kemi*, *16*, 614-617

IARC (1974) *IARC Monographs on the Evaluation of Carcinogenic Risk of Chemicals to Man*, Vol. 5, *Some Organochlorinic Pesticides*, Lyon, pp. 211-218

IARC (1987a) *IARC Monographs on the Evaluation of Carcinogenic Risks to Humans*, Suppl. 7, *Overall Evaluations of Carcinogenicity: An Updating of* IARC Monographs *Volumes 1 to 42*, Lyon, pp. 194-195

IARC (1987b) *IARC Monographs on the Evaluation of Carcinogenic Risks to Humans*, Suppl. 7, *Overall Evaluations of Carcinogenicity: An Updating of* IARC Monographs *Volumes 1 to 42*, Lyon, p. 71

IARC (1987c) *IARC Monographs on the Evaluation of Carcinogenic Risks to Humans*, Suppl. 7, *Overall Evaluations of Carcinogenicity: An Updating of* IARC Monographs *Volumes 1 to 42*, Lyon, pp. 220-222

IRPTC/UNEP (1990) *Data Profiles*, Geneva

Jackson, R.J. & Goldman, L. (1986) Aldicarb poisoning. Reply to a Letter. *J. Am. med. Assoc.*, *256*, 3218

Jackson, R.J., Stratton, J.W., Goldman, L.R., Smith, D.F., Pond, E.M., Epstein, D., Neutra, R.R., Kelter, A. & Kizer, K.W. (1986) Aldicarb food poisoning from contaminated melons— California. *J. Am. med. Assoc.*, *256*, 175-176

Knaak, J.B., Tallant, M.J. & Sullivan, L.J. (1966) The metabolism of 2-methyl-2-(methylthio)-propionaldehyde O-(methylcarbamoyl)oxime in the rat. *J. agric. Food Chem.*, *14*, 573-578

Lee, M.H. & Ransdell, J.F. (1984) A farmworker death due to pesticide toxicity: a case report. *J. Toxicol. environ. Health*, *14*, 239-246

Marshall, E. (1985) The rise and decline of Temik. *Science*, *229*, 1369-1371

Meister, R.T., ed. (1990) *Farm Chemical Handbook '90*, Willoughby, OH, Meister Publishing Co., pp. E-10, C-402, C-279—C-280

Minister of National Health and Welfare (1987) *Guidelines for Canadian Drinking Water Quality*, Ottawa

Mitchell, A.D., Rudd, C.J. & Caspary, W.J. (1988) Evaluation of the L5178Y mouse lymphoma cell mutagenesis assay: intralaboratory results for sixty-three coded chemicals tested at SRI International. *Environ. mol. Mutagenesis, 12* (Suppl. 13), 37-101

Mortensen, M.L. (1986) Management of acute childhood poisoning caused by selected insecticides and herbicides. *Pediatr. Clin. North Am., 33*, 421-445

Moye, H.A. & Miles, C.J. (1988) Aldicarb contamination of groundwater. *Rev. environ. Contam. Toxicol., 105*, 99-146

Myhr, B.C. & Caspary, W.J. (1988) Evaluation of the L5178Y mouse lymphoma cell mutagenesis assay: intralaboratory results for sixty-three coded chemicals tested at Litton Bionetics, Inc. *Environ. mol. Mutagenesis, 12* (Suppl. 13), 103-194

Narang, A.S. & Eadon, G. (1982) Use of XAD-2 macroreticular resin for the recovery of aldicarb and its metabolites in drinking water. *Int. J. environ. anal. Chem., 11*, 167-174

Olson, L.J., Erickson, B.J., Hinsdil, R.D., Wyman, J.A., Porter, W.P., Binning, L.K., Bidgood, R.C. & Nordheim, E.V. (1987) Aldicarb immunomodulation in mice: an inverse dose-response to parts per billion levels in drinking water. *Arch. environ. Contam. Toxicol., 16*, 433-439

Payne, L.K., Jr & Weiden, M.H.J. (1965) 2-Hydrocarbylthiosulfinyl and sulfonylalkanal carbamoyloximes. *US Patent 3,217,037* (to Union Carbide Co., NY)

Peoples, S.A., Maddy, K.T. & Smith, C.R. (1978) Occupational exposure to Temic (aldicarb) as reported by California physicians for 1974-1976. *Vet. hum. Toxicol., 20*, 321-324

Rashid, K.A. & Mumma, R.O. (1986) Screening pesticides for their ability to damage bacterial DNA. *J. environ. Sci. Health, B21*, 319-334

Rhone-Poulenc Ag Co. (1987) *Material Safety Data Sheet: Aldicarb, Technical Grade*, Research Triangle Park, NC

Rhone-Poulenc Ag Co. (1989) *Product Label Guide*, Research Triangle Park, NC, pp. 324-350

Rhone-Poulenc Ag Co. (1990a) *Material Safety Data Sheet: Temik® Brand 10G Aldicarb Pesticide for Agricultural Use (Gypsum)*, Research Triangle Park, NC

Rhone-Poulenc Ag Co. (1990b) *Material Safety Data Sheet: Temik® Brand 15G Aldicarb Pesticide (Gypsum)*, Research Triangle Park, NC

Rhone-Poulenc Ag Co. (1990c) *Material Safety Data Sheet: Temik® Brand TSX Granular Pesticide*, Research Triangle Park, NC

Risher, J.F., Mink, F.L. & Stara, J.F. (1987) The toxicologic effects of the carbamate insecticide aldicarb in mammals: a review. *Environ. Health Perspect., 72*, 267-281

Romine, R.R. (1974) Aldicarb. In: Zweig, G., ed., *Analytical Methods for Pesticides and Plant Growth Regulators*, Vol. VII, New York, Academic Press, pp. 147-162

Royal Society of Chemistry (1986) *European Directory of Agrochemical Products*, Vol. 3, *Insecticides, Acaricides, Nematicides*, Cambridge, pp. 4-10

Royal Society of Chemistry (1989) *The Agrochemicals Handbook* [Dialog Information Services (File 306)], Cambridge

Sharaf, A.A., Temtamy, S.A., de Hondt, H.A., Belal, M.H. & Kassam, E.A. (1982) Effect of aldicarb (Temik) a carbamate insecticide on chromosomes of the laboratory rat. *Egypt. J. genet. Cytol., 11*, 135-144

Shirazi, M.A., Erickson, B.J., Hinsdill, R.D. & Wyman, J.A. (1990) An analysis of risk from exposure to aldicarb using immune response of nonuniform populations of mice. *Arch. environ. Contam. Toxicol., 19*, 447-456

Sterling, G.H. (1983) Poisoning by cholinesterase-inhibiting insecticides. *Am. Fam. Physician*, *27*, 159-162

Sterman, A.B. & Varma, A. (1983) Evaluating human neurotoxicity of the pesticide aldicarb: when man becomes the experimental animal. *Neurobehav. Toxicol. Teratol.*, *5*, 493-495

Supak, J.R., Swoboda, A.R. & Dixon, J.B. (1977) Volatilization and degradation losses of aldicarb from soils. *J. environ. Qual.*, *6*, 413-417

Thomas, P.T., Ratajczak, H.V., Eisenberg, W.C., Furedi-Machacek, M., Ketels, K.V. & Barbera, P.W. (1987) Evaluation of host resistance and immunity in mice exposed to the carbamate pesticide aldicarb. *Fundam. appl. Toxicol.*, *9*, 82-89

US Environmental Protection Agency (1975) *Substitute Chemical Program: Initial Scientific and Minieconomic Review of Aldicarb* (EPA 540/1-75-013; NTIS PB-243-743), Washington DC

US Environmental Protection Agency (1976) Infrared spectra of pesticides. In: *Manual of Chemical Methods for Pesticides and Devices*, Arlington, VA, Association of Official Analytical Chemists

US Environmental Protection Agency (1984) *Pesticide Fact Sheet Number 19: Aldicarb* (PB 87-10881), Washington DC, Office of Pesticide Programs

US Environmental Protection Agency (1987) *Aldicarb*, Washington DC, Health Advisory Office of Drinking Water

US Environmental Protection Agency (1988) *Aldicarb* (Special Review, Technical Support Document), Washington DC, Office of Pesticides and Toxic Substances

US Environmental Protection Agency (1989a) Method 531.1 Measurement of *N*-methylcarbamoyl-oximes and *N*-methylcarbamates in water by direct aqueous injection HPLC with post column derivatization. In: *Methods for the Determination of Organic Compounds in Drinking Water* (EPA-600/4-88-039; US NTIS PB89-220461), Cincinnati, OH, Environmental Monitoring Systems Laboratory, pp. 357-378

US Environmental Protection Agency (1989b) Aldicarb; tolerances for residues. *US Code fed. Regul.*, *Title 40*, Part 180.269, pp. 324-325

US Environmental Protection Agency (1989c) Aldicarb. Tolerances for pesticides in animal feed. *US Code fed. Regul.*, *Title 40*, Part 185.150, p. 440

US Environmental Protection Agency (1991) National primary drinking water regulations—monitoring for synthetic organic chemicals; MCLGs and MCLs for aldicarb, aldicarb sulfoxide, aldicarb sulfone, pentachlorophenol and barium. *Fed. Reg.*, *56*, 3600-3614

US Food and Drug Administration (1989a) *Pesticide Analytical Manual*, Vol. II, Washington DC, US Department of Health and Human Services

US Food and Drug Administration (1989b) Residues in foods—1988. *J. Assoc. Off. Anal. Chem.*, *72*, 133A-142A

US National Cancer Institute (1979) *Bioassay of Aldicarb for Possible Carcinogenicity* (Carcinogenesis Technical Report Series No. 136; DHEW Publ. No. (NIH) 79-1391), Washington DC, US Government Printing Office

WHO (1990) *The WHO Recommended Classification of Pesticides by Hazard and Guidelines to Classification 1990-91*, Geneva

WHO (1991) *Aldicarb* (Environmental Health Criteria No. 121), Geneva

Williams, S., ed. (1984) *Official Methods of Analysis of the Association of Official Analytical Chemists*, 14th ed., Washington DC, Association of Official Analytical Chemists, p. 137

Worthing, C.R. & Walker, S.B., eds (1987) *The Pesticide Manual—A World Compendium*, 8th ed., Thornton Heath, British Crop Protection Council, pp. 7-8

Zaki, M.H., Moran, D. & Harris, D. (1982) Pesticides in groundwater: the aldicarb story in Suffolk County, NY. *Am. J. public Health*, 72, 1391-1395

Zeiger, E., Anderson, B., Haworth, S., Lawlor, T. & Mortelmans, K. (1988) *Salmonella* mutagenicity tests: IV. Results from the testing of 300 chemicals. *Environ. mol. Mutagenesis, 11* (Suppl. 12), 1-158

CHLORDANE AND HEPTACHLOR

Chlordane and heptachlor were considered together because of their close structural similarity and because technical-grade products each contain approximately 20% of the other compound.

These substances were considered by a previous Working Group, in 1978 (IARC, 1979). Since that time, new data have become available, and these have been incorporated into the monograph and taken into consideration in the present evaluation.

1. Exposure Data

1.1 Chemical and physical data

1.1.1 *Synonyms, structural and molecular data*

Table 1. Chemical Abstract Services Registry numbers, names and synonyms

Name	CAS Reg. Nos[a]	Chem. Abstr. names[b] and synonyms
Chlordane	57-74-9 (39400-80-1; 53637-13-1)	ENT 9932; **1,2,4,5,6,7,8,8-octachloro-2,3,3a,4,7,7a-hexa-hydro-4,7-methano-1H-indene;** 1,2,4,5,6,7,8,8-octachloro-2,3,3a,4,7, 7a-hexahydro-4,7-methanoindene (IUPAC); octachloro-4,7-methanotetrahydroindane; 1,2,4,5,6,7,8,8-octachloro-3a,4,7,7a-tetrahydro-4,7-methanoindan; OMS 1437
Technical-grade chlordane	12789-03-6	
cis-Chlordane	5103-71-9 (22212-52-8; 26703-86-6; 28140-46-7)	α-Chlordan; α-chlordane; *cis*-chlordan; **(1α,2α,3aα,4β,·7β,7aα)-1,2,4,5,6,7,8,8-octachloro-2,3,3a,4,7,7a-hexahydro-4,7-methano-1H-indene;** 1α,2α,4β,5,6,7β,8,8-octachloro-3aα,4,7,7aα-tetrahydro-4,7-methanoindan
trans-Chlordane	5103-74-2 (17436-70-3; 28181-89-7)	β-Chlordan; β-chlordane; *trans*-chlordan; **(1α,2β,3aα,4β,7β,·7aα)-1,2,4,5,6,7,8,8-octachloro-2,3,3a,4,7,7a-hexahydro-4,7-methano-1H-indene;** 1β,2α,4α,5,6,7α,8,8-octachloro-3aβ,4,7,7aβ,4,7,7aβ-tetrahydro-4,7-methanoindan
γ-Chlordane	5566-34-7	γ-Chlordan; **2,2,4,5,6,7,8,8-octachloro-2,3,3a,4,7,7a-hexa-hydro-4,7-methano-1H-indene;** 2,2,4,5,6,7,8,8-octachloro-3a,4,7,7a-tetrahydro-4,7-methanoindan stereoisomer
Heptachlor	76-44-8 (23720-59-4; 37229-06-4)	3-Chlorochlordene; E 3314; ENT 15 152; **1,4,5,6,7,8,8-hepta-chloro-3a,4,7,7a-tetrahydro-4,7-methano-1H-indene;** 1,4,5,6,7,8,8-heptachloro-3a,4,7,7a-tetrahydro-4,7-methano-indene (IUPAC); OMS 193

Table 1 (contd)

Name	CAS Reg. Nos[a]	Chem. Abstr. names[b] and synonyms
Heptachlor epoxide	1024-57-3 (4067-30-5; 24699-42-1; 24717-72-4; 28044-82-8; 66240-71-9)	ENT 25584; epoxyheptachlor; 1,4,5,6,7,8,8-heptachloro-2,3-epoxy-3a,4,7,7a-tetrahydro-4,7-methanoindan; (1aα, 1bβ,2α,5α,5aβ,6β,6aα)-2,3,4,5,6,7,7-**heptachloro-1a,1b,5,5a,6,6a-hexahydro-2,5-methano-2H-indeno(1,2-b)-oxirene**; heptachlor *cis*-oxide

[a]Replaced CAS Registry number(s) in parentheses
[b]In bold

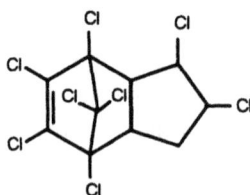
Chlordane

$C_{10}H_6Cl_8$ Mol. wt: 409.8

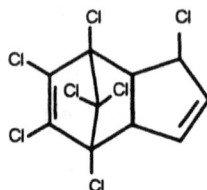
Heptachlor

$C_{10}H_5Cl_7$ Mol. wt: 373.5

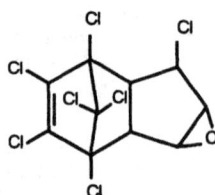
Heptachlor epoxide

$C_{10}H_5Cl_7O$ Mol. wt: 389.4

1.1.2 *Chemical and physical properties*

Chlordane

  (a) *Description*: Light-yellow to amber-coloured, viscous liquid (technical product) (WHO, 1988a)
  (b) *Boiling-point*: 175°C at 1 mm Hg [0.13 kPa] (pure material) (Royal Society of Chemistry, 1989)

(c) *Melting-point*: 106-107°C (α-isomer); 104-105°C (γ-isomer) (WHO, 1988)

(d) *Spectroscopy data*: Infrared (prism [534]; grating [41094P]) spectroscopy data have been reported (Sadtler Research Laboratories, 1980).

(e) *Solubility*: Practically insoluble in water (0.1 mg/l at 25°C) but soluble in most organic solvents (e.g., acetone, ethanol, kerosene, trichloroethylene) (Worthing & Walker, 1987)

(f) *Volatility*: Vapour pressure, 1×10^{-5} mm Hg [0.13×10^{-5} kPa] at 25°C (pure); 4.6×10^{-4} mm Hg [0.61×10^{-4} kPa] at 25°C (technical product) (Royal Society of Chemistry, 1989)

(g) *Stability*: Decomposed by alkalis, with loss of chlorine; ultra-violet irradiation induces a change in the skeletal structure and of the chlorine content; corrosive to iron, zinc and various protective coatings (Royal Society of Chemistry, 1989)

(h) *Conversion factor for airborne concentrations*[1]: mg/m^3 = 16.76 × ppm

Heptachlor

(a) *Description*: White crystalline solid with mild odour of camphor (Worthing & Walker, 1987; WHO, 1988b)

(b) *Boiling-point*: 135-145°C at 1-1.5 mm Hg [0.13-0.210 kPa] (US Environmental Protection Agency, 1986a)

(c) *Melting-point*: 95-96°C (pure compound) (Worthing & Walker, 1987)

(d) *Spectroscopy data*: Infrared (prism [74915]; grating [74915]) and nuclear magnetic resonance (proton [47772]) spectral data have been reported (Sadtler Research Laboratories, 1990).

(e) *Solubility*: Practically insoluble in water (56 μg/l at 25-29°C); fairly soluble in organic solvents: acetone (750 g/l), benzene (1060 g/l), ethanol (45 g/l) and xylene (1020 g/l) (WHO, 1988b)

(f) *Volatility*: Vapour pressure, 4×10^{-4} mm Hg [0.5×10^{-4} kPa] at 25°C (Worthing & Walker, 1987; WHO, 1988b)

(g) *Stability*: Stable in daylight, air, moisture and moderate heat (160°C); corrosive to metals; susceptible to epoxidation; slowly loses hydrogen chloride in alkaline media (WHO, 1988b; Royal Society of Chemistry, 1989)

(h) *Conversion factor for airborne concentrations*[1]: mg/m^3 = 15.28 × ppm

Heptachlor epoxide

(a) *Description*: Solid (Agency for Toxic Substances and Disease Registry, 1989a)

(b) *Melting-point*: 160-161.5°C (US Environmental Protection Agency, 1987a)

(c) *Spectroscopy data*: Infrared (prism [74932]; grating [74932]) and nuclear magnetic resonance (proton [47783]) spectral data have been reported (Sadtler Research Laboratories, 1990).

(d) *Solubility*: Practically insoluble in water (0.35 mg/l at 25°C) (US Environmental Protection Agency, 1987a)

(e) *Conversion factor for airborne concentrations*[1]: mg/m^3 = 15.93 × ppm

---

[1]Calculated from: mg/m^3 = (molecular weight/24.45) × ppm, assuming standard temperature (25°C) and pressure (760 mm Hg [101.3 kPa])

1.1.3 *Trade names, technical products and impurities*

Some examples of trade names are:

Chlordane: Aspon; Belt; CD 68; Chlordan; Chlorindan; Chlor Kil; Chlorotox; Corodane; Cortilan-neu; Dowchlor; Gold Crest; HCS 3260; Intox; Kypchlor; M 140; Niran[2]; Octachlor; Oktaterr; Ortho-Klor[2]; Starchlor; Sydane; Synklor; Tat Chlor 4; Termex; Topichlor; Toxichlor; Unexan-Koeder; Velsicol 1068

Heptachlor: Aahepta; Agroceres; Arbinex 30TN; Basaklor; Drinox; GPKh; Hepta; Heptachlorane; Heptagran; Heptagranox; Heptamak; Heptamul; Heptasol; Heptox; Rhodiachlor; Soleptax; Velsicol 104

Heptachlor epoxide: GPKh epoxide; HCE; Hepox; Heptepoxide; Velsicol 53-CS-17

The term chlordane commonly refers to a complex mixture of chlordane isomers, other chlorinated hydrocarbons and by-products, and at least 26 different components have been identified (WHO, 1988a). Technical-grade chlordane contains 60-75% of chlordane isomers (Royal Society of Chemistry, 1989), the major components being two stereoisomers (*cis* and *trans*, or α and γ), the nomenclature of which has been confused in the literature. The α or *cis*-isomer is described above under [5103-71-9]; the *trans*-isomer [5103-74-2], also usually known as the γ-isomer, is occasionally referred to as β-chlordane (the term γ-chlordane has been assigned by the Chemical Abstracts Service to the 2,2,4,5,6,7,8,8-octachloro-isomer [5566-34-7]). The remainder of the technical grade comprises other congeners (each $\leq 7\%$) and heptachlor. One description of the approximate composition of technical chlordane is as follows: *trans*-chlordane, 24%; *cis*-chlordane, 19%; chlordene isomers, 21.5%; heptachlor, 10%; nonachlor, 7%; octachlorocyclopentene, 1%; hexachlorocyclopentadiene, 1%; other, 16.5% (Brooks, 1974). Several reviews give details of the composition of technical-grade chlordane (Cochrane & Greenhalgh, 1976; Sovocool *et al.*, 1977; Miyazaki *et al.*, 1985; Buchert *et al.*, 1989).

Chlordane has been available in various formulations, including 5-30% granules, oil solutions containing 2-300 g/litre chlordane and emulsifiable concentrates containing 400-900 g/litre (Worthing & Walker, 1987; WHO, 1988a; Royal Society of Chemistry, 1986).

Technical-grade heptachlor contains about 72% heptachlor and 28% related compounds (20-22% γ-chlordane and 4-8% γ-nonachlor). Formulations have included emulsifiable concentrates, wettable powders, dusts and granules containing various concentrations of active material (Izmerov, 1982; Worthing & Walker, 1987; WHO, 1988b). In the USSR, the hexachlorocyclopentadiene content of heptachlor is limited by law to less than 2% (Izmerov, 1982). Heptachlor is registered in Czechoslovakia for formulation in combination with thiram (see IARC, 1976) (Royal Society of Chemistry, 1986).

1.1.4 *Analysis*

Determination of chlordane residues is difficult because of the complex nature of the components and the fact that each component degrades independently. Resulting residues may bear little relation to the proportions in the technical product. Extraction from crops, other plant products, dairy products, plants and oils has been achieved with an 80-100%

---

[2]Discontinued

efficiency using acetonitrile for extraction, petroleum ether for partitioning and clean-up on a Florisil column. Gel-permeation chromatography can also be used for clean-up, particularly of human adipose tissue. The method of choice for the qualitative and quantitative estimation of chlordane isomers and heptachlor is gas chromatography with electron-capture detection. Gas chromatographic analyses can be confirmed by gas chromatography–mass spectrometry, a method that can also provide better determination of some of the components, such as heptachlor epoxide. Analysis for total organically bound chlorine remains the preferred method for determination of technical-grade chlordane and heptachlor and of the active ingredient in formulations (WHO, 1988a,b).

Selected methods for the analysis of chlordane, heptachlor and heptachlor epoxide in various matrices are given in Table 2. Several reviews are available on the analysis of chlordane, heptachlor and heptachlor epoxide in technical products, formulations and as residues in various matrices, including titrimetric, colorimetric, spectrophotometric, infrared spectroscopic and gas chromatographic methods (Bowery, 1964; Raw, 1970; Izmerov, 1982; WHO, 1984a,b; Williams, 1984a,b; Anon., 1985; Worthing & Walker, 1987; Agency for Toxic Substances and Disease Registry, 1989a,b; Royal Society of Chemistry, 1989; Fendick et al., 1990).

Table 2. Methods for the analysis of chlordane, heptachlor and heptachlor oxide

Sample matrix	Sample preparation	Assay procedure[a]	Limit of detection[b]	Reference
Air	Collect vapours on polyurethane foam; extract with 5% diethyl ether in hexane	GC/ECD	NR	US Environmental Protection Agency (1988a)
	Collect vapours on Chromosorb 102; desorb with toluene	GC/ECD	0.1 μg/sample	Taylor (1979); Eller (1989)
Water	Extract with hexane; inject extract	GC/ECD	0.14, 0.003, 0.004 μg/l (0.006, 0.012 μg/l)[c]	US Environmental Protection Agency (1988b)
	Extract with dichloromethane; dry, concentrate (packed column)	GC/MS	NR, 1.9, 2.2 μg/l	US Environmental Protection Agency (1986b)
	Extract with dichloromethane; isolate; extract; dry; concentrate with methyl tert-butyl ether (capillary column)	GC/ECD	0.0015[c], 0.01, 0.015 μg/l	US Environmental Protection Agency (1988c)
	Extract by passing sample through liquid-solid extractor; elute with dichloromethane; conc. by evaporation (capillary column)	GC/MS	0.2, 0.1 μg/l[c], 0.04, 0.2 μg/l (0.3 g/l)[d]	US Environmental Protection Agency (1988d)
Waste-water	Extract with dichloromethane; dry; exchange to hexane	GC/ECD	0.014, 0.03, 0.083 μg/l	US Environmental Protection Agency (1986c, 1989a)

Table 2 (contd)

Sample matrix	Sample preparation	Assay procedure[a]	Limit of detection[b]	Reference
Waste-water (contd)	Extract with dichloromethane; dry; concentrate (packed column)	GC/MS	NR, 1.9 2.2 µg/l	US Environmental Protection Agency (1989b)
Formulations (chlordane)	Dissolve in toluene or benzene, then toluene; extract with 0.1N silver nitrate solution	TCM	NR	Williams (1984a)
Formulations (chlordane)	Dissolve in methanol/benzene or extract with pentane; dissolve; add Davidow reagent[e], boil; cool; read absorbance at 550 nm	Colorimetric	NR	Williams (1984a)
Formulations (heptachlor)	Dissolve in acetic acid; add silver nitrate or extract with pentane; dissolve	ACM	NR	Horwitz (1975)
	Dissolve in carbon disulfide or extract with pentane; dissolve	GC/FID	NR	Horwitz (1975)
Selected vegetables	Extract with pentane; clean-up on Florex column; evaporate to dryness; react with Polen-Silverman reagent[f]; read absorbance at 560 nm for heptachlor and at 410 nm for heptachlor oxide	Colorimetric	– 0.02, 0.02-0.04 ppm (mg/kg)	US Food and Drug Administration (1989)
Soil, sediment, wastes	Mix with anhydrous sodium sulfate; extract using Soxhlet or sonication process; clean-up using Florisil column or gel-permeation (packed column)	GC/MS	NR, 1.9, 2.2 µg/kg	US Environmental Protection Agency (1986b)
	Mix with anhydrous sodium sulfate; extract using Soxhlet or sonication process; clean-up using Florisil column or gel-permeation (capillary column)	GC/MS	NR	US Environmental Protection Agency (1986d)

[a]Abbreviations: ACM, active chlorine method; GC/ECD, gas chromatography/electron capture detection; GC/FID, gas chromatography/flame ionization detection; GC/MS, gas chromatography/mass spectrometry; TCM, total chlorine method

[b]The limits of detection are presented for chlordane, heptachlor and heptachlor epoxide, respectively; NR, not reported

[c]Detection limit(s) for α- and γ-chlordane

[d]trans-Nonachlor

[e]Diethanolamine-potassium hydroxide solution

[f]Prepared by dissolving potassium hydroxide in distilled water, cooling to room temperature, adding butyl Cellosolve and monoethanolamine and diluting to 1 litre with butyl Cellosolve. This solution, after standing several days, is decanted from any sediment and diluted with an equal volume of benzene.

1.2 Production and use

The discovery, chemistry and uses of chlordane and heptachlor and the problems associated with their technical-grade products have been reviewed (Brooks, 1974).

1.2.1 *Production*

Chlordane was first produced commercially in the USA in 1947. In 1974, production in the USA amounted to 9500 tonnes (WHO, 1988a); the US Environmental Protection Agency estimated that approximately 1600-1800 tonnes of chlordane were used in 1986. From 1 July 1983, the only use of chlordane approved in the USA was in the control of underground termites, but this use was prohibited in April 1988. The amounts of chlordane both produced and used have decreased considerably in recent years (US Environmental Protection Agency, 1987b; Agency for Toxic Substances and Disease Registry, 1989b).

Heptachlor was isolated from technical-grade chlordane in 1946. Production of heptachlor in the USA was 2700 tonnes in 1971, 900 tonnes in 1974, 590 tonnes in 1978, 180 tonnes in 1980 and 45 tonnes in 1982. Sales of heptachlor in the USA were voluntarily stopped by the sole US producer in August 1987, and since April 1988, heptachlor can no longer be used for the underground control of termites in the USA (WHO, 1988a; Agency for Toxic Substances and Disease Registry, 1989b). Chlordane and heptachlor are currently produced by one company in the USA; heptachlor epoxide is not produced commercially in the USA.

Chlordene, the starting material for the synthesis of both chlordane and heptachlor, is prepared by the Diels-Alder condensation of hexachlorocyclopentadiene with cyclopentadiene (Agency for Toxic Substances and Disease Registry, 1989b). Chlordane is prepared by the Lewis-acid catalysed addition of chlorine to chlordene (WHO, 1984a), whereas heptachlor is prepared by the free-radical chlorination of chlordene (Sittig, 1980).

Heptachlor epoxide can be prepared from heptachlor in a one-step oxidation. It is a metabolite as well as an environmental oxidation product of heptachlor (Anon., 1985).

1.2.2 *Use*

Chlordane has been used as an insecticide since the 1950s. It is a versatile, broad-spectrum, contact insecticide and has been used mainly for nonagricultural purposes (primarily for the protection of structures, but also on lawn and turf, ornamental trees and drainage ditches). It has also been used on maize, potatoes and livestock (WHO, 1984a). The use pattern for chlordane in the USA in the mid 1970s was as follows: 35% used by pest control operators, mostly on termites; 28% on agricultural crops, including maize and citrus; 30% for home lawn and garden use; and 7% on turf and ornamental plants (Agency for Toxic Substances and Disease Registry, 1989b). Since the mid-1970s, the use of chlordane has been increasingly restricted in many countries (WHO, 1988a). By 1980, less than 4500 tonnes of chlordane were being used yearly in the USA, mostly for termite control (Esworthy, 1985). By 1986, use had been reduced to 1800 tonnes (US Environmental Protection Agency, 1987b). In Japan, where chlordane was used exclusively for termite control, it was prohibited in 1986 (Takamiya, 1990).

Heptachlor was first introduced as a contact insecticide in the USA in 1952 for foliar, soil and structural application. It has also been used in the control of malaria. It is a nonsystemic internal and contact insecticide (WHO, 1988b). The use pattern for heptachlor in the USA in the mid-1970s was as follows: 58% on maize, 27% by pest control operators, 13% as seed treatment and 2% for miscellaneous uses, including fire ant control, use on pineapples and possibly on citrus (IARC, 1979). In 1970, the use of heptachlor throughout the world was as follows: Africa, 5%; Asia, 15%; Canada and the USA, 5%; Europe, 60%; and South America, 15% (WHO, 1988b). For example, in the Republic of Korea, average use of heptachlor was about 33 tonnes per year over the period 1962-79 (Lee, 1982). The use of heptachlor has been increasingly restricted in many countries; it is now confined almost exclusively to the control of soil insects and termites (WHO, 1988b). By 1986, less than 340 tonnes of heptachlor were used in the USA, mainly for termite control (US Environmental Protection Agency, 1987a).

1.3 Occurrence

The environmental occurrence and fate of chlordane and heptachlor have been reviewed (WHO, 1984a,b; Fendick *et al.*, 1990).

1.3.1 *Air*

Treatment for termite control in the USA in 1978, by subslab injection of 2% chlordane or exterior ditching of apartment blocks, produced high indoor air concentrations (0.4-263.5 $\mu g/m^3$) within one year; the levels after two years were 0-37.9 $\mu g/m^3$. Termite treatments in the USA in 1970 produced air concentrations within houses of 14.5-37.8 $\mu g/m^3$ (Livingston & Jones, 1981). Other US houses treated for termites with an emulsion containing 0.54% chlordane, 0.76 ppm diazinon and 0.93 ppm malathion resulted in airborne household dust containing 30 ppm (503 mg/m^3) chlordane and traces of the other pesticides (Vinopal & Olds, 1977).

1.3.2 *Water*

An episode of chlordane contamination of a segment of a municipal water system occurred in 1976 in Chattanooga, TN (USA), resulting in a concentration of chlordane in the water of up to 1200 mg/l (0.12%) (*sic*). The contamination probably occurred through careless handling of a concentrated chlordane solution, and a period of negative water pressure during dilution of the concentrate may have caused back-siphonage into the water system (Harrington *et al.*, 1978). Another public water supply was contaminated in Pittsburgh, PA: Levels of up to 6600 ppb ($\mu g/l$) chlordane were found in tap-water; six months later, the level was < 1 ppb (< 1 $\mu g/l$) (Anon., 1981).

After chlordane was applied to the surface of a lake, the concentration in the water was 4-5.5 $\mu g/l$ after seven days and 0.008-0.011 $\mu g/l$ after 421 days. The concentration in the lake sediments reached 20-30 $\mu g/kg$ during the first 279 days and 10 $\mu g/kg$ 421 days after application. Chlordane is not expected to leach since it is insoluble in water and should be adsorbed on the soil surface (US Environmental Protection Agency, 1986e).

1.3.3 *Soil*

Application of chlordane at 9 kg/ha (active ingredient) to turf over a sandy loam soil resulted in residues of 1.6-2.1 mg/kg in the root zone (0-1 cm depth) and < 0.3 mg/kg in the soil zone (1-3.5 cm depth). Total residues after 56 days had declined to 69% of the dose originally applied. In studies in Maryland, USA, where chlordane was applied to sandy loam soil at rates of 56, 112 and 224 kg/ha, 83% of that applied was still present after one year and 45% remained after 15 years (US Environmental Protection Agency, 1986e).

Heptachlor is stable to light and moisture, and volatilization is the major mechanism of transport of topically applied material. Its half-time in soil in temperate regions ranges between 0.75 and 2 years, depending on soil type and may be less in tropical regions. Residues have been detected in soil 14 years after initial use (WHO, 1984b).

A survey on cropland soils in 37 states of the USA in 1971 revealed heptachlor residues in 4.9% of samples at a maximum of 1.37 mg/kg; heptachlor epoxide was detected in 6.9% of the samples at a maximum level of 0.43 mg/kg (Carey et al., 1978).

1.3.4 Food

Many studies were carried out during the 1970s in Canada, the United Kingdom, the USA and other countries on the occurrence of pesticide residues in foods. Generally, residues of chlordane were seldom found. For example, in a market basket survey in the USA from 1963 to 1969, chlordane residues were found in less than 1% of samples at levels of 1-5 μg/kg (WHO, 1984a).

Significant levels were found in meat, milk and eggs, as a result of residues in feed crops or direct applications to cattle and poultry (as reported by the WHO, 1984a). In a study on eggs in Canada, trans-chlordane was found in 78% of samples, at a mean level of 2 μg/kg fresh weight, and cis-chlordane in 81% of the eggs, at a mean level of 1 μg/kg (Mes et al., 1974). In another study (Herrick et al., 1969), no residue was found in the eggs of chickens fed chlordane in the diet at 0.08 mg/kg for one week.

In analyses of cows' milk in the USA, 87% of samples contained chlordane, at levels ranging from 0.02 to 0.06 mg/l (IARC, 1979). In another study, the milk of cows grazing on pastures to which chlordane had been applied at 0.55 kg/ha contained an average chlordane concentration of 0.03 mg/litre; no residue was found at lower treatment levels (WHO, 1984a). Chlordane was also found in Canadian meat samples at levels ranging from 0 to 106 μg/kg in beef, 0 to 32 μg/kg in pork and 0 to 70 μg/kg in fowl (Saschenbrecker, 1976).

Of 1171 samples of fruits, meats, dairy products, grains and wine analysed for chlordane as part of the Canadian national surveillance programme (1984-89), none contained residues. Of 1227 samples of fruits, vegetables, meats, dairy products and wine analysed for heptachlor and its epoxide, four contained residues (2/21 carrots and 2/100 cucumbers), at levels of 0.01-0.02 mg/kg (Government of Canada, 1990).

In Brazil, 1998 samples of cattle meat, 102 samples of horse meat and 158 samples of corned beef and roast beef were analysed for heptachlor/heptachlor epoxide and oxychlordane/transnonaclor in 1984 and 1985; no residue was reported (limit of detection, 0.02 mg/kg) (Codex Committee on Pesticide Residues, 1989).

The daily human intake of heptachlor epoxide in the USA was calculated to be 0.29-0.64 μg/day during 1971-74 (as reported by the WHO, 1984b). The daily intake of heptachlor epoxide from food in 1965 in the USA was estimated as 2 μg/day; in 1970, this figure was 1 μg/day (Duggan & Corneliussen, 1972).

Market basket surveys carried out in 1972-73 in the USA showed maximum values for heptachlor epoxide ranging from trace to 2 μg/kg (Johnson & Manske, 1976). In a study done in 1966-67 in the United Kingdom, the heptachlor epoxide content in the total diet was, in general, less than 0.5 µg/kg; heptachlor was not detected (Abbott *et al.*, 1969). In a series of studies of total diets in the USA, heptachlor epoxide was found in small amounts in fish, poultry, meat and dairy products, and in trace amounts in fruits, vegetables, oils and cereals. The maximum values in poultry, meat and fish ranged from trace to 2 µg/kg (Johnson & Manske, 1976).

Heptachlor was not found in foods examined between August 1972 and July 1973 in a total-diet study conducted by the US Food and Drug Administration (Johnson & Manske, 1976). In a study (reported by WHO, 1984b) conducted in 20 cities in the USA in 1974-75, only 3 of 12 food classes contained detectable residues of heptachlor epoxide. Levels ranged from 0.6-3 µg/kg. A study (reported by WHO, 1984b) that started in 1974 in the USA revealed residues of heptachlor and heptachlor epoxide at the mean levels shown in Table 3.

Table 3. Heptachlor and heptachlor epoxide levels in food[a]

Residue	Level (µg/kg wet weight)				
	Pork	Horse meat	Chicken	Beef	Turkey
Heptachlor	1.25	1.06	3.27	0.10	0.65
Heptachlor epoxide	1.95	5.28	9.58	0.50	6.66

[a]As reported by WHO (1984b)

Within the framework of the Joint FAO/WHO Food Contamination Monitoring Programme, the levels of heptachlor and heptachlor epoxide residues in various food samples in 1980-82 were reported from Austria, Canada, Denmark, Guatemala, Japan, the Netherlands and the USA. On a fat basis, the median levels ranged from 0 (not detected) in butter and cattle fat in Denmark to 13 µg/l in cows' milk in Japan. Median levels in the products ranged from 0 (not detected) in hens' eggs in Denmark to 4 µg/kg in fresh onions in Guatemala. The median levels of heptachlor epoxide on a fat basis ranged from 0 (not detected) in butter and pasteurized cows' milk to 0.30 µg/l in raw cows' milk in Germany (WHO, 1983).

Heptachlor and/or heptachlor epoxide was present in 32% of 590 fish samples in the USA in 1967-68, at levels of 0.01-8.46 mg/kg (Henderson *et al.*, 1969). Fish have been shown to accumulate heptachlor and heptachlor epoxide: 0.008 mg/kg was found after exposure to a concentration of 0.06 µg/l water. Residues of heptachlor plus heptachlor epoxide were found at 0.001-0.026 mg/kg (on a fibre basis) and < 0.01-0.8 (on a tissue basis) (Hannon *et al.*, 1970). The average concentration of heptachlor and heptachlor epoxide in oysters in the USA was < 0.01 mg/kg (Bugg *et al.*, 1967).

In a German study reported by WHO (1984b), heptachlor and heptachlor epoxide residues were determined in cheese, butter, pasteurized milk and human milk. The average total residue in milk and milk products was less than 0.05 mg/kg, but the levels in human milk were about 10 times higher, with heptachlor at 0.1 mg/kg and heptachlor epoxide at 0.34 mg/kg in milk fat.

1.3.5 Other

The occurrence of chlordane and heptachlor and their metabolites in human tissues and biological fluids is reviewed in section 4.1.1.

Members of families living on dairy farms who consumed milk and milk products contaminated with heptachlor were compared with a group of unexposed people. The cows' milk contained levels of heptachlor epoxide ranging up to 89.2 ppm (mg/l; lipid basis). After 33 farms in Arkansas and five in Missouri and Oklahoma had been placed in quarantine, the level of heptachlor epoxide in milk was 12.6 ppm (mg/l; lipid basis). Heptachlor epoxide and oxychlordane were detected in the serum of 23.1% of the exposed persons and trans-nonachlor in 30.8%, versus 3.7, 4.0 and 6.5%, respectively, in the control group. The mean levels (0.81, 0.70 and 0.79 µg/l) of heptachlor epoxide, oxychlordane and trans-nonachlor were significantly different from those found in the control group (Stehr-Green et al., 1986).

1.4 Regulations and guidelines

The FAO/WHO Joint Meeting on Pesticide Residues evaluated chlordane at its meetings in 1965, 1967, 1969, 1970, 1972, 1974, 1977, 1982, 1984 and 1986 (FAO/WHO, 1965, 1968, 1970, 1971, 1973, 1975, 1978, 1983, 1985, 1987). In 1970, it re-established residue tolerances for food at 0.02-0.5 mg/kg for the sum of cis- and trans-isomers of chlordane and oxychlordane. In 1986, an acceptable daily intake in food of 0.0005 mg/kg bw was established (FAO/WHO, 1987).

The FAO/WHO Joint Meeting on Pesticide Residues evaluated heptachlor at its meetings in 1965, 1966, 1967, 1968, 1969, 1970, 1974, 1975, 1977 and 1987 (FAO/WHO, 1965, 1967, 1968, 1969, 1970, 1971, 1975, 1976, 1978, 1988). In 1970, an acceptable daily intake in food of 0.0005 mg/kg bw was established (Codex Committee on Pesticide Residues, 1990).

European Community legislation prohibits the marketing and use of plant protection products containing chlordane. The use of chlordane in agriculture is prohibited in several countries, including those of the Community, Argentina, Chile, Ecuador, Japan, Singapore, Switzerland, Sweden, the USA and Yugoslavia (WHO, 1988a) as well as Finland and the USSR. The use of chlordane is restricted in Cyprus and Venezuela. It must be registered for import, export or manufacture in India (WHO, 1988a). In Canada, since 1985, the registration of chlordane limits it to use as a restricted class termiticide. Chlordane has not been used in Norway since 1968.

European Community legislation prohibits the marketing and use of plant protection products containing heptachlor. The use of heptachlor in agriculture is prohibited in several countries, including those of the Community, Argentina, Cyprus, Ecuador, Singapore, the USA (with some exceptions, e.g., fire ants; US Environmental Protection Agency, 1987b) and Yugoslavia. Chile and Venezuela restricted its use in agriculture; its use is permitted in agriculture but prohibited in domestic sanitation in Brazil (WHO, 1988b). It has never been registered for use in Norway. The only accepted uses of heptachlor in Finland are as a termiticide in particle-board and in the plywood industry (for exported materials) and as a laboratory chemical. The registration of heptachlor in Canada was discontinued in 1985.

Maximum residue levels have been established by the Codex Alimentarius Commission for chlordane (sum of *cis*- and *trans*-chlordane or, in the case of animal products, sum of *cis*- and *trans*-chlordane and 'oxychlordane' (fat-soluble residue)) in or on the following commodities (in mg/kg): 0.05 for cottonseed oil (crude), linseed oil (crude), meat (fat), poultry meat (fat), soya bean oil (crude); and 0.02 for almonds, cottonseed oil (edible), eggs, fruit, hazelnuts, maize, oats, pecans, rice (polished), rye, sorghum, soya bean oil (refined), vegetables, walnuts, wheat (Codex Committee on Pesticide Residues, 1990).

Maximum residue limits have been established by the Codex Alimentarius Commission for heptachlor (sum of heptachlor and heptachlor epoxide (fat-soluble residue)) in or on the following commodities (in mg/kg): 0.5 for soya bean oil (crude); 0.2 for carrots, meat (fat), poultry meat (fat); 0.05 for eggs, vegetables (except carrots, soya beans, sugar beets and tomatoes); 0.02 for cereal grains, cottonseed, soya beans (immature seeds), soya bean oil (refined), tomatoes; 0.01 for citrus fruit, pineapples; and 0.006 for milk (Codex Committee on Pesticide Residues, 1990).

WHO (1988c) recommended guideline limit values of 0.3 μg/l for chlordane (total of isomers) and 0.1 μg/l for heptachlor and heptachlor epoxide in drinking-water. In Mexico, maximum permissible concentrations of chlordane in ambient water are 0.002 mg/l for coastal and estuarine waters and 0.003 mg/l for water treated for drinking; those of heptachlor in ambient water are 0.2 μg/l for coastal waters, 0.002 mg/l for estuarine waters and 0.018 mg/l for water treated for drinking (WHO, 1988a,b). The US Environmental Protection Agency has established a National Ambient Water Quality Criterion for heptachlor of 0.28 μg/l (Agency for Toxic Substances and Disease Registry, 1989a).

Chlordane and heptachlor epoxide were included in the 1987 Canadian guidelines for drinking-water quality for re-evaluation; the maximum acceptable concentrations in 1978 were 0.007 mg/l and 0.003 mg/l, respectively. Heptachlor was also included in the 1987 Canadian guidelines for drinking-water quality, with an interim maximum acceptable concentration of 0.28 mg/l (Ritter & Wood, 1989).

Treatment of root crops and soil with heptachlor is prohibited in the USSR, and it cannot be applied in water-catchment areas with a large number of open water reservoirs. The maximum allowable concentration of heptachlor in water used for drinking and domestic water supplies is 0.05 mg/l; that in the atmosphere of populated areas is 0.001 mg/m^3 for a maximum single concentration and 0.0002 mg/m^3 for a daily average concentration (Izmerov, 1982).

National and regional pesticide residue limits for chlordane, heptachlor and heptachlor epoxide in foods are presented in Tables 4 and 5. Tables 6 and 7 present occupational exposure limits and guidelines for chlordane and heptachlor in several countries. Because of potentially continuous household exposure, the Committee on Toxicology of the US National Academy of Sciences (1979) recommended a maximum acceptable level of 5 μg/m^3 chlordane in residences.

Table 4. National and regional pesticide residue limits for chlordane in foods[a]

Country or region	Residue limits (mg/kg)	Commodities
Australia	0.2	Mammalian meat (fat basis)
	0.1	Sugar beets
	0.05	Cottonseed oil (crude), cucurbits, fish, linseed oil (crude), milk (fat basis), milk products (fat basis), soya bean oil (crude)
	0.02	Cereal grains, citrus, cottonseed oil (edible), eggs, fruit (pome, stone), pineapples, soya bean oil (edible), vegetables (except cucurbits)
Austria	0.05[b]	Meat, animal fats (edible), milk
	0.02	Eggs (without shell)
Belgium	0.05[c]	Meat, poultry, hare, fowl, game, meat products, animal fats
	0.005	Eggs
	0.002	Milk and milk products
	0 (0.05)[d,e]	All foodstuffs of vegetable origin
	0 (0.02)[c,e]	All other foodstuffs of animal origin
Canada	0.1[f]	Butter, cheese, milk and other dairy products, meat and meat by-products (cattle, goats, hogs, poultry sheep)
Chile	0.5[d]	Soya bean oil (unrefined)
	0.3[d]	Potatoes, sugar beets
	0.2[d]	Lettuce
	0.05[c,d]	Maize, milk and dairy products (fat basis), carcasses (fat basis), poultry (fat basis), rice (polished), wheat
	0.02	Citrus fruit, eggs, tomatoes
Czechoslovakia	0.3[d]	Sugar beets
	0.2[d]	Pineapples
	0.1[c,d]	All spices, cereals (raw), maize (roasted, sweet), cucumbers, egg-plant, green peppers, leaf vegetables, pumpkin, squash, tomatoes, watermelons
Denmark	0.05[c]	Fat from meat
	0.02[c,d]	Berries and small fruit, carrots, cereals, eggs, fruit (citrus, pome, stone, other), other root vegetables and onions
	0.01[d]	Potatoes
	0.002[c]	Milk, milk products and dairy products
European Community	0.05[g]	Fat contained in meat, preparations of meat, offal and animal fats
	0.02[g]	Barley, buckwheat, grain sorghum, maize, millet, oats, paddy rice, rye, triticale, wheat, other cereals
	0.002[g]	Raw cows' milk and whole-cream cows' milk
Finland	0.1[h]	Fish, crustaceans, shellfish and their products
France	0.05[g]	Fruit, vegetables
	0.02	Cereal grains
Germany	0.2	Tobacco products
	0.05[i]	Meat, meat products, edible animal fats, milk, dairy products (all on fat basis), spices, tea, tea-like products
	0.02[i]	Cereals, eggs (without shell), egg products
	0.01[i]	Other foodstuffs of animal and plant origin
Hungary	0.02	Imported products

Table 4 (contd)

Country or region	Residue limits (mg/kg)	Commodities
India	0.3[d]	Sugar beets
	0.2[d]	Vegetables
	0.1[d]	Fruit
	0.05[d]	Foodgrains, milk and milk products (fat basis)
Israel	0.5	Linseed oil (crude), soya bean oil (crude)
	0.3	Potatoes, radishes, sugar beets, sweet potatoes, turnips
	0.2	Asparagus, broccoli, Brussels' sprouts, cabbage, cauliflower, celery, lettuce, mustard greens, spinach
	0.1	Almonds, bananas, cottonseed oil (crude), cucumbers, figs, filberts, guavas, mangoes, melons, olives, papayas, passion fruit, peanuts, pecans, pineapples, pomegranates, pumpkins, squash, strawberries, walnuts, watermelons
	0.05	Carcass meat (fat basis), maize, milk and milk products (fat basis), oats, poultry (fat basis), rice (polished), rye, wheat, sorghum
	0.02	Beans, cottonseed oil (edible), eggplant, eggs (without shell), fruit (citrus, pome, stone), peas, peppers, pimentos, soya bean oil (edible), tomatoes, other foodstuffs
Italy	0.2[j]	Tobacco (dried)
	0.05[j]	Aromatic and medicinal herbs, teas
	0.02[j]	Coffee
Kenya	0.5	Linseed oil (crude), soya bean oil (crude)
	0.3	Parsnips, potatoes, radishes, rutabagas, sugar beets, sweet potatoes, turnips
	0.2	Asparagus, broccoli, Brussels' sprouts, cabbage, cauliflower, celery, lettuce, mustard greens, spinach, Swiss chard
	0.1	Almonds, bananas, cantaloupes, cottonseed oil (crude), cucumbers, figs, filberts, guavas, mangoes, olives, papayas, passion fruit, pecans, pineapples, pomegranates, pumpkin, squash, strawberries, walnuts, watermelons
	0.05	Milk and milk products (fat basis), meat and poultry (fat basis), sorghum
	0.02	Beans, collards, cottonseed oil (edible), eggplant, eggs (without shell), fruit (citrus, pome, stone), maize, oats, peas, popcorn, rice (polished), rye, soya bean oil (edible), tomatoes, wheat
Luxembourg	0.05[k]	Animal fats (except butyric fats), meat and meat products (fat basis), milk and milk products (fat basis), poultry and poultry products (fat basis)
	0.02[k]	Eggs (without shell)
Netherlands	0.1[g]	Cucumbers, melons, pineapples
	0.05[g]	Potatoes, other dairy products (fat basis)
	0.02[g]	Other fruit, other vegetables, pulses, plant oil
	0.002[g]	Milk
	0 (0.02)[l]	Other plant products
Romania	0.05	Meat, milk and milk products
Spain	0.05[g]	Spices, tea and similar products
	0.02[g]	Cereal grains
	0.01[g]	Other plant products

Table 4 (contd)

Country or region	Residue limits (mg/kg)	Commodities
Sweden	0.1[d]	Fruits, vegetables
	0.02	Cereals, hulled grain, flakes and flour made from cereals
	0.01	Potatoes
United Kingdom	0.05[c,d]	Meat, fat and preparations of meats (fat basis), dairy produce (> 2% fat)
	0.02	Apples, bananas, barley, blackcurrants, beans, Brussels' sprouts, cabbage, carrots, celery, cauliflower, cucumbers, eggs (birds' eggs in shell (other than eggs for hatching) and whole egg products and egg yolk products (whether fresh, dried or otherwise prepared)), grapes, leeks, lettuce, maize, mushrooms, nectarines, oats, onions, oranges, paddy rice, peaches, pears, peas, plums, potatoes, raspberries, rye, strawberries, swedes, tomatoes, turnips, wheat, other cereals, other citrus
	0.002	Milk (fresh raw cows' milk and fresh whole cream cows' milk expressed as whole milk)
USA	0.3[m]	Animal fat (rendered), fish (edible portion)
	0.1[m]	Animal feed (processed), asparagus, bananas, beans, beetroot (with or without tops), beetroot greens, berries (except cranberries, currants, elderberries, gooseberries, and olallie berries), *Brassica* (cole) leafy vegetables (except broccoli raab, Chinese mustard cabbage, and rape greens), carrots, celery, citrus fruit, maize, cucumbers, eggplant, lettuce, melons, okra, onions, papayas, parsnips, peanuts, peas, peppers, pineapples, pome fruit (except crabapples and loquats), potatoes, radishes (with or without tops), radish tops, rutabagas (with or without tops), rutabaga tops, small fruit, spinach, squash, stone fruit (except chickasaw, damson and Japanese plums), sweet potatoes, Swiss chard, tomatoes, turnips (with or without tops), turnip greens
Yugoslavia	0.05	Meat and meat products (fat basis), vegetables
	0.02	Fruit, grain

[a]From Health and Welfare Canada (1990); US Food and Drug Administration (1990)
[b]Chlordane and oxychlordane (total calculated as chlordane)
[c]Sum of *cis*- and *trans*-chlordane and oxychlordane (usually for animal products)
[d]Sum of *cis*- and *trans*-chlordane (usually for plant products)
[e]Residues should not be present; the value in parentheses indicates the lower limit for residue determination according to the standard method of analysis, this limit having being used to reach the no-residue conclusion.
[f]Calculated on the fat content; including the metabolite oxychlordane
[g]Sum of *cis*- and *trans*-isomers and oxychlordane expressed as chlordane
[h]Sum of *cis*- and *trans*-chlordane, oxychlordane and *trans*-nonachlor
[i]Chlordane and oxychlordane (calculated as chlordane) for animal products; chlordane for plant products
[j]Includes isomers and/or metabolites; active substance revoked
[k]Singly or combined, including oxychlordane, expressed as chlordane
[l]Residues shall be absent, while the value in parentheses is the highest concentration at which this requirement is still deemed to have been met.
[m]Recommended action levels

Table 5. National and regional pesticide residue limits for heptachlor in foods[a]

Country or region	Residue limits (mg/kg)	Commodities
Argentina	0[b]	Cereals, fruit, garden vegetables, oilseeds
Australia	0.5[c]	Soya bean oil (crude)
	0.2[c]	Carrots, meat fat
	0.15[c]	Milk and milk products (fat basis)
	0.05[c]	Eggs, fish, vegetables (except carrots, tomatoes)
	0.02[c]	Cereal grains, cottonseed, soya bean oil (edible), soya beans, sugar-cane, tomatoes
	0.01[c]	Citrus fruit, pineapples
Austria	0.01[c]	All foodstuffs of animal origin
Belgium	0.2[c]	Meat, poultry, hare, fowl, game, meat products, animal fats
	0.1	Herbal teas, spices and dried herbs, teas
	0.02[c]	Eggs
	0.01	Grains
	0.004[c]	Milk and milk products
	0 (0.01)[d]	Other foodstuffs of animal and vegetable origin
Brazil	0.2	Carrots, tomatoes
	0.01	Milk and milk products (fat basis)
	0.05	Eggs (without shell), vegetables
	0.02	Maize, meat (fat basis), rice
	0.01	Bananas, sugar-cane
Canada	0.2[e]	Meat, meat by-products, fat (cattle, goats, hog, poultry, sheep)
	0.1[e]	Butter, cheese, milk, other dairy products
Chile	0.2[c]	Carcasses (fat), carrots, poultry (fat)
	0.15	Milk and milk products (fat)
	0.05	Eggs, garden vegetables, sugar beets
	0.02	Cereals (raw), tomatoes
	0.01	Citrus fruit
Czechoslovakia	0.5[c]	Soya bean oil (crude)
	0.2[c]	Meat (fat basis)
	0.15[c]	Milk and milk products (fat basis)
	0.05[c]	Eggs (egg white, yolk, without shell), vegetables
	0.02[c]	Cereals (raw), cottonseed, soya bean oil (edible), soya beans, tomatoes
	0.01[c]	Citrus fruit, pineapples
Denmark	0.2[c]	Meat fat
	0.05	Carrots, eggs
	0.01	Cereals, onions, potatoes, other vegetables
	0.004	Milk, milk products, dairy products
European Community	0.2[c]	Meat fat, preparations of meat, offal and animal fats
	0.01	Barley, buckwheat, grain sorghum, maize, millet, oats, paddy rice, rye, triticale, wheat, other cereals
	0.004	Raw cows' milk, whole-cream cows' milk

Table 5 (contd)

Country or region	Residue limits (mg/kg)	Commodities
Finland	0.1^c	Fish, crustaceans, shellfish and their products
	0.05^c	Other crops and foodstuffs
France	0.01^c	Cereal grains, fruit, vegetables
Germany	0.2^c	Meat, meat products, edible animal fats (all on fat basis), tobacco products
	0.1^c	Milk, dairy products, spices, tea, tea-like products
	0.05^c	Eggs (without shell), egg products
	0.01^c	Other foodstuffs of animal and plant origin
Hungary	0.05^f	Brussels' sprouts, beetroot, cabbage, carrots, cauliflower, celery, celery leaf, celery leaf (dried), garlic, horseradish, kohlrabi, lettuce, onion (red), parsley, parsley root, radishes, savoy, sorrel, spinach
	0.02^f	Grains (barley, oats, rye, wheat), maize, rice (brown, polished), sorghum, soya bean oil, soya beans, tomatoes, triticale
	0.01^f	Lemons, oranges, pineapples
India	0.15^c	Milk and milk products (fat basis)
	0.05	Vegetables
	0.01	Food grains
	0.002	Milled food grains
Ireland	0.2^c	Carrots
	0.05	Other vegetables
	0.02	Tomatoes
	0.01	Other food products
Israel	0.5	Soya bean oil (crude)
	0.2	Carcass meat (cattle, goats, pigs, poultry, sheep) (fat basis), carrots
	0.15	Milk and milk products (fat basis)
	0.05	Eggs (without shell), sugar beets, vegetables (except where otherwise specified)
	0.02	Cottonseed, raw cereals (barley, corn, oats, rice, wheat), soya bean oil (edible), soya beans, tomatoes
	0.01	Citrus fruit, pineapples
Italy	0.01^c	Fruit, garden vegetables
Kenya	0.5	Soya bean oil (crude)
	0.2	Carrots, fat or meat and poultry
	0.15	Milk and milk products (fat basis)
	0.05	Eggs (without shell), vegetables (except where otherwise specified)
	0.02	Cereals (raw), cottonseed, soya bean oil (edible), soya beans, tomatoes
	0.01	Citrus fruit

Table 5 (contd)

Country or region	Residue limits (mg/kg)	Commodities
Luxembourg	0.2^g	Meat and meat products (fat basis), poultry and poultry products (fat basis), animal fats (except butyric fats)
	0.15^g	Milk and milk products (fat basis)
	0.05^g	Eggs (without shell), nursing foods used in feeds
	0.03^g	Other foods used in feeds
	0.02^g	Natural foods used in feeds (except animal fats)
Netherlands	0.5^c	Eggs (fat basis)
	0.2^c	Game and fowl, meat, poultry meat (all on fat basis)
	0.1^c	Tea
	0.05^c	Potatoes, other vegetables
	0.02^c	Cottonseed, soya beans, tomatoes, plant oil and fat
	0.01^h	Citrus fruit, pineapples
	0.004^c	Milk
	0 (0.01)^i	Other crops or foodstuffs
Peru	0.5	Soya bean oil (raw)
	0.2	Carrots, meat (fat basis), poultry (fat basis)
	0.15	Milk and milk products (fat basis)
	0.05	Eggs (without shell)
	0.02	Cereals (raw), cottonseed, soya bean oil (edible), soya beans, tomatoes
	0.01	Beets, citrus fruit, pineapples
Romania	0.20	Meat
	0.10	Milk and milk products
	0.05	Eggs (without shell)
Spain	0.10^c	Spices, tea and similar products
	0.01^c	Other plant products
Sweden	0.1^c	Butter, cheese
	0.05^c	Eggs, fruit, vegetables
	0.02^c	Meat raw material
	0.01^c	Cereal and hulled grain, flakes and flour made from cereals, potatoes
	0.005	Milk
Switzerland	0.2^c	Meat and meat products (except fish and fish based products) (fat basis)
	0.125^c	Milk and milk products (fat basis)
	0.05^c	Cocoa butter and bulk cocoa (fat basis)
	0.02^c	Cereals
	0.01^c	Eggs, vegetables
	0.002^c	Cereal products, infant and baby foods (expressed as food as consumed: milk products and other products [limit value: 0.006 mg/kg]

Table 5 (contd)

Country or region	Residue limits (mg/kg)	Commodities
Thailand	0.3^c	Aquatic animal products, meat, milk
	0.1^c	Vegetables
	0.05^c	Eggs, fruit, pulses
	0.03^c	Cereals
	0.02^c	Fat and oil from animals and vegetables
United Kingdom	0.2^c	Carrots, meat, fat and preparations of meats (fat basis)
	0.1^c	Dairy produce (> 2% fat)
	0.05^c	Beans, Brussels' sprouts, cabbage, cauliflower, celery, cucumbers,
	0.02^c	eggs (birds' eggs in shell (other than eggs for hatching) and whole
	0.01^c	egg products and egg yolk products (whether fresh, dried, or otherwise prepared)), leeks, lettuce, mushrooms, onions, peas, potatoes, swedes, turnips
	0.02^c	Tomatoes
	0.01^c	Apples, bananas, barley, blackcurrants, grapes, maize, nectarines, oats, oranges, paddy rice, peaches, pears, plums, raspberries, rye, strawberries, wheat, other cereals, other citrus
	0.004	Milk (fresh raw cows' milk and fresh whole-cream cows' milk expressed as whole milk)
USA	0.3^j	Fish and shellfish
	$0.2^{c,j}$ (fat basis)	Cattle, goats, horses, sheep, swine, poultry, rabbits
	$0.1^{c,j}$ (fat basis)	Milk
	$0.02^{c,j}$	Fat, meat and meat by-products, cucurbit vegetables, quinces, cucumbers, melons, pumpkins, squash (winter or summer), pineapple
	$0.01^{c,j}$	Artichokes, asparagus, *Brassica* (cole) leafy vegetables, bulb vegetables, cereal grains, citrus fruits, leafy vegetables (except *Brassica*), non-grass animal feeds, pome fruits, small fruits and berries, stone fruits, processed animal feed, eggs, figs, fruiting vegetables except cucurbits, grass forage, fodder and hay, legume vegetables, root and tuber vegetables, beans (except snap beans), eggplant, okra, pimentoes, leafy vegetables, salsify tops, pears, rice grain, small fruits, blackberries, blueberries, boysenberries, dewberries, peppers, raspberries, tomatoes, alfalfa, apples, barley, lima beans, snap beans, beetroot, sugar beets, blackeyed peas, Brussels' sprouts, cabbage, carrots, cauliflower, cherries, clover, sweet clover, cottonseed, cowpeas, grapes, grass (pasture), grass (range), kohlrabi, lettuce, maize, oats, onions, peaches, peanuts, peas, potatoes, radishes, rutabagas, rye, sorghum (grain milo), sugar-cane, sweet potatoes, tomatoes, turnips (including tops)

Table 5 (contd)

Country or region	Residue limits (mg/kg)	Commodities
USSR	None	All food products
Yugoslavia	0.1[c]	Meat and meat products (fat basis)
	0.05[c]	Eggs (without shell) and egg products, milk and milk products (fat basis)

[a]From Health and Welfare Canada (1990)

[b]Residue below the sensitivity limit of the test method; calculated as heptachlor and its epoxide

[c]Including heptachlor epoxide

[d]Residues should not be present; the value in parentheses indicates the lower limit for residue determination according to the standard method of analysis, this limit having being used to reach the no-residue conclusion

[e]Calculated on fat content; including heptachlor epoxide

[f]Heptachlor epoxide only

[g]Singly or combined, including heptachlor epoxide, expressed as heptachlor

[h]A pesticide may be used on an eating or drinking ware or raw material without a demonstrable residue remaining behind; the value listed is considered the highest concentration at which this requirement is deemed to have been met.

[i]Residues shall be absent; the value in parentheses is the highest concentration at which this requirement is still deemed to have been met.

[j]Recommended action levels, tolerances revoked (US Food and Drug Administration, 1990)

Table 6. Occupational exposure limits for chlordane[a]

Country	Year	Concentration (mg/m³)	Interpretation[b]
Austria	1987	0.5	TWA
Belgium	1987	0.5 (s)[c]	TWA
Denmark	1988	0.5 (s)	TWA
Germany	1989	0.5 (s)	TWA
India	1987	0.5 (s)	TWA
		2 (s)	STEL
Indonesia	1987	0.5	TWA
Italy	1985	0.5 (s)	TWA
Mexico	1987	0.5 (s)	TWA
Netherlands	1987	0.5 (s)	TWA
Romania	1975	0.3	Average
		0.6	Maximum
Switzerland	1987		TWA
United Kingdom	1987	0.5 (s)	TWA
		2 (s)	STEL (10 min)
USA			
ACGIH	1989	0.5 (s)	TWA
OSHA	1989	0.5 (s)	TWA
USSR	1987	0.01 (s)	MAC

Table 6 (contd)

Country	Year	Concentration (mg/m³)	Interpretation[b]
Venezuela	1987	0.5	TWA
		2	Ceiling
Yugoslavia	1987	0.5	TWA

[a]From Cook (1987); Arbejdstilsynet (1988); American Conference of Governmental Industrial Hygienists (ACGIH) (1989); Deutsche Forschungsgemeinschaft (1989); US Occupational Safety and Health Administration (1989)
[b]MAC, maximum allowable concentration; TWA, time-weighted average; STEL, short-term exposure level
[c]Skin irritant notation

Table 7. Occupational exposure limits for heptachlor[a]

Country	Year	Concentration (mg/m³)	Interpretation[b]
Austria	1987	0.5 (s)[c]	TWA
Belgium	1987	0.5 (s)	TWA
Bulgaria	1984	0.1 (s)	TWA
Denmark	1988	0.5 (s)	TWA
Germany	1989	0.5 (s)	TWA
Finland	1987	0.5 (s)	TWA
		1.5 (s)	STEL
Indonesia	1987	0.5 (s)	TWA
Mexico	1987	0.5 (s)	TWA
Netherlands	1987	0.5 (s)	TWA
Romania	1985	0.3	Average
		0.6	Maximum
Switzerland	1987	0.5 (s)	TWA
UK	1987	0.5 (s)	TWA
		2 (s)	STEL (10 mn)
USA			
ACGIH	1989	0.5 (s)	TWA
OSHA	1989	0.5 (s)	TWA
USSR	1987	0.01 (s)	MAC
Venezuela	1987	0.5 (s)	TWA
		1.5 (s)	Ceiling
Yugoslavia	1987	0.5	TWA

[a]From Cook (1987); Arbejdstilsynet (1988); American Conference of Governmental Industrial Hygienists (ACGIH) (1989); Deutsche Forschungsgemeinschaft (1989); US Occupational Safety and Health Administration (OSHA) (1989)
[b]MAC, maximum allowable concentration; TWA, time-weighted average; STEL, short-term exposure level
[c]Skin irritant notation

2. Studies of Cancer in Humans

2.1 Case reports

Infante *et al.* (1978) reported five cases of neuroblastoma in children, which were associated with pre- and postnatal exposure to chlordane for termite control, as well as three cases of aplastic anaemia and three of acute leukaemia associated with exposure to chlordane or heptachlor. Three of the patients with blood dyscrasia had also been exposed to other pesticides.

Four cases of leukaemia were among 25 cases of blood dyscrasia associated with exposure to chlordane/heptachlor (Epstein & Ozonoff, 1987) (see also Table 19).

A two-month-old neonate with a gliosarcoma was reported to have been exposed to heptachlor during prenatal development through contamination 'at unacceptable levels' of milk drunk by her mother (Chadduck *et al.*, 1987). [Details of the contamination were not given.]

2.2 Cohort studies

Three studies analysed the mortality experience of workers at two US plants—one producing chlordane and the other producing heptachlor (Ditraglia *et al.*, 1981). Exposures to other chemicals, including chlorine and dicyclopentadiene (chlordane plant) as well as endrin, chlorine, chlorendic anhydride, hexachlorocyclopentadiene and vinyl chloride (heptachlor plant) were also reported. As the bases of these studies overlap substantially, they do not provide independent information on the carcinogenicity of chlordane/-heptachlor. Table 8 shows the population enrolled in each study and the results obtained with regard to mortality from lung cancer.

Wang and MacMahon (1979a) evaluated the mortality experience of white male workers employed for three months or more at the two plants between 1946 or 1952 and 1976. The identities of 1403 of the 1685 men were established (83%); 104 deaths were determined through social security records and nine from other sources. The chlordane plant had been the place of employment for 570 of the identified men and 76 of the deaths. Expected deaths were calculated on the basis of national rates. There were 24 observed cancer deaths, with 29.3 expected (standardized mortality ratio [SMR], 0.82; 95% confidence interval [CI], 0.54-1.2). An excess of lung cancer was observed (12 observed, 9.0 expected; SMR, 1.3; 95% CI, 0.73-2.3). Seven lung cancers were observed (6.1 expected) in the chlordane plant and five (2.9 expected) in the heptachlor/endrin plant. Risks did not increase with duration of employment at the plants, but SMRs were higher for men aged < 35 years at entry (7 observed, 2.6 expected) and aged > 35 years at death (5 observed, 6.3 expected).

Another investigation included white men employed for at least six months between 1946 or 1951 and 1964, who were followed up to 1976. In the first plant, there were 327 workers, nine (3%) of whom were lost to follow-up; in the second there were 305 men, with 16 (5%) lost to follow-up. Expected deaths were calculated according to US white male mortality rates. There were 11 (SMR, 0.69; 95% CI, 0.35-1.2) and six (0.91; 0.33-2.0) cancer deaths, respectively. Mortality from respiratory cancers was slightly elevated in each plant:

Table 8. Cohort studies on white male workers in US plants producing chlordane and heptachlor

Reference	Plant	Enrolled population	Criteria for inclusion (months of employment)	Years of recruitment	Years of follow-up	Observed no. of lung cancer deaths	SMR	95% confidence interval
Wang & MacMahon (1979a)	Chlordane	570[a]	3	1946-76	1946-76	7	1.2	0.46-2.4
	Heptachlor	835[a]	3	1952-76	1952-76	5	1.7	0.57-4.1
Ditraglia et al. (1981)	Chlordane	327	6	1946-64	1946-76	6	1.1	0.40-2.4
	Heptachlor	305	6	1951-64	1951-76	3	1.2	0.25-3.6
Shindell & Ulrich (1986); Shindell (1987)	Chlordane	706[b]	3	1946-85	1946-85	12	0.86	0.4-1.5

[a]Two people employed in both plants

[b]87 women and 7 nonwhite men were also studied but not included in the calculation

six cases (1.1; 0.40-2.4) and three cases (1.2; 0.25-3.6), respectively. Mortality from stomach cancer was elevated (three deaths; 3.0; 0.61-8.9) among workers in the chlordane plant (Ditraglia *et al.*, 1981).

An analysis of the mortality of workers of each sex and all races who were employed for at least three months between 1946 and 1985 in the factory producing chlordane was carried out by Shindell and Ulrich (1986). Mortality was followed up to mid-1985. This study included 706 white men (of whom three were untraced) and 94 others (7 blacks and 87 women; all traced); the results given here are for white men only. Expected numbers were based on US mortality rates. There were 37 cancer deaths (40.6 expected; SMR, 0.91 [95% CI, 0.6-1.3]). The SMR for lung cancer was 0.86. The observed and expected numbers of deaths are not given, but 12 deaths from respiratory cancer are indicated in a figure giving the numbers of lung cancer deaths by years of employment; however, denominators were not provided. This lapse was pointed out in a letter by Infante and Freeman (1987). In a reply, Shindell (1987) reported 12 respiratory cancer deaths and 14.4 expected [SMR, 0.8; 0.4-1.5] and 25 other cancer deaths with 26.2 expected [1.0; 95% CI, 0.6-1.4]. No trend with duration of employment was seen for respiratory cancer.

Cancer risks have also been evaluated among cohorts of pesticide applicators engaged in termite control, in which chlordane has been the chemical most widely used until recently. Subjects may also have had contact with other pesticides.

The study of Wang and MacMahon (1979b) of the mortality experience of a cohort of over 16 000 urban applicators, described in detail in the monograph on occupational exposures in spraying and application of insecticides (p. 60), was extended (MacMahon *et al.*, 1988), to give a maximal period of follow-up of 18 years. A significant excess of lung cancer (SMR, 1.4; 90% CI, 1.1-1.6) was observed, along with nonsignificant excesses for cancers of the skin (1.3; 0.65-2.2) and bladder (1.2; 0.50-2.5). The risk for lung cancer was lower among termite control operators (0.97 [0.7-1.3]), the group who probably had more contact with chlordane, than among other employees (1.6; 1.3-1.9). Risks for cancers of the skin and bladder were about the same for the two groups. The risk for lung cancer did not rise with increasing duration of employment.

In another investigation of commercial applicators, also described in the monograph on occupational exposures (p. 62), an overall excess of lung cancer (SMR, 1.4 [95% CI, 0.9-1.9]) occurred among licensed pesticide applicators in Florida (Blair *et al.*, 1983). The risk for lung cancer death rose to nearly three fold among those licensed for 20 years or more: the SMRs were 1.0 [95% CI, 0.6-1.7] for < 10 years, 1.6 [0.8-2.8] for 10-19 years and 2.9 [1.2-5.6] for > 20 years. Excesses, based on small numbers of deaths, were also seen for leukaemia [1.3; 0.4-3.4] and for cancers of the skin [1.3; 0.2-4.8], bladder [1.6; 0.3-4.6] and brain (2.0 [0.6-4.7]). People working for firms certified for treatment of termites had an SMR of 1.4 [0.9-2.1] for lung cancer; other pest control workers had an SMR of 1.2 [0.6-2.2].

[Although none of these cohort investigations had access to information on tobacco use, smoking is probably not the explanation for the positive results because there was no excess mortality from emphysema or nonmalignant respiratory disease and because smoking is unlikely to explain the trend with duration of employment in the study of Florida applicators.]

2.3 Case-control studies

Two population-based case-control interview studies in the USA—one of soft-tissue sarcomas and non-Hodgkin's lymphoma and one of leukaemia—provide estimates of the risks for cancer associated with exposure to chlordane/heptachlor. Both are described in detail in the monograph on occupational exposures in spraying and application of insecticides (pp. 67 and 68).

An excess of non-Hodgkin's lymphoma (odds ratio, 1.6; 95% CI, 0.7-3.8) but no excess of soft-tissue sarcoma (0.96; 0.2-4.8) was associated with possible exposure to chlordane in the study from Washington State (Woods *et al.*, 1987). Adjustment for selected chemical exposures by regression analysis did not change the risk estimates substantially. In an additional report from Washington State in which the analysis was restricted to farmers (Woods & Polissar, 1989), the odds ratio for non-Hodgkin's lymphoma in relation to exposure to chlordane was 1.6 (0.5-5.1).

In the study of leukaemia in Iowa and Minnesota (Brown *et al.*, 1990), farmers who reported use of chlordane on crops had a slight deficit (odds ratio, 0.7; 95% CI, 0.3-1.6), while those who reported use of chlordane on animals had a slight excess (1.3; 0.7-2.3). Among farmers using chlordane on animals, the risks rose inconsistently with frequency of use, from an odds ratio of 1.1 (0.4-2.8) for < 5 days per year, to no exposed case and five exposed controls for 5-9 days per year, to an odds ratio of 3.2 (0.9-11.0) for > 10 days per year. This risk estimate was not adjusted for other agricultural exposures.

Cohort and case-control studies on chlordane and heptachlor are summarized in Table 9 (see also Table 8).

Table 9. Studies of populations exposed to chlordane/heptachlor

Reference and design	Cancer	No. of cases	Relative risk	95% CI	Comments
MacMahon *et al.* (1988) Cohort	*Entire cohort of applicators*				Pesticide applicators; chlordane use for termites a component; 90% CI
	Lung	108	1.4	1.1-1.6	
	Skin	9	1.3	0.65-2.2	
	Bladder	5	1.2	0.50-2.5	
	Lymphatic and haematopoietic	25	1.0	0.67-1.4	
	Termite control operators only				90% CI
	Lung	30	0.97	[0.7-1.3]	
	Skin	3	1.2	[0.4-2.9]	
	Bladder	2	1.3	[0.3-3.9]	
Blair *et al.* (1983) Cohort	Lung	34	1.4	[0.9-1.9]	Pesticide applicators; chlordane use for termites a component; lung cancer risk among employees of firms licensed to treat termites was 1.4
	Skin	2	[1.3]	[0.2-4.8]	
	Bladder	3	[1.6]	[0.3-4.6]	
	Brain	5	2.0	[0.6-4.7]	
	Leukaemia	4	[1.3]	[0.3-3.4]	
Woods *et al.* (1987) Case-control	Soft-tissue sarcoma	Not reported	0.96	0.2-4.8	Author indicates that 1.6% of study population was possibly exposed to chlordane
	Non-Hodgkin's lymphoma	Not reported	1.6	0.7-3.8	

Table 9 (contd)

Reference and design	Cancer	No. of cases	Relative risk	95% CI	Comments
Woods & Polissar (1989) Case-control	Non-Hodgkin's lymphoma	Not reported	1.6	0.5-5.1	Farmers only
Brown et al. (1990) Case-control	Leukaemia Leukaemia	7 19	0.7 1.3	0.3-1.6 0.7-2.3	Used on plants Used on animals

3. Studies of Cancer in Experimental Animals

The carcinogenicity of chlordane and heptachlor/heptachlor epoxide in experimental animals has been reviewed (US Environmental Protection Agency, 1986a).

Selected histopathological materials from several of the carcinogenicity studies on chlordane/heptachlor and/or heptachlor epoxide which were reviewed in a previous monograph (IARC, 1979) were re-evaluated by a panel of pathologists (Pesticide Information Review and Evaluation Committee) convened by the US National Academy of Sciences (1977) at the request of the US Environmental Protection Agency. The intent was to provide uniform diagnosis of hepatocellular neoplasms which had been diagnosed under several different classification systems for liver neoplasia by the original investigators or, in some cases, a second review panel of pathologists. The review panel diagnosed hepatocellular tumour and hepatocellular carcinoma and nodule change or nodule according to the definitions given in Annex 1 to this monograph (p. 177).

3.1 Oral administration

3.1.1 *Mouse*

Epstein (1976) and the US Environmental Protection Agency (1986a) reported a previously unpublished study by the Food and Drug Administration, carried out in 1965, in which three groups of 100 male and 100 female C3H mice [age unspecified] were fed 0 or 10 mg/kg of diet *heptachlor* or *heptachlor epoxide* [purity unspecified] for 24 months. A review of the histopathology of liver samples from this study by the panel of the US National Academy of Sciences (1977) indicated a significant increase in the incidence of hepatocellular carcinomas in females but not in males given heptachlor, and in both males and females given heptachlor epoxide (Table 10).

In an unpublished study conducted by the International Research and Development Corporation in 1973 and reported by Epstein (1976), groups of 100 male and 100 female Charles River CD-1 mice, seven weeks of age, were fed *a mixture of 75% heptachlor epoxide and 25% heptachlor* [purity unspecified] at levels of 0, 1, 5 or 10 mg/kg of diet for 18 months. Excluding 10 animals sacrificed from each group for interim study at six months, mortality at 18 months was 34-49%, with the exception of males and females receiving the 10 mg/kg diet level, which had mortalities of approximately 70%; in addition, comparatively large numbers

Table 10. Tumour incidence in C3H mice treated with heptachlor and heptachlor epoxide[a]

Treatment	Males		Females	
	Hepatocellular carcinomas	Hepatocellular carcinomas and nodules	Hepatocellular carcinomas	Hepatocellular carcinomas and nodules
Controls	29/77	48/77	5/53	11/53
Heptachlor (10 mg/kg diet)	35/85	72/85 ($p = 0.001$)	18/80 ($p = 0.04$)	61/80 ($p < 0.001$)
Heptachlor epoxide (10 mg/kg diet)	42/78 ($p = 0.031$)	71/78 ($p < 0.001$)	34/83 ($p < 0.001$)	75/83 ($p < 0.001$)

[a]From National Academy of Sciences (1977)

of animals from all groups were lost to histology by autolysis. A review of the histopathology of liver samples from this study by the panel of the US National Academy of Sciences (1977) indicated a significant increase in the combined incidence of hepatocellular carcinomas and nodules in the high-dose groups (Table 11).

Table 11. Tumour incidence in CD-1 mice treated with a mixture of heptachlor and heptachlor epoxide[a]

Concentration (mg/kg diet)	Males		Females	
	Hepatocellular carcinomas	Hepatocellular carcinomas and nodules	Hepatocellular carcinomas	Hepatocellular carcinomas and nodules
Controls	1/59	2/59	1/74	1/74
1	1/58	1/58	0/71	0/71
5	2/66	4/66	1/65	3/65
10	1/73	27/73 ($p < 0.001$)	4/52	16/52 ($p < 0.001$)

[a]From National Academy of Sciences (1977)

In an unpublished study conducted by the International Research and Development Corporation in 1973 and reported by Epstein (1976), groups of 100 male and 100 female Charles River CD-1 mice, six weeks of age, were fed 0, 5, 25 or 50 mg/kg of diet *technical-grade chlordane* [purity unspecified] for 18 months. Excluding 10 animals sacrificed from each group for interim study at six months, mortality at 18 months was 27-49%, with the exception of males and females receiving the 50 mg/kg diet level, in which mortalities of 86 and 76%, respectively, were seen; in addition, a relatively large number of animals were lost by autolysis. A review of of the histopathology of liver samples from this study by the panel of the US National Academy of Sciences (1977) indicated a significant increase in the incidence of hepatocellular carcinomas in mid-dose males and in mid-dose and high-dose females (Table 12).

Table 12. Tumour incidence in CD-1 mice treated with chlordane[a]

Concentration (mg/kg diet)	Males		Females	
	Hepatocellular carcinomas	Hepatocellular carcinomas and nodules	Hepatocellular carcinomas	Hepatocellular carcinomas and nodules
Control	1/33	4/33	0/44	1/44
5	1/55	11/55	0/61	0/61
25	11/51 ($p = 0.015$)	30/51 ($p < 0.001$)	11/51 ($p < 0.001$)	23/51 ($p < 0.001$)
50	7/44	25/44 ($p < 0.001$)	6/40 (($p = 0.009$)	22/40 ($p < 0.001$)

[a]From National Academy of Sciences (1977)

Groups of 50 male and 50 female B6C3F$_1$ hybrid mice, five weeks of age, were fed *analytical-grade chlordane* (consisting of 94.8% chlordane (71.7% *cis*-chlordane and 23.1% *trans*-chlordane), 0.3% heptachlor, 0.6% nonachlor, 1.1% hexachlorocyclopentadiene, 0.25% chlordene isomers and other chlorinated compounds) for 80 weeks. Males received initial levels of 20 and 40 mg/kg of diet and females 40 and 80 mg/kg of diet; time-weighted average dietary concentrations were 30 and 56 mg/kg of diet for males and 30 and 64 mg/kg of diet for females. There were 20 male and 20 female matched controls and 100 male and 80 female pooled controls. Survivors were killed at 90 weeks. Survival in all groups was relatively high: over 60% in treated males, over 80% in treated females and over 90% in male and female controls (US National Cancer Institute, 1977a). A review of the histopathology of liver samples from this study by the panel of the US National Academy of Sciences (1977) indicated a significant increase in the incidence of hepatocellular carcinomas by linear trend analysis in males and females given diets containing chlordane, and a significant increase in the combined incidence of hepatocellular carcinomas and 'nodular changes' in high-dose males and females (Table 13).

Table 13. Tumour incidence in B6C3F$_1$ mice treated with chlordane or heptachlor[a]

Treatment	Males		Females	
	Hepatocellular carcinomas	Hepatocellular carcinomas and nodules	Hepatocellular carcinomas	Hepatocellular carcinomas and nodules
Controls	2/20	5/20	1/19	1/19
Chlordane (low)	4/45	16/45	0/46	2/46
Chlordane (high)	12/46 ($p = 0.031$) (trend)	30/46 ($p = 0.003$)	7/47 ($p = 0.018$) (trend)	20/47 ($p = 0.002$)
Controls	2/19	5/19	0/10	1/10
Heptachlor (low)	3/45	14/45	0/44	3/44
Heptachlor (high)	2/45	24/45 ($p = 0.042$)	2/42	21/42 (($p = 0.022$)

[a]From National Academy of Sciences (1977)

Groups of 50 male and 50 female $B6C3F_1$ hybrid mice, five weeks of age, were fed *technical-grade heptachlor* (72% heptachlor, 18% *trans*-chlordane, 2% *cis*-chlordane, 2% nonachlor, 1% chlordene, 0.2% hexachlorobutadiene) in the diet for 80 weeks. Males received initial dietary concentrations of 10 and 20 mg/kg of diet and time-weighted average concentrations of 6 and 14 mg/kg of diet; females received initial concentrations of 20 and 40 mg/kg of diet and time-weighted average concentrations of 9 and 18 mg/kg of diet. Initial dose levels were reduced during the experiment due to adverse toxic effects. Matched controls consisted of 20 males and 20 females; and pooled controls consisted of 100 males and 80 females. Survival in all groups was relatively high: over 70% of treated and control males and 60% of treated and control females were still alive at 90 weeks. Survival of female mice showed a significant trend to lower survival in treated groups compared to that of controls (US National Cancer Institute, 1977b). A review of the histopathology of liver samples from this study by the panel of the US National Academy of Sciences (1977) indicated a significant increase in the combined incidence of hepatocellular carcinomas and 'nodular changes' ($p < 0.05$) in males and females receiving the high dose (Table 13).

Groups of 80 male and 80 female Charles River (ICR) (SPF) mice, five weeks of age, were fed diets containing 0, 1, 5 or 12.5 mg/kg of diet *'technical chlordane'* (containing unspecified amounts of *cis*- and *trans*-chlordane, isomers of chlordene, heptachlor and nonachlor) for 104 weeks. Eight males and eight females from each group were killed for evaluation at 52 weeks. Survival of treated groups did not differ from that of controls: at 104 weeks, males: 28 controls, 21 low-dose, 32 mid-dose and 29 high-dose; females: 30 controls, 35 low-dose, 38 mid-dose and 37 high-dose. The incidence of hepatocellular adenomas was significantly increased in male mice receiving the high dose (control, 12/79; low-dose, 14/79; mid-dose, 14/80; high-dose, 27/80; $p < 0.01$). The number of high-dose male mice with haemangiomas of the liver was also significantly increased (control, 4/79; low-dose, 1/79; mid-dose, 8/80; high-dose, 14/80; $p < 0.05$) [The authors described haemangiomas as 'benign tumors of vascular cells associated with the liver adenomas'.] (Khasawinah & Grutsch, 1989a). [The Working Group noted that hepatocellular adenocarcinomas were apparently also diagnosed in all groups of treated and control male mice, but the incidences of these tumours were not reported specifically. The combined incidences of hepatocellular adenomas and adenocarcinomas in male mice could not be determined from the report, and the incidences of hepatocellular neoplasms were not given for female mice.]

3.1.2 Rat

Epstein (1976) reported on an unpublished study, carried out in 1955, in which groups of 20 male and 20 female CF rats, 10 weeks of age, were administered 0, 1.5, 3, 5, 7 or 10 mg/kg of diet *heptachlor* [purity unspecified] by spraying alcoholic solutions onto Purina Chow pellets, for 110 weeks. Mortality in all test groups was stated to be random. No increase in the incidence of liver tumours was found in treated animals. [The Working Group noted the small number of animals and the uncertain concentrations of heptachlor in the feed.]

Epstein (1976) reported on another unpublished study by the same laboratory, carried out in 1959, in which groups of 25 male and 25 female CFN rats, seven weeks of age, were fed 0.5, 2.5, 5.0, 7.5 or 10.0 mg/kg of diet *heptachlor epoxide* [purity unspecified] by spraying alcoholic solutions on Purina Chow pellets, for 108 weeks. Survival at that time was over 45%

in treated and control groups. A review of the histopathology of liver samples from this study by the panel of the US National Academy of Sciences (1977) found no increase in the incidence of liver tumours in treated animals. [The Working Group noted the small number of animals and the uncertain concentrations of heptachlor epoxide in the feed.]

A group of 95 male and female suckling Wistar rats were administered 10 mg/kg bw *heptachlor* (97% pure) in corn oil by gavage on five successive occasions at two-day intervals starting at 10 days of age; 19 male and 27 female controls received corn oil alone. Excluding nine male and 20 female treated animals that were sacrificed for interim histology at 60 weeks, survival in treated and control groups was high and comparable. The numbers of tumours in treated and control groups were comparable; 'lipomatous' renal tumours were noted in two females treated with heptachlor (Cabral *et al.*, 1972). [The Working Group noted the small number of doses administered and the short duration of treatment.]

Groups of 50 male and 50 female Osborne-Mendel rats, five weeks of age, were administered *analytical-grade chlordane* (see p. 142) in the diet for 80 weeks at initial dose levels of 400 and 800 mg/kg of diet for males and 200 and 400 mg/kg of diet for females. These were reduced during the experiment due to adverse toxic effects, and the time-weighted average dietary concentrations were 204 and 407 mg/kg of diet for males and 121 and 242 mg/kg of diet for females. There were 10 male and 10 female matched controls and 60 male and 60 female pooled controls. Survivors were killed at 109 weeks, at which time approximately 50% of treated and control males and 60% of treated females and 90% of control females were still alive. In treated females, there was an increase in the incidence of follicular-cell thyroid neoplasms (6/32 high-dose, $p < 0.05$; 4/43 low-dose, 3/58 pooled controls; $p = 0.03$, trend test). There was also an increase in the incidence of malignant fibrous histiocytomas [site unspecified] in treated males: 7/44 in high-dose animals ($p < 0.05$), 1/44 in low-dose animals and 2/58 in pooled controls (US National Cancer Institute, 1977a). [The Working Group noted the short duration of treatment.]

Groups of 50 male and 50 female Osborne-Mendel rats, five weeks of age, were fed *technical-grade heptachlor* (see p. 143) in the diet for 80 weeks. Males received initial dietary concentrations of 80 and 160 mg/kg of diet and time-weighted average concentrations of 39 and 78 mg/kg of diet; females received initial concentrations of 40 and 80 mg/kg of diet and time-weighted average concentrations of 26 and 51 mg/kg of diet. Matched controls consisted of 10 males and 10 females; and pooled controls consisted of 60 males and 60 females. At 110 weeks, 60-75% of all treated and control groups were still alive. Thyroid follicular-cell neoplasms occurred in 14/38 high-dose females and 3/58 controls ($p < 0.01$) and in 9/38 low-dose males and 4/51 controls ($p < 0.05$); the incidence in high-dose males was 3/38 (US National Cancer Institute, 1977b). [The Working Group noted the short duration of treatment.]

Groups of 80 male and 80 female Fischer 344 (SPF) rats, five weeks of age, were fed diets containing 0, 1, 5 or 25 mg/kg of diet *technical-grade chlordane* (containing unspecified amounts of *cis*- and *trans*-chlordane, isomers of chlordene, heptachlor and nonachlor) for 130 weeks. Eight males and nine females in each group were killed for evaluation at 26 and 52 weeks. Survival at 130 weeks was: males—13 controls, 20 low-dose, 11 mid-dose and nine high-dose; females—23 controls, 24 low-dose, 28 mid-dose and 24 high-dose. Survival in all groups was greater than 65% at 104 weeks. The incidence of hepatocellular nodules as diagnosed by the original pathologist was increased in treated male rats, with an incidence of 1/80 controls, 2/80 low-dose, 3/80 mid-dose and 9/80 high-dose males, the latter being significantly different from that in controls ($p < 0.05$). A group of seven other pathologists re-evaluated selected liver sections and observed increased incidences of hepatocellular adenomas: in 2/64 controls, 4/64 low-dose, 2/64 mid-dose and 7/64 high-dose males ($p = 0.018$ trend test) (Khasawinah & Grutsch, 1989b).

3.2 Administration with known carcinogens

Chlordane (25 and 50 mg/kg diet) or heptachlor (5 and 10 mg/kg diet) was fed in the diet for 25 weeks at concentrations of 5-50 mg/kg to groups of 40 male B6C3F$_1$ mice previously treated with N-nitrosodiethylamine at 20 mg/l in drinking-water for 14 weeks. An increase in the incidence and multiplicity of liver adenomas and carcinomas was seen over that observed in untreated mice or mice receiving treatment with N-nitrosodiethylamine only (Williams & Numoto, 1984).

4. Other Relevant Data

The toxicology of chlordane and heptachlor has been reviewed (FAO/WHO, 1964, 1965, 1967, 1968, 1971, 1978, 1983; WHO, 1984a,b; FAO/WHO, 1987; US Public Health Service, 1989a,b).

4.1 Absorption, distribution, metabolism and excretion

4.1.1 *Humans*

The main components of technical-grade chlordane—chlordane, heptachlor and *trans*-nonachlor—have all been identified in human tissues following a variety of exposures, indicating that all are absorbed (see Tables 14-16). *trans*- and *cis*-Chlordane are metabolized to oxychlordane, and heptachlor is metabolized to heptachlor epoxide; a minor component of technical-grade chlordane, *trans*-nonachlor, has been found in human plasma and milk as a major residue of technical-grade chlordane. Being lipophilic, these compounds are stored mainly in the adipose tissue. Elimination takes place *via* both urine (Curley & Garrettson, 1969) and faeces (Garrettson *et al.*, 1985). Breast milk is a supplementary excretory route in lactating women (WHO, 1984a,b).

A positive relationship was found in pest control operators between blood levels of total chlordane (*trans*-nonachlor, oxychlordane and heptachlor epoxide) and the conditions of spraying technical-grade chlordane: total amount of chlordane sprayed ($r = 0.68$), number of spraying days in the last year ($r = 0.78$) and particularly in the last three months ($r = 0.81$). Blood levels are reported in Table 14 (Saito *et al.*, 1986).

Levels of chlordane residue determined after accidental ingestion of chlordane preparations are summarized in Table 15.

Table 14. Compounds derived from technical-grade chlordane in the blood of 51 pest control operators[a]

Compound	Positive samples (%)	Level (μg/l)	
		Mean	Range
Total chlordane	37	0.89	ND-5.6
Oxychlordane	22	0.29	ND-1.5
Heptachlor epoxide	20	0.29	ND-1.6
trans-Nonachlor	37	0.55	ND-2.9

[a]From Saito *et al.* (1986)

Table 15. Total chlordane levels in human tissue after accidental ingestion of technical-grade chlordane

Time after event	Chlordane (μg/g)			Estimated half–time (days)	Reference
	Adipose tissue	Serum	Tissues: serum		
> 3 h	3.12	2.71	[1.15:1]	21	Curley & Garrettson (1969)
8 days	–	–	147:1		
3 months	25.53	0.017	1470:1		
First day	–	3.4	–	88	Aldrich & Holmes (1969)
3 days	–	0.138	–		
130 days	–	0.03	–		
Third day	–	[0.103]	–	–	Olanoff *et al.* (1983)
After 49 days	–	0.039	–		
After 58 days			–		
oxychlordane	0.51				
trans-nonachlor	1.88				
heptachlor epoxide	2.62				

–, not reported

Heptachlor epoxide was the first among the materials derived from technical chlordane to be analysed routinely in human adipose tissue. Residues in humans originate from the use of technical-grade chlordane in agriculture and households. Studies on the storage of heptachlor epoxide and oxychlordane in the adipose tissue of the general population in different countries are summarized in Table 16. *trans*-Nonachlor has also been identified in the adipose tissue of people representative of the general population of the USA (Sovocool & Lewis, 1975).

The presence of heptachlor epoxide in the adipose tissue of stillborns (Wassermann *et al.*, 1974) and in the blood of newborns (cord blood) (D'Ercole *et al.*, 1976) demonstrates placental transfer of heptachlor and/or heptachlor epoxide.

Table 16. Storage of heptachlor epoxide and oxychlordane in the adipose tissue of the general population

Country	No. of samples	Heptachlor epoxide (µg/g)		Oxychlordane (µg/g)		Reference
		Mean	Range	Mean	Range	
USA	25	0.24	0.03–1.45			Hayes et al. (1965)
Italy	18	0.46	0.01–1.50			Paccagnella et al. (1967)
United Kingdom	248	0.04	0.0–0.40			Abbott et al. (1968)
Netherlands	11	0.01	0.004–0.03			de Vlieger et al. (1968)
USA	64	0.10[a]	0.03–0.61			Zavon et al. (1969)
France	98	0.28	[ND – ~ 1.6 men];			Fournier et al. (1972)
		0.36	([ND – ~ 0.65 women)			
United Kingdom	201	0.03	0.0–0.14			Abbott et al. (1972)
Japan	241	0.02	< 0.01–0.2			Curley et al. (1973)
USA	27			0.14	0.03–0.40	Biros & Enos (1973)
				77.8% positive		
Israel	53[b]	0.015	0.0001–0.132			Wassermann et al. (1974)

[a]On lipid basis
[b]Results cited for age group 25-44 years; total number of samples, 307; age range, stillborn—≥ 70 years

Components of technical-grade chlordane and their metabolites are excreted in human milk in quantities that vary with agricultural and household use, dietary habits, individual phenotype and time of milk sampling. In Israel, the mean levels of heptachlor epoxide in the milk of 29 women 2-4 days after delivery were 9.1 µg/litre in whole milk and 720 µg/kg fat. The values were 9.8 µg/litre in women aged 20-29 and 7.2 µg/litre in those aged 30-39 (Polishuk et al., 1977). [The number of positive samples was not given, and the means are presumed to be for all samples tested.] The levels of heptachlor epoxide in the breast milk in 50 women in Switzerland were < 10-110 µg/kg fat with a mean value of 30 µg/kg fat (Schuepbach & Egli, 1979). A total of 1436 samples of breast milk were analysed in a study in the USA; the mean level of oxychlordane was 96 µg/kg fat in 1061 positive samples, and the mean level of heptachlor epoxide was 91 µg/kg fat in 906 positive samples. In a subset of 288 samples from southeastern USA, oxychlordane was found at 116 µg/kg fat in 239 samples and heptachlor epoxide at 128 µg/kg fat in 221 samples (Savage et al., 1981). In 29 positive samples analysed in Japan, cis-chlordane was found at geometric mean levels of 3.08 µg/kg fat and 0.09 µg/litre whole milk; trans-chlordane at 1.20 µg/kg fat and 0.04 µg/litre whole milk; oxychlordane at 11.5 µg/kg fat and 0.39 µg/litre whole milk; heptachlor epoxide at 20 µg/kg fat and 0.66 µg/litre whole milk; trans-nonachlor at 15.7 µg/kg fat and 0.55 µg/litre whole milk; and cis-nonachlor at 4.0 µg/kg fat and 0.14 µg/litre whole milk (Tojo et al., 1986). Analysis of samples from 155 primipara mothers in Finland in 1984-85 showed fat contents of 410 µg/kg total chlordane (cis- and trans-chlordane, oxychlordane and trans-nonachlor) (20 positive samples), 100 µg/kg cis-chlordane (8), 200 µg/kg trans-chlordane (9), 70 µg/kg heptachlor (16), 230 µg/kg oxychlordane (6), 100 µg/kg heptachlor epoxide (9) and 760 µg/kg trans-nonachlor (7) (Mussalo-Rauhamaa et al., 1988). In women who followed a strict vegetarian diet, the mean levels of heptachlor epoxide in milk were 1-2% of the average for the US general population (Hergenrather et al., 1981). In a Japanese study, the level of total chlordane in milk was higher in eight women with a high frequency of fish intake than in four with a low frequency of intake (2.53 ng/ml versus 1.25 ng/ml) (Tojo et al., 1986). Curley and Kimbrough (1969) found traces of heptachlor epoxide in milk during lactation. A downward trend in level with progression of the lactation period was reported by Mes et al. (1984) for oxychlordane and trans-nonachlor and by Klein et al. (1986) for heptachlor epoxide.

4.1.2 Experimental systems

The metabolism of chlordane (WHO, 1984a; Nomeir & Hajjar, 1987) and of heptachlor (WHO, 1984b; Fendick et al., 1990) has been reviewed.

Chlordane is readily absorbed from the gastrointestinal tract in rats and mice (Barnett & Dorough, 1974; Tashiro & Matsumura, 1977; Ewing et al., 1985), from the skin of rats (Ambrose et al., 1953) and from the respiratory system in rats (Nye & Dorough, 1976).

Heptachlor is readily absorbed via most routes of exposure and is readily metabolized to heptachlor epoxide by mammals (US Public Health Service, 1989a; Fendick et al., 1990). Heptachlor epoxide is stored mainly in fat but also in liver, kidney and muscle in rats and dogs. In rats fed 30 mg/kg diet heptachlor for 12 weeks, maximal heptachlor epoxide concentrations occurred in fat within two to four weeks; 12 weeks after cessation of exposure, heptachlor epoxide had completely disappeared from the adipose tissue (Radomski &

Davidow, 1953). Heptachlor is also stored in fat as heptachlor epoxide in steers (Bovard *et al.*, 1971) and laying hens (Kan & Tuinstra, 1976). Heptachlor epoxide and a hydrophilic metabolite, 1-*exo*-hydroxy-2,3-epoxychlordene, were excreted in the faeces and urine of rats and rabbits treated with heptachlor (Klein *et al.*, 1968). Another metabolite, a dehydrogenated derivative of 1-hydroxy-2,3-epoxychlordene, has been isolated from rat faeces (Matsumura & Nelson, 1971).

Following uptake of chlordane after oral administration to rats, it was rapidly distributed, with the highest levels in fat and lower levels in other organs in the following order: liver, kidney, brain and muscle. Treatment with *trans*-chlordane resulted in slightly higher tissue concentrations than that with *cis*-chlordane. Patterns of distribution were similar following single and repeated oral dosing (Barnett & Dorough, 1974).

The major route of metabolism of chlordane in treated animals is *via* oxychlordane. Heptachlor is a minor metabolite of both optical isomers of chlordane. *cis*- and *trans*-Chlordane give rise qualitatively to the same metabolites (Tashiro & Matsumura, 1977). Four metabolic pathways for the metabolism of chlordane have been proposed (Nomeir & Hajjar 1987, Fig. 1):

(i)   hydroxylation to form 3-hydroxychlordane followed by dehydration to form the postulated precursor of oxychlordane, 1,2-dichlorochlordene;

(ii)   dehydrochlorination to form heptachlor with the subsequent formation of heptachlor epoxide and various hydroxylation products;

(iii)   dechlorination to monochlorodihydrochlordene;

(iv)   replacement of chlorine atoms by hydroxyl groups with the formation of mono-, di- and trihydroxy metabolites that are excreted or conjugated with glucuronic acid.

Human liver preparations have little capability to convert *trans*-nonachlor (a minor component of technical-grade chlordane) to *trans*-chlordane in comparison to rat liver prepared similarly (Tashiro & Matsumura, 1978).

Phenobarbital pretreatment significantly enhanced the metabolism of heptachlor in rats, causing a 6- to 11-fold increase in the formation of heptachlor epoxide in liver (Miranda *et al.*, 1973). In liver microsomes from rats and humans, heptachlor epoxide constituted 85.8% of the metabolized heptachlor in rats but only 20.4% in the human liver microsome system. Other metabolites identified in the human liver microsome system were 1-hydroxy-2,3-epoxychlordene (5%), 1-hydroxychlordene (4.8%) and 1,2-dihydroxydi-hydrochlordene (0.1%); 68.6% was unmetabolized heptachlor (Tashiro & Matsumura, 1978).

Rats and mice eliminated 80–$\geq$ 90% of single oral doses of ^{14}C-labelled chlordane within seven days (Barnett & Dorough, 1974; Tashiro & Matsumura, 1977; Ewing *et al.*, 1985). Most of the radiolabel was eliminated in faeces. C57Bl/6JX mice showed two distinct excretory patterns: the vast majority were high excretors, their elimination rate during the first day after dosing being 20 times faster than that of the low excretors (Ewing *et al.*, 1985).

Mice were given repeated doses of technical-grade chlordane (containing 5.88% *trans*- and 1.45% *cis*-nonachlor) in olive oil by gavage at 0.48 mg/mouse every other day for 29 days. No increase in body burden of *trans*- or *cis*-chlordane was noted; rather, the levels decreased continuously, indicating that chlordane induced its own metabolism. The levels of *trans*- and

Fig. 1. Metabolic pathways of chlordane (from Nomeir & Hajjar, 1987)

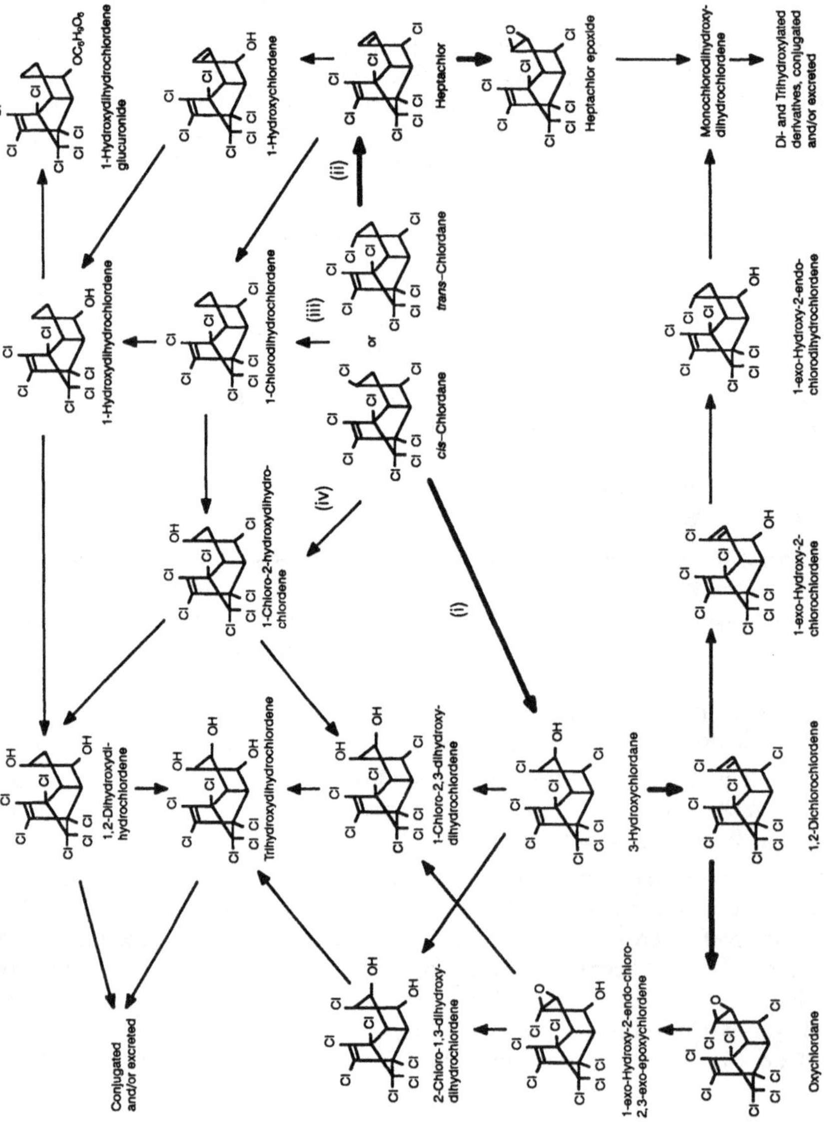

cis-nonachlor and of oxychlordane, however, increased throughout the study period (Hirasawa & Takizawa, 1989).

In cows fed hay containing heptachlor over 30 days, heptachlor epoxide was present in the milk from 10 days after the start of feeding (Huber & Bishop, 1961).

4.2 Toxic effects

4.2.1 *Humans*

Case reports and epidemiological studies of poisoning with technical-grade chlordane and heptachlor following both occupational exposures and exposure of the general population are summarized in Table 17.

4.2.2 *Experimental systems*

Chlordane

The toxic effects of chlordane have been reviewed (WHO, 1984a).

The acute oral LD_{50} of chlordane in peanut oil was 335 (299-375) mg/kg bw for male and 430 (391-473) for female Sherman rats (Gaines, 1960). The LD_{50} values for *cis*- and *trans*-chlordane were reported to be similar (392 and 327 mg/kg bw, respectively). The major metabolite, oxychlordane, was reported to have an LD_{50} in rats of 19.1 mg/kg bw, and several other metabolites had LD_{50} values > 4600 mg/kg bw. The signs associated with acute chlordane poisoning include ataxia, convulsions, respiratory failure and cyanosis, followed by death (WHO, 1984a).

Oral doses of chlordane of 50 mg/kg bw per day for 15 days resulted in convulsions and death in rats, whereas doses of 25 mg/kg bw per day had no such effect (Ambrose *et al.*, 1953).

In long-term studies (see section 3), chlordane caused tremor in female rats fed the high dose during one week, decreased body weight gains in high-dose animals and increased liver weights (US National Cancer Institute, 1977; Khasawinah & Grutsch, 1989b). In mice (Khasawinah & Grutsch, 1989a), the liver was the target organ for non-neoplastic toxicity; the serum levels of aspartate transferase and alanine transferase were elevated in animals of each sex, and liver weights were increased in males fed 12.5 mg/kg of diet. Increased liver-cell volume was seen in males and females fed 5 or 12.5 mg/kg, whereas hepatocyte degeneration and necrosis were seen only in treated males. Chlordane induced hepatic drug-metabolizing enzymes in experimental animals (WHO, 1984a) and enhanced oestrone metabolism in rats and mice (Welch *et al.*, 1971).

Mice treated with chlordane at doses of 0.1-8 mg/kg bw for 14 days showed a dose-related increase in cell-mediated immunity, as evaluated *in vitro*. Expression of delayed hypersensitivity and the antibody response to sheep red blood cells *in vivo* were unaltered (Johnson *et al.*, 1986).

Wistar rats and cynomolgus monkeys were exposed to chlordane by inhalation at concentrations close to 0.1, 1 and 10 mg/m^3 for 8 h per day on five days per week for 90 days (Khasawinah *et al.*, 1989). In rats, the liver was the main target organ, and liver weights were significantly increased in animals of each sex exposed to 10 mg/m^3. Histopathological changes, such as centrilobular hepatocyte enlargement, were observed in males and females at 1 and 10 mg/m^3. In male rats, increased weight of the follicular thyroid epithelium was

Table 17. Case reports, health surveys and epidemiological studies of cases of poisoning with technical-grade chlordane and technical-grade heptachlor

Population	Clinical features	Reference
34 workers manufacturing and formulating chlordane, aldrin, dieldrin	No evidence of adverse health effects	Princi & Spurbeck (1951)
24 workers employed for 2 months to 5 years in a plant manufacturing chlordane	No evidence of adverse health effects	Alvarez & Hyman (1953)
A female worker spilled a mixture of pesticides (including chlordane) on her clothing	Confusion, generalized convulsions, death; congestion of brain, lung and stomach mucosa	Derbes et al. (1955)
Suicide of a 32-year-old woman who ingested a 5% chlordane talc formulation; estimated ingested dose of chlordane: 6 g (104 mg/kg bw)	Vomiting, dry cough, agitation and restlessness, haemorrhagic gastritis, bronchopneumonia, muscle twitching, convulsions, death after 9.5 days	Derbes et al. (1955)
15 workers exposed for 1-15 years to chlordane during manufacture	No evidence of adverse health effects	Fishbein et al. (1964)
A 20-month-old boy drank an unknown quantity of a 74% technical-grade chlordane formulation	Vomiting 45 min after ingestion and seizures; serum alkaline phosphatase and thymal turbidity levels slightly elevated after 3 months	Curley & Garrettson (1969)
A 4-year-old girl ingested an unknown amount of 45% chlordane	Convulsions, increased excitability, loss of coordination, dyspnoea, tachycardia	Aldrich & Holmes (1969)
A segment of a municipal water system in Chattanooga, TN (USA), 1976, was contaminated with chlordane, initially up to 1200 mg/l; 1-3 days later, 0.0001-92.5 mg/l. Of 105 residents in affected houses, 71 reported contact with contaminated water	13/71 (18%) described mild symptoms compatible with chlordane exposure (gastrointestinal and/or neurological)	Harrington et al. (1978)
Case reports of blood dyscrasias associated with exposure to chlordane or heptachor alone or in combination with other agents	25 previously reported and 6 new cases include 22 aplastic anaemia, 3 acute leukaemia, 2 leukopenia and 1 each hypoplastic anaemia, haemolytic anaemia, megaloblastic anaemia and thrombocytopenia	Infante et al. (1978)
Workers employed for more than 3 months in the manufacture of chlordane and heptachlor, 1946-76 [study population overlaps with that of Shindell & Ulrich, 1986]	17 deaths from cerebrovascular disease observed versus 9.3 expected	Wang & MacMahon (1979a)

Table 17 (contd)

Population	Clinical features	Reference
Cohort of 16 126 men employed as pesticide applicators for 3 months or more in 1967, 1968 and 1976, including group of 6734 termite control operators	All deaths, 311 (SMR, 84); cerebrovascular disease among termite control operators (SMR, 39)	Wang & MacMahon (1979b)
A 62-year-old man accidentally ingested ~300 ml of 75% chlordane	Unresponsive to verbal commands, generalized tonic seizures, profuse diarrhoea, transient increase in liver enzymes; recovery by 2 months	Olanoff et al. (1983)
A 59-year-old man with a history of Alzheimer's disease inadvertently drank from a bottle containing a chlordane formulation	Rapid occurrence of convulsions, death, despite cardiopulmonary resuscitation and treatment	Kutz et al. (1983)
A 30-year-old woman exposed to chlordane through excessive household use	Numbness around mouth and nose and in arm used for spraying; nausea, vomiting, persistent fatigue and anorexia, menometrorrhagia; irregular theta discharges on EEG	Garrettson et al. (1985)
Workers employed in the manufacture of chlordane for 3 months or more, in 1946–85 [study population overlaps with that of Wang & MacMahon, 1979a]	20 deaths from cerebrovascular disease observed versus 11.7 expected	Shindell & Ulrich (1986)
45 members of dairy-farm families who consumed milk and milk products contaminated with heptachlor metabolites	No heptachlor-related metabolic effect observed in routine liver function tests or specific assays for hepatic enzyme induction	Stehr-Green et al. (1986)
25 case reports of blood dyscrasias associated with exposure to chlordane and heptachlor; of 16 cases for which exposure data available, 75% involved home and garden applications and 25% professional applicators	Aplastic anaemia, thrombocytopenic purpura, leukaemia, pernicious anaemia, megaloblastic anaemia	Epstein & Ozonoff (1987)
261 residents of 85 households treated with chlordane for termite control	Headache in 22% of cases; sore throat and respiratory infections in 16%; fatigue, 14%; sleeping difficulties, blurred vision and fainting also frequent	Menconi et al. (1988)

observed in 11/35 animals at 10 mg/m^3. A dose-related increased in cytochrome P450 concentration and microsomal protein was evident in each sex throughout the dose range studied. Essentially all of the observed changes were reversed within 90 days after cessation of exposure. No significant finding was noted in male or female monkeys exposed to up to 10 mg/m^3; however, cytochrome P450 and microsomal protein were not measured.

Chlordane at 200 μM stimulated protein kinase C *in vitro* in preparations from mouse brain, liver and epidermis. The stimulation was calcium- and phospholipid-dependent and could be inhibited by quercetin, a known inhibitor of protein kinase C activity (Moser & Smart, 1989).

Heptachlor

The toxic effects of heptachlor have been reviewed (WHO, 1984b; Fendick *et al.*, 1990).

The acute oral LD$_{50}$ of heptachlor in peanut oil was 100 (74-135) mg/kg bw for male and 162 (140-188) mg/kg bw for female Sherman rats (Gaines, 1960). The signs associated with acute heptachlor poisoning include hyperexcitability, tremors, convulsions and paralysis. Liver damage may occur as a late manifestation (WHO, 1984b).

Heptachlor epoxide has a higher acute toxicity than the parent compound, e.g., the oral LD$_{50}$ of the epoxide in rats was 62 mg/kg bw (Sperling & Ewinike, 1969), and the intravenous lethal doses for heptachlor and heptachlor epoxide in mice were 40 and 10 mg/kg bw, respectively (WHO, 1984b).

Daily oral doses of pure heptachlor at 50 and 100 mg/kg bw were lethal to rats after 10 days. In animals given 5 mg/kg bw, hyperreflexia, dyspnoea and convulsions occurred, and pathological changes were observed in the liver, kidney and spleen (Pelikan *et al.*, 1968).

As reported in a review, rats were fed heptachlor epoxide in the diet at concentrations varying from 5 to 300 mg/kg for two years. All animals given 80 mg/kg in the diet or more were reported to have died within 20 weeks, and all female rats given 40 mg/kg in the diet died within 54 weeks, whereas male mortality was unaffected. Liver weights were increased in males at dietary levels higher than 10 mg/kg and in females from 5 mg/kg upwards (WHO, 1984b). Dogs given 5 mg/kg bw heptachlor per day orally died within 21 days (Lehman, 1952).

Heptachlor induced hepatic drug-metabolizing enzymes (for review, see Fendick *et al.*, 1990) and enhanced oestrone metabolism in rats (Welch *et al.*, 1971). Dietary levels of 2 mg/kg heptachlor given for two weeks induced aniline hydroxylase and aminopyrine demethylase in rats (Den Tonkelaar & Van Esch, 1974). It inhibited oxidative phosphorylation in rat liver mitochondria (Nelson, 1975) and (at 200 μM) stimulated protein kinase C *in vitro* in preparations from mouse brain (Moser & Smart, 1989).

4.3 Reproductive and prenatal effects

4.3.1 Humans

An ecological study was done to compare the incidence rates of 37 congenital malformations in Hawaii and in the USA as a whole (Le Marchand *et al.*, 1986), following contamination of milk on Oahu Island by heptachlor. Milk contamination occurred between the autumn of 1980 and December 1982 and was traced to contaminated foliage of pineapple plants used as cattle feed. Data on birth defects were obtained from the Birth Defects

Monitoring Program, which covers 62-76% of all births in Hawaii. Temporal and geographical comparisons were made (Table 18). Increased incidence rates were reported on Oahu for cardiovascular malformations and hip dislocation: In 1978-80, the incidence rates for cardiovascular malformations were 63.2/10 000 births on Oahu Island and 24.9 on the other Hawaian islands; in 1981-83, these rates were 76.2 and 24.4, respectively. For hip dislocation, the only increase occurred in 1981-83: rates were 42.2/10 000 on Oahu and 22.4 on the other islands. All of the increased rates for Oahu were statistically significant ($p < 0.01$). The authors noted that the increase in cardiovascular malformations and hip dislocation began in 1978-80, which included only the first few months of contamination. [The Working Group noted that the incidence rates for hip dislocation were unstable.]

Table 18. Incidence rates per 10 000 births of cardiovascular malformations and hip dislocation on Oahu Island and on the other Hawaiian islands, 1970-83[a]

Defect	Oahu				Other islands			
	1970-74	1975-77	1978-80	1981-83	1970-74	1975-77	1978-80	1981-83
Cardiovascular malformations	38.3	33.6	63.2	76.2	21.3	23.4	24.9	24.4
Hip dislocation	12.6	8.8	29.3	42.2	9.9	30.8	31.1	22.4

[a]From Le Marchand et al. (1986)

4.3.2 Experimental systems

The reproductive effects of chlordane and heptachlor/heptachlor epoxide have been reviewed (WHO, 1984a,b; US Public Health Service, 1989a,b).

Smith et al. (1970) found little effect of heptachlor on the hatchability of hens' eggs treated at doses below 1.5 mg/egg.

Incubation of sea-urchin embryos at the two-cell stage in the presence of heptachlor at 0.02 mM/litre (~7 ppm) until controls had developed up to the pluteus stage resulted in impaired development of the fertilized eggs; no living embryo was formed. When embryos were incubated in sea-water containing heptachlor for only 2 h, no effect on embryonic development was observed. When heptachlor was added 15 min before fertilization and the eggs allowed to incubate in the medium for an additional 15 min, the effect of heptachlor on fertilization and development to the two-cell stage was delayed; 7% reached the two-cell stage (Bresch & Arendt, 1977).

Rats treated with 320 mg/kg [0.032%] chlordane in their diet had substantially impaired fertility and reduced survival of the offspring (Ambrose et al., 1953).

Pregnant CD-1 mice were treated with chlordane orally at a dose of 50 mg/kg bw on gestation days 8-12. Although 3/25 animals died, no effect was observed on number of live pups or pup weight on postnatal days 1 and 3 (Chernoff & Kavlock, 1983).

Spyker Cranmer et al. (1978) explored the effect of chlordane on endocrine function in mice. Mice were treated orally with 0.16 or 8.0 mg/kg bw from mating to parturition on day 22 of gestation. During the first week of life, 55% of offspring born to mothers receiving 8.0 mg/kg died. At 101 days of age, there was no difference in plasma or adrenal corticosterone levels or adrenal weight between control and treated female offspring; male offspring of dams treated at the lower dose, however, appeared to have increased levels of plasma corticosterone and increased adrenal weight.

In a continuation of this study, Cranmer *et al*. (1984) evaluated plasma corticosterone concentrations over the lifespan of mice treated prenatally throughout gestation with chlordane at 0.16 or 8.0 mg/kg bw per day. At 400 days, plasma corticosterone levels were increased among male mice treated at either level. There was no difference in the corticosterone levels at 800 days in the lower-dose group (no male offspring from the higher-dose group was available for sacrifice at 800 days). Among female mice, cortico-sterone levels were elevated only at 400 days among those treated at 0.16 mg/kg.

Spyker Cranmer *et al*. (1982) evaluated cell-mediated and humoral immune response in adult BALB/c mice treated *in utero* with chlordane at 0.16 or 8.0 mg/kg bw per day from mating throughout gestation. Cell-mediated immunity (measured by contact hyper-sensitivity) was decreased in a dose-dependent manner in offspring at 101 days; no difference in humoral immune response was seen between treated and control mice.

Menna *et al*. (1985) explored the effect of prenatal exposure to chlordane on response to influenza A virus infection. BALB/c mice were treated orally with chlordane at doses of 0.16, 2.0, 4.0 and 8.0 mg/kg from mating to day 19, and at 38 days of age the mice were inoculated with influenza type A/PR/8/34(HON1) at three different rates. Survival was enhanced following the challenge, and antiviral titres were higher in mice treated with chlordane *in utero* than in controls.

Cytotoxic T lymphocyte activity was unchanged in 100-day-old mice treated with chlordane *in utero*, but natural killer cell activity was increased, only in female offspring. By 200 days of age, natural killer cell activity had declined in treated male and female offspring (Blaylock *et al*., 1990). Prenatal treatment with chlordane also substantially decreased the number of granulocyte/macrophage and splenic colony forming units at both 100 and 200 days of age. The number of bone-marrow cells in these mice was unchanged at 100 days of age (Barnett *et al*., 1990).

4.4 Genetic and related effects (see Tables 19 and 20 and Appendices 1 and 2)

4.4.1 *Humans*

No data were available to the Working Group.

4.4.2 *Experimental systems*

Chlordane induced neither DNA damage nor point mutation in bacteria. It caused gene conversion in *Saccharomyces cerevisiae* and mutation in plants. In cultured mammalian cells, it did not induce unscheduled DNA synthesis but did induce gene mutations at the *tk* and Na^+/K^+ ATPase loci. It inhibited gap-junctional intercellular communication in cultured mammalian cells. In cultured human cells, conflicting results were obtained for unscheduled DNA synthesis; evidence was obtained for sister chromatid exchange induction but not for the induction of gene mutation. Sister chromatid exchange was induced in intestinal cells of *Umbra limi* (mud-minnow) *in vivo*. No dominant lethal effect was found in mice.

Heptachlor did not induce DNA damage or point mutation in bacteria or gene conversion in *Saccharomyces cerevisiae*. It induced mutation and chromosomal aberrations

Table 19. Genetic and related effects of chlordane

Test system	Result[a] Without exogenous metabolic system	Result[a] With exogenous metabolic system	Dose[b] LED/HID	Reference
ECB, Chromosome breakage, plasmid DNA *in vitro*	–	0	100.0000	Griffin & Hill (1978)
SAD, *Salmonella typhimurium* TA1538/1978, differential toxicity	–	0	2000.0000	Rashid & Mumma (1986)
BSD, *Bacillus subtilis rec* strains, differential toxicity	–	–	50.0000	Matsui et al. (1989)
ERD, *Escherichia coli* WP2, differential toxicity	–	0	2000.0000	Rashid & Mumma (1986)
ERD, *Escherichia coli* K12, differential toxicity	–	0	2000.0000	Rashid & Mumma (1986)
SA0, *Salmonella typhimurium* TA100, reverse mutation	0	–	2500.0000	Simmon et al. (1977)
SA0, *Salmonella typhimurium* TA100, reverse mutation	–	–	0.0000	Probst et al. (1981)
SA0, *Salmonella typhimurium* TA100, reverse mutation	–	–	0.0000	Gentile et al. (1982)
SA0, *Salmonella typhimurium* TA100, reverse mutation	–	–	500.0000	Mortelmans et al. (1986)
SA5, *Salmonella typhimurium* TA1535, reverse mutation	0	–	2500.0000	Simmon et al. (1977)
SA5, *Salmonella typhimurium* TA1535, reverse mutation	–	–	0.0000	Probst et al. (1981)
SA5, *Salmonella typhimurium* TA1535, reverse mutation	–	–	0.0000	Gentile et al. (1982)
SA5, *Salmonella typhimurium* TA1535, reverse mutation	–	–	500.0000	Mortelmans et al. (1986)
SA7, *Salmonella typhimurium* TA1537, reverse mutation	0	–	2500.0000	Simmon et al. (1977)
SA7, *Salmonella typhimurium* TA1537, reverse mutation	–	–	0.0000	Probst et al. (1981)
SA7, *Salmonella typhimurium* TA1537, reverse mutation	–	–	0.0000	Gentile et al. (1982)
SA7, *Salmonella typhimurium* TA1537, reverse mutation	–	–	500.0000	Mortelmans et al. (1986)
SA8, *Salmonella typhimurium* TA1538, reverse mutation	0	–	2500.0000	Simmon et al. (1977)
SA8, *Salmonella typhimurium* TA1538, reverse mutation	–	–	0.0000	Probst et al. (1981)
SA8, *Salmonella typhimurium* TA1538, reverse mutation	–	–	0.0000	Gentile et al. (1982)
SA9, *Salmonella typhimurium* TA98, reverse mutation	0	–	2500.0000	Simmon et al. (1977)
SA9, *Salmonella typhimurium* TA98, reverse mutation	–	–	0.0000	Probst et al. (1981)
SA9, *Salmonella typhimurium* TA98, reverse mutation	–	–	0.0000	Gentile et al. (1982)
SA9, *Salmonella typhimurium* TA98, reverse mutation	–	–	500.0000	Mortelmans et al. (1986)
SAS, *Salmonella typhimurium* G46, reverse mutation	–	–	0.0000	Probst et al. (1981)
SAS, *Salmonella typhimurium* C3076, reverse mutation	–	–	0.0000	Probst et al. (1981)
SAS, *Salmonella typhimurium* D3052, reverse mutation	–	–	0.0000	Probst et al. (1981)
EC2, *Escherichia coli* WP2, reverse mutation	–	–	0.0000	Probst et al. (1981)

Table 19 (contd)

Test system	Result[a] Without exogenous metabolic system	Result[a] With exogenous metabolic system	Dose[b] LED/HID	Reference
ECW, *Escherichia coli* WP2 *uvr*A−, reverse mutation	−	−	0.0000	Probst et al. (1981)
SCG, *Saccharomyces cerevisiae*, gene conversion	0	+	6.6000	Gentile et al. (1982)
PLM, *Zea mays*, forward mutation	+	0	0.0000	Gentile et al. (1982)
*, DNA synthesis inhibition, mouse lymphoma cells	−	0	4.0000	Brubaker et al. (1970)
URP, Unscheduled DNA synthesis, rat hepatocytes	−	0	4.0000	Maslansky & Williams (1981)
UIA, Unscheduled DNA synthesis, mouse hepatocytes	−	0	4.0000	Maslansky & Williams (1981)
UIA, Unscheduled DNA synthesis, hamster hepatocytes	−	0	4.0000	Maslansky & Williams (1981)
URP, Unscheduled DNA synthesis, mouse hepatocytes	−	0	41.0000	Probst et al. (1981)
G9O, Gene mutation, *V79* Chinese hamster cells, Na$^+$/K$^+$ ATPase locus	+	0	4.0000	Ahmed et al. (1977a)
G9H, Gene mutation, V79 Chinese hamster cells, *hprt* locus	−	0	1.6000	Tsushimoto et al. (1983)
G5T, Gene mutation, mouse lymphoma L5178Y cells, *tk* locus	+	0	25.0000	McGregor et al. (1988)
GIA, Gene mutation, rat liver epithelial cells, *hprt* locus	−	0	41.0000	Telang et al. (1982)
GIA, Gene mutation, *V79* Chinese hamster cells, diphtheria toxin resistance	−	0	1.6000	Tsushimoto et al. (1983)
SVA, Sister chromatid exchange, *Umbra limi* intestinal cells *in vivo*	+	0	0.0002	Vigfusson et al. (1983)
UHF, Unscheduled DNA synthesis, human fibroblasts	+	−	0.4000	Ahmed et al. (1977b)
UHT, Unscheduled DNA synthesis, HeLa cells	−	0	16.0000	Brandt et al. (1972)
GIH, Gene mutation, human fibroblasts	−	−	41.0000	Tong et al. (1981)
SHL, Sister chromatid exchanges, human lymphoid cells *in vitro*	+	+	41.0000	Sobti et al. (1983)
DLM, Dominant lethal test, mice	−	0	240.0000 × 1 i.p.	Epstein et al. (1972)
DLM, Dominant lethal test, mice	−	0	75.0000 × 5 p.o.	Epstein et al. (1972)
DLM, Dominant lethal test, mice	−	0	100.0000 × 1 i.p.	Arnold et al. (1977)
DLM, Dominant lethal test, mice	−	0	100.0000 × 1 p.o.	Arnold et al. (1977)
ICR, Inhibition of metabolic cooperation, rat liver epithelial cells	+	0	0.2000	Telang et al. (1982)

Table 19 (contd)

Test system	Result[a]		Dose[b] LED/HID	Reference
	Without exogenous metabolic system	With exogenous metabolic system		
ICR, Inhibition of metabolic cooperation in V79 cells	(+)	0	1.6000	Tsushimoto et al. (1983)
ICR, Inhibition of metabolic cooperation mouse hepatocytes	+	0	20.0000	Ruch et al. (1990)
ICR, Inhibition of metabolic cooperation rat hepatocytes	+	0	20.0000	Ruch et al. (1990)

*Not displayed on profile

[a] +, positive; (+), weakly positive; −, negative; 0, not tested; ?, inconclusive (variable response in several experiments within an adequate study)

[b] In-vitro tests, μg/ml; in-vivo tests, mg/kg bw

Table 20. Genetic and related effects of heptachlor

Test system	Result[a]		Dose[b] LED/HID	Reference
	Without exogenous metabolic system	With exogenous metabolic system		
ECB, Breakage of plasmid DNA in vitro	–	0	100.0000	Griffin & Hill (1978)
SAD, Salmonella typhimurium TA1538/1978, differential toxicity	–	0	2000.0000	Rashid & Mumma (1986)
ERD, Escherichia coli WP2, differential toxicity	–	0	2000.0000	Rashid & Mumma (1986)
BSD, Bacillus subtilis rec strains, differential toxicity	–	–	356.0000	Matsui et al. (1989)
ERD, Escherichia coli K12, differential toxicity	–	0	2000.0000	Rashid & Mumma (1986)
SA0, Salmonella typhimurium TA100, reverse mutation	0	–	2500.0000	Simmon et al. (1977)
SA0, Salmonella typhimurium TA100, reverse mutation	–	–	0.0000	Probst et al. (1981)
SA0, Salmonella typhimurium TA100, reverse mutation	–	(+)[c]	5.0000	Gentile et al. (1982)
SA0, Salmonella typhimurium TA100, reverse mutation	–	–	2500.0000	Moriya et al. (1983)
SA0, Salmonella typhimurium TA100, reverse mutation	–	–	167.0000	Zeiger et al. (1987)
SA0, Salmonella typhimurium TA100, reverse mutation	–	–	500.0000	Mersch-Sundermann et al. (1988)
SA2, Salmonella typhimurium TA102, reverse mutation	–	–	500.0000	Mersch-Sundermann et al. (1988)
SA5, Salmonella typhimurium TA1535, reverse mutation	0	–	500.0000	Marshall et al. (1976)
SA5, Salmonella typhimurium TA1535, reverse mutation	0	–	2500.0000	Simmon et al. (1977)
SA5, Salmonella typhimurium TA1535, reverse mutation	–	–	0.0000	Probst et al. (1981)
SA5, Salmonella typhimurium TA1535, reverse mutation	–	(+)[c]	10.0000	Gentile et al. (1982)
SA5, Salmonella typhimurium TA1535, reverse mutation	–	–	2500.0000	Moriya et al. (1983)
SA5, Salmonella typhimurium TA1535, reverse mutation	–	–	167.0000	Zeiger et al. (1987)
SA7, Salmonella typhimurium TA1537, reverse mutation	–	–	500.0000	Marshall et al. (1976)
SA7, Salmonella typhimurium TA1537, reverse mutation	0	–	2500.0000	Simmon et al. (1977)
SA7, Salmonella typhimurium TA1537, reverse mutation	–	–	0.0000	Probst et al. (1981)
SA7, Salmonella typhimurium TA1537, reverse mutation	–	–	2500.0000	Moriya et al. (1983)
SA7, Salmonella typhimurium TA1537, reverse mutation	–	–	167.0000	Zeiger et al. (1987)
SA8, Salmonella typhimurium TA1538, reverse mutation	–	–	500.0000	Marshall et al. (1976)
SA8, Salmonella typhimurium TA1538, reverse mutation	0	–	2500.0000	Simmon et al. (1977)
SA8, Salmonella typhimurium TA1538, reverse mutation	–	–	0.0000	Probst et al. (1981)

Table 20 (contd)

Test system	Result[a]		Dose[b] LED/HID	Reference
	Without exogenous metabolic system	With exogenous metabolic system		
SA8, *Salmonella typhimurium* TA1538, reverse mutation	–	–	2500.0000	Moriya *et al.* (1983)
SA9, *Salmonella typhimurium* TA98, reverse mutation	0	–	2500.0000	Simmon *et al.* (1977)
SA9, *Salmonella typhimurium* TA98, reverse mutation	–	–	0.0000	Probst *et al.* (1981)
SA9, *Salmonella typhimurium* TA98, reverse mutation	–	(+)[c]	5.0000	Gentile *et al.* (1982)
SA9, *Salmonella typhimurium* TA98, reverse mutation	–	–	2500.0000	Moriya *et al.* (1983)
SA9, *Salmonella typhimurium* TA98, reverse mutation	–	–	167.0000	Zeiger *et al.* (1987)
SA9, *Salmonella typhimurium* TA98, reverse mutation	–	–	500.0000	Mersch–Sundermann *et al.* (1988)
SAS, *Salmonella typhimurium* TA1536, reverse mutation	–	–	500.0000	Marshall *et al.* (1976)
SAS, *Salmonella typhimurium* G46, reverse mutation	–	–	0.0000	Probst *et al.* (1981)
SAS, *Salmonella typhimurium* C3076, reverse mutation	–	–	0.0000	Probst *et al.* (1981)
SAS, *Salmonella typhimurium* D3052, reverse mutation	–	–	0.0000	Probst *et al.* (1981)
SAS, *Salmonella typhimurium* TA97, reverse mutation	–	–	500.0000	Mersch–Sundermann *et al.* (1988)
EC2, *Escherichia coli* WP2, reverse mutation	–	–	0.0000	Probst *et al.* (1981)
EC2, *Escherichia coli* WP2 *hcr*, reverse mutation	–	–	2500.0000	Moriya *et al.* (1983)
ECW, *Escherichia coli* WP2 *uvrA*−, reverse mutation	–	–	0.0000	Probst *et al.* (1981)
SCG, *Saccharomyces cerevisiae*, gene conversion	–	–	0.0000	Gentile *et al.* (1982)
PLM, *Zea mays*, forward mutation	+	0	0.0000	Gentile *et al.* (1982)
PLC, *Lens* sp, chromosomal aberrations,	+	0	1000.0000	Jain (1988)
PLC, *Pisum* sp, chromosomal aberrations,	+	0	1000.0000	Jain (1988)
PLC, *Tradescantia*, micronuclei	+	0	1.8800	Sandhu *et al.* (1989)
DMX, *Drosophila melanogaster*, sex–linked recessive lethal mutations	–	0	5.0000 (feeding solutions)	Benes & Sram (1969)
URP, Unscheduled DNA synthesis, rat hepatocytes	–	0	3.7000	Maslansky & Williams (1981)
UIA, Unscheduled DNA synthesis, mouse hepatocytes	–	0	3.7000	Maslansky & Williams (1981)

Table 20 (contd)

Test system	Result[a] Without exogenous metabolic system	With exogenous metabolic system	Dose[b] LED/HID	Reference
UIA, Unscheduled DNA synthesis, hamster hepatocytes	–	0	3.7000	Maslansky & Williams (1981)
UIA, Unscheduled DNA synthesis, mouse hepatocytes	–	0	3.7000	Probst et al. (1981)
G5T, Gene mutation, mouse lymphoma L5178Y cells, tk locus	+	0	25.0000	McGregor et al. (1988)
GIA, Gene mutation, rat liver epithelial cells, hprt locus	–	0	37.0000	Telang et al. (1982)
UHF, Unscheduled DNA synthesis, human fibroblasts	–	+	37.0000	Ahmed et al. (1977b)
*, Inhibition of DNA synthesis, testicular cells in mice	–	0	40.0000	Seiler (1977)
DLM, Dominant lethal test, mice	–	0	24.0000	Epstein et al. (1972)
DLM, Dominant lethal test, mice	–	0	15.0000 × 1 p.o.[d]	Arnold et al. (1977)
DLM, Dominant lethal test, mice	–	0	15.0000 × 1 i.p.[d]	Arnold et al. (1977)
ICR, Inhibition of metabolic cooperation, V79 cells	+	0	10.0000	Kurata et al. (1982)
ICR, Inhibition of metabolic cooperation, rat liver epithelial cells	+	0	0.0400	Telang et al. (1982)
ICR, Inhibition of metabolic cooperation, rat hepatocytes	+	0	20.0000	Ruch et al. (1990)
ICM, Inhibition of metabolic cooperation, mouse hepatocytes	+	0	20.0000	Ruch et al. (1990)

*Not displayed on profile

[a]+, positive; (+), weakly positive; –, negative; 0, not tested; ?, inconclusive (variable response in several experiments within an adequate study)

[b]In-vitro tests, μg/ml; in-vivo tests, mg/kg bw

[c]Plant activation

[d]25:75 mixture of heptachlor:heptachlor epoxide; not displayed on profile

in plants but not in *Drosophila melanogaster*. Heptachlor did not induce unscheduled DNA synthesis in cultured rodent cells, but did so in human fibroblasts. It induced gene mutation at the *tk* but not at the *hprt* locus in rodent cells. Heptachlor inhibited gap-junctional intercellular communication in cultured mammalian cells. It did not inhibit DNA synthesis in mouse testicular cells and did not induce dominant lethal effects in mice *in vivo*,

5. Summary of Data Reported and Evaluation

5.1 Exposure data

Chlordane has been used since the 1950s as a broad-spectrum contact insecticide, mainly for nonagricultural purposes and to a lesser extent on crops and on livestock. Since the mid-1970s, its use has generally been restricted to underground control of termites.

Heptachlor has been used since the 1950s as an insecticide in agriculture and in the control of termites and soil insects. Like chlordane, its use is now largely restricted to subsoil treatment for termites.

Chlordane and heptachlor have been formulated as granules, emulsifiable concentrates and solutions.

Both compounds can persist in soil for many years. Human exposure to chlordane and heptachlor occurs mainly during their application and in the air of buildings where they have been applied for termite control. When these compounds were used on crops, exposure may have occurred at much lower levels as a result of consumption of foods containing residues.

5.2 Carcinogenicity in humans

Case reports of leukaemia and other blood dyscrasias have been associated with exposure to chlordane/heptachlor, primarily in domestic situations.

Mortality from lung cancer was slightly elevated in two cohort studies of pesticide applicators and one of chlordane/heptachlor manufacturers. Termite control operators probably have greater exposure to chlordane than other pesticide applicators; however, in one study of applicators, the excess occurred only among workers who were not engaged in termite control. In the other study of applicators, the relative risk for lung cancer among workers engaged in termite control was similar to that of workers engaged in other pest control. Inconsistencies in these findings make it difficult to ascribe the excesses to exposure to chlordane.

Small excess risks for other cancers, including leukaemia, non-Hodgkin's lymphoma and soft-tissue sarcoma and cancers of the brain, skin, bladder and stomach were observed, with little consistency among studies.

5.3 Carcinogenicity in experimental animals

Chlordane, technical-grade chlordane, heptachlor, technical-grade heptachlor, heptachlor epoxide and a mixture of heptachlor and heptachlor epoxide have been tested for carcinogenicity by oral administration in several strains of mice and rats. These studies uniformly demonstrate increases in the incidence of hepatocellular neoplasms in mice of each sex. Increases in the incidence of thyroid follicular-cell neoplasms were observed in rats treated with chlordane and technical-grade heptachlor. An increased incidence of malignant fibrous histiocytomas was observed in one study in male rats treated with chlordane. A small increase in the incidence of liver adenomas was seen in one study in male rats treated with technical-grade chlordane.

5.4 Other relevant data

Metabolites of chlordane and heptachlor, like those of other chlorinated hydrocarbons, accumulate in human fat. Chlordane and heptachlor induce liver microsomal enzymes. The liver is the target organ for chronic toxicity.

No data were available on the genetic and related effects of chlordane or heptachlor in humans.

Chlordane and heptachlor did not cause dominant lethal effects in mice. Both compounds inhibited gap-junctional intercellular communication and induced gene mutation in rodent cells but did not induce unscheduled DNA synthesis. In plants, heptachlor induced mutation and chromosomal aberrations. Neither chlordane nor heptachlor was mutagenic to bacteria and neither damaged bacterial or plasmid DNA.

5.5 Evaluation[1]

There is *inadequate evidence* in humans for the carcinogenicity of chlordane and of heptachlor.

There is *sufficient evidence* in experimental animals for the carcinogenicity of chlordane and of heptachlor.

Overall evaluations

Chlordane *is possibly carcinogenic to humans (Group 2B).*

Heptachlor *is possibly carcinogenic to humans (Group 2B).*

6. References

Abbott, D.C., Goulding, R. & Tatton, J. O'G. (1968) Organochlorine pesticide residues in human fat in Great Britain. *Br. med. J.*, *iii*, 146–149

Abbott, D.C., Holmes, D.C. & Tatton, J.O'G. (1969) Pesticide residues in the total diet in England and Wales, 1966–1967. II. Organochlorine pesticide residues in the total diet. *J. Sci. Food Agric.*, *20*, 245–249

Abbott, D.C., Collins, G.B. & Goulding, R. (1972) Organochlorine pesticide residues in human fat in the United Kingdom 1969–1971. *Br. med. J.*, *ii*, 553–556

Agency for Toxic Substances and Disease Registry (1989a) *Toxicological Profile for Heptachlor/-Heptachlor Epoxide* (Report No. ATSDR/TP–88/16; US NTIS PB89-194492), Washington DC, US Public Health Service, US Environmental Protection Agency

Agency for Toxic Substances and Disease Registry (1989b) *Toxicological Profile for Chlordane* (Report No. ATSDR/TP–89/06; US NTIS PB90–168709), Washington DC, US Public Health Service, US Environmental Protection Agency

---

[1]For definition of the italicized terms, see Preamble, pp. 26-28.

Ahmed, F.E., Lewis, N.J. & Hart, R.W. (1977a) Pesticide induced ouabain resistant mutants in Chinese hamster V79 cells. *Chem.-biol. Interactions, 19*, 369-374

Ahmed, F.E., Hart, R.W. & Lewis, N.J. (1977b) Pesticide induced DNA damage and its repair in cultured human cells. *Mutat. Res., 42*, 161-174

Aldrich, F.D. & Holmes, J.H. (1969) Acute chlordane intoxication in a child. Case report with toxicological data. *Arch. environ. Health, 19*, 129-132

Alvarez, W.C. & Hyman, S. (1953) Absence of toxic manifestations in workers exposed to chlordane. *Arch. ind. Hyg. occup. Med., 19*, 480-483

Ambrose, A.M., Christensen, H.E., Robbins, D.J. & Rather, L.J. (1953) Toxicological and pharmacological studies on chlordane. *Arch. ind. Hyg. occup. Med., 8*, 197-210

American Conference of Governmental Industrial Hygienists (1989) *Threshold Limit Values and Biological Exposure Indices for 1989-1990*, Cincinnati, OH, pp. 16, 25

Anon. (1981) Chlordane contamination of a public water supply—Pittsburgh, Pennsylvania. *Morb. Mortal. Wkly Report, 30*, 571-572, 577-578

Anon. (1985) Epoxy heptachlor. *Dangerous Prop. ind. Mater. Rep., 5*, 63-74

Arbejdstilsynet (Labour Inspection) (1988) *Graensevaerdier for Stoffer og Materialen* (Limit Values for Compounds and Materials) (No. 3.1.0.2), Copenhagen, pp. 14, 20 (in Danish)

Arnold, D.W., Kennedy, G.L., Jr, Keplinger, M.L., Calandra, J.C. & Calo, C.J. (1977) Dominant lethal studies with technical chlordane, HCS-3260 and heptachlor: heptachlor epoxide. *J. Toxicol. environ. Health, 2*, 547-555

Barnett, J.R. & Dorough, H.W. (1974) Metabolism of chlordane in rats. *J. agric. Food Chem., 22*, 612-619

Barnett, J.B., Blaylock, B.L., Gandy, J., Menna, J.H., Denton, R. & Soderberg, L.S.F. (1990) Long-term alteration of adult bone marrow colony formation by prenatal chlordane exposure. *Fundam. appl. Toxicol., 14*, 688-695

Benes, V. & Sram, R. (1969) Mutagenic activity of some pesticides in *Drosophila melanogaster. Ind. Med., 38*, 442-444

Biros, F.J. & Enos, H.F. (1973) Oxychlordane residues in human adipose tissue. *Bull. environ. Contam. Toxicol., 10*, 257-260

Blair, A., Grauman, D.J., Lubin, J.H. & Fraumeni, J.F., Jr (1983) Lung cancer and other causes of death among licensed pesticide applicators. *J. natl Cancer Inst., 71*, 31-37

Blaylock, B.L., Soderberg, L.S.F., Gandy, J., Menna, J.H., Denton, R. & Barnett, J.B. (1990) Cytotoxic T-lymphocyte and NK responses in mice treated prenatally with chlordane. *Toxicol. Lett., 51*, 41-49

Bovard, K.P., Fontenot, J.P. & Priode, B.M. (1971) Accumulation and dissipation of heptachlor residues in fattening steers. *J. anim. Sci., 33*, 127-132

Bowery, T.G. (1964) Heptachlor. In: Zweig, G., ed., *Analytical Methods for Pesticides, Plant Growth Regulators, and Food Additives*, Vol. II, *Insecticides*, New York, Academic Press, pp. 245-256

Brandt, W.N., Flamm, W.G. & Bernheim, N.J. (1972) The value of hydroxyurea in assessing repair synthesis of DNA in HeLa cells. *Chem.-biol. Interactions, 5*, 327-339

Bresch, H. & Arendt, U. (1977) Influence of different organochlorine pesticides on the development of sea urchin embryo. *Environ. Res., 13*, 121-128

Brooks, G.T. (1974) *Chlorinated Insecticides*, Vol. 1, *Technology and Application*, Cleveland, OH, CRC Press, pp. 85-158

Brown, L.M., Blair, A., Gibson, R., Everett, G.D., Cantor, K.P., Schuman, L.M., Burmeister, L.F., Van Lier, S.F. & Dick, F. (1990) Pesticide exposures and other agricultural risk factors for leukemia among men in Iowa and Minnesota. *Cancer Res.*, *50*, 6585-6591

Brubaker, P.E., Flamm, W.G. & Bernheim, N.J. (1970) Effect of γ-chlordane on synchronized lymphoma cells and inhibition of cell division. *Nature*, *226*, 548-549

Buchert, H., Class, T. & Ballschmiter, K. (1989) High resolution gas chromatography of technical chlordane with electron capture- and mass selective detection. *Fresenius Z. anal. Chem.*, *333*, 211-217

Bugg, J.C., Jr, Higgins, J.E. & Robertson, E.A., Jr (1967) Chlorinated pesticide levels in the eastern oyster (*Crassostrea virginica*) from selected areas of the South Atlantic and Gulf of Mexico. *Pestic. Monit. J.*, *1*, 9-12

Cabral, J.R., Testa, M.C. & Terracini, B. (1972) Absence of long-term effects of the administration of heptachlor to suckling rats (Ital.). *Tumori*, *58*, 49-53

Carey, A.E., Gowen, J.A., Tai, H, Mitchell, W.G. & Wiersma, G.B. (1978) Pesticide residue levels in soils and crops, 1971. National Soils Monitoring Program (III). *Pestic. Monit. J.*, *12*, 117-136

Chadduck, W.M., Gollin, S.M., Gray, B.A., Norris, J.S., Araoz, C.A. & Tryka, A.F. (1987) Gliosarcoma with chromosome abnormalities in a neonate exposed to heptachlor. *Neurosurgery*, *21*, 557-559

Chernoff, N. & Kavlock, R.J. (1983) A teratology test system which utilizes postnatal growth and viability in the mouse. *Environ. Sci. Res.*, *27*, 417-427

Cochrane, W.P. & Greenhalgh, R. (1976) Chemical composition of technical chlordane. *J. Assoc. off. anal. Chem.*, *59*, 696-702

Codex Committee on Pesticide Residues (1989) *Codex Alimentarius* (Document 14), Geneva

Codex Committee on Pesticide Residues (1990) *Guide to Codex Maximum Limits for Pesticide Residues*, Part 2 (CAC/PR 2—1990; CCPR Pesticide Classification No 012 & 043), The Hague

Cook, W.A., ed. (1987) *Occupational Exposure Limits—Worldwide*, Washington DC, American Industrial Hygiene Association, pp. 118, 132, 141, 171, 191

Cranmer, J.M., Cranmer, M.F. & Goad, P.T. (1984) Prenatal chlordane exposure: effects on plasma corticosterone concentrations over the lifespan of mice. *Environ. Res.*, *35*, 204-210

Curley, A. & Garrettson, L.K. (1969) Acute chlordane poisoning. Clinical and chemical studies. *Arch. environ. Health*, *18*, 211-215

Curley, A. & Kimbrough, R.D. (1969) Chlorinated hydrocarbon insecticides in plasma and milk of pregnant and lactating women. *Arch. environ. Health*, *18*, 156-164

Curley, A., Burse, V.W., Jennings, R.W., Villanueva, E.C., Tomatis, L. & Akazaki, K. (1973) Chlorinated hydrocarbon pesticides and related compounds in adipose tissue from people of Japan. *Nature*, *242*, 338-340

Den Tonkelaar, E.M. & Van Esch, G.J. (1974) No-effect levels of organochlorine pesticides based on induction of microsomal liver enzymes in short-term toxicity experiments. *Toxicology*, *2*, 371-380

Derbes, V.J., Dent, J.H., Forrest, W.W. & Johnson, M.F. (1955) Fatal chlordane poisoning. *J. Am. med. Assoc.*, *158*, 1367-1369

D'Ercole, A.J., Arthur, R.D., Cain, J.D. & Barrentine, B.F. (1976) Insecticide exposure of mothers and newborns in a rural agricultural area. *Pediatrics*, *57*, 869-874

Deutsche Forschungsgemeinschaft (1989) *Maximum Concentrations at the Workplace and Biological Tolerance Values for Working Materials 1989* (Report No. 25), Weinheim, VCH Verlagsgesellschaft, pp. 25, 40

Ditraglia, D., Brown, D.P., Namekata, T. & Iverson, N. (1981) Mortality study of workers employed at organochlorine pesticide manufacturing plants. *Scand. J. Work Environ. Health*, 7 (Suppl. 4), 140-146

Duggan, R.E. & Corneliussen, P.E. (1972) Dietary intake of pesticide chemicals in the United States (III), June 1968-April 1970. *Pestic. Monit. J.*, 5, 331-341

Eller, P.M. (1989) *NIOSH Manual of Analytical Methods*, 3rd ed., 3rd Suppl. (DHHS (NIOSH) Publ. No. 84-100), Washington DC, US Government Printing Office, pp. 5510-1—5510-4

Epstein, S.S. (1976) Carcinogenicity of heptachlor and chlordane. *Sci. total Environ.*, 6, 103-154

Epstein, S.S. & Ozonoff, D. (1987) Leukemias and blood dyscrasias following exposure to chlordane and heptachlor. *Teratog. Carcinog. Mutagenesis*, 7, 527-540

Epstein, S.S., Arnold, E., Andrea, J., Bass, W. & Bishop, Y. (1972) Detection of chemical mutagens by the dominant lethal assay in the mouse. *Toxicol. appl. Pharmacol.*, 23, 288-325

Esworthy, R.F. (1985) *Preliminary Quantitative Usage Analysis of Chlordane*, Washington DC, US Environmental Protection Agency, Office of Pesticide Programs

Ewing, A.D., Kadry, A.M. & Dorough, H.W. (1985) Comparative disposition and elimination of chlordane in rats and mice. *Toxicol. Lett.*, 26, 233-239

FAO/WHO (1964) *Evaluation of the Toxicity of Pesticide Residues in Food. Report of a Joint Meeting of the FAO Committee on Pesticides in Agriculture and the WHO Expert Committee on Pesticide Residues* (FAO Meeting Report No. PL/1963/13; WHO/Food Add./23), Rome

FAO/WHO (1965) *Evaluation of the Toxicity of Pesticide Residues in Food. Report of a Joint Meeting of the FAO Committee on Pesticides in Agriculture and the WHO Expert Committee on Pesticide Residues* (FAO Meeting Report No. PL/1965/10/1; WHO/Food Add. 27.65), Rome

FAO/WHO (1967) *Evaluation of the Toxicity of Pesticide Residues in Food. Report of a Joint Meeting of the FAO Committee on Pesticides in Agriculture and the WHO Expert Committee on Pesticide Residues* (FAO Meeting Report No. PL:CP/15; WHO/Food Add./67.32), Rome

FAO/WHO (1968) *Evaluation of the Toxicity of Pesticide Residues in Food. Report of a Joint Meeting of the FAO Committee on Pesticides in Agriculture and the WHO Expert Committee on Pesticide Residues* (FAO Meeting Report No. PL:1967/M/11/1; WHO/Food Add./68.30), Rome

FAO/WHO (1969) *1968 Evaluations of Some Pesticide Residues in Food* (FAO Meeting Report. No. PL-1968/M/9/1; WHO/Food Add./69.35), Rome

FAO/WHO (1970) *1969 Evaluations of Some Pesticide Residues in Food* (FAO/PL: 1969/M/17/1, WHO/Food Add. 170.38), Geneva

FAO/WHO (1971) *Evaluation of the Toxicity of Pesticide Residues in Food. Report of a Joint Meeting of the FAO Committee on Pesticides in Agriculture and the WHO Expert Committee on Pesticide Residues* (AGP:1970/M/12/1; WHO/Food Add./71.42), Rome

FAO/WHO (1973) *1972 Evaluations of Some Pesticide Residues in Food* (WHO Pesticide Residue Series No. 2), Geneva

FAO/WHO (1975) *1974 Evaluations of Some Pesticide Residues in Food* (WHO Pesticide Residue Series No. 4), Geneva

FAO/WHO (1976) *1975 Evaluations of Some Pesticide Residues in Food* (WHO Pesticide Residue Series No. 5), Geneva

FAO/WHO (1978) *Pesticide Residues in Food: 1977 Evaluations* (FAO Plant Production and Protection Paper 10 Sup.), Rome

FAO/WHO (1979) *Pesticide Residues in Food—1978 Evaluations. Report of the Joint Meeting of the FAO Panel of Experts on Pesticide Residues and Environment and the WHO Expert Group on Pesticide Residues* (FAO Plant Production and Protection Paper 15), Rome

FAO/WHO (1983) *Pesticide Residues in Food—1982 Evaluations. Data and Recommendations of the Joint Meeting of the FAO Panel of Experts on Pesticide Residues in Food and the Environment and the WHO Expert Group on Pesticide Residues* (FAO Plant Production and Protection Paper 49), Rome

FAO/WHO (1985) *Pesticide Residues in Food—1984. Report of the Joint Meeting of the FAO Panel of Experts on Pesticide Residues in Food and the Environment and a WHO Expert Group on Pesticide Residues* (FAO Plant Production and Protection Paper 77), Rome

FAO/WHO (1987) *Pesticide Residues in Food—1986. Report of the Joint Meeting of the FAO Panel of Experts on Pesticide Residues in Food and the Environment and a WHO Expert Group on Pesticide Residues* (FAO Plant Production and Protection Paper 77), Rome

FAO/WHO (1988) *Pesticide Residues in Food—1987. Report of the Joint Meeting of the FAO Panel of Experts on Pesticide Residues in Food and the Environment and a WHO Expert Group on Pesticide Residues* (FAO Plant Production and Protection Paper 86/1), Rome

Fendick, E.A., Mather-Mihaich, E., Houck, K.A., St Clair, M.B., Faust, J.B., Rockwell, C.H. & Owens, M. (1990) Ecological toxicology and human health effects of heptachlor. *Rev. environ. Contam. Toxicol.*, *111*, 61-142

Fishbein, W.I., White, J.V. & Isaacs, H.J. (1964) Survey of workers exposed to chlordane. *Ind. Med. Surg.*, *33*, 726-727

Fournier, E., Treich, I., Campagne, L. & Capelle, N. (1972) Organochlorine pesticides in human adipose tissue in France (Fr.). *J. eur. Toxicol.*, *1*, 11-26

Gaines, T.B. (1960) The acute toxicity of pesticides to rats. *Toxicol. appl. Pharmacol.*, *2*, 88-89

Garrettson, L.K., Guzelian, P.S. & Blanke, R.V. (1985) Subacute chlordane poisoning. *Clin. Toxicol.*, *22*, 565-571

Gentile, J.M., Gentile, G.J., Bultman, J., Sechriest, R., Wagner, E.D. & Plewa, M.J. (1982) An evaluation of the genotoxic properties of insecticides following plant and animal activation. *Mutat. Res.*, *101*, 19-29

Government of Canada (1990) *Report on National Surveillance Data from 1984/85 to 1988/89*, Ottawa

Griffin, D.E., III & Hill, W.E. (1978) In vitro breakage of plasmid DNA by mutagens and pesticides. *Mutat. Res.*, *52*, 161-169

Hannon, M.R., Greichus, Y.A., Applegate, R.L. & Fox, A.C. (1970) Ecological distribution of pesticides in Lake Poinsett, South Dakota. *Trans. Am. Fish. Soc.*, *99*, 496-500

Harrington, J.M., Baker, E.L., Jr, Folland, D.S., Saucier, J.W. & Sandifer, S.H. (1978) Chlordane contamination of a municipal water system. *Environ. Res.*, *15*, 155-159

Hayes, W.J., Jr, Dale, W.E. & Burse, V.W. (1965) Chlorinated hydrocarbon pesticides in the fat of people in New Orleans. *Life Sci.*, *4*, 1611-1615

Health and Welfare Canada (1990) *National Pesticide Residue Limits in Foods*, Ottawa, Bureau of Chemical Safety, Food Directorate, Health Protection Branch

Henderson, C., Johnson, W.L. & Inglis, A. (1969) Organochlorine insecticide residues in fish (National Pesticide Monitoring Program). *Pestic. Monit. J.*, *3*, 145-171

Hergenrather, J., Hlady, G., Wallace, B. & Savage, E. (1981) Pollutants in breast milk of vegetarians (Letter to the Editor). *New Engl. J. Med.*, *304*, 792

Herrick, G.M., Fry, J.L., Fong, W.G. & Golden, D.C. (1969) Insecticide residues in eggs resulting from the dusting and short-term feeding of low levels of chlorinated hydrocarbon insecticides to hens. *J. agric. Food Chem.*, *17*, 291-295

Hirasawa, F. & Takizawa, Y. (1989) Accumulation and declination of chlordane congeners in mice. *Toxicol. Lett.*, *47*, 109-117

Horwitz, W., ed. (1975) *Official Methods of Analysis of the Association of Official Analytical Chemists*, 12th ed., Washington DC, Association of Oficial Analytical Chemists, pp. 112-113

Huber, J.T. & Bishop, J.L. (1961) Secretion of heptachlor epoxide in the milk of cows fed field-cured hay from soils treated with heptachlor. *J. Dairy Sci.*, *45*, 79-81

IARC (1976) *IARC Monographs on the Evaluation of Carcinogenic Risks of Chemicals to Man*, Vol. 12, *Some Carbamates, Thiocarbamates and Carbazides*, Lyon, pp. 225-236

IARC (1979) *IARC Monographs on the Evaluation of the Carcinogenic Risk of Chemicals to Humans*, Vol. 20, *Some Halogenated Hydrocarbons*, Lyon, pp. 45-65, 129-154

Infante, P.F. & Freeman, C. (1987) Cancer mortality among workers exposed to chlordane. *J. occup. Med.*, *29*, 908-909

Infante, P.F., Epstein, S.S. & Newton, W.A., Jr (1978) Blood dyscrasias and childhood tumors and exposure to chlordane and heptachlor. *Scand. J. Work Environ. Health*, *4*, 137-150

Izmerov, N.F., ed. (1982) *International Register of Potentially Toxic Chemicals. Scientific Reviews of Soviet Literature on Toxicity and Hazards of Chemicals: Heptachlor* (Issue 3), Moscow, Centre of International Projects, United Nations Environment Programme

Jain, A.K. (1988) Cytogenetic effects of heptachlor on *Lens* and *Pisum* species. *Geobios*, *15*, 61-69

Johnson, R.D. & Manske, D.D. (1976) Pesticide residues in total diet samples (IX). *Pestic. Monit. J.*, *9*, 157-169

Johnson, K.W., Holsapple, M.P. & Munson, A.E. (1986) An immunotoxicological evaluation of gamma-chlordane. *Fundam. appl. Toxicol.*, *6*, 317-326

Kan, C.A. & Tuinstra, L.G.M.T. (1976) Accumulation and excretion of certain organochlorine insecticides in broiler breeder hens. *J. agric. Food Chem.*, *24*, 775-778

Khasawinah, A.M. & Grutsch, J.F. (1989a) Chlordane: 24-month tumorigenicity and chronic toxicity test in mice. *Regul. Toxicol. Pharmacol.*, *10*, 244-254

Khasawinah, A.M. & Grutsch, J.F. (1989b) Chlordane: thirty-month tumorigenicity and chronic toxicity test in rats. *Regul. Toxicol. Pharmacol.*, *10*, 95-109

Khasawinah, A.M., Hardy, C.J. & Clark, G.C. (1989) Comparative inhalation toxicity of technical chlordane in rats and monkeys. *J. Toxicol. environ. Health*, *28*, 327-347

Klein, W., Korte, F., Weisgerber, I., Kaul, R., Mueller, W. & Djirsarai, A. (1968) The metabolism of endrin, heptachlor and telodrin (Ger.). *Qual. Plant Mater. Veg.*, *15*, 225-238

Klein, D., Dillon, J.C., Jirou-Najou, J.L., Gagey, M.J. & Debry, G. (1986) Kinetics of the elimination of organochlorine compounds during the first week of breast feeding (Fr.). *Food chem. Toxicol.*, *24*, 869-873

Kurata, M., Hirose, K. & Umeda, M. (1982) Inhibition of metabolic cooperation in Chinese hamster cells by organochlorine pesticides. *Gann*, *73*, 217-221

Kutz, F.W., Strassman, S.C., Sperling, J.F., Cook, B.T., Sunshine, I. & Tessari, J. (1983) A fatal chlordane poisoning. *J. Toxicol. clin. Toxicol.*, *20*, 167-174

Lee, S.-R. (1982) Overall assessment of organochlorine insecticide residues in Korean foods (Korean). *Korean J. Food Sci. Technol.*, *14*, 82-93

Lehman, A.J. (1952) Chemicals in foods: a report to the Association of Food and Drug Officials on current developments. Part II. Pesticides. Section III: Subacute and chronic toxicity. *Q. Bull. Assoc. Food Drug Off. US*, *16*, 47-53

Le Marchand, L., Kolonel, L.N., Siegel, B.Z. & Dendle, W.H., III (1986) Trends in birth defects for a Hawaiian population exposed to heptachlor and for the United States. *Arch. environ. Health*, *41*, 145-148

Livingston, J.M. & Jones, C.R. (1981) Living area contamination by chlordane used for termite treatment. *Bull. environ. Contam. Toxicol.*, *27*, 406-411

MacMahon, B., Monson, R.R., Wang, H.H. & Zheng, T. (1988) A second follow-up of mortality in a cohort of pesticide applicators. *J. occup. Med.*, *30*, 429-432

Marshall, T.C., Dorough, H.W. & Swim, H.E. (1976) Screening of pesticides for mutagenic potential using *Salmonella typhimurium* mutants. *J. agric. Food Chem.*, *24*, 560-563

Maslansky, C.J. & Williams, G.M. (1981) Evidence for an epigenetic mode of action in organochlorine pesticide hepatocarcinogenicity: a lack of genotoxicity in rat, mouse and hamster hepatocytes. *J. Toxicol. environ. Health*, *8*, 121-130

Matsui, S., Yamamoto, R. & Yamada, H. (1989) The *Bacillus subtilis*/microsome rec-assay for the detection of DNA damaging substances which may occur in chlorinated and ozonated waters. *Water Sci. Technol.*, *21*, 875-887

Matsumura, F. & Nelson, J.O. (1971) Identification of the major metabolic product of heptachlor epoxide in rat feces. *Bull. environ. Contam. Toxicol.*, *5*, 489-492

McGregor, D.B., Brown, A., Cattanach, P., Edwards, I., McBride, D., Riach, C. & Caspary, W.J. (1988) Responses of the L5178Y tk$^+$/tk$^-$ mouse lymphoma cell forward mutation assay: III. 72 coded chemicals. *Environ. mol. Mutagenesis*, *12*, 85-154

Menconi, S., Clark, J.M., Langenberg, P. & Hryhorczuk, D. (1988) A preliminary study of potential human health effects in private residences following chlordane applications for termite control. *Arch. environ. Health*, *43*, 349-352

Menna, J.H., Barnett, J.B. & Soderberg, L.S.F. (1985) Influenza type A virus infection of mice exposed in utero to chlordane: survival and antibody studies. *Toxicol. Lett.*, *24*, 45-52

Mersch-Sundermann, V., Dickgiesser, N., Hablizel, U. & Gruber, B. (1988) Examination of the mutagenicity of organic microcontaminants on the environment. I. The mutagenicity of selected herbicides and insecticides in the *Salmonella*-microsome test (Ames test) in relation to the pathogenetic potency of contaminated ground- and drinking-water (Ger.). *Zbl. Bakt. Hyg. B.*, *186*, 247-260

Mes, J., Coffin, D.E. & Campbell, D. (1974) Polychlorinated biphenyl and organochlorine pesticide residues in Canadian chicken eggs. *Pestic. Monit. J.*, *8*, 8-11

Mes, J., Doyle, J.A., Adams, B.R., Davies, D.J. & Turton, D. (1984) Polychlorinated biphenyls and organochlorine pesticides in milk and blood of Canadian women during lactation. *Arch. environ. Contam. Toxicol.*, *13*, 217-223

Miranda, C.L., Webb, R.E. & Ritchey, S.J. (1973) Effect of dietary protein quality, phenobarbital and SKF 525-A on heptachlor metabolism in the rat. *Pestic. Biochem. Physiol.*, *3*, 456-461

Miyazaki, T., Yamagishi, T. & Matsumoto, M. (1985) Isolation and structure elucidation of some components in technical grade chlordane. *Arch. environ. Contam. Toxicol.*, *14*, 475-483

Moriya, M., Ohta, T., Watanabe, K., Miyazawa, T., Kato, K. & Shirasu, Y. (1983) Further mutagenicity studies on pesticides in bacterial reversion assay systems. *Mutat. Res.*, *116*, 185-216

Mortelmans, K., Haworth, S., Lawlor, T., Speck, W., Tainer, B. & Zeiger, E. (1986) *Salmonella* mutagenicity tests: II. Results from the testing of 270 chemicals. *Environ. Mutagenesis*, *8* (Suppl. 7), 1-119

Moser, G.J. & Smart, R.C. (1989) Hepatic tumor-promoting chlorinated hydrocarbons stimulate protein kinase C activity. *Carcinogenesis*, *10*, 851-856

Mussalo-Rauhamaa, H., Pyysalo, H. & Antervo, K. (1988) Relation between the content of organochlorine compounds in Finnish human milk and characteristics of the mothers. *J. Toxicol. environ. Health*, *25*, 1-19

Nelson, B.D. (1975) The action of cyclodiene pesticides on oxidative phosphorylation in rat liver mitochondria. *Biochem. Pharmacol.*, 24, 1485-1490

Nomeir, A.A. & Hajjar, N.P. (1987) Metabolism of chlordane in mammals. *Rev. environ. Contam. Toxicol.*, 100, 1-22

Nye, D.E. & Dorough, H.W. (1976) Fate of insecticides administered endotracheally to rats. *Bull. environ. Contam. Toxicol.*, 15, 291-296

Olanoff, L.S., Bristow, W.J., Colcolough, J., Jr & Reigart, J.R. (1983) Acute chlordane intoxication. *J. Toxicol. clin. Toxicol.*, 20, 291-306

Paccagnella, B., Prati, L. & Cavazzini, G. (1967) Organic chloro-derived insecticides in the adipose tissue of people living in the province of Ferrara (Ital.). *Nuovi Ann. Ig. Microbiol.*, 18, 17-26

Pelikan, Z., Halacka, K., Polster, M. & Cerny, E. (1968) Long-term intoxication of rats by small doses of heptachlor (Fr.). *Arch. belg. Méd. trav. Méd. leg.*, 26, 529-538

Polishuk, Z.W., Ron, M., Wassermann, M., Cucos, S., Wassermann, D. & Lemesch, C. (1977) Organochlorine compounds in human blood plasma and milk. *Pestic. Monit. J.*, 10, 121-129

Princi, F. & Spurbeck, G.H. (1951) A study of workers exposed to the insecticides chlordan, aldrin, dieldrin. *Arch. ind. Hyg. occup. Med.*, 3, 64-72

Probst, G.S., McMahon, R.E., Hill, L.E., Thompson, C.Z., Epp, J.K. & Neal, S.B. (1981) Chemically-induced unscheduled DNA synthesis in primary rat hepatocyte cultures: a comparison with bacterial mutagenicity using 218 compounds. *Environ. Mutagenesis*, 3, 11-32

Radomski, J.L. & Davidow, B. (1953) The metabolite of heptachlor, its estimation, storage and toxicity. *J. Pharmacol. exp. Ther.*, 107, 266-272

Rashid, K.A. & Mumma, R.O. (1986) Screening pesticides for their ability to damage bacterial DNA. *J. environ. Sci. Health*, B21, 319-334

Raw, G.R., ed. (1970) *CIPAC Handbook*, Vol. 1, Cambridge, Collaborative International Pesticides Analytical Council, pp. 420-427

Ritter, L. & Wood, G. (1989) Evaluation and regulation of pesticides in drinking water: a Canadian approach. *Food Add. Contam.*, 6, S87-S94

Royal Society of Chemistry (1986) *European Directory of Agrochemical Products*, Vol. 3, *Insecticides, Acaricides, Nematicides*, Cambridge, pp. 112, 331-332

Royal Society of Chemistry (1989) *The Agrochemicals Handbook* [Dialog Information Services (File 306)], Cambridge

Ruch, R.J., Fransson, R., Flodstrom, S., Warngard, L. & Klaunig, J.E. (1990) Inhibition of hepatocyte gap junctional intercellular communication by endosulfan, chlordane and heptachlor. *Carcinogenesis*, 11, 1097-1101

Sadtler Research Laboratories (1980) *The Standard Spectra, 1980, Cumulative Index*, Philadelphia, PA

Sadtler Research Laboratories (1990) *The Sadtler Standard Spectra, 1981-1990, Supplementary Index*, Philadelphia, PA

Saito, I., Kawamura, N., Uno, K., Hisanaga, N., Takeuchi, Y., Ono, Y., Iwata, M., Gotoh, M., Okutani, H., Matsumoto, T., Fukaya, Y., Yoshitomi, S. & Ohno, Y. (1986) Relationship between chlordane and its metabolites in blood of pest control operators and spraying conditions. *Int. Arch. occup. environ. Health*, 58, 91-97

Sandhu, S.S., Ma, T.-H., Peng, Y. & Zhou, X. (1989) Clastogenicity evaluation of seven chemicals commonly found at hazardous industrial waste sites. *Mutat. Res.*, 224, 437-445

Saschenbrecker, P.W. (1976) Levels of terminal pesticide residues in Canadian meat. *Can. vet. J.*, 17, 158-163

Savage, E.P., Keefe, T.J., Tessari, J.D., Wheeler, H.W., Applehans, F.M., Goes, E.A. & Ford, S.A. (1981) National study of chlorinated hydrocarbon insecticide residues in human milk, USA. I. Geographic distribution of dieldrin, heptachlor, heptachlor epoxide, chlordane, oxychlordane and mirex. *Am. J. Epidemiol.*, *113*, 413-422

Schuepbach, M.R. & Egli, H. (1979) Organochlorine pesticides and polychlorinated biphenyls in human milk (Ger.). *Mitt. Geb. Lebensmitteluntersuch. Hyg.*, *70*, 451-463

Seiler, J.P. (1977) Inhibition of testicular DNA synthesis by chemical mutagens and carcinogens. Preliminary results in the validation of a novel short-term test. *Mutat. Res.*, *46*, 305-310

Shindell, S. (1987) Cancer mortality among workers exposed to chlordane. (Reply to a letter to the Editor). *J. occup. Med.*, *29*, 909-911

Shindell, S. & Ulrich, S. (1986) Mortality of workers employed in the manufacture of chlordane: an update. *J. occup. Med.*, *28*, 497-501

Simmon, V.F., Kauhanen, K. & Tardiff, R.G. (1977) Mutagenic activity of chemicals identified in drinking water. *Dev. Toxicol. Environ. Sci.*, *2*, 249-258

Sittig, M., ed. (1980) *Pesticide Manufacturing and Toxic Materials Control Encyclopedia*, Park Ridge, NJ, Noyes Data Corp., pp. 445-448

Smith, S.I., Weber, C.W. & Reid, B.L. (1970) The effect of injection of chlorinated hydrocarbon pesticides on hatchability of eggs. *Toxicol. appl. Pharmacol.*, *16*, 179-185

Sobti, R.C., Krishan, A. & Davies, J. (1983) Cytokinetic and cytogenetic effect of agricultural chemicals on human lymphoid cells in vitro. II. Organochlorine pesticides. *Arch. Toxicol.*, *52*, 221-231

Sovocool, G.W. & Lewis, R.G. (1975) The identification of trace levels of organic pollutants in human tissues: compounds related to chlordane/heptachlor exposure. *Trace Subst. environ. Health*, *9*, 265-280

Sovocool, G.W., Lewis, R.G., Harless, R.L., Wilson, N.K. & Zehr, R.D. (1977) Analysis of technical chlordane by gas chromatography/mass spectrometry. *Anal. Chem.*, *49*, 734-740

Sperling, F. & Ewinike, H. (1969) Changes in LD$_{50}$ of parathion and heptachlor after turpentine pretreatment (Abstract No. 24). *Toxicol. appl. Pharmacol.*, *14*, 622

Spyker Cranmer, J., Avery, D.L., Grady, R.R. & Kitay, J.I. (1978) Postnatal endocrine dysfunction resulting from prenatal exposure to carbofuran, diazinon or chlordane. *J. environ. Pathol. Toxicol.*, *2*, 357-369

Spyker Cranmer, J.M., Barnett, J.B., Avery, D.L. & Cranmer, M.F. (1982) Immunoteratology of chlordane: cell-mediated and humoral immune responses in adult mice exposed *in utero*. *Toxicol. appl. Pharmacol.*, *62*, 402-408

Stehr-Green, P.A., Schilling, R.J., Burse, V.W., Steinberg, K.K., Royce, W., Wohlleb, J.C. & Donnell, H.D. (1986) Evaluation of persons exposed to dairy products contaminated with heptachlor (Letter to the Editor). *J. Am. med. Assoc.*, *256*, 3350-3351

Takamiya, K. (1990) Interruption of chronic chlordane exposure and plasma residue levels in occupational workers. *Bull. environ. Contam. Toxicol.*, *44*, 905-909

Tashiro, S. & Matsumura, F. (1977) Metabolic routes of *cis*- and *trans*-chlordane in rats. *J. agric. Food Chem.*, *25*, 872-880

Tashiro, S. & Matsumura, F. (1978) Metabolism of *trans*-nonachlor and related chlordane components in rat and man. *Arch. environ. Contam. Toxicol.*, *7*, 113-127

Taylor, D.G. (1979) *NIOSH Manual of Analytical Methods*, 2nd ed., Vol. 5 (DHEW (NIOSH) Publ. No. 79/141; US NTIS PB83-105445), Cincinnati, OH, National Institute for Occupational Safety and Health, pp. S287-1—S287-9

Telang, S., Tong, C. & Williams, G.M. (1982) Epigenetic membrane effects of a possible tumor promoting type on cultured liver cells by the non-genotoxic organochlorine pesticides chlordane and heptachlor. *Carcinogenesis*, 3, 1175-1178

Tojo, Y., Wariishi, M., Suzuki, Y. & Nishiyama, K. (1986) Quantitation of chlordane residues in mother's milk. *Arch. environ. Contam. Toxicol.*, 15, 327-332

Tong, C., Fazio, M. & Williams, G.M. (1981) Rat hepatocyte-mediated mutagenesis of human cells by carcinogenic polycyclic aromatic hydrocarbons but not organochlorine pesticides. *Proc. Soc. exp. Biol. Med.*, 167, 572-575

Tsushimoto, G., Chang, C.C., Trosko, J.E. & Matsumura, F. (1983) Cytotoxic, mutagenic, and cell-cell communication inhibitory properties of DDT, lindane and chlordane on Chinese hamster cells *in vitro. Arch. environ. Contam. Toxicol.*, 12, 721-730

US Environmental Protection Agency (1986a) *Carcinogenicity Assessment of Chlordane and Heptachlor/Heptachlor Epoxide*, Washington DC, Office of Health and Environmental Assessment

US Environmental Protection Agency (1986b) Method 8250. Gas chromatography/mass spectrometry for semivolatile organics: packed column technique. In: *Test Methods for Evaluating Solid Waste—Physical/Chemical Methods*, 3rd ed. (US EPA No. SW-846), Washington DC, Office of Solid Waste and Emergency Response

US Environmental Protection Agency (1986c) Method 8080. Organochlorine pesticides and PCBs. In: *Test Methods for Evaluating Solid Waste—Physical/Chemical Methods*, 3rd ed. (US EPA No. SW-846), Washington DC, Office of Solid Waste and Emergency Response

US Environmental Protection Agency (1986d) Method 8270. Gas chromatography/mass spectrometry for semivolatile organics: capillary column technique. In: *Test Methods for Evaluating Solid Waste—Physical/Chemical Methods*, 3rd ed. (US EPA No. SW-846), Washington DC, Office of Solid Waste and Emergency Response

US Environmental Protection Agency (1986e) *Guidance for the Registration of Pesticide Products Containing Chlordane as Active Ingredient*, Washington DC

US Environmental Protection Agency (1987a) *Heptachlor and Heptachlor Epoxide*, Washington DC, Office of Drinking Water

US Environmental Protection Agency (1987b) *Chlordane, Heptachlor, Aldrin and Dieldrin* (Technical Report Document), Washington DC, Office of Pesticides and Toxic Substances

US Environmental Protection Agency (1988a) Method TO-10. Method for the determination of organochlorine pesticides in ambient air using low volume polyurethane foam (puf) sampling with gas chromatography/electron capture detector (GC/ECD). In: *Compendium of Methods for the Determination of Toxic Organic Compounds in Ambient Air* (US EPA Report No. EPA-600/4-89-017; US NTIS PB90-116989), Research Triangle Park, NC, Atmospheric Research and Exposure Assessment Laboratory

US Environmental Protection Agency (1988b) Method 505. Analysis of organohalide pesticides and commercial polychlorinated biphenyl (PCB) products in water by microextraction and gas chromatography. In: *Methods for the Determination of Organic Compounds in Drinking Water* (EPA Report No. EPA-600/4-88-039; US NTIS PB89-220461), Cincinnati, OH, Environmental Monitoring Systems Laboratory, pp. 109-141

US Environmental Protection Agency (1988c) Method 508. Determination of chlorinated pesticides in water by gas chromatography with an electron capture detector. In: *Methods for the Determination of Organic Compounds in Drinking Water* (EPA Report No. EPA-600/4-88-039; US NTIS PB89-220461), Cincinnati, OH, Environmental Monitoring Systems Laboratory, pp. 171-198

US Environmental Protection Agency (1988d) Method 525. Determination of organic compounds in drinking water by liquid-solid extraction and capillary column gas chromatography/mass spectrometry. In: *Methods for the Determination of Organic Compounds in Drinking Water* (EPA Report No. EPA-600/4-88-039; US NTIS PB89-220461), Cincinnati, OH, Environmental Monitoring Systems Laboratory, pp. 325-356

US Environmental Protection Agency (1989a) Method 608—organochlorine pesticides and PCBs. *US Code fed. Regul., Title 40*, Part 136, Appendix A, pp. 354-374

US Environmental Protection Agency (1989b) Method 625—base/neutrals and acids. *US Code fed. Regul., Title 40*, Part 136, Appendix A, pp. 447-474

US Food and Drug Administration (1989) *Pesticide Analytical Manual*, Vol. II, *Methods Which Detect Multiple Residues*, US Department of Health and Human Services

US Food and Drug Administration (1990) Action levels for residues of certain pesticides in food and feed. *Fed. Reg., 55*, 14359-14363

US National Academy of Sciences (1977) *An Evaluation of the Carcinogenicity of Chlordane and Heptachlor*, Washington DC

US National Academy of Sciences (1979) *Chlordane in Military Family Housing*, Washington DC, Committee on Toxicology

US National Cancer Institute (1977a) *Bioassay of Chlordane for Possible Carcinogenicity* (Technical Report Series No. 8; DHEW Publ. No. (NIH) 77-808), Washington DC, Department of Health, Education, and Welfare

US National Cancer Institute (1977b) *Bioassay of Heptachlor for Possible Carcinogenicity* (Technical Report Series No. 9; DHEW Publ. No. (NIH) 77-809), Washington DC, US Government Printing Office

US Occupational Safety and Health Administration (1989) Air contaminants—permissible exposure limits. *US Code fed. Regul., Title 29*, Part 1910.1000

US Public Health Service (1989a) *Agency for Toxic Substances and Disease Registry Toxicological Profile for Heptachlor/Heptachlor Epoxide* (Report No. ATSDR/TP-88/16; US NTIS PB89-194492), Washington DC

US Public Health Service (1989b) *Agency for Toxic Substances and Disease Registry Toxicological Profile for Chlordane* (Report No. ATSDR/TP-89/06; US NTIS PB90-168709), Washington DC

Vigfusson, N.V., Vyse, E.R., Pernsteiner, C.A. & Dawson, R.J. (1983) In vivo induction of sister-chromatid exchange in *Umbra limi* by the insecticides endrin, chlordane, diazinon and guthion. *Mutat. Res., 118*, 61-68

de Vlieger, M., Robinson, J., Baldwin, M.K., Crabtree, A.N. & van Dijk, M.C. (1968) The organochlorine insecticide content of human tissues. *Arch. environ. Health, 17*, 759-767

Vinopal, J.H. & Olds, K.L. (1977) *Investigation of Suspected Non-occupational Human Intoxication/Chlordane Termite Treatment, Fort Monmouth, New Jersey, May-June 1977* (US AEHA-44-0957-77), Washington DC, National Technical Information Service

Wang, H.H. & MacMahon, B. (1979a) Mortality of workers employed in the manufacture of chlordane and heptachlor. *J. occup. Med., 21*, 745-748

Wang, H.H. & MacMahon, B. (1979b) Mortality of pesticide applicators. *J. occup. med., 21*, 741-744

Wassermann, M., Tomatis, L., Wassermann, D., Day, N.E., Groner, Y., Lazarovici, S. & Rosenfeld, D. (1974) Epidemiology of organochlorine insecticides in the adipose tissue of Israelis. *Pestic. Monit. J., 8*, 1-7

Welch, R.M., Levin, W., Kuntzman, R., Jacobson, M. & Conney, A.H. (1971) Effect of halogenated hydrocarbon insecticides on the metabolism and uterotropic action of estrogens in rats and mice. *Toxicol. appl. Pharmacol.*, *19*, 234-246

WHO (1983) *Summary of 1980-1981 Monitoring Data Received from the Collaborating Centres of the Joint FAO/WHO Food Contamination Monitoring Programme* (EFP/83.57), Geneva

WHO (1984a) *Chlordane* (Environmental Health Criteria 34), Geneva

WHO (1984b) *Heptachlor* (Environmental Health Criteria 38), Geneva

WHO (1988a) *Chlordane Health and Safety Guide* (Health and Safety Guide No. 13), Geneva

WHO (1988b) *Heptachlor Health and Safety Guide* (Health and Safety Guide No. 14), Geneva

WHO (1988c) *Introduction to National Seminars on Drinking Water Quality* (WHO/PEP/88.10), Geneva

Williams, S., ed. (1984a) *Official Methods of Analysis of the Association of Official Analytical Chemists*, 14th ed., Washington DC, Association of Official Analytical Chemists, pp. 111-113

Williams, S., ed. (1984b) *Official Methods of Analysis of the Association of Official Analytical Chemists*, 14th ed., Washington DC, Association of Official Analytical Chemists, pp. 533-543

Williams, G.M. & Numoto, S. (1984) Promotion of mouse liver neoplasms by the organochlorine pesticides chlordane and heptachlor in comparison to dichlorodiphenyltrichloroethane. *Carcinogenesis*, *5*, 1689-1696

Woods, J.S. & Polissar, L. (1989) Non-Hodgkin's lymphoma among phenoxy herbicide-exposed farm workers in western Washington State. *Chemosphere*, *18*, 401-406

Woods, J.S., Polissar, L., Severson, R.K., Heuser, L.S. & Kulander, B.G. (1987) Soft tissue sarcoma and non-Hodgkin's lymphoma in relation to phenoxyherbicide and chlorinated phenol exposure in western Washington. *J. natl Cancer Inst.*, *78*, 899-910

Worthing, C.R. & Walker, S.B., eds (1987) *The Pesticide Manual—A World Compendium*, 8th ed., Thornton Heath, British Crop Protection Council, pp. 145-146, 455-456

Zavon, M.R., Tye, R. & Latorre, L. (1969) Chlorinated hydrocarbon insecticide content of the neonate. *Ann. N.Y. Acad. Sci.*, *160*, 196-200

Zeiger, E., Anderson, B., Haworth, S., Lawlor, T., Mortelmans, K. & Speck, W. (1987) *Salmonella* mutagenicity tests: III. Results from the testing of 255 chemicals. *Environ. Mutagenesis*, *9* (Suppl. 9), 1-110

Annex 1.

Criteria for classification of rodent hepatocellular neoplasms[a]

Hepatocellular carcinoma: focal thickening of hepatocellular plates producing trabeculae that are at least 4-5 cells thick, or the presence of papillary formations with finger-like projection of hepatocytes completely surrounded by endothelial cells. Cytological variation is frequently prominent, with a high nucleus: cytoplasm ratio; but the cells may at times resemble normal hepatocytes. Infiltration of the surrounding parenchyma is rare but indicates malignancy.

Basophilic nodules: hepatocyte plates 1-3 cells thick, characterized by intense cytoplasmic staining with haematoxylin. Most of the cells are small and rather uniform, but some show a significant degree of cytological variation. These nodules are characterized by increased cell number with compression of surrounding parenchyma.

Hyperplastic nodules: several cytological variants exist. In the mouse, these nodules frequently show considerable megalocytosis with numerous, often bizarre mitotic figures. A feature common to all of them is hyperplasia with compression of the surrounding parenchyma and 2-cell-thick hepatocyte plates. Swelling of individual hepatocytes is often prominent in these nodules. Portal triads are absent.

Nodules showing features indicative of carcinoma: histological changes may not be diagnostic of carcinoma, but the presence of a combination of several features strongly suggests transition to hepatocellular carcinoma. These features may include a suspicion of trabeculae formation, basophilic cytoplasmic changes, the formation of 'nodules within nodules' (clusters of hepatocytes within hyperplastic nodules showing different cytological features), a peculiar 'packing' phenomenon with close compression of many hepatocytes or marked cytological atypia with the presence of unusually large numbers of mitotic cells.

---

[a]Elaborated by the Pesticide Information Review and Evaluation Committee convened by the US National Academy of Sciences (1977)

DDT AND ASSOCIATED COMPOUNDS

These substances were considered by previous Working Groups, in 1973 (IARC, 1974) and 1987 (IARC, 1987a). Since that time, new data have become available, and these have been incorporated into the monograph and taken into consideration in the present evaluation.

1. Exposure Data

1.1 Chemical and physical data

1.1.1 *Synonyms, structural and molecular data*

Table 1. Chemical Abstract Services Registry numbers, names and synonyms

Name	CAS Reg. Nos	Chem. Abstr. names[a] and synonyms
para,para' -DDT	50-29-3	α,α-Bis(*para*-chlorophenyl)-β,β,β-trichloroethane; 1,1-bis(*para*-chlorophenyl)-2,2,2-trichloroethane; 2,2-bis(*para*-chlorophenyl)-1,1,1-trichloro-ethane; 1,1-bis(4-chlorophenyl)-2,2,2-trichloroethane; DDT; 4,4'-DDT; *para,para'*-dichlorodiphenyltrichloroethane; 4,4'-dichlorodiphenyltrichloroethane; *para,para'*-dichlorodiphenyltrichloromethylmethane; ENT 1506; OMS 0016; 1,1,1-trichloro-2,2-bis(*para*-chlorophenyl)ethane; 1,1,1-trichloro-2,2-bis(4,4'-dichlorodiphenyl)ethane; 2,2,2-trichloro-1,1-bis(4-chlorophenyl)ethane; 1,1,1-trichloro-2,2-bis(4-chlorophenyl)ethane (IUPAC); trichlorobis(4'-chlorophenyl)ethane; **1,1'-(2,2,2-trichloro-ethylidene)bis(4-chlorobenzene)**
ortho,para' -DDT	789-02-6	2-(2-Chlorophenyl)-2-(4-chlorophenyl)-1,1,1-trichloroethane; **1-chloro-2-(2,2,2-trichloro-1-(4-chlorophenyl)ethyl)-benzene**; 2,4'-DDT; 1,1,1-trichloro-2-(*ortho*-chlorophenyl)-2-(*para*-chlorophenyl)ethane; 1,1,1-trichloro-2-(2-chlorophenyl)-2-(4-chlorophenyl)ethane (IUPAC)
para,para' -TDE	72-54-8	1,1-Bis(*para*-chlorophenyl)-2,2-dichloroethane; 1,1-bis(4-chlorophenyl)-2,2-dichloroethane; 2,2-bis(*para*-chlorophenyl)-1,1-dichloroethane; 2,2-bis(4-chlorophenyl)-1,1-dichloroethane; DDD; *para,para'*-DDD; 4,4'-DDD; 1,1-dichloro-2,2-bis(*para*-chlorophenyl)ethane; 1,1-dichloro-2,2-bis(4-chlorophenyl)ethane (IUPAC), dichlorodiphenyl dichloroethane; *para, para'*-dichlorodiphenyldichloroethane; *para, para'*-dichlorodiphenyl-2,2-dichloroethylene; **1,1'-(2,2-dichloroethylidene)-bis(4-chlorobenzene)**; TDE
ortho,para' -TDE	53-19-0	**1-Chloro-2-[2,2-dichloro-1-(4-chlorophenyl)ethyl]-benzene**; 2-(2-chlorophenyl)-2-(4-chlorophenyl-1,1-dichloroethane; *ortho,para'*-DDD; 1,1-dichloro-2-(*ortho*-chlorophenyl)-2-(*para*-chlorophenyl)ethane; 2,4'-dichlorodiphenyldichloroethane

Table 1 (contd)

Name	CAS Reg. Nos	Chem. Abstr. names[a] and synonyms
para,para'-DDE	72-55-9	**2,2-Bis(4-chlorophenyl)-1,1-dichloroethene**; 1,1-bis(*para*-chloro-phenyl)-2,2-dichloroethylene; 2,2-bis(4-chlorophenyl)-1,1-dichloro-ethylene; DDE; 4,4'-DDE; 1,1-dichloro-2,2-bis(*para*-chloro-phenyl)-ethylene; *para,para'*-dichlorodiphenyldichloroethylene; 1,1-dichloro-2,2-di(4-chlorophenyl)ethylene (IUPAC); **1,1'-(dichloro-ethenylidene)-bis(4-chlorobenzene)**

[a]In bold

$C_{14}H_9Cl_5$ (*para,para'*-DDT)   Mol. wt: 354.5

$C_{14}H_9Cl_5$ (*ortho,para'*-DDT)   Mol. wt: 354.5

$C_{14}H_{10}Cl_4$ (*para,para'*-TDE)   Mol. wt: 320.0

$C_{14}H_{10}Cl_4$ (*ortho,para'*-TDE)   Mol. wt: 320.0

$C_{14}H_8Cl_4$ (*para,para'*-DDE)   Mol. wt: 318.0

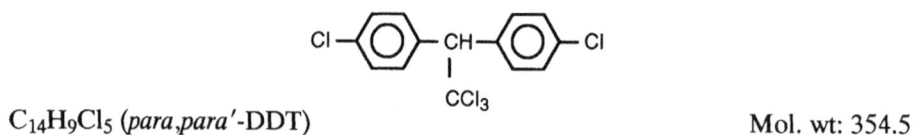

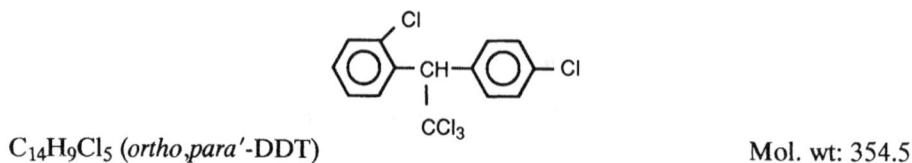

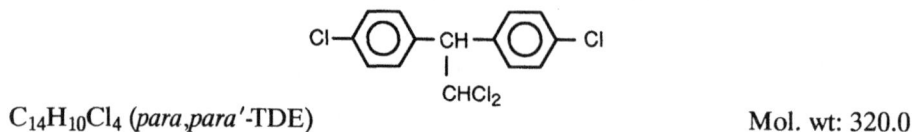

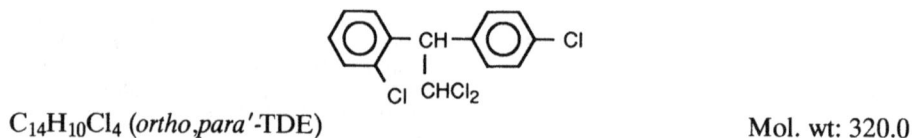

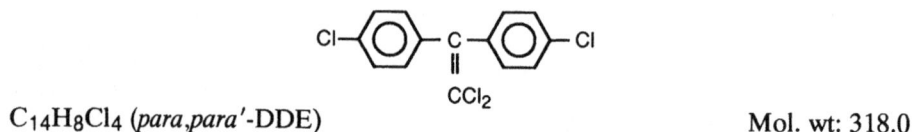

1.1.2 *Chemical and physical properties*

From Agency for Toxic Substances and Disease Registry (1989), unless otherwise noted

para,para'-DDT

(a) *Description*: Colourless crystalline solid, odourless or with weak aromatic odour
(b) *Boiling-point*: 260°C
(c) *Melting-point*: 108-109°C

(d) *Spectroscopy data*: Infrared (prism [27, 127, 15542]; grating [15014, 36866]), ultraviolet [47, 4655, 36806] and nuclear magnetic resonance (proton [15, V620, 23171, 34386]; C-13 [2410, 4401]) spectral data have been reported (Sadtler Research Laboratories, 1980, 1990).

(e) *Solubility*: Practically insoluble in water (0.0034 mg/l at 25°C); at 27-30°C, soluble in acetone (58 g/100 ml), benzene (78 g/100 ml), cyclohexanone (116 g/100 ml), diethyl ether (28 g/100 ml) (Budavari, 1989), chloroform (96 g/100 ml) (WHO, 1989) and other organic solvents (Brooks, 1974)

(f) *Volatility*: Vapour pressure, 5.5×10^{-6} mm Hg [0.73×10^{-6} kPa] at 20°C

(g) *Stability*: Stable to oxidation; corrosive to iron; dehydrochlorinated at temperatures above its melting point to the non-insecticidal DDE, a reaction catalysed by iron (III) or aluminium chlorides, by ultraviolet light and, in solution, by alkali (Worthing & Walker, 1987)

(h) *Octanol/water partition coefficient (P)*: log P, 6.19

(i) *Conversion factor for airborne concentrations*[1]: $mg/m^3 = 14.5 \times ppm$

ortho,para'-DDT

(a) *Description*: White, crystalline solid (WHO, 1989)

(b) *Melting-point*: 74-75°C

(c) *Spectroscopy data*: Infrared (prism [46974]; grating [31974]), ultraviolet [23375] and nuclear magnetic resonance (proton [19449]) spectral data have been reported (Sadtler Research Laboratories, 1980).

(d) *Solubility*: Slightly soluble in water (0.085 mg/l at 25°C); soluble in lipids and most organic solvents (IARC, 1974)

(e) *Volatility*: Vapour pressure, 5.5×10^{-6} mm Hg [0.73×10^{-6} kPa] at 30°C (Brooks, 1974)

(f) *Stability*: Stable to concentrated sulfuric acid (IARC, 1974)

(g) *Conversion factor for airborne concentrations*[1]: $mg/m^3 = 14.5 \times ppm$

para,para'-TDE

(a) *Description*: Colourless, odourless crystalline solid

(b) *Boiling-point*: 193°C at 1 mm Hg [0.13 kPa]

(c) *Melting-point*: 109-110°C

(d) *Spectroscopy data*: Infrared (prism [18450]; grating [36636]), ultraviolet [5898] and nuclear magnetic resonance (proton [2040]; C-13 [1284]) spectral data have been reported (Sadtler Research Laboratories, 1980).

(e) *Solubility*: Slightly soluble in water (0.160 mg/l at 25°C)

(f) *Volatility*: Vapour pressure, 10.2×10^{-7} mm Hg [1.36×10^{-7} kPa] at 30°C

(g) *Stability*: Similar to that of *para,para'*-DDT but more slowly hydrolysed by alkalis (IARC, 1974)

(h) *Octanol/water partition coefficient (P)*: log P, 6.20

(i) *Conversion factor for airborne concentrations*[1]: $mg/m^3 = 13.09 \times ppm$

---

[1]Calculated from: $mg/m^3 = $ (molecular weight/24.45) $\times$ ppm, assuming standard temperature (25°C) and pressure (760 mm Hg [101.3 kPa])

ortho,para'-TDE

    (*a*) *Description*: Colourless crystals

    (*b*) *Melting-point*: 76-78°C

    (*c*) *Conversion factor for airborne concentrations*[1]: mg/m^3 = 13.09 × ppm

para,para'-DDE

    (*a*) *Description*: White, crystalline solid

    (*b*) *Melting-point*: 88.4-90°C

    (*c*) *Spectroscopy data*: Infrared (prism [27905]; grating [3631]), ultraviolet [10847] and nuclear magnetic resonance (proton [498]; C-13 [6360]) spectral data have been reported (Sadtler Research Laboratories, 1980)

    (*d*) *Solubility*: Slightly soluble in water (0.12 mg/l at 25°C); soluble in lipids and most organic solvents (IARC, 1974)

    (*e*) *Volatility*: Vapour pressure, 6.5 × 10^{-6} mm Hg [0.87 × 10^{-6} kPa] at 20°C

    (*f*) *Stability*: Stable to concentrated sulfuric acid; may be oxidized to *para,para'*-dichlorobenzophenone, catalysed by ultraviolet radiation (IARC, 1974)

    (*g*) *Octanol/water partition coefficient (P)*: log P, 7.00

    (*h*) *Conversion factor for airborne concentrations*[1]: mg/m^3 = 13.01 × ppm

1.1.3 *Trade names, technical products and impurities*

    Some examples of trade names are:

***para,para'*-DDT**: Aavero-extra; Agritan; Anofex; Arkotine; Azotox M 33; Benzochloryl; Bosan supra; Bovidermol; Chlorophenothane; Chlorphenotoxum; Citox; Clofenotane; Deoval; Detox; Detoxan; Dibovin; Dicophane; Dinocide; Dodat; Dykol; ENT-1506; Estonate; Genitox; Gesafid; Gesarol; Guesapon; Guesarol; Gyron; Hildit; Ivoran; Ixodex; Mutoxan; Neocid; Neocidol; Parachlorocidum; PEB1; Pentachlorin; Penticidum; Zerdane

    ***para,para'*-TDE**: Dilene; ME 1700; Rhothane

    ortho,para'-TDE: Chloditan; Mitotan; CB313; Lysodren

    The WHO specification for technical DDT intended for use in public health programmes requires that the product contain 49-51% total organic chlorine, 9.5-11.5% hydrolysable chlorine and a minimum of 70% *para,para'*-DDT (WHO, 1985).

    A typical sample of technical DDT had the following constituents: *para,para'*-DDT, 77.1%; *ortho,para'*-DDT, 14.9%; *para,para'*-TDE, 0.3%; *ortho,para'*-TDE, 0.1%; *para,para'*-DDE, 4%, *ortho,para'*-DDE, 0.1%; and unidentified products, 3.5% (WHO, 1989). Another analysis showed the following approximate composition (%): *para,para'*-DDT, 63-77; *ortho,para'*-DDT, 8-21; *para,para'*-TDE, 0.3-4.0; *ortho,para'*-TDE, 0.04; 1-(*ortho*-chlorophenyl)ethyl-2-trichloro-*para*-chlorobenzene sulfonate, 0.1-1.9; 2-trichloro-1-(*para*-chlorophenyl)ethanol, 0.2; bis(*para*-chlorophenyl)sulfone, 0.03-0.6; α-chloro-α-(*para*-chlorophenyl)acetamide, 0.01; α-chloro-α-(chlorophenyl) acetamide, 0.01; chlorobenzene, 0.3; *para*-dichlorobenzene (see IARC, 1987b), 0.1; 1,1,1,2-tetrachloro-2-(*para*-chlorophenyl)-ethane, trace; sodium *para*-chlorobenzenesulfonate, 0.02; ammonium *para*-chlorobenzene-

---

[1]Calculated from: mg/m^3 = (molecular weight/24.45) × ppm, assuming standard temperature (25°C) and pressure (760 mm Hg [101.3 kPa])

sulfonate, 0.01; inorganics, 0.01-0.1; and unidentified components and losses, 5.1-10.6 (Bhuiya & Rothwell, 1969).

Technical DDT has been formulated in almost every conceivable form, including solutions in xylene (see IARC, 1989a) and petroleum distillates (see IARC, 1989b), emulsifiable concentrates, water-wettable powders, granules, aerosols, smoke candles, charges for vaporizers and lotions. Aerosols and other household formulations are often combined with synergized pyrethrins (WHO, 1989).

Technical TDE has been formulated as solutions in aromatic solvents, wettable powders and dusts (Brooks, 1974).

1.1.4 *Analysis*

Selected methods for the analysis of DDT and its metabolites in various media are summarized in Table 2. Reviews of analytical methods for DDT and metabolites in various media have been reported (Brooks, 1974; Horwitz, 1975a,b,c,d; WHO, 1979; Williams, 1984a; Rovinsky *et al.*, 1988; Agency for Toxic Substances and Disease Registry, 1989).

Table 2. Methods for the analysis of DDT and metabolites

Sample matrix	Sample preparation	Assay procedure[a]	Limit of detection[b]	Reference
Air	Collect vapours on glass-fibre filter with polyurethane foam; extract with 5% ether in hexane	GC/ECD	> 1 ng/m^3	US Environmental Protection Agency (1988a)
	Collect vapours on polyurethane foam; extract with 5% diethyl ether in hexane	GC/ECD	NR	US Environmental Protection Agency (1988b)
	Collect vapours on glass-fibre filter; extract with isooctane	GC/ECD	NR	Taylor (1977)
Water	Extract with dichloromethane; isolate extract, dry and concentrate with methyl *tert*-butyl ether	GC/ECD	0.0025, 0.01, 0.06 μg/l	US Environmental Protection Agency (1988c)
Waste-water	Extract with dichloromethane; dry; exchange into hexane	GC/ECD	0.011, 0.004, 0.012 μg/l	US Environmental Protection Agency (1986a, 1989a)
	Extract with dichloromethane; dry and concentrate (packed column)	GC/MS	2.8, 5.6 4.7 μg/l	US Environmental Protection Agency (1989b)
Formulations	Extract with carbon disulfide and sodium sulfate; compare with reference spectrum at 9.4-10.2 μm	IR	NR	Williams (1984b)
Food (high moisture, non-fatty)	Blend with acetone; extract with petroleum ether/dichloromethane; dry; concentrate in petroleum ether and acetone	GC/HECD	NR	Williams (1985)

Table 2 (contd)

Sample matrix	Sample preparation	Assay procedure[a]	Limit of detection[b]	Reference
Soil, sediment, wastes	Mix with anhydrous sodium sulfate; extract using Soxhlet or sonication; clean-up using Florisil column or gel-permeation (packed column)	GC/MS	2.8, 5.6, 4.7 µg/l	US Environmental Protection Agency (1986b)
	Mix with anhydrous sodium sulfate; extract using Soxhlet or sonication; clean-up using Florisil column or gel-permeation (capillary column)	GC/MS	NR	US Environmental Protection Agency (1986c)

[a]Abbreviations: GC/ECD, gas chromatography/electron capture detection; GC/HECD, gas chromatography/ Hall electrolytic conductivity detector; GC/MS, gas chromatography/mass spectrometry; IR, infrared spectroscopy
[b]The limits of detection are presented for 4,4'-TDE, 4,4'-DDE and 4,4'-DDT, respectively; NR, not reported

1.2 Production and use

The discovery, chemistry and uses of DDT and problems associated with its use have been reviewed (Brooks, 1974; Mellanby, 1989).

1.2.1 *Production*

Technical-grade DDT is made by condensing chloral hydrate with chlorobenzene in the presence of sulfuric acid. To prepare *ortho,para'*-DDT, an excess of chlorobenzene is condensed with 1-(2-chlorophenyl)-2,2,2-trichloroethanol in the presence of a mixture of 96% sulfuric acid and 25% oleum at 60°C (Brooks, 1974).

DDT was first synthesized in 1874, but it was not until 1939 that its insecticidal properties were discovered. By 1943, low-cost production methods had been developed, and commercial production had begun. At the height of DDT production, about 400 000 tonnes were used annually worldwide, but this decreased to approximately 200 000 tonnes in 1971. Peak production in the USA occurred in 1963, when 80 000 tonnes were produced. After restrictions were introduced in the USA in 1969 (Brooks, 1974), production of DDT in 1971 in that country was estimated to be 2000 tonnes. In 1985, approximately 300 tonnes of DDT were exported. In 1989, there were three producers, but no data were available on the current production of DDT in the USA (Agency for Toxic Substances and Disease Registry, 1989). DDT is produced currently by one company each in Italy, India and Indonesia (Meister, 1990) and in China.

TDE was introduced commercially in Germany in 1945 under the trade name Rhothane. The commercial preparation of TDE from the ethyl acetal of dichloroacetaldehyde and chlorobenzene usually gives a technical product consisting mainly of the *para,para'*-isomer, with 7-8% of the *ortho,para'*-isomer (Brooks, 1974; IARC, 1974).

1.2.2 *Use*

DDT is a nonsystemic contact and stomach insecticide with a broad spectrum of insecticidal activity (Worthing & Walker, 1987). DDT has been used primarily in the prevention of malaria, yellow fever and sleeping sickness. In 1971, approximately 50% of production was used for these purposes (IARC, 1974).

DDT was used extensively for the control of malaria, typhus and other insect-transmitted disease during the Second World War. It has been used worldwide in agriculture in the control of insects. In 1972, 4500-6400 tonnes of DDT were used in the USA; use on cotton crops was estimated to account for 67-90% of the total use, with the remainder primarily on peanut and soya bean crops. Since 1973, use of DDT in the USA has been limited to the control of public health problems. It was estimated in 1973 that more than 2 million tonnes of DDT had been used for insect control since 1940, about 80% of that in agriculture. DDT was once registered for use on 334 commodities in the USA (Agency for Toxic Substances and Disease Registry, 1989).

Even before 1963, some restrictions had been placed on the use of DDT, mainly to minimize residues in food and in the feed of animals that produce milk and meat. Another important reason for reducing the use of DDT was the increasing resistance of pests. Although many pests of public health importance became resistant to DDT in some or all of their range, resistance among vectors of malaria was less marked. Because malaria control constitutes such a large segment of vector control, the use of DDT for vector control has tended to remain stable, while its use in agriculture has continued to decline, especially in temperate climates (WHO, 1979).

DDT was introduced in India for use in public health and agriculture in 1948. Since then, nearly 250 000 tonnes have been used, of which only 50 000 tonnes were in agriculture. The use of DDT in India over a 20-year period is given in Table 3 (Mehrotra, 1985). India banned the use of DDT for agricultural purposes in 1989 (County NatWest WoodMac, 1990).

Table 3. Total use of DDT (in thousands of tonnes) in India during 1960-84[a]

Type of use	1960	1966	1970	1975	1976	1977	1978	1979	1980	1984
Public health	21.0	2.7	6.2	7.3	7.3	9.0	6.8	6.5	8.5	12.0
Agriculture	0.6	2.4	2.4	2.5	1.3	2.5	4.7	4.2	4.0	2.0

[a]From Mehrotra (1985)

About 12 000 tonnes of DDT were used in Iraq by the agricultural authorities between 1960 and 1978 (Al-Omar et al., 1985). In Pakistan, the yearly agricultural use of DDT (active ingredient) during the period 1977-81 ranged from 40 to 100 tonnes (Baloch, 1985). In one province in Indonesia, a large-scale malaria control programme was begun in 1952. Between 1952 and 1980, yearly usage of DDT (active ingredient) was as high as [1400 tonnes] [calculated by the Working Group from a graph] (Bang et al., 1982).

TDE is a nonsystemic contact and stomach insecticide, which does not have the broad-spectrum insecticidal activity of DDT but has equal or greater potency against the larvae of some mosquitoes and lepidoptera (Brooks, 1974). It has had limited use as a pesticide (Agency for Toxic Substances and Disease Registry, 1989). In 1971, 110 tonnes of TDE were used by farmers in the USA, 67% of which was on tobacco (US National Cancer Institute, 1978).

The pure *ortho,para'*-TDE isomer, which must be specially synthesized, has been used in the treatment of adrenocortical carcinoma (Bergenstal *et al.*, 1960) and of the overproduction of adrenal cortical steroids (Wallace *et al.*, 1961; Bledsoe *et al.*, 1964; Southern *et al.*, 1966).

1.3 Occurrence

The physiochemical properties of DDT and its metabolites enable organisms to take them up readily. As these compounds are resistant to breakdown, they are readily adsorbed by sediments and soils, which can act as both sinks and long-term sources of exposure. Organisms can accumulate these chemicals from the surrounding medium and from food. Uptake from water is generally more important for aquatic organisms, whereas food provides the major source in terrestrial fauna.

Earlier data on occurrence were summarized in the previous monograph on DDT (IARC, 1974). Environmental aspects of DDT and its derivatives were reviewed (WHO, 1989). The occurrence of DDT and its metabolites in human tissues and fluids is discussed in section 4.1.1.

1.3.1 *Soil*

The absorption of DDT was greatest in muck soil and least in sandy loam soil and was closely related to the organic matter content of the soil, the major fraction identified with absorption being the humic material. The degree of sorption is strongly associated with the degree of humidification (WHO, 1989).

After application to the soil surface, 50% of DDT was lost within 16-20 days, with an estimated time for 90% loss of 1.5-2 years. When it was mixed into the soil, the half-time of DDT was 5-8 years, and it was estimated that 90% would be lost in 25-40 years (Wheatley, 1965).

In a study to determine the ability of river sediments to degrade DDT, labelled material was added to sediments in the laboratory or on mud flats in the United Kingdom. Incubation *in situ* over 46 days led to very little metabolism of DDT; some *para,para'*-TDE was produced, but metabolism did not proceed further. In the laboratory, however, a greater amount of degradation occurred over 21 days. Investigations of the microbial population of the sediment showed that some organisms were capable of degrading DDT (Albone *et al.*, 1972).

When cotton plants in Kenya were sprayed at 1.05 or 2.52 kg active ingredient/ha, and soil and leaf samples were taken, the half-times for *para,para'*-DDT in soil for the two rates were 18.5 and 2.2 days, respectively. The low persistence of surface-applied DDT in tropical climates represents a totally different situation from that reported for temperate climates. With a soil temperature of over 65°C by mid-afternoon, the loss was attributed to volatilization. Residues on cotton foliage had a similarly short half-time of 4.8 days. The metabolite *para,para'*-DDE was slightly more persistent, with a half-time of 8.8 days (Foxall & Maroko, 1984). In a review of DDT residues in Indian soils in cotton-growing areas, the half-time of DDT was about three months, as compared to 4-30 years in temperate regions (Mehrotra, 1985).

1.3.2 Plants

[14]C-Labelled DDT was applied to loam and sandy soils at 4 and 2 mg/kg and oats were grown in the treated soils for 13 days. Of the total DDT applied, 95% was recovered from the loam and 84% from the sandy soil, showing that little metabolism had taken place. DDE was detected in both soils, together with very small amounts of other metabolites. Very little DDT was detected in oat roots grown on loam (0.2%); uptake was greater (4.6%) in the roots of oats grown on sand. No label was detected in the plant tops (Fuhremann & Lichtenstein, 1980).

DDT was not translocated into foliage of alfalfa after application to soil (Ware *et al.*, 1970), or into soya beans (Eden & Arthur, 1965). Only trace amounts of DDT or its metabolites were found in stored carrots, radishes and turnips which had been grown in soils containing up to 15 mg/kg DDT (Harris & Sans, 1967).

1.3.3 Food

Residues were found in 36 of 1535 samples analysed for DDT as part of a Canadian national surveillance programme in 1984-89. The highest levels were found in carrots (12/75 samples), cheese (10/94) and grapes (7/129). The levels ranged from 0.01 to a maximum of 0.6 mg/kg (Government of Canada, 1990).

In Brazil, the average levels of DDT in 1998 samples of cattle meat were 0.04-0.13 mg/kg, those in 102 samples of horse meat, 0.01-0.02 mg/kg and those in corned beef and roast beef, 0.03-0.04 mg/kg (Codex Committee on Pesticide Residues, 1989).

para,para'-DDE was detected in 408 of 19 851 food and animal feed samples analysed in the USA during the period 1982-86; 288 samples contained less than 0.05 mg/kg (maximum, 2.0 mg/kg) (Luke *et al.*, 1988).

1.3.4 Fish

Small fish take up more DDT from water than larger fish of the same species: a range in weight of mosquito fish between 70 and 1000 mg led to a four-fold difference in DDT uptake over 48 h (Murphy, 1971).

Rainbow trout were exposed to concentrations of DDT in water of 176, 137 and 133 ng/l at 5, 10 and 15°C, respectively. Whole-body residues of DDT after 12 weeks of exposure were 3.8, 5.9 and 6.8 mg/kg for the three temperatures, indicating increased uptake by fish with temperature (WHO, 1989).

Fish accumulate DDT from food in a dose-dependent manner. Rainbow trout fed diets containing 0.2 or 1.0 mg/kg DDT retained more than 90% of the dietary intake over a 90-day exposure. The time for 50% elimination was estimated at 160 days. There was a straight-line relationship between exposure time and body burden of total DDT, with no tendency for residues to reach a plateau within 45 days of feeding. The fish had accumulated 1.1 μg/kg from food containing 0.58 μg/kg DDT, 11 μg/kg from food containing 9.0 μg/kg and 110 μg/kg from food containing 93 μg/kg at the end of the experiment (WHO, 1989).

1.4 Regulations and guidelines

Sweden was the first country to ban the use of DDT, in 1970 (WHO, 1979). Many other countries subsequently restricted its use, although DDT continues to be used in some circumstances, for the control of vector-borne diseases.

DDT and its metabolites were included in the 1987 Canadian guidelines for drinking-water quality for re-evaluation; the 1978 maximum acceptable concentration was 30 µg/l (Ritter & Wood, 1989).

The FAO/WHO Joint Meeting on Pesticide Residues evaluated DDT at its meetings in 1963, 1965, 1966, 1967, 1968, 1969, 1977, 1979, 1980, 1983 and 1984 (FAO/WHO, 1964, 1965, 1967a,b, 1968a,b, 1969, 1970a,b, 1978, 1980a,b, 1981, 1984, 1985). In 1963, an acceptable daily intake in food of 0.005 mg/kg bw was established (FAO/WHO, 1964); this was raised to 0.01 mg/kg bw in 1965. In 1967, the level was extended to metabolites. The acceptable daily intake was lowered to 0.005 mg/kg bw in 1969 and was raised to 0.02 mg/kg bw in 1984 (FAO/WHO, 1985).

Maximum residue levels were established by the Codex Alimentarius Commission for DDT (as the sum of *para,para'*-DDT, *ortho,para'*-DDT, *para,para'*-DDE and *para,para'*-TDE (fat-soluble residue)) in or on the following (in mg/kg): meat (fat), 5; fruit and vegetables, 1; eggs, 0.5; cereal grains, 0.1; milks, 0.05 (Codex Committee on Pesticide Residues, 1990).

National and regional pesticide residue limits for DDT and its metabolites in foods are presented in Table 4. Table 5 presents occupational exposure limits and guidelines for DDT in some countries. The maximum allowable concentrations in the USSR are 0.001 mg/m^3 for average daily exposure to DDT in the atmospheric air of populated areas, 0.005 mg/m^3 for a single exposure in the same areas, 0.1 mg/l for DDT in water for drinking and domestic purposes and 1 mg/kg for DDT in soil (Izmerov, 1983).

Table 4. National and regional pesticide residue limits for DDT in foods[a]

Country or region	Residue limits (mg/kg)	Commodities
Australia	5	Fat (meat, poultry)
	1.25	Goat milk (fat basis), milk (fat basis), milk products (fat basis)
	1	Edible oils, fish, fruit, margarine, vegetables
	0.5	Eggs
	0.1	Cereal grains
Austria	3[b]	Fish
	1.0[b]	Cocoa nibs, spices, tea, tea-like products, unroasted coffee
	0.5[b]	Eggs (without shell), other foodstuffs of animal origin
	0.1[b]	Oilseeds
Belgium	1[c]	Meat, poultry, hare, fowl, game, meat products, animal fats
	0.1[c]	Eggs, fruit, vegetables
	0.04[c]	Milk and milk products
	0 (0.05)[c,d]	Other foodstuffs of animal and vegetable origin
Canada	5[e]	Fish
	1.0	Butter, cheese, milk and other dairy products, meat, fat and meat by-products (cattle, hogs, poultry, sheep)
	0.5	Eggs, fresh vegetables

Table 4 (contd)

Country or region	Residue limits (mg/kg)	Commodities
Chile	7^c	Apples, carcasses (fat), garden vegetables, peaches, pears, poultry (fat)
	3.5	Cherries, citrus fruit, plums
	1.25	Milk and dairy products (fat)
	1.0	Vegetables (root, tuber)
	0.5	Eggs
China	≤ 1.0	Fish (including other seafood products)
	≤ 0.2	Processed foodstuffs
	≤ 0.1	Fruit, vegetables
Czechoslovakia	2^e	Animal fats (fat basis), fish, meat
	1.25	Milk and milk products (fat basis) (imported)
	0.5	Eggs (without shell) (imported and domestic)
	0.4	Milk and milk products (fat basis)
	0.1	Fruit, potatoes, vegetables
Denmark	5^c	Fish liver
	2	Fish and fish products
	1	Fat from meat
	0.5	Eggs
	0.2	Berries and small fruit, carrots, fruit (citrus, pome, stone, other), onions, potatoes, vegetables (leafy, other root)
	0.05	Cereals
	0.04	Milk, milk products, dairy products
European Community	1.0^b	Fat contained in meat, preparations of meat, offal and animal fats
	0.1	Other crop and food products
	0.05	Barley, buckwheat, grain sorghum, maize, millet, oats, paddy rice, rye, triticale, wheat, other cereals
	0.04	Raw cows' milk and whole-cream cows' milk
Finland	3^c	Codliver oil
	0.5	Crustaceans, fish, shellfish and their products (excluding codliver oil), other crops and food products
	0.1	Cereal grains
France	0.1^c	Fruit, vegetables
	0.05^c	Cereal grains
Germany	10^b	Tobacco products
	5^f	Fish liver and roe products
	3.5	Eel, salmon and sturgeon, as well as products thereof (except roe)
	2^g	Other fish and other cold-blooded animals, seafood as well as products thereof (except liver and roe)
	1.0	Meat, meat products, edible animal fats (fat basis)
	1.0^b	Spices, raw coffee, tea, tea-like products
	1.0^f	Milk, dairy products
	0.5^f	Eggs (without shell), egg products
	0.1^f	Citrus juice, fruit, oilseed, vegetables
	0.05^g	Other foodstuffs of plant origin
Hungary	0.1^c	Crops, food

Table 4 (contd)

Country or region	Residue limits (mg/kg)	Commodities
India	7^h	Fish, meat, poultry (whole product)
	3.5^h	Fruit, vegetables (including potatoes)
	1.25^h	Milk, milk products (fat basis)
	0.5^h	Eggs (without shell)
Ireland	0.1^c	All crop and food products
Israel	3	Apples, apricots, carcass meat (in fat), cherries, fruit (citrus, tropical), peaches, pears, plums, other small fruit not mentioned in list (except strawberries), poultry (in fat), vegetables
	0.25	Milk products (fat basis)
	1.0	Cottonseed, nuts (shelled), strawberries
	0.5	Eggs (without shell)
	0.05	Milk (fat basis)
Italy	$1.0^{c,i}$	Aromatic and medicinal herbs, tea
	0.1	Coffee, fruit, garden vegetables
Japan	0.2	Apples, asparagus, baby kidney beans, baby peas, burdock, cabbage, cauliflower, celery, cherries, Chinese white cabbage, cucumbers, eggplant, garden radish, garden radish leaves, grapes, Irish potatoes, lettuce, loquats, mandarins, oranges, peaches, pears (Bartlett, Japanese), persimmon, pumpkin, soft greens, Spanish paprika, spinach, strawberries, summer oranges (peel, pulp), sweet potatoes, taro, tea, tomatoes, trefoil, turnip, turnip leaves, watermelons, white muskmelons
Kenya	7	Apples, apricots, meat (fat basis), peaches, pears, poultry (fat basis), small fruit (except strawberries), vegetables (except root)
	3.5	Cherries, fruit (citrus, tropical), plums
	1.25	Milk products (fat basis)
	1.0	Maize, millet, nuts (shelled), root vegetables, sorghum, strawberries, sunflower seeds (entire), wheat grain
	0.5	Eggs (without shell), whole milk
Luxembourg	5^j	Fish eggs, liver products
	3.5^j	Eel, salmon and sturgeon and derived products (except fish eggs)
	3^j	Animal fats (except butyric fats), meat and meat products, poultry and poultry products
	2^j	Other fish, crustaceans, molluscs and derived products (except fish eggs and liver)
	1.25^j	Milk and milk products
	0.5^j	Eggs (without shell), animal fats and fish meal (used as animal feed)
	0.2^j	Other foodstuffs (used as animal feed)
	0.1^j	Vegetable fats (used as animal feed), supplementary feed for lactating animals
	0.05	Natural foods (used as animal feed)
	0.03	Cereals (used as animal feed)

Table 4 (contd)

Country or region	Residue limits (mg/kg)	Commodities
Mexico	7	Beans, chili peppers, grapes, lettuce, pineapples, tomatoes
	6	Soya bean oil (processed)
	4	Cottonseed
	3.5	Avocado, carrots, citrus fruit, maize, papayas
	1.5	Soya beans
	1.0	Artichokes, asparagus, broccoli, cabbage, celery, okra, onions, potatoes, radishes, spinach, sweet potatoes
	0.5	Apples, cucumbers, eggplant, guavas, mangoes, melons, peaches, peanuts, pears, peas, squash, strawberries
Netherlands	5[c]	Eggs (fat basis)
	1[c]	Meat, poultry meat, other animal products (fat basis), tea
	0.5[c]	Cocoa butter (wring/refined)
	0.1[c]	Fruit, plant oil and fat, vegetables, tropical seed (fat basis)
	0.05[c]	Other foodstuffs
	0.04[c]	Milk
	0.02[c]	Other cocoa (fat basis)
New Zealand	5[e]	Meat fat in any foodstuff
	2[e]	Fruit, vegetables
	1.25[e]	Milk fat in any foodstuff
	0.5[e]	Eggs
Peru	7[h]	Fruit (drupe, pome), meat (fat basis), poultry (fat basis)
	3.5[h]	Fruit (citrus, tropical)
	1.25[h]	Milk and milk products (fat basis)
	1.0[h]	Walnuts (shelled)
	0.5[h]	Eggs (without shell)
Romania	5	Meat (cattle, goats, sheep)
	3	Meat (pigs, poultry)
	1.25	Milk and milk products
Singapore	0.2	Fat (cattle, hogs, sheep), other foodstuffs
	0.005	Milk
South Africa	3[c]	Carcass meat (fat basis)
	0.5[c]	Eggs (without shell)
	0.05[c]	Milk (fat basis)
Spain	1.0[c]	Coffee, spices, tea and similar products
	0.1[c]	Fruit, vegetables (except potatoes)
	0.05[c]	Potatoes, other plant products
Sweden	5[c]	Fishery products
	1.0[c]	Butter, cheese, fruit, vegetables
	0.5[c]	Eggs, raw meat
	0.05[c]	Cereals and hulled grain, flakes and flour made from cereals, milk, potatoes

Table 4 (contd)

Country or region	Residue limits (mg/kg)	Commodities
Switzerland	1.0[c]	Meat and meat products (except fish and fish-based products (fat basis)), tea and tea plants
	0.5[c]	Eggs
	0.25[c]	Cocoa butter and bulk cocoa (fat basis)
	0.125[c]	Milk and milk products (fat basis)
	0.1[c]	Cereal, fruit, vegetables
	0.01[c]	Cereal products
	0.02[c]	Infant and baby foods (as consumed); other products [limit value, 0.06]
	0.005[c]	Infant and baby foods (as consumed); milk products [limit value, 0.015]
Thailand	7	Fruit
	6	Fat and oil from animals and vegetables
	5	Aquatic animal products, meat
	2	Vegetables
	1.5	Eggs, pulses
	1.0	Milks
	0.5	Cereals
United Kingdom	1[b]	Bananas, oranges, other citrus, meat, fat and preparations of meats (fat basis), dairy produce (> 2% fat)
	0.5	Eggs (birds' eggs in shell (other than eggs for hatching) and whole egg products and egg yolk products (whether fresh, dried or otherwise prepared))
	0.1	Apples, blackcurrants, beans, Brussels' sprouts, cabbage, carrots, celery, cauliflower, cucumbers, grapes, leeks, lettuce, mushrooms, nectarines, onions, peaches, pears, peas, plums, potatoes, raspberries, strawberries, swedes, tomatoes, turnips
	0.05	Barley, maize, oats, paddy rice, rye, wheat, other cereals
	0.04	Milk (fresh raw cows' milk and fresh whole-cream cows' milk expressed as whole milk)
USA[k]	5	Fat of meat (cattle, goats, hogs, horses, sheep), fish
	3	Carrots
	1.25	Manufactured dairy products
	1.0	Beans (cocoa, whole raw), peppermint oil, potatoes, soya bean oil (crude), spearmint oil, sweet potatoes
	0.5	Artichokes, asparagus, barley grain (food, feed), broccoli, Brussels' sprouts, cabbage, cauliflower, celery, collards, eggs, endives (escarole), hay, kale, kohlrabi, lettuce, maize grain (food, feed), milo sorghum grain (food, feed), mushrooms, mustard greens, oat grain (food, feed), peppermint hay, rice grain (food, feed), rye grain (food, feed), spearmint hay, spinach, Swiss chard, tomato pomace (dried, for use in dog and cat food), wheat grain (food, feed)
	0.2	Apricots, avocadoes, beans, beans (dried), beets (roots, tops), cherries, guavas, mangoes, nectarines, okra, onions (dry bulb), papayas, parsnips (roots, tops), peaches, peanuts, peas, pineapples, plums (fresh prunes), radishes (roots, tops), rutabagas (roots, tops), soya beans, (dry), turnips (roots, tops)

Table 4 (contd)

Country or region		Residue limits (mg/kg)	Commodities
USA (contd)		0.1	Apples, blackberries, blueberries (huckleberries), boysenberries, citrus fruit, maize (fresh sweet plus cob with husk removed), cottonseed, cranberries, cucumbers, currants, dewberries, eggplant, gooseberries, hops (fresh), loganberries, melons, pears, peppers, pumpkins, quinces, raspberries, squash, squash (summer), strawberries, youngberries
		0.05	Grapes, hops (dried), tomatoes, lettuces
USSR	DDT	0.7	Tobacco products
		0.5	Fruit, vegetables
		Not permitted	All other food products including milk, meat, butter, eggs, garden strawberries and raspberries
	TDE	7	Fruits, vegetables
		3.5	Grain
Yugoslavia		2.0[e]	Vegetable oil (refined, unrefined) and their products (fat basis)
		1.0[e]	Venison, fish (fat basis)
		0.5[e]	Meat and meat products (cattle, hogs, poultry, sheep (fat basis), milk and milk products (fat basis)
		0.1[e]	Eggs (without shell) and egg products, fruit, vegetables, other food commodities
		0.03[e]	Cereals
		0.01[e]	Processed cereals

[a]From Health and Welfare Canada (1990)
[b]DDT, DDE, TDE and their isomers (total calculated as DDT)
[c]Sum of *para,para'*-DDT, *ortho,para'*-DDT, *para,para'*-DDE and *para,para'*-TDE
[d]Residues should not be present; the value in parentheses indicates the lower limit for residue determination according to the standard method of analysis, this limit having being used to reach the no-residue conclusion
[e]Including TDE and DDE
[f]TDE and isomers
[g]DDE (total calculated as DDT)
[h]Limits apply to DDT, TDE and DDE singly or in any combination
[i]Active substance revoked; EEC value for fruit and garden vegetables
[j]DDT, TDE, DDE (singly or combined, expressed as DDT)
[k]Recommended action levels, tolerances revoked (US Food and Drug Administration, 1990)

WHO (1984) recommended a guideline value of 1 µg/l for DDT (total isomers) in drinking-water, and the US Environmental Protection Agency (1980) established an ambient water quality criteria for DDT of 2.85 µg/l.

Table 5. Occupational exposure limits for DDT[a]

Country	Year	Concentration (mg/m^3)	Interpretation[b]
Austria	1987	1 (s)[c]	TWA
Belgium	1987	1	TWA
Bulgaria	1987	0.1	TWA
China	1987	0.3	TWA
Denmark	1988	1	TWA
Finland	1987	1 (s)	TWA
		3 (s)	STEL
Germany	1989	1 (s)	TWA
Hungary	1987	0.1 (s)	TWA
		0.5 (s)	STEL
India	1987	1	TWA
		3	STEL
Indonesia	1987	1 (s)	TWA
Italy	1987	1	TWA
Mexico	1987	1	TWA
Netherlands	1986	1	TWA
Poland	1987	0.1	TWA
Romania	1987	0.7 (s)	Average
		1 (s)	Maximum
Switzerland		1 (s)	TWA
United Kingdom	1987	1	TWA
		3	STEL (10 min)
USA			
ACGIH	1989	1	TWA
OSHA	1989	1 (s)	TWA
USSR	1987	0.1 (s)	MAC
Venezuela	1987	1	TWA
		3	Ceiling
Yugoslavia	1987	0.1 (s)	TWA

[a]From Arbeidsinspectie (1986); Cook (1987); Health and Safety Executive (1987); Työsuojeluhallitus (1987); Arbejdstilsynet (1988); American Conference of Governmental Industrial Hygienists (ACGIH) (1989); Deutsche Forschungsgemeinschaft (1989); US Occupational Safety and Health Administration (OSHA) (1989)
[b]MAC, maximum allowable concentration; TWA, time-weighted average; STEL, short-term exposure level
[c]Skin irritant notation

2. Studies of Cancer in Humans

2.1 Cohort studies

Venous blood samples were sought from 1708 adults in Charleston, SC, USA, enrolled in a prospective cohort study (Boyle, 1970; Keil *et al.*, 1984) in 1974-75 (468 white men, 602 white women, 310 black men and 328 black women) and were obtained for 919 subjects (304 white men, 327 white women, 204 black men and 84 black women) (Austin *et al.*, 1989).

para,para'-DDT and *para,para'*-DDE levels in the blood specimens were analysed, and total serum DDT was estimated; the mean serum DDT level was 48 ppb (μg/l) with a standard deviation of 36 ppb (μg/l). When the 919 subjects were traced through 1984, 209 were found to be deceased and 700 still alive; 10 were lost to follow-up. National and state age-, sex- and race-specific mortality rates for 1980 were used for external comparisons. In internal comparisons, the rates for persons in the upper (> 52 ppb) and middle (31-52 ppb) terciles of serum DDT levels were compared to those in the lowest tercile (0-31 ppb). These relative mortality rates were adjusted for differences in age, race, sex, years of schooling and smoking using a proportional hazards model. Mean levels were slightly higher among men than women (by 6%), among blacks than whites (by 14%) and among nonsmokers than smokers [% not given]. Compared to the general population, mortality from respiratory cancer was slightly higher among the cohort than expected (standardized mortality ratio (SMR), 1.2; 21 deaths; 95% confidence interval (CI), 0.76-1.9). Relative rates for total mortality by serum DDT levels were 1.2 (72 deaths; 0.8-1.7) for the middle tercile and 1.2 (80 deaths; 0.9-1.8) for the upper tercile (57 deaths for the lowest tercile). The trend was not significant. Relative mortality rates for respiratory cancer by tercile were 1.5 (7 deaths; 95% CI, 0.5-4.9) and 1.8 (7 deaths; 95% CI, 0.5-6.2) (5 deaths for the lowest tercile) with a non-significant trend.

Mortality was evaluated among workers employed at three manufacturing plants in Michigan and Arkansas, USA, and one research establishment in Michigan, where potential exposure to brominated chemicals existed (Wong *et al.*, 1984). Workers employed in the plants between 1935 and 1976 were identified from personnel records. Of the 3612 male workers identified, 33 were excluded because their dates of birth were not available, leaving 3579 for analysis (2806 alive as of 31 December 1976), 578 deceased (541 with death certificates) and 195 with unknown vital status. SMRs for the cohort were calculated using US white male rates to generate expected numbers. Race was not available on all employment records, but, according to the company, few blacks had worked at the plants. DDT had been produced at one time in one of the plants, and 740 workers were identified as having worked in DDT production departments. Mortality from all causes combined among these workers was about the same as expected (SMR, 0.99; 112 deaths; 95% CI, 0.82-1.2), as was mortality from all cancers (SMR, 0.95; 19 deaths; 95% CI, 0.57-1.5). Cancers for which the rates were slightly elevated, with more than one death, included leukaemia (SMR, 2.1; 2 deaths; 95% CI, 0.24-7.6) and lung (1.5; 9 deaths; 0.68-2.8). Many of the workers with potential exposure to DDT also had potential exposure to other chemicals, including inorganic brominated compounds. Information on smoking was not available for the entire cohort (see General Remarks for a discussion). In a nested case-control study of respiratory cancer, the 46 workers from the entire cohort who had died from respiratory cancer were each matched to two workers who had died from other causes (except cancer, nonmalignant respiratory disease or unknown causes) on plant, age at death and time of hiring. Information was sought on detailed work history and smoking history from employment records and other sources; information obtained on smoking was incomplete (20% were ascertained to be smokers, but no information was available on the remainder) and was not considered further. On the basis of detailed work histories, 10 cases and 25 controls were judged to have been exposed to DDT (odds ratio, 0.74 [95% CI, 0.3-1.7]).

Ditraglia *et al.* (1981) studied 354 workers at a plant in California, USA, that had produced DDT exclusively since 1947. (Three plants that produced other organochlorine pesticides were also studied, but the results presented here are restricted to the DDT plant.) All workers employed for at least six months prior to 31 December 1964 were included. Vital status as of 31 December 1976 was ascertained for 90% of the cohort: 278 were alive and 42 were dead; those whose vital status was unknown were assumed to be alive as of the closing date of the study. Mortality among the cohort was compared to that of US white males, adjusted for age and calendar time. Fewer cancers occurred than expected (SMR, 0.68; 6 deaths; 95% CI, 0.25-2.5). For respiratory cancer, an SMR of 1.3 was obtained (4 deaths, 95% CI, 0.34-3.2). Observed SMRs for all cancers combined by years since first employment at the plant were none for < 10 years, one (3.7 expected) for 10-19 years and five (3.8 expected) for 20 or more years.

Subjects enrolled in 1971-73 in a national programme to monitor the health effects of exposures to pesticides were followed to 1977 to ascertain mortality and morbidity (details of the design of this study are presented in the monograph on occupational exposures in spraying and application of insecticides, p. 62) (Morgan *et al.*, 1980). Blood samples were obtained from each of the 3669 volunteers on their entry into the study and analysed for serum DDT and DDE levels. The geometric mean for volunteers who developed cancer was similar to that of those who did not (43 ppb and 45 ppb, respectively). [Relative risks for cancer were not presented by serum DDT and DDE level.]

Cohort studies on DDT are summarized in Table 6.

Table 6. Cohort studies of populations exposed to DDT

Reference	Cancer site	No. of cases	Relative risk	95% CI	Comments
Austin *et al.* (1989)	Respiratory cancer	5 (low DDT) 7 (medium) 7 (high)	1.0 1.5 1.8	 0.5-4.9 0.5-6.2	Exposure levels based on serum levels of DDT (*p* for trend = 0.34) Respiratory cancer in total cohort: SMR, 1.2
Wong *et al.* (1984)	Lung Leukaemia [Lymphomas	9 2 1	1.5 2.1 0.7	0.68-2.8 0.24-7.6 0.0-5.8]	Workers at a DDT manufacturing plant; also exposed to other pesticides Nested case-control analysis gave odds ratio = 0.74 for DDT exposure
Ditraglia *et al.* (1981)	Respiratory system Lymphatic and haematopoietic system	4 0	1.3 -	0.34-3.2 -	Workers at a DDT manufacturing plant; no death from skin, brain, bladder cancer or leukaemia

2.2 Case-control studies

2.2.1 *Based on measured levels in tissues*

Caldwell *et al.* (1981) compared serum levels of DDT in 10 children with colorectal cancer diagnosed between 1974 and 1976 and 24 controls without a malignancy who had visited a health clinic. The cases were aged 14-19 years and the controls, 5-18 years. One case was deleted because no information on exposure could be found. The mean serum level of DDT was 65.6 ppb (µg/l) for the remaining cases and 28.3 ppb for the 24 controls. When two cases with very high levels (in excess of 200 ppb) were excluded, the mean level was 22.9 ppb.

Unger and Olsen (1980) analysed the levels of polychlorinated biphenyls and DDE in adipose tissue from people in Denmark who had died of cancer. In an extension of this study (Unger *et al.*, 1982), adipose tissue was obtained *post mortem* from 51 cancer cases and 63 noncancer cases between 1978 and 1980. Ten of the patients had died from cancer of the gut, 13 from lung cancer and the remainder from various other types. The controls had died of apoplexy (11), coronary or vascular disease (28) and various other diseases. Mean levels of DDE were higher (5.5 ppm) among the cancer cases than among the controls (3.4 ppm). Mean levels of polychlorinated biphenyls were also higher among the cancer cases than among the noncancer cases (10.2 ppm and 6.1 ppm, respectively). [The Working Group noted that it was difficult to separate the effects of the two compounds in the published reports.]

Breast fat tissue was obtained from 14 patients with breast cancer and 21 patients with other breast disorders who were undergoing breast surgery. Mean DDE levels were similar in the cancer cases (1.23 ppm) and the controls (1.25 ppm) (Unger *et al.*, 1984).

[Measurement of tissue levels of DDT provides information on individual exposure to DDT, but the Working Group was concerned that levels determined after diagnosis of cancer, particularly in serum, may be affected by the disease process.]

2.2.2 *Lymphatic and haematopoietic tissues*

The risk for non-Hodgkin's lymphoma from exposure to DDT was evaluated in a population-based case-control study in Washington State, USA (Woods *et al.*, 1987). The design of this investigation is given in detail in the monograph on occupational exposures in spraying and application of insecticides (p. 67). A total of 576 patients with non-Hodgkin's lymphoma and 694 controls were interviewed to obtain information on pesticide use. The odds ratio for non-Hodgkin's lymphoma was 1.8 (95% CI, 1.0-3.2) among those reporting use of DDT. Adjustment for other agricultural exposures did not substantially change this estimate. When the analysis was restricted to farmers (Woods & Polissar, 1989), the odds ratio for exposure to DDT was 1.7 (95% CI, 0.9-3.3).

In the case-control study on leukaemia in Iowa and Minnesota, USA, described in detail in the monograph on occupational exposures in spraying and application of insecticides (p. 68), the odds ratio for leukaemia was 1.2 (95% CI, 0.7-1.8) for use of DDT on crops and 1.3 (1.0-1.8) for use on animals. The odds ratio for leukaemia rose with frequency of reported use of DDT on animals from 0.6 (95% CI, 0.3-1.4; 7 cases) for fewer than five days of use per year, 1.1 (0.4-2.7; 7 cases) for 5-9 days, to 2.1 (1.1-3.9; 21 cases) for 10 or more days. No such pattern was evident for use of DDT on crops. Elevated risks for both chronic lymphatic and chronic myeloid leukaemia were found among farmers who used DDT: the odds ratios were 1.5 (0.9-2.3; based on 36 cases) and 1.9 (0.9-4.2; 10 cases), respectively (Brown *et al.*, 1990).

Cases of chronic lymphatic leukaemia diagnosed in five hospitals in Sweden between 1964 and 1984 in patients who survived after 1981 were compared with population controls living in the catchment areas of the hospitals. The study design is described in the monograph on occupational exposures in spraying and application of insecticides (p. 68). Results of a stratified analysis based on a confounder score including age, sex, exposure to fresh wood, solvents, exhausts, DDT, horses and employment as farmer were presented. Exposure to DDT was reported by six cases and four controls; the odds ratio was 6.0 (95% CI, 1.5-23) (Flodin *et al.*, 1988). [The Working Group noted the limitation of inclusion of prevalent cases because of the potential influence on recall of exposure.]

A study on Hodgkin's disease and B-cell non-Hodgkin's lymphomas was conducted in one of the areas included in the study summarized above (Persson *et al.*, 1989) and described in the monograph on occupational exposures in spraying and application of insecticides (p. 69). The same criteria were applied for selection of cases, and the same series of controls was used. Logistic regression analysis was carried out including sex, age, occupation in farming, exposure to fresh wood and all exposures resulting in a crude odds ratio greater than 2.0. Exposure to DDT was reported by three patients with Hodgkin's disease, none with non-Hodgkin's lymphoma and three controls. The odds ratio for Hodgkin's disease was 7.5 (90% CI, 0.8-70) [The limitation of the study by Flodin *et al.* (1988) noted above also applies to this study.]

In the case-control study of malignant lymphomas in northern Sweden described in the monograph on occupational exposures in spraying and application of insecticides (p. 69) (Hardell *et al.*, 1981), 22 cases and 26 controls reported exposure to DDT [odds ratio, 1.8; 95% CI, 1.0-3.2]. Seven cases and 11 controls reported exposure to DDT and not to phenoxyacetic acid herbicides [odds ratio, 1.6; 95% CI, 0.6-4.1]. Information was not presented separately for Hodgkin's disease and non-Hodgkin's lymphoma.

Case-control studies on cancers of lymphatic and haematopoietic tissues and exposure to DDT are summarized in Table 7.

2.2.3 *Soft-tissue sarcoma*

Four population-based case-control studies in Sweden assessed the risk of soft-tissue sarcoma, primarily in association with exposure to phenoxyacetic acid herbicides and chlorophenols (Hardell & Sandström, 1979; Eriksson *et al.*, 1981; Hardell & Eriksson, 1988; Eriksson *et al.*, 1990a). The studies are described in detail in the monograph on occupational exposures in spraying and application of insecticides (pp. 69-70). In the first study, in northern Sweden, four cases and 14 controls reported exposure to DDT (crude odds ratio, 1.2 [95% CI, 0.4-3.7] (Hardell & Sandström, 1979). In the second study, in southern Sweden, seven cases and 11 controls reported exposure to DDT [crude odds ratio 1.3; 95% CI, 0.5-3.4] (Eriksson *et al.*, 1981). In the third study, in northern Sweden, six cases, 19 population-based controls and eight cancer controls reported exposure to DDT [crude odds ratio, 1.9; 95% CI, 0.7-5.0 (population controls); crude odds ratio, 2.7; 95% CI, 0.9-7.8 (cancer controls)]. One case, 10 population-based controls and three cancer controls

Table 7. Case-control studies of cancers of lymphatic and haematopoietic tissues containing information of exposure to DDT

Reference Location	Cancer site	No. of exposed cases/ controls	Relative risk	95% CI	Comments
Woods et al. (1987); Woods & Polissar (1989) Washington State, USA	Non-Hodgkin's lymphoma	Not reported	1.8	1.0-3.2	Not adjusted for other agricultural exposures
		Not reported	1.7	0.9-3.3	Farmers only
Persson et al. (1989) Sweden	Non-Hodgkin's lymphoma	0/3	–	–	Adjusted for some other agricultural exposures
	Hodgkin's disease	3/3	7.5	0.8-70	90% CI
Hardell et al. (1981) Northern Sweden	Malignant lymphoma	22/26	[1.8]	[1.0-3.2]	Crude risk calculated from data in paper. Not adjusted for other agricultural exposures.
		7/11	[1.6]	[0.6-4.1]	Crude risk for DDT, without exposure to phenoxyacetic acid herbicides
Brown et al. (1990) Iowa and Minnesota, USA	Leukaemia	35/75	1.2	0.7-1.8	DDT used on crops
		80/149	1.3	1.0-1.8	DDT used on animals Not adjusted for other agricultural exposures; risks increased with duration of use[a]
	Chronic lymphatic leukaemia	36	1.5	0.9-2.3	DDT used on crops and animals[b]
	Chronic myeloid leukaemia	10	1.9	0.9-4.2	
Flodin et al. (1988) Sweden	Chronic lymphatic leukaemia	6/4	6.0	1.5-23	Adjusted for other agricultural exposures

[a]Increased risks reported also in association with exposure to other insecticides
[b]No data provided for other subtypes of leukaemia

reported exposure to DDT without exposure to phenoxyacetic acid herbicides [crude odds ratio, 0.6 (95% CI, 0.1-5.0)] for population controls and [1.2 (95% CI, 0.1-12.1)] for cancer controls (Hardell & Eriksson, 1988). In the fourth study, from central Sweden, exposure to DDT was reported by 22 cases and 33 controls (odds ratio, 0.61; 95% CI, 0.34-1.1) (Eriksson et al., 1990a).

In the case-control study on soft-tissue sarcomas in Kansas, USA, also described in the monograph on occupational exposures (p. 66), an odds ratio of 2.3 (95% CI, 0.9-5.6, based on 10 exposed cases and 28 exposed controls) was reported for use of DDT on animals (Hoar Zahm et al., 1988). In the population-based case-control study of soft-tissue sarcoma in

Washington State, USA (Woods *et al.*, 1987) (see p. 67), the odds ratio for soft-tissue sarcoma was 1.1 (0.4-3.2).

Case-control studies on soft-tissue sarcoma and exposure to DDT are summarized in Table 8.

Table 8. Case-control studies of soft-tissue sarcoma containing information on exposure to DDT

Reference Location	No. of exposed cases/ controls	Relative risk	95% CI	Comments
Hardell & Sandström (1979) Sweden	4/14	1.2	[0.4-3.7]	Not adjusted for other agricultural exposures
Eriksson *et al.* (1981) Sweden	7/11	[1.3]	[0.5-3.4]	Crude risk calculated from data in paper; not adjusted for other agricultural exposures
Hardell & Eriksson (1988) Sweden	6/19 6/8	[1.9][a] [2.7][b]	[0.7-5.0] [0.9-7.8]	Crude risk calculated from data in paper; not adjusted for other agricultural exposures
	1/10 1/3	[0.6][a] [1.2][b]	[0.1-5.0] [0.1-12.1]	Crude risk for exposure to DDT and not phenoxyacetic acids
Eriksson *et al.* (1990a) Sweden	22/33	0.61	0.34-1.1	Not adjusted for other agricultural exposures
Hoar Zahm *et al.* (1988) Kansas, USA	10/28	2.3	0.9-5.6	DDT on animals[c]; not adjusted for other agricultural exposures
Woods *et al.* (1987) Washington, USA	Not reported	1.1	0.4-3.2	Not adjusted for other agricultural exposures

[a]Population controls
[b]Cancer controls
[c]No data provided for DDT use on crops

2.2.4 *Other cancers*

A proportionate analysis of occupational mortality in Washington State, USA, identified a 30% increased risk for respiratory cancer among orchardists (Milham, 1983), and a case-control study was thus undertaken in Washington State in 1968-80 (Wicklund *et al.*, 1988). The design of the study is described in the monograph on occupational exposures in spraying and application of insecticides (p. 70). A total of 89 cases and 89 controls were assumed to have had exposure to DDT. When men exposed to DDT but not to lead arsenate were considered, there were 33 cases and 29 controls, and the odds ratio (adjusted for smoking) was 0.91 (95% CI, 0.40-2.1). [The Working Group noted that the unexposed group included men for whom details on exposure to DDT were not available, which may have biased the odds ratio towards the null.]

Two case-control studies in Sweden examined the risks for colon cancer (Hardell, 1981) and nasal and nasopharyngeal cancer (Hardell *et al.*, 1982), primarily in relation to exposure to phenoxyacetic acid herbicides and chlorophenols. These studies are described in the monograph on occupational exposures (p. 71). Odds ratios for exposure to DDT, without controlling for other agricultural exposures, were [0.8; 0.4-1.7] for colon cancer and [1.2; 95% CI, 0.5-2.9] for nasal and nasopharyngeal cancer. In the study of colon cancer, exposure to DDT was also analysed after excluding subjects who had been exposed to phenoxyacetic acids and chlorophenols; the odds ratio was [0.5; 0.2-1.6].

Men aged 25-80 who had been diagnosed with liver cancer between 1974 and 1981 and reported to the Department of Oncology, Umeå, Sweden, were included in another case-control study (Hardell *et al.*, 1984), described in the monograph on occupational exposures (p. 71). Odds ratios for exposure to DDT, without controlling for other agricultural exposures, were [0.4; 95% CI, 0.1-1.1] for exposure to DDT in farming and [1.3; 0.4-4.0] for exposure to DDT in forestry.

These studies are summarized in Table 9.

Table 9. Case-control studies of other cancers containing information of DDT exposure

Reference Location	Cancer	No. of exposed cases/ controls	Relative risk	95% CI	Comments
Hardell (1981) Sweden	Colon	9/40	[0.8]	[0.4-1.7]	Crude risk calculated from data in paper; not adjusted for other agricultural exposures
	Colon	3/21	[0.5]	[0.2-1.6]	Crude risk calculated from data in paper; for exposure to DDT and not phenoxyacetic acids or chlorophenols
Hardell *et al.* (1982) Sweden	Nose, naso-pharynx	6/40	[1.2]	[0.5-2.9]	Crude risk calculated from data in paper; not adjusted for other agricultural exposures
Hardell *et al.* (1984) Sweden	Primary liver	4/20	[0.4]	[0.1-1.1]	Crude risk calculated from data in paper; not adjusted for other agricultural exposures; farmers
	Primary liver	5/8	[1.3]	[0.4-4.0]	Crude risk calculated from data in paper; not adjusted for other agricultural exposures; foresters
Wicklund *et al.* (1988) USA	Respiratory	33/29	0.9	0.40-2.1	Both cases and controls were orchard workers

3. Studies of Cancer in Experimental Animals

The carcinogenicity of DDT in experimental animals has been reviewed (Cabral, 1985).

The Working Group was aware of studies of *para,para'*-DDT by oral and subcutaneous administration and by skin application in mice, rats, hamsters and trout by Bennison and Mostofi (1950; mice, skin), Halver (1967; trout), Weisburger and Weisburger (1968; rat, oral), Gargus *et al.* (1969; mice, subcutaneous), the US National Technical Information Service (1968) and Innes *et al.* (1969; mice; *para,para'*-TDE, oral and subcutaneous; DDT, subcutaneous), Agthe *et al.* (1970; hamster, oral), Shabad *et al.* (1973; mice, oral) and Lacassagne and Hurst (1965; rat; *ortho,para'*-TDE, oral). These were considered in the previous IARC monograph (IARC, 1974). Studies of oral administration of DDT to mice (Del Pup *et al.*, 1978; Reuber, 1979; Lipsky *et al.*, 1989) and rats (Shivapurkar *et al.*, 1986) were considered but are not summarized here since they do not contribute to an evaluation of carcinogenicity.

Because of the large number of studies, histopathological findings are summarized for some studies in Table 10 at the end of this section (p. 209).

3.1 Oral administration

3.1.1 *Mouse*

In a screening study on about 70 compounds, groups of 18 male and 18 female (C57Bl/6 × C3H/Anf)F_1 and (C57Bl/6 × AKR)F_1 mice, seven days old, were given daily single doses of 46.4 mg/kg bw (maximum tolerated dose) *para,para'*-DDT [purity unspecified] by stomach tube, followed by daily administration of the same absolute amount until 28 days of age, at which time the mice were transferred to a diet containing 140 mg/kg *para,para'*-DDT. Animals were killed at 81 weeks of age. About 30% of females of both strains died during the treatment. Hepatomas were found in male and female mice of each strain, and malignant lymphomas were found in (C57Bl/6 × AKR)F_1 females (see Table 10) (US National Technical Information Service, 1968; Innes *et al.*, 1969).

In a five-generation study, originally designed to investigate the effects of DDT on behaviour, one treated and one control group of BALB/c mice were taken from each of the five generations and studied for tumour incidence. A total of 683 mice received a diet containing 2.8-3 mg/kg *para,para'*-DDT ([purity unspecified] melting-point, 108-109 °C), and 406 received a control diet. Lung carcinomas were observed in 116 of the treated mice and in five controls [$p < 0.001$]. [The incidence of lung adenomas was not reported, although the authors noted an average incidence of 5% in their colony of mice.] The incidence of leukaemias was 85/683 in treated mice (64 in females) and 10/406 in controls [$p < 0.001$] (see Table 10) (Tarján & Kemény, 1969).

In a two-generation dose-response study, 939 treated and 242 control CF-1 mice were fed dietary concentrations of 0 or 2, 10, 50 or 250 mg/kg technical-grade DDT (73-78% *para,para'*-DDT, 20% *ortho,para'*-DDT, 1% *meta,para'*-DDT, 0.5-1.5% *para,para'*-TDE and 0.5% *para,para'*-DDE), starting at 6-7 weeks of age for the parent (P) generation and continuing in the P and offspring (F_1) for life. There was excess mortality from week 60 onwards among mice of the P and F_1 generations that had received 250 mg/kg of diet DDT.

Only the incidence of liver-cell tumours was increased by exposure to DDT: males, 25/113 (controls), 57/124, 52/104, 67/127, 82/103 in treated groups; females, 4/111 (controls), 4/105, 11/124, 13/104, 60/90 in treated groups. The excess of liver-cell tumours over that in controls in mice of each sex fed 250 mg/kg of diet DDT was significant ($p < 0.01$). The excess over that in controls of liver-cell tumours in males fed 2, 10 or 50 mg/kg of diet was significant ($p < 0.01$) in animals surviving more than 70 weeks. In females, all liver-cell tumours were found after 100 weeks of age, and the excess over that controls was significant ($p < 0.05$) in the group fed 50 mg/kg diet DDT and ($p < 0.01$) in the group fed 250 mg/kg of diet DDT. Four liver-cell tumours, all occurring in DDT-treated mice, gave metastases. No remarkable difference was observed between P and F_1 mice in this study (Tomatis et al., 1972).

In a continuation of this study (Turusov et al., 1973), the effects of the same doses of DDT were studied in six consecutive generations of CF-1 mice (including the first two generations described by Tomatis et al., 1972). The experiment involved a total of 2764 exposed and 668 control animals. Exposure to all four levels of DDT significantly increased the incidence of liver-cell tumours (hepatomas) in males; in females, hepatoma incidence increased considerably after exposure to 250 mg/kg (see Table 10). No progressive increase in hepatoma incidence from generation to generation was noted in treated mice. Malignant hepatoblastomas were observed at a slightly increased incidence in DDT-treated male mice: 3/328 in control males, 5/354, 14/362, 12/383 and 25/350 in 2, 10, 50 and 250 ppm DDT-treated males, respectively [positive trend, $p < 0.001$]. Ten of 56 hepatoblastomas found in DDT-treated mice metastasized to the lungs. DDT did not alter significantly the tumour incidence at sites other than the liver.

In a two-generation study, 515 female and 430 male BALB/c mice were administered dietary concentrations of 0, 2, 20 or 250 mg/kg technical-grade DDT (70-75% para,para'-DDT, 20% ortho,para'-DDT and 0.2-4% para,para'-TDE) for life. In females, the survival rates were comparable in all groups; in males, early deaths occurred in all groups as a consequence of fighting and (at the high dose) because of toxicity. In animals that survived more than 60 weeks, only liver-cell tumours were found in excess, and only at 250 mg/kg of diet was the increase significant (see Table 10) (Terracini et al., 1973a). Confirmatory results were obtained in two subsequent generations of BALB/c mice fed DDT, although F_1, F_2 and F_3 mice, which were exposed to DDT both in utero and after birth for life, developed more liver tumours than did P mice, which were exposed to DDT only after weaning (Terracini et al., 1973b).

Groups of 30-32 CF-1 mice of each sex were fed diets containing 50 or 100 mg/kg para,para'-DDT (purity, > 99.5%) for two years. A control group of 47 mice of each sex was available. A significant increase in the incidence of liver-cell tumours was observed in treated males and females (see Table 10) (Walker et al., 1973).

In a subsequent study, 30 male and 30 female CF-1 mice were fed 100 mg/kg of diet para,para'-DDT (> 99.5% pure) for 110 weeks. The animals were not sent for autopsy until the intra-abdominal masses reached a size that caused the animals to become anorexic or clinically affected. A significant increase ($p < 0.01$) in the incidence of liver tumours (23/30 males and 26/30 females compared with 11/45 and 10/44 controls, respectively) was observed within 26 months (see Table 10) (Thorpe & Walker, 1973).

Groups of 30 male and 30 female Swiss inbred mice, six weeks of age, were held as untreated controls or were given technical-grade DDT (70.5% *para ,para'*-DDT, 21.3% *ortho ,para'*-DDT) orally as 100 mg/kg of diet DDT or by daily gavage of 0.25 mg DDT in olive oil for 80 weeks. Survival (37-54%) and weight gains were not affected by treatment. The incidence of lymphomas was significantly increased ($p < 0.05$) in treated males and females (see Table 10) (Kashyap *et al.*, 1977). [The Working Group noted the small number of animals used.]

Groups of 50 male and 50 female B6C3F$_1$ mice, six weeks old, were fed diets containing technical-grade DDT (principal component, about 70%, assumed to be *para ,para'*-DDT) for 78 weeks and were then held for 14 or 15 additional weeks before terminal sacrifice. Groups of 20 mice were fed a control diet for 91 or 92 weeks. Initially, males received diets containing 10 or 20 mg/kg and females received diets containing 50 or 100 mg/kg DDT; after nine weeks, these concentrations were gradually increased up to 25 and 50 mg/kg of diet for males and 100 and 200 mg/kg of diet for females because of the absence of toxicity. The time-weighted average dietary concentrations were 22 and 44 mg/kg of diet for males and 87 and 175 mg/kg of diet for females. Survival in all groups of male mice was poor, possibly due to fighting. Survival of male mice at week 70 was 12/20 control, 20/50 low-dose and 37/50 high-dose animals; terminal survival of female mice was 20/20 control, 45/50 low-dose and 36/50 high-dose animals. There was no difference in body weight gain between treated and control mice. The incidence of malignant lymphoma was increased in females (control, 0/20; low-dose, 3/49; high-dose, 7/46 [$p < 0.05$, trend test]) (see Table 10) (US National Cancer Institute, 1978). [The Working Group noted that females received four times higher doses than males.]

3.1.2 *Rat*

In two two-year experiments started at an interval of one year, 228 Osborne-Mendel rats, three weeks of age, received diets containing technical-grade DDT (81.8% *para ,para'*-DDT, 18.2% *ortho ,para'*-DDT) as a powder or as a solution in corn oil at concentrations of 0 (24 males and 12 females), 100 (12 males), 200 (24 males and 12 females), 400 (24 males and 12 females), 600 (24 males and 24 females) or 800 (36 males and 24 females) mg/kg of diet. Of the 192 rats exposed to DDT, 111 died before 18 months of treatment; only 14 rats given 800, 23 rats given 600, 14 given 400, 24 given 200, six given 100 mg/kg of diet and 20 controls were alive at this time. Tumour incidences were not given for each dose level. Among the 81 rats that survived at least 18 months, four had 'low-grade' hepatic-cell carcinomas (measuring 0.5-1.2 cm), and 11 showed nodular adenomatous hyperplasia (nodules measuring up to 0.3 cm). No liver lesion was found in control rats. Hepatic-cell tumours were reported to occur spontaneously in 1% of the rats of this colony and nodular adenomatous hyperplasia was reported to be rare (Fitzhugh & Nelson, 1947). [The Working Group noted the inadequate reporting.] An unspecified amount of histopathological material from this study was reviewed by Reuber (1978), who confirmed the presence of neoplastic liver lesions in treated animals.

In two experiments reported from the same institution, groups of 30 male and 30 female Osborne-Mendel rats were exposed from weaning for at least two years to either 80 or 200 mg/kg of diet DDT [purity unspecified] and were compared to two control groups of 30 animals of each sex. Undifferentiated bronchogenic carcinomas were seen in 2/120 controls (two experiments combined), in 8/60 rats (males and females combined) fed 80 mg/kg of diet DDT, and in none of the animals receiving 200 mg/kg of diet DDT. One hepatoma occurred in a control female in one experiment and another in a female given 200 mg/kg of diet DDT. Incidences of other tumours were similar in control and treated rats (see Table 10) (Radomski et al., 1965; Deichmann et al., 1967).

Groups of 36 or 37 male and 35 female outbred Wistar rats, seven weeks of age, were fed a control diet or a diet containing 500 mg/kg of diet technical-grade DDT (70-75% para,para'-DDT, 20% ortho,para'-DDT, 0.2-4% para,para'-TDE) until 152 weeks of age. Survival was not affected by the treatment and was greater than 50% at 100 weeks in all groups. Body weight gains were decreased by 10-20% in the treated groups as compared to the controls. The average dose of DDT was 34.1 mg/kg bw per day in males and 37.0 mg/kg bw per day in females. The incidence of liver-cell tumours (neoplastic nodules) was increased in treated males (9/37; controls, 0/36) [$p = 0.001$] and females (15/35; controls, 0/35) [$p < 0.001$] (see Table 10) (Rossi et al., 1977).

Groups of 50 male and 50 female Osborne-Mendel rats, seven weeks of age, were fed diets containing technical-grade DDT (principal component, 70%, assumed to be para,para'-DDT) for 78 weeks and killed at 111 weeks. The initial concentrations of DDT were 420 or 840 mg/kg of diet for males and 315 or 630 mg/kg of diet for females; these concentrations were subsequently increased to 500 and 1000 and then decreased to 250 and 500 mg/kg of diet for males and were decreased to 158 and 315 mg/kg of diet for females when signs of toxicity (tremors) appeared. The time-weighted average concentrations were 321 and 642 mg/kg of diet for males and 210 and 420 mg/kg of diet for females. Groups of 20 males and 20 females received a control diet. Body weights of high-dose rats were lower than those of controls by as much as 15% during the study. Survival was not affected by the treatment. There was no increase in the incidence of tumours that could be attributed to treatment with DDT (US National Cancer Institute, 1978). [The Working Group noted the short duration of treatment.]

Groups of 38 male and 38 female MRC Porton rats, six to seven weeks of age, were fed control diet or a diet containing 500 mg/kg technical-grade DDT (78.9% para,para'-DDT, 16.7% ortho,para'-DDT, 1.6% para,para'-DDE, 0.6% para,para'-TDE, 0.2% ortho,para'-DDE, 0.1% ortho,para'-TDE and 1.9% unknown) for 144 weeks. Groups of 30 male and 30 female rats received diets containing 125 or 250 mg/kg of diet DDT. Survival and body weight gains were not significantly different between treated and control groups; survival at 80 weeks was greater than 70% in all groups except that of high-dose males (61%). The incidence of liver-cell tumours was significantly increased in female rats (0/38 control, 2/30 low-dose, 4/30 mid-dose, 7/38 high-dose; $p < 0.001$, trend test). Liver-cell nodules [hyperplastic] or foci of cellular alteration occurred significantly more frequently ($p < 0.05$) in low- and mid-dose females than in controls. Residues of DDT, TDE and DDE in liver, determined in three male and three female high-dose rats killed at 52 weeks, were on average 2.5 times higher in females than males (Cabral et al., 1982a).

3.1.3 *Hamster*

Groups of 30-40 male and 29-40 female outbred Syrian golden hamsters, five weeks old, were fed for life on diets containing 0, 125, 250 or 500 mg/kg of diet technical-grade DDT (78.9% *para,para'*-DDT, 16.7% *ortho,para'*-DDT, 1.6% *para,para'*-DDE, 0.6% *para,para'*-TDE, 0.2% *ortho,para'*-DDE, 0.1% *ortho,para'*-TDE and 1.9% unknown). Survival and body weight gains were comparable between treated and control animals. The experiment was terminated at 120 weeks when the last survivor was killed. There was no significant difference in tumour incidence in the various groups; however, a significant trend was observed for tumours of the adrenal cortex (mostly adenomas) in males: 3/40 control, 4/30 low-dose, 6/31 mid-dose and 8/39 high-dose [$p = 0.04$] (Cabral *et al.*, 1982b).

Groups of 45 or 48 male and 46 or 48 female Syrian golden hamsters, eight weeks old, were fed diet containing 0 or 1000 mg/kg DDT (70-75% *para,para'*-DDT, 20% *ortho,para'*-DDT, 0.2-4% *para,para'*-TDE) until 128 weeks of age. Survival was 60% or greater in all groups at 80 weeks. Adrenal gland tumours ('mainly cortical adenomas') occurred in 14/35 treated males compared to 8/31 male controls [$p > 0.05$] and in 10/36 treated females compared to 2/42 female controls [$p < 0.01$] (see Table 10) (Rossi *et al.*, 1983).

Groups of 30 male and 30 female hamsters [strain unspecified] were given diets containing 0, 250, 500 or 1000 mg/kg technical-grade DDT for 18 months. No difference in body weight gains between groups was observed. Mean survival time ranged from 13 to 14.9 months in male and female control groups, to 17.3 and 17.1 months in high-dose male and female groups. The incidence of lymphosarcomas was reduced from 50% in male controls and 41% in female controls to 0 in the high-dose groups of each sex (Graillot *et al.*, 1975). [The Working Group noted the short duration of treatment.]

3.2 Skin application

Mouse: Groups of 30 male and 30 female Swiss inbred mice, six weeks of age, were held as untreated controls or were administered 0.25 mg/animal technical-grade DDT (70.5% *para,para'*-DDT, 21.3% *ortho,para'*-DDT) in 0.1 ml olive oil twice weekly by skin application for 80 weeks. Survival (40-57%) and weight gains were not affected by treatment, and no increase in tumour incidence was observed (Kashyap *et al.*, 1977). [The Working Group noted the short duration of treatment.]

3.3 Subcutaneous and/or intramuscular injection

Mouse: Groups of 30 male and 30 female Swiss inbred mice, six weeks of age, were held as untreated controls or received twice-monthly subcutaneous injections of 0.25 mg/animal technical-grade DDT (70.5% *para,para'*-DDT, 21.3% *ortho,para'*-DDT) in 0.1 ml olive oil for 80 weeks. Survival (40-57%) and weight gain were not affected by treatment. The incidence of liver-cell carcinomas was 7/26 in treated females and 0/20 in control females [$p = 0.01$] (see Table 10) (Kashyap *et al.*, 1977).

3.4 Studies with known carcinogens

Rat: Dietary intake of DDT was found to promote 2-acetylaminofluorene-induced tumorigenesis in rat liver, in a way similar to that of phenobarbital (Peraino *et al.*, 1975). It also significantly shortened the latent period for the appearance of mammary tumours in rats treated with 2-acetamidophenanthrene (Scribner & Mottet, 1981).

3.5 Carcinogenicity of metabolites

TDE

Mouse: A group of 60 male and 60 female CF-1 mice, 6-7 weeks old, was fed a diet containing 250 mg/kg *para,para'*-TDE (99% pure) until 130 weeks of age; 100 males and 90 females served as controls. The incidence of hepatomas was significantly increased in treated males, and the incidences of lung tumours were significantly increased in males and females compared with controls (see Table 10) (Tomatis *et al.*, 1974).

Groups of 50 male and 50 female B6C3F$_1$ mice, six weeks of age, were fed diets initially containing 315 or 630 mg/kg technical-grade TDE (principal component, 60%, assumed to be *para,para'*-TDE, 19 unidentified impurities) for 78 weeks and were killed at 90 weeks. The dietary concentrations were increased to 425 and 850 mg/kg due to lack of toxicity. The time-weighted average dietary concentrations were 411 and 822 mg/kg of diet. Further groups of 20 males and 20 females were fed control diets. Body weight gain of high-dose females was somewhat reduced late in the study. Survival was not affected by treatment; terminal survival was 13/20 control, 30/50 low-dose and 27/50 high-dose males and 18/20 control, 41/50 low-dose and 44/50 high-dose females. There was no significant increase in the incidence of hepatocellular carcinomas (see Table 10) (US National Cancer Institute, 1978). [The Working Group noted the short duration of treatment.]

Rat: Groups of 50 male and 50 female Osborne-Mendel rats, seven weeks of age, were fed diets containing technical-grade TDE (principal component, 60%, assumed to be *para,para'*-TDE, 19 unidentified impurities) for 78 weeks and were killed at 111 weeks. The initial dietary concentrations for male rats of 1400 or 2800 mg/kg were increased to 1750 and 3500 mg/kg due to lack of toxicity. Females received diets containing 850 or 1700 mg/kg of diet throughout the study. The time-weighted average concentrations given to males were 1647 and 3294 mg/kg of diet. Further groups of 20 males and 20 females were fed control diets. Body weight gains were substantially reduced in high-dose rats and somewhat reduced in low-dose rats compared to controls. Survival was not affected by treatment. Increased incidences of tumours of the thyroid gland were seen in animals of each sex, but significance was reached only for follicular-cell adenomas and carcinomas combined in low-dose males ($p < 0.05$) (see also Table 10) (US National Cancer Institute, 1978).

DDE

Mouse: A group of 60 male and 60 female CF-1 mice, 6-7 weeks old, was fed a diet containing 250 mg/kg *para,para'*-DDE (99% pure) until 130 weeks of age. A group of 100 males and 90 females was used as controls. An increased incidence of hepatomas was found in treated males and treated females compared with controls (see Table 10) (Tomatis *et al.*, 1974).

Groups of 50 male and 50 female B6C3F$_1$ mice, six weeks of age, were fed diets containing *para,para'*-DDE (> 95% pure) for 78 weeks and were killed at 92 weeks. The initial dietary concentrations of 125 and 250 mg/kg of diet were increased during the study to 150 and 300 mg/kg due to lack of toxicity. When toxicity became apparent, the concentrations in the diet were held constant, but the high-dose diets were replaced by control diet every fifth week for the duration of the treatment period. The time-weighted average dietary concentrations were 148 and 261 mg/kg of diet for males and females, respectively. Further groups of 20 males and 20 females were fed control diets. Body weight gain was reduced somewhat in treated females compared to controls. At 70 weeks survival was 5/20 control, 35/50 low-dose and 31/50 high-dose males; at 75 weeks, survival in females was 19/20 control, 47/50 low-dose and 28/50 high-dose animals. The incidences of hepatocellular carcinoma were 0/19 control, 7/41 low-dose and 17/47 high-dose males and 0/19 control, 19/47 low-dose and 34/48 high-dose females ($p < 0.001$ for both low- and high-dose female mice and $p = 0.001$ for high-dose males) (see Table 10) (US National Cancer Institute, 1978). [The Working Group noted the low survival and the frequent changes in dietary concentrations of DDE.]

Rat: Groups of 50 male and 50 female Osborne-Mendel rats, seven weeks of age, were fed diets containing *para,para'*-DDE (> 95% pure) for 78 weeks and were killed at 111 weeks. The initial dietary concentrations of 675 or 1350 mg/kg for male rats and of 375 or 750 mg/kg for females were reduced to 338 and 675 mg/kg of diet for males and 187 and 375 for females due to the onset of toxic signs. Additionally, the high-dose diets were replaced by control diet every fifth week during the latter part of the study. The time-weighted average concentrations were 437 and 839 mg/kg of diet for males and 242 and 462 mg/kg of diet for females. Further groups of 20 males and 20 females were fed control diets. Body weight gains were somewhat reduced in treated male and high-dose female rats compared to controls. Survival at 92 weeks was 16/20 control, 34/50 low-dose and 26/50 high-dose males and 20/20 control, 42/50 low-dose and 36/50 high-dose females. No increase in tumour incidence was observed (US National Cancer Institute, 1978). [The Working Group noted the short duration of treatment.]

Hamster: Groups of 40-47 male and 43-46 female Syrian golden hamsters, eight weeks old, were fed a control diet or a diet containing 500 or 1000 mg/kg *para,para'*-DDE (purity, 99%) until 128 weeks of age. Survival was 50% or greater in all groups at 80 weeks. There were significantly ($p < 0.05$) increased incidences of liver-cell tumours (neoplastic nodules) in both groups of treated males and females: males—control, 0/10; low-dose, 7/15; and high-dose, 8/24; females—control, 0/31; low-dose, 4/26; and high-dose, 5/24 (Rossi *et al.*, 1983).

4. Other Relevant Data

The toxicokinetics of DDT has been reviewed (WHO, 1979; FAO/WHO, 1964, 1965, 1967b, 1968b, 1970b, 1980a; Hayes, 1982; FAO/WHO, 1985; Agency for Toxic Substances and Diseases Registry, 1989).

4.1 Absorption, distribution, metabolism and excretion

4.1.1 *Humans*

DDT is absorbed by all routes; its fate and its metabolism in man was studied in volunteers receiving known quantities of technical-grade DDT (77% *para,para'*, 23% *ortho,para'*), *para,para'*-2,2-bis(*para*-chlorophenyl)acetic acid (DDA), *para,para'*-TDE or *para,para'*-DDE (Roan, 1970; Morgan & Roan, 1971; Roan *et al.*, 1971). DDT, TDE or DDA ingested at 5, 10 or 20 mg per day for 21-183 days was partly excreted as DDA in urine—most

Table 10. Summary of selected experimental carcinogenicity studies

Reference	Species/strain	Sex	Dose schedule	Experimental parameter/observation	Group 0	1	2	3	4	Statistical trend
DDT										
Innes et al. (1969)	Mouse (C57Bl/6 × C3H/Anf)F_1	M	Gavage/day 28 days; in diet to 81 weeks of age	Dose (gavage; mg/kg bw)	0	46.4				
				Dose (mg/kg of diet)	0	140				
				Hepatoma	8/79	11/18**				NA
		F	Gavage/day 28 days; in diet to 81 weeks of age	Dose (gavage; mg/kg bw)	0	46.4				
				Dose (mg/kg of diet)	0	140				
				Hepatoma	0/87	4/18**				NA
	Mouse (C57Bl/6 × AKR)F_1	M	Gavage/day 28 days; in diet to 81 weeks of age	Dose (gavage; mg/kg bw)	0	46.4				
				Dose (mg/kg of diet)	0	140				
				Hepatoma	5/90	7/18**				NA
		F	Gavage/day 28 days; in diet to 81 weeks of age	Dose (gavage; mg/kg bw)	0	46.4				
				Dose (mg/kg of diet)	0	140				
				Hepatoma	1/82	1/18				
				Lymphoma	4/82	6/18**				NA
Tarján & Kemény (1969)		M & F	5-generation	Dose (mg/kg diet)	0	2.8–3				
				Lung carcinomas	5/406	116/683***				
				Leukaemia	10/406	85/683				
				Lymphosarcomas	1/406	15/683				NA
Turusov et al. (1973)	Mouse CF-1	M	Diet multi-generation	Dose (mg/kg diet)	0	2	10	50	250	
				Liver-cell tumours	97/328	179/354**	181/362**	214/383**	301/350**	[p < 0.001]
				Hepatoblastomas	3/328	5/354	14/362*	12/383*	25/350**	[p < 0.001]
		F	Diet multi-generation	Liver-cell tumours	16/340	12/339	32/355*	43/328**	192/293**	[p < 0.001]
Terracini et al. (1973a)	Mouse BALB/c	M	Diet for lifespan 2-generation	Dose (mg/kg of diet)	0	2	20	250		
				Liver-cell tumours[a]	1/62	3/48	0/48	14/31**		[p < 0.001]
				Malignant lymphoma	6/107	5/112	4/106	1/106		[p = 0.04]
		F	Diet for lifespan 2-generation	Dose (mg/kg of diet)	0	2	20	250		
				Liver-cell tumours[a]	0/124	0/130	1/126	71/115**		[p < 0.001]

Table 10 (contd)

Reference	Species/strain	Sex	Dose schedule	Experimental parameter/observation	Group 0	1	2	3	4	Statistical trend
Walker et al. (1973)	Mouse CF-1	M	Diet for 2 years	Dose (mg/kg of diet)	0	50	100			
				Liver-cell tumours	6/47	12/32*	17/32**			[$p < 0.001$]
		F	Diet for 2 years	Dose (mg/kg of diet)	0	50	100			
				Liver-cell tumours	8/47	15/30**	24/32**			[$p < 0.001$]
Thorpe & Walker (1973)	Mouse CF-1	M	Diet for 110 weeks	Dose (mg/kg of diet)	0	100				
				Liver-cell tumours	11/45	23/30**				NA
				Malignant lymphoma	16/45	4/30				[$p < 0.05$]
		F	Diet for 110 weeks	Dose (mg/kg of diet)	0	100				
				Liver-cell tumours	10/44	26/30**				NA
				Malignant lymphoma	16/44	6/30				
Kashyap et al. (1977)	Mouse Swiss	M	Diet or gavage for 80 weeks	Dose (mg/kg of diet) (mg/animal)	Untreated 0	Diet 100	Gavage 0.25			
				Lymphoma	2/26	8/27*	6/24			NS
				Lung adenoma	4/26	8/27	7/24			
		F	Diet or gavage for 80 weeks	Dose (mg/kg of diet) (mg/animal)	0	100	0.25			
				Lymphoma	2/20	8/22*	8/24			NS
				Lung adenoma	1/20	3/22	5/24			
US National Cancer Institute (1978)	Mouse B6C3F1	F	Diet for 78-92 weeks	Dose (mg/kg of diet)	0	87	175			
				Survival (70 weeks)	20/20	45/50	36/50			
				Lymphoma	0/20	3/49	7/46	NS		
Radomski et al. (1965); Deichmann et al. (1967)	Rat Osborne-Mendel	M & F	Diet for 2 years	Dose (mg/kg of diet)	0	80	200			
				Lung carcinoma	2/120	8/60*	0/60			$p < 0.05$
		F	Diet for 2 years	Dose (mg/kg of diet)	0	80	200			
				Hepatoma	1/30	0/30	1/30			
Rossi et al. (1977)	Rat Wistar	M	Diet until 152 weeks of age	Dose (mg/kg of diet)	0	500				
				Liver-cell tumours	0/36	9/37**		NA		
		F	Diet until 152 weeks of age	Dose (mg/kg of diet)	0	500				
				Liver-cell tumours	0/35	15/35***		NA		

Table 10 (contd)

Reference	Species/ strain	Sex	Dose schedule	Experimental parameter/ observation	Group 0	1	2	3	4	Statistical trend
Cabral et al. (1982a)	Rat MRC Porton	F	Diet for 144 weeks	Dose (mg/kg of diet) Liver-cell tumours	0 0/38	125 2/30	250 4/30	500 7/38		$p < 0.001$
Cabral et al. (1982b)	Hamster Syrian golden	M	Diet for 120 weeks	Dose (mg/kg of diet) Adrenal cortex tumour (mostly adenomas)	0 3/40	125 4/30	250 6/31	500 8/39		[$p = 0.04$]
		F		Adrenal cortex tumour	0/39	0/28	1/28	3/40		NS
Rossi et al. (1983)	Hamster Syrian golden	M	Diet until 128 weeks of age	Dose (mg/kg of diet) Adrenal cortex tumour (mostly adenomas)	0 8/31	1000 14/35				NA
		F		Adrenal cortex tumour	2/42	10/36**				NA
Kashyap et al. (1977)	Mouse Swiss	F	Subcutaneous	Dose (mg/animal) Liver-cell carcinomas	0 0/20	0.25 7/26				[$p = 0.01$]
TDE										
Tomatis et al. (1974)	Mouse CF-1	M	Diet until 130 weeks of age	Dose (mg/kg of diet) Liver-cell tumours Lung tumours	0 33/98 53/98	250 31/59** 51/59**				NA
		F	Diet until 130 weeks of age	Dose (mg/kg of diet) Liver-cell tumours Lung tumours	0 1/90 37/90	250 1/59 43/59**				NA
US National Cancer Institute (1978)	Mouse B6C3F$_1$	M	Diet for 78 weeks	Dose (mg/kg of diet) Hepatocellular carcinoma	0 2/18	411 12/44	822 14/50			NS
		F	Diet for 78 weeks	Dose (mg/kg of diet) Hepatocellular carcinoma	0 0/20	411 2/48	822 3/47			NS
National Cancer Institute (1978)	Rat Osborne-Mendel	M	Diet for 78 weeks	Dose (mg/kg of diet) Follicular-cell adenoma and carcinoma	0 1/19	1647 16/49*	3294 11/49			$p = 0.03$
		F	Diet for 78 weeks	Dose (mg/kg of diet) Follicular-cell adenoma and carcinoma	0 2/19	850 11/48	1700 6/50			NS

Table 10 (contd)

Reference	Species/strain	Sex	Dose schedule	Experimental parameter/observation	0	1	2	3	4	Statistical trend
DDE										
Tomatis et al. (1974)	Mouse CF-1	M	Diet until 110 weeks of age	Dose (mg/kg of diet)	0	250				NA
				Liver-cell tumours	33/98	39/53**				
		F	Diet until 110 weeks of age	Dose (mg/kg of diet)	0	250				NA
				Liver-cell tumours	1/90	54/55***				
US National Cancer Institute (1978)	Mouse B6C3F$_1$	M	Diet for 78 weeks	Dose (mg/kg of diet)	0	148	261			$p < 0.001$
				Survival at 70 weeks	5/20	35/50	31/50			
				Hepatocellular carcinoma	0/19	7/41	17/47*			
		F	Diet for 78 weeks	Dose (mg/kg of diet)	0	148	261			$p < 0.001$
				Survival at 75 weeks	19/20	47/50	28/50			
				Hepatocellular carcinoma	0/19	19/47***	34/48***			
Rossi et al. (1983)	Hamster Syrian golden	M	Diet until 128 weeks of age	Dose (mg/kg of diet)	0	500	1000			NA
				Liver-cell tumours	0/10	7/15*	8/24*			
		F	Diet until 128 weeks of age	Dose (mg/kg of diet)	0	050	1000			NA
				Liver-cell tumours	0/31	4/26*	5/24*			

NA, not applicable; NS, not statistically significant
*$p < 0.05$
**$p < 0.01$
***$p < 0.001$
[a]In mice that died after 60 weeks

rapidly following DDA ingestion and least following DDT. Urinary excretion of DDA began within 24 h of ingestion of DDT, TDE or DDA. Urinary DDA returned to its predose level two to three days after its administration but continued to be excreted slightly above the predose level for more than four months following termination of ingestion of TDE or DDT. DDE failed to produce any increase in DDA excretion (Roan *et al.*, 1971). Dechlorination of DDT (administered to volunteers at 5, 10 or 20 mg day for 183 days) led to conversion to TDE (measured in serum and adipose tissue) and further metabolism to the readily excreted DDA. Dehydrochlorination of DDT yielded DDE, a stable metabolite. In two subjects who ingested technical-grade DDT, the conversion of *para,para'*-DDT to *para,para'*-DDE was limited, as assessed by measuring DDE concentrations in serum and adipose tissue (Morgan & Roan, 1971). After oral administration of technical-grade DDT at 10 or 20 mg per day for six months, the level of *ortho,para'*-DDT was reported to decline more rapidly than that of *para,para'*-DDT. After the treatment period, excretion of DDA declined sharply, despite a very slow decrease in serum and adipose tissue levels of DDT (Roan, 1970).

A positive dose-related correlation between exposure to DDT and urinary excretion of DDA has been observed (Perini & Ghezzo, 1970; Wolfe & Armstrong, 1971), indicating that the urinary level of DDA could be used as a monitoring test of the extent of recent exposure to DDT.

As discussed in section 1.3, DDT and its metabolites tend to accumulate in the human body as well as in the environment (WHO, 1979, 1989), and DDT and/or its metabolites have been determined in several human organs and maternal milk. As use of DDT was either banned or restricted during the 1970s throughout the world, temporal changes occurred in some pharmacokinetic parameters of DDT in the general population. Some examples in various countries are shown in Tables 11-13.

4.1.2 *Experimental systems*

The metabolism of DDT has been reviewed (WHO, 1979; Lund, 1989; Agency for Toxic Substances and Disease Registry, 1989).

Several metabolic pathways leading from DDT to DDA have been proposed, and those suggested for the degradation of DDT, including areas at which reactive metabolites may be involved, are given in Figure 1. The biological half-time for DDT is about one month in dogs (Deichmann *et al.*, 1969), two months in hens (Lillard & Noles, 1973), three months in monkeys (Durham *et al.*, 1963) and approximately five weeks in rats (Datta & Nelson, 1968). In the latter species, the half-time was reduced to five days under conditions of starvation for three days followed by a restricted diet (Mitjavila *et al.*, 1981). Most species, including humans but with the exception of rhesus monkeys, store DDE more tenaciously than they do DDT (WHO, 1979). DDA is the major and final water-soluble metabolite in the urine of rats, mice and rabbits (Reif & Sinsheimer, 1975; Gold & Brunk, 1982; White & Sweeney, 1945).

In the main pathway from *para,para'*-DDT *via para,para'*-TDE to *para,para'*-DDA, the formation of two reactive intermediates is postulated, i.e., a free radical and an acid chloride (Baker & Van Dyke, 1984; Gold & Brunk, 1984). Both intermediates are probably capable of binding covalently to cellular macromolecules. Other reactive intermediates in the metabolism of DDT include side-chain epoxides of DDE, 1-chloro-2,2-bis(*para*-chloro-phenyl)ethene and 1,1-bis(*para*-chlorophenyl)ethene (Planche *et al.*, 1979; Gold *et al.*, 1981;

**Table 11. Temporal trends in total DDT
levels in human adipose tissue (mg/kg) in the
US population (range of reported values)[a]**

Period	DDT (mg/kg)
1955-65	6.7-19.9
1965-72	5.5-23.2
1975-88	1[b]-4.3

[a]From WHO (1979); Adeshina & Todd (1990)
[b]North Texas only

**Table 12. Temporal trends in total DDT levels in human
blood in different populations (mean or range of means)[a]**

Country	Period[b]	DDT (μg/l)[c]
Brazil	1973	45
	[late 1970s][d]	30
Canada	[early 1970s][d]	32
	[early 1980s][d]	2-3
India	1975	166-683
	1979-80	26.2

[a]From Agarwal et al. (1976); WHO (1979); Procianoy & Schvartsman
(1981); Saxena et al. (1983); Mes et al. (1984)
[b]In square brackets, approximate date (dates not given in article)
[c]Reported as μg/l or approximated from concentrations given in paper

**Table 13. Temporal trends in concentrations of DDT-
derived material in human milk[a]**

Country	Period	mg/l[b]
France	1971-73	0.11
	1979	0.001
Sweden	1967	0.1
	1978-79	0.06

[a]From Luquet et al. (1974); WHO (1979); Hofvander et al. (1981);
Klein et al. (1986)
[b]Reported as mg/l or approximated from concentrations in paper

Fawcett et al., 1987). Ring epoxides (arenoxides) may lead to the formation of the methyl
sulfone of DDE (Jensen & Jansson, 1976; Lund, 1989).

    In a study in mice pretreated for five months with DDE and subsequently given
radiolabelled DDE, however, most of the radiolabel in urine, faeces and liver was bound to
unchanged DDE and one phenolic metabolite (Gold & Brunk, 1986). The authors concluded
that there was no indication for the metabolism of DDE to a reactive electrophilic species.

Fig. 1. Compilation of metabolic pathways proposed for DDT in rodents; asterisks indicate where reactive intermediates are suggested to be formed[a]

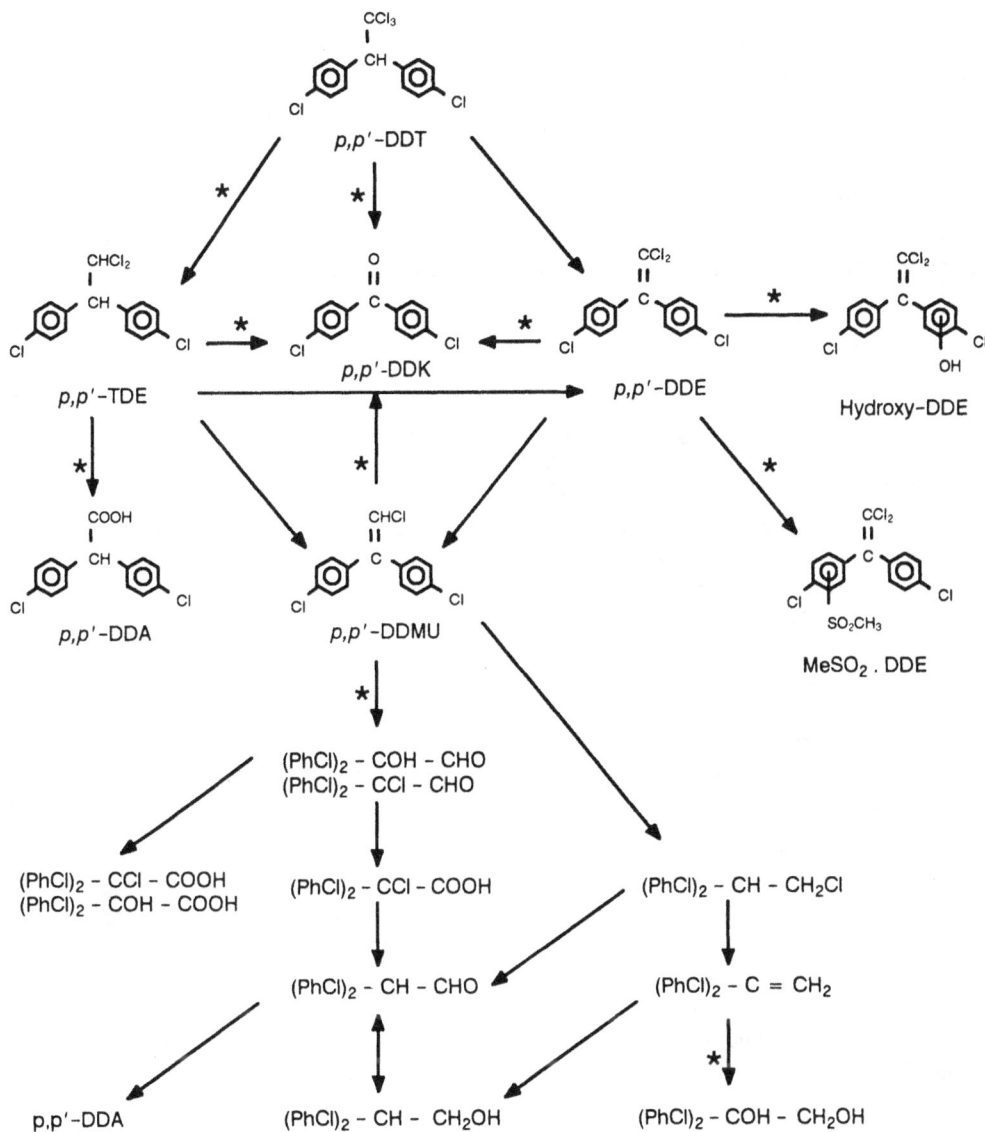

[a]From Lund (1989); p,p'-DDK, bis(4-chlorophenyl)ketone; DDA, para,para'-2,2-bis(para-chloro-phenyl)acetic acid; DDMU, 1-chloro-2,2-bis(para-chlorophenyl)ethene; PhCl, 4-chlorophenyl

Several studies have indicated that the metabolic pathways are similar in various species including humans (Reif & Sinsheimer, 1975; Gingell, 1976; Fawcett *et al.*, 1987). Hamsters differ from mice, however, in that after dietary treatment with *para,para'*-DDT, they do not excrete DDE in the urine; furthermore, the relative DDE tissue levels in hamsters are much lower than those in mice (Gingell & Wallcave, 1974; Gingell, 1976). The metabolism of DDT is promoted by DDT itself in hamsters but not in mice (Gingell & Wallcave, 1974). Monkeys fed diet containing up to 5000 ppm (mg/kg) of *para,para'*-DDT stored little or no DDE in body fat, but when DDE itself was fed (at 200 ppm in the diet), DDE was readily accumulated in body fat (Durham *et al.*, 1963).

ortho,para'-TDE was bound irreversibly in the alveolar and bronchiolar areas of rabbit and mouse lung (Lund *et al.*, 1986; Lund, 1989). 3-Methylsulfonyl-DDE was bound covalently in the zona fasciculata of the mouse adrenal cortex, causing necrotic changes (Lund *et al.*, 1988).

4.2 Toxic effects

4.2.1 *Humans*

Signs and symptoms reported following acute intoxication by DDT include nausea, vomiting, paraesthesia, dizziness, ataxia, confusion, tremor and, in severe cases, convulsions (WHO, 1979; Hayes, 1982).

Increased serum levels of triglyceride, cholesterol and γ-glutamyl transpeptidase were associated with increased serum levels of DDT in a largely black, agricultural US community, where over a period of years fish had been consumed that was contaminated with DDT, as they were caught from a river in which DDT wastes from a nearby manufacturing plant had accumulated in sediments. Serum levels of DDT were several fold higher than the US average (Kreiss *et al.*, 1981).

Therapeutic use of *ortho,para'*-TDE for Cushing's syndrome and adrenocortical carcinoma at doses of 1-12 g per day for up to 34 months was associated with fatigue, nausea, anorexia, vomiting and diarrhoea (Southern *et al.*, 1966; Hoffman & Mattox, 1972; Luton *et al.*, 1979).

4.2.2 *Experimental systems*

The acute toxicity of DDT is high in insects (LD_{50}, 14 mg/kg bw) and less pronounced in mammals (oral LD_{50}, 150-400 mg/kg bw; Fahmy *et al.*, 1973; Hrdina *et al.*, 1975; Lund, 1989). The oral LD_{50}s in rats of DDE, TDE and DDA are lower (880-1240, > 4000 and 600-1900 mg/kg bw, respectively) (WHO, 1979).

Acute intoxication with DDT elicits symptoms mainly from the central nervous system, and death is usually caused by respiratory arrest. Large doses of DDT cause focal necrosis of liver cells in several species (WHO, 1979).

Long-term studies of oral administration of DDT have been performed in rats, mice, hamsters, dogs and monkeys (reviewed by the Agency for Toxic Substances and Disease Registry, 1989). The liver is one of the main target organs, and hepatic effects range from increased liver weights to cellular necrosis. As reported by the Agency for Toxic Substances and Disease Registry (1989), the no-observed-adverse-effect level for hepatic effects in a study by the US National Cancer Registry (1978) was 32 mg/kg bw per day for 78 weeks in rats, and that in a study by Durham *et al.* (1963) was 8 mg/kg bw per day when given to rhesus monkeys for 3.5-7.5 years.

Effects on the central nervous system such as tremors and hyperactivity are also associated with chronic exposure to DDT. As reported by the Agency for Toxic Substances and Disease Registry (1989), tremors were apparent with doses of 10.5 mg/kg bw per day in the study of the US National Cancer Institute (1978) in rats; in a study by Cabral *et al.* (1982b), it was reported that hamsters showed no clinical sign of neurotoxicity at doses up to 40 mg/kg bw per day for life.

DDT and its derivatives induce a variety of microsomal enzymes in rodents and primates, mainly involving cytochrome P450-related enzymes (WHO, 1979; Campbell *et al.*, 1983). In rats, DDT increased the hepatic activity of microsomal drug hydroxylation and glucuronidation (Vainio, 1974, 1975). Species differences in isozyme-specific induction by DDT and its derivatives may contribute to species differences in the toxicology of these compounds. In the livers of partially hepatectomized rats treated *in vivo* with *N*-nitrosodiethylamine, DDT induced the metabolism of pentoxy- and benzyloxyresorufin, markers of cytochrome P450b isozymes, but not of ethoxyresorufin, a marker of the cytochrome P450c-d isozymes (Flodström *et al.*, 1990). Ioannides *et al.* (1984) also showed that DDT has no significant effect on ethoxyresorufin *O*-deethylase in rat liver or kidney [described in the paper in terms of the former terminology as cytochrome P448 activity]. Mice appear to be relatively resistant to induction of hepatic microsomal enzymes by DDT (Chhabra & Fouts, 1973).

ortho,para'-DDT has oestrogenic activity in rats, while *para,para'*-DDT has less and TDE and DDE have little or no activity (Welch *et al.*, 1969; Robison *et al.*, 1985a).

Feeding of *para,para'*-DDT to Wistar rats at 100 mg/kg of diet significantly suppressed both humoral and cell-mediated immune responses after 18-22 weeks (Banerjee, 1987).

DDT also enhanced the incidence of γ-glutamyltranspeptidase-positive enzyme-altered foci *in vivo* in partially hepatectomized, *N*-nitrosodiethylamine-initiated male Sprague-Dawley rats that received 1000 ppm (mg/kg) DDT in the diet for 11 weeks. It induced significantly more foci per cubic centimetre and a larger percentage of liver tissue occupied by focus tissue than was seen in a vehicle-treated group. The related compound, fenarimol, caused no significant change in the incidence of foci, although it induced cytochrome P450-related enzyme activities similar to those induced by DDT (Flodström *et al.*, 1990). Induction of altered foci by DDT has also been demonstrated using other protocols (Ito *et al.*, 1983).

DDT at 200 μM stimulated protein kinase C activity *in vitro* in preparations from mouse brain (Moser & Smart, 1989). In contrast, DDT (at 25 μM) did not stimulate protein kinase C activity in hamster V-79 cells (utilized for studies on cell-cell communication), nor could any binding of DDT to the phorbol ester receptor be demonstrated (Wärngård *et al.*, 1989). Furthermore, cytosolic calcium was not involved in the DDT-induced loss of gap-junctional intercellular communication in rat liver WB-F344 cells (Fransson *et al.*, 1990). Co-administration of quercetin with DDT *in vivo* did not prevent the development of preneoplastic enzyme-altered foci in the livers of rats that had undergone a partial hepatectomy and been initiated with *N*-nitrosodiethylamine (Wärngård *et al.*, 1989).

4.3 Reproductive and prenatal effects

4.3.1 *Humans*

In one study of 101 spontaneous abortions in Florida, USA (28 in whites and 73 in blacks) and 152 normal pregnancies (45 in whites and 107 blacks), blood was collected and analysed for the concentration of DDT. The women investigated lived in an area where DDT was used extensively for industrial and residential pest control. No difference was found between the two groups. No confounding was apparently exerted by age or parity (O'Leary *et al.*, 1970). [The Working Group noted that the levels of exposure may have been low and homogeneous.]

In a study in Brazil, 54 maternal-infant pairs were divided into two groups: term deliveries (30 pairs) and pre-term deliveries (24). None of the mothers had had known occupational exposure or domiciliary use of DDT, but all lived in an area highly conta-minated with DDT. Maternal blood and cord blood were collected at the time of delivery, and DDT metabolites were measured. No difference was found in the concentration of DDT metabolites between mothers in the two groups, and there was no correlation between DDT levels in the neonates and their gestational ages; however, a significant correlation was detected between low birth weight and DDT levels in neonates ($p < 0.05$). The authors interpreted those findings as indicating that the most important factor determining the cord blood level of DDT is the amount of fetal adipose tissue (Procianoy & Schvartsman, 1981).

In a study from Israel, mean serum levels of total DDT were 71.1 ppb ($\mu g/l$) in 17 women who gave birth prematurely and 26.5 ppb in a group of 10 women with term deliveries (Wassermann *et al.*, 1982).

In a study in North Carolina, USA, birthweight, head circumference, neonatal jaundice and neurological and behavioural changes were determined in 912 infants born between 1978 and 1982 and followed to 1985. Blood samples from the mothers and the babies and samples of placenta and milk or colostrum were collected and analysed for the concentration of DDE. DDE levels in milk fat at birth were presented in categories ranging from 0 to ≥ 6 ppm ($\mu g/kg$). No association was found between DDE concentrations and birthweight, head circumference and hyperbilirubinaemia; a statistically significant association was detected between the levels and hyporeflexia, measured in the babies through a reflex score (Rogan *et al.*, 1986).

4.3.2 *Experimental systems*

The effects of DDT on reproduction and development have been reviewed (Ware, 1975; Agency for Toxic Substances and Disease Registry, 1989).

Because they have weak oestrogenic effects, DDT and its metabolites have been investigated for reproductive and developmental effects (Bitman & Cecil, 1970; Bustos *et al.*, 1988; Mason & Schulte, 1981; Robison *et al.*, 1985a,b; Uphouse & Williams, 1989). Studies by Deichmann and Keplinger (1966) [abstract] and Deichmann *et al.* (1971) suggested impaired reproduction. Gellert *et al.* (1974) and Gellert and Heinrichs (1975) demonstrated altered reproductive function in rats treated perinatally with DDT or metabolites.

Treatment of 10-day old NMRI mice with DDT or its metabolite, 2,2-bis(4-chloro-phenyl)ethanol-palmitic acid, at doses as low as 1.4 $\mu mol/kg$ bw (0.5 mg/kg bw for DDT) resulted in changes in behaviour (such as disruption of a nonassociative learning process).

DDT treatment also resulted in changes in acetylcholine metabolism in the brain in adulthood (Eriksson *et al.*, 1990b).

Developmental effects, such as decreased survival of neonatal rats, were observed after feeding technical-grade DDT to rats at 200 ppm (mg/kg) in the diet. Premature puberty was seen in dogs fed 5 mg/kg per day (Ottoboni, 1969; Ottoboni *et al.*, 1977). Del Pup *et al.* (1978) examined the effect of technical-grade DDT (100 ppm [mg/kg] in the diet) on stable mouse populations, each containing about 400 animals. During the 70-week treatment with DDT, no alteration in viability index (survival at day 4:survival at day 1) was observed; however, a decrease in the lactation index (survival at day 30:survival at day 4) was noted. The no-observed-adverse-effect level for developmental effects was reported to be 1 mg/kg bw per day for all three studies (Agency for Toxic Substances and Disease Registry, 1989).

Tarján and Kemény (1969) conducted five-generation studies in BALB/c mice by feeding them DDT (mostly *para,para'*-) at 2.8-3.0 ppm [mg/kg] in the diet. No effect on number of pregnancies, births, litters, offspring or weanling survival was noted.

Male rats were given DDT at either 500 mg/kg bw on days 4 and 5 of life or 200 mg/kg bw per day from day 4 to day 23 of life by gavage. Testicular weight was decreased by both treatments, as was tubular diameter. Spermatogenesis and fertility were also impaired (Krause *et al.*, 1975).

Dean *et al.* (1980) examined the effect of a single injection of DDT (8% (w/v) DDT (95% *para,para'*-) [40 mg] in 0.5 ml arachis oil, intraperitoneally) on gestational day 13 on the androgen status of two-, four-, six-, eight- and ten-day-old male rats. Cross-fostering of litters from treated and control rats suggested that substantial amounts of DDT were transferred to the pups during lactation. Neonatal exposure to DDT increased hepatic metabolism of testosterone without altering circulating testosterone levels or testicular synthesis of testosterone.

Preimplantation treatment of New Zealand white rabbits with DDT decreased the size of the conceptus by approximately 60% and decreased the weight of 28-day-old fetuses, of fetal brain and of fetal kidney. It also altered the protein profile of the yolk sac fluids, as demonstrated by polyacrylamide gel electrophoresis (Fabro *et al.*, 1984).

Early studies on reproductive effects suggested that DDT affects avian eggshell thickness (Bitman *et al.*, 1969). These studies demonstrated that administration of *ortho,para'*- or *para,para'*-DDT in the diet at 100 ppm (mg/kg) decreased egg weight, eggshell thickness and the percentage of calcium in the shells. A series of studies conducted since that time further defined the effect of DDT and its metabolites on eggshell thickness (see WHO, 1979, for review).

Swartz (1984) evaluated the effect on DDT on the chick embryo, with specific attention to gonadal development. DDT at 5, 10 or 20 mg was injected into the yolk sac of eggs, which were incubated for five or 12 days before examination. After five days of incubation, no difference in the number of primordial germ cells was observed in treated or control chicks; after 12 days of incubation, however, there were differences in the morphology and histochemistry of the chick gonads.

Treatment of quail eggs with an aqueous suspension of DDT over five generations produced a progressive decrease over generations in the number of germ cells in the gonad of the chicks (David, 1977). Shellenberger (1978) observed no effect of *para,para'*-DDT at 5 or 50 ppm (mg/kg) in the diet on quail growth or reproduction over four generations and no effect on growth, egg production, hatchability or fertility.

Bryan *et al.* (1989) examined the effect of *ortho,para'*-DDT (1-10 mg) and *para,para'*-DDT (1-10 mg) on Japanese quail following treatment *in ovo* beginning on day 1 of incubation. Neither *ortho,para'*- nor *para,para'*-DDT affected hatchability, survival to day 16 post-hatching or the numbers of malpositioned or malformed chicks at doses up to 10 mg/egg. A dose-dependent increase in the percentage of chicks with ataxia and tremor and embryos that pipped but did not emerge was observed when eggs were treated with *para,para'*-DDT. Survival to five weeks of age was decreased in chicks treated with 6.25 mg *ortho,para'*-DDT and above and with 1.75 mg *para,para'*-DDT and above. Feather morphology was altered in more than 50% of birds treated with 6.25 mg *ortho,para'*-DDT and above and 1.75 mg *para,para'*-DDT and above. Ovipositions and the percentage hatched were decreased by exposure to 5 mg *ortho,para'*- and 1.75 mg *para,para'*-DDT. Reproductive behaviour was altered by treatment with 6.25 mg *ortho,para'*- but not with 1.75 mg *para,para'*-DDT.

Jelinek *et al.* (1985) found an increased incidence of malformations in a chick embryo screening test. Fry and Toone (1981) injected DDT into gulls' eggs at concentrations comparable to those found in contaminated eggs in the 1970s (2-100 ppm [mg/kg] per whole egg). Treatment induced abnormal development of gonadal tissues, with formation of ovarian tissue and oviducts in male embryos.

4.4 Genetic and related effects (see also Tables 14-17 and Appendices 1 and 2)

4.4.1 Humans

Blood samples were taken from 50 workers in three pesticide plants in Brazil who were of similar socioeconomic status and were either directly or indirectly exposed to DDT. They were divided into two groups on the basis of their type of employment and DDT plasma levels: 20 people in a 'control group' had a DDT plasma level of 0.275 µg/ml (range, 0.03-1.46 µg/ml), and 30 people in an 'exposed group' had a plasma level of 0.993 µg/ml (range, 0.16-3.25 µg/ml). The frequencies of cells with chromatid aberrations was 8.8% in the control group and 12.0% in the exposed group ($p < 0.05$, analysis of variance); there was no difference in the frequency of cells with chromosome-type aberrations (Nazareth Rabello *et al.*, 1975). [The Working Group noted that smoking was not controlled for and that details of the choice of the original controls were not given. Furthermore, a 72-h culture time was used, and only 50 metaphases per individual were analysed, thus weakening the significance of the results.]

4.4.2 Experimental systems

DDT

DDT did not induce DNA damage in either bacteria or cultured rodent and human cells. It did not induce gene mutation in bacteria, fungi or insects, in rodent host-mediated assays or in the mouse spot test *in vivo*. Gene mutation was not induced in Chinese hamster V79 cells at the *hprt* locus. Tests for the induction of aneuploidy in insects gave conflicting results, while one study in *Drosophila melanogaster* showed that DDT induced dominant lethality in insects.

Conflicting results were obtained in tests for chromosomal aberration in cultured rodent and human cells.

Inhibition of gap-junctional intercellular communication (as measured by inhibition of metabolic cooperation or dye transfer) was found consistently in rodent and human cells following treatment with DDT. In corroboration of these findings, exposure of rats to DDT *in vivo* reduced the number of gap junctions. Conflicting results were obtained in cell transformation assays.

In a study *in vivo*, positive results were reported for chromosomal aberrations in mouse bone-marrow cells. The Working Group noted that an additional study, reported from the same laboratory, was inadequate for evaluation because of the small number of control animals (Larsen & Jalal, 1974). Negative results were obtained in the same tests in the rat. A weak positive response was seen for induction of chromosomal aberrations in mouse spermatocytes in a single study. Dominant lethal tests in mice and rats gave equivocal results. No significant effect on sperm morphology was observed in several studies; but, in a single study in rats, significant changes were found.

para,para'-TDE

para,para'-TDE was not mutagenic to bacteria, and an unspecified isomer of TDE did not induce unscheduled DNA synthesis in primary cultures of mouse, rat or Syrian hamster hepatocytes. *para,para'*-TDE weakly induced chromosomal aberrations in rodent cells. In a single study, it inhibited gap-junctional intercellular communication in cultured rodent cells. In one study, it did not induce transformation in mouse embryo cells.

ortho,para'-TDE

ortho,para'-TDE did not induce mutation in *Salmonella typhimurium*. An unspecified isomer of TDE did not induce unscheduled DNA synthesis in primary cultures of rat, mouse or Syrian hamster hepatocytes. Equivocal results were obtained for induction of chromosomal aberrations in cultured rodent cells. In a single study, it did not induce transformation in mouse embryo cells.

para,para'-DDE

para,para'-DDE did not induce DNA damage in bacteria or mutation in bacteria or yeast. It induced intrachromosomal rearrangements in yeast. [The Working Group noted that this is a newly developed, not yet validated assay system involving DNA rearrangement in an integrated recombinant plasmid.] *para,para'*-DDE did not induce unscheduled DNA synthesis in primary cultures of rat, mouse or hamster hepatocytes. It induced gene mutation in insects and rodent cells. Weak positive results were obtained in a single study for sister chromatid exchange and in the majority of studies on chromosomal aberrations in rodent cells.

In single studies, *para,para'*-DDE inhibited gap-junctional intercellular communication between cultured rodent cells, but it did not induce transformation of mouse embryo cells.

Table 14. Genetic and related effects of DDT

Test system	Result[a]		Dose[b] LED/HID	Reference
	Without exogenous metabolic system	With exogenous metabolic system		
ECB, Breakage in plasmid DNA *in vitro*	–	0	100.0000	Griffin & Hill (1978)
BSD, *Bacillus subtilis rec* strains, differential toxicity	–	–	72.6000	Matsui et al. (1989)
ERD, *Escherichia coli*, WP2, differential toxicity	–	0	2000.0000	Rashid & Mumma (1986)
ERD, *Escherichia coli* K–12, differential toxicity	–	0	2000.0000	Rashid & Mumma (1986)
ERD, *Escherichia coli* WP2, differential toxicity	–	–	2000.0000	De Flora et al. (1984)
SAD, *Salmonella typhimurium* TA1538/1978, differential toxicity	–	0	2000.0000	Rashid & Mumma (1986)
SA0, *Salmonella typhimurium* TA100, reverse mutation	–	–	170.0000	Bartsch et al. (1980)
SA0, *Salmonella typhimurium* TA100, reverse mutation	–[c]	–	177.0000	Planche et al. (1979)
SA0, *Salmonella typhimurium* TA100, reverse mutation	0	–	35.0000	Probst et al. (1981)
SA0, *Salmonella typhimurium* TA100, reverse mutation	–	–	2500.0000	Simmon et al. (1977)
SA0, *Salmonella typhimurium* TA100, reverse mutation	–	–	2500.0000	Moriya et al. (1983)
SA0, *Salmonella typhimurium* TA100, reverse mutation	–	–	2500.0000	Byeon et al. (1976)
SA0, *Salmonella typhimurium* TA100, reverse mutation	0	–	500.0000	Glatt & Oesch (1987)
SA0, *Salmonella typhimurium* TA100, reverse mutation	–	–	250.0000	Bruce & Heddle (1979)
SA0, *Salmonella typhimurium* TA100, reverse mutation	–	–	370.0000	Van Dijck & Van de Voorde (1976)
SA0, *Salmonella typhimurium* TA100, reverse mutation	–	–	177.0000	Nishimura et al. (1982)
SA0, *Salmonella typhimurium* TA100, reverse mutation	–	–	500.0000	De Flora et al. (1989)
SA5, *Salmonella typhimurium* TA1535, reverse mutation	–	–	2500.0000	Moriya et al. (1983)
SA5, *Salmonella typhimurium* TA1535, reverse mutation	–	–	1250.0000	Marshall et al. (1976)
SA5, *Salmonella typhimurium* TA1535, reverse mutation	–	–	35.0000	Probst et al. (1981)
SA5, *Salmonella typhimurium* TA1535, reverse mutation	–	–	2500.0000	Byeon et al. (1976)
SA5, *Salmonella typhimurium* TA1535, reverse mutation	0	–	2500.0000	Simmon et al. (1977)
SA5, *Salmonella typhimurium* TA1535, reverse mutation	0	–	500.0000	Glatt & Oesch (1987)
SA7, *Salmonella typhimurium* TA1537, reverse mutation	–	–	1250.0000	Marshall et al. (1976)
SA7, *Salmonella typhimurium* TA1537, reverse mutation	–	–	35.0000	Probst et al. (1981)
SA7, *Salmonella typhimurium* TA1537, reverse mutation	0	–	2500.0000	Simmon et al. (1977)
SA7, *Salmonella typhimurium* TA1537, reverse mutation	–	–	2500.0000	Moriya et al. (1983)

Table 14 (contd)

Test system	Result[a] Without exogenous metabolic system	With exogenous metabolic system	Dose[b] LED/HID	Reference
SA7, *Salmonella typhimurium* TA1537, reverse mutation	0	–	500.0000	Glatt & Oesch (1987)
SA7, *Salmonella typhimurium* TA1537, reverse mutation	–	–	250.0000	Bruce & Heddle (1979)
SA8, *Salmonella typhimurium* TA1538, reverse mutation	–	–	1250.0000	Marshall et al. (1976)
SA8, *Salmonella typhimurium* TA1538, reverse mutation	–	–	2500.0000	Moriya et al. (1983)
SA8, *Salmonella typhimurium* TA1538, reverse mutation	–	–	35.0000	Probst et al. (1981)
SA8, *Salmonella typhimurium* TA1538, reverse mutation	–	–	2500.0000	Byeon et al. (1976)
SA8, *Salmonella typhimurium* TA1538, reverse mutation	0	–	2500.0000	Simmon et al. (1977)
SA8, *Salmonella typhimurium* TA1538, reverse mutation	0	–	500.0000	Glatt & Oesch (1987)
SA9, *Salmonella typhimurium* TA98, reverse mutation	–	–	170.0000	Bartsch et al. (1980)
SA9, *Salmonella typhimurium* TA98, reverse mutation	–[c]	–	177.0000	Planche et al. (1979)
SA9, *Salmonella typhimurium* TA98, reverse mutation	–	–	35.0000	Probst et al. (1981)
SA9, *Salmonella typhimurium* TA98, reverse mutation	–	–	2500.0000	Moriya et al. (1983)
SA9, *Salmonella typhimurium* TA98, reverse mutation	0	–	2500.0000	Simmon et al. (1977)
SA9, *Salmonella typhimurium* TA98, reverse mutation	–	–	2500.0000	Byeon et al. (1976)
SA9, *Salmonella typhimurium* TA98, reverse mutation	0	–[d]	500.0000	Glatt & Oesch (1987)
SA9, *Salmonella typhimurium* TA98, reverse mutation	–	–	250.0000	Bruce & Heddle (1979)
SA9, *Salmonella typhimurium* TA98, reverse mutation	–	–	370.0000	Van Dijck & Van de Voorde (1976)
SA9, *Salmonella typhimurium* TA98, reverse mutation	–	–	177.0000	Nishimura et al. (1982)
SA9, *Salmonella typhimurium* TA98, reverse mutation	0	–	500.0000	De Flora et al. (1989)
SAS, *Salmonella typhimurium* TA92, reverse mutation	–	–	500.0000	Glatt & Oesch (1987)
SAS, *Salmonella typhimurium* TA1536, reverse mutation	–	–	1250.0000	Marshall et al. (1976)
SAS, *Salmonella typhimurium* C3076, reverse mutation	–	–	35.0000	Probst et al. (1981)
SAS, *Salmonella typhimurium* D3052, reverse mutation	–	–	35.0000	Probst et al. (1981)
SAS, *Salmonella typhimurium* G46, reverse mutation	–	–	35.0000	Probst et al. (1981)
SAS, *Salmonella typhimurium* TA1978, reverse mutation	–	–	370.0000	Van Dijck & Van de Voorde (1976)

Table 14 (contd)

Test system	Result[a] Without exogenous metabolic system	With exogenous metabolic system	Dose[b] LED/HID	Reference
ECW, *Escherichia coli* WP *uvrA*, reverse mutation	–	–	35.0000	Probst *et al.* (1981)
ECW, *Escherichia coli* WP2 *uvrA*, reverse mutation	0	–	500.0000	Glatt & Oesch (1987)
EC2, *Escherichia coli* WP2, reverse mutation	–	–	35.0000	Probst *et al.* (1981)
EC2, *Escherichia coli* WP2 *hcr*, reverse mutation	–	–	2500.0000	Moriya *et al.* (1983)
ANN, *Aspergillus nidulans*, aneuploidy	–	0	990.0000	Crebelli *et al.* (1986)
ANF, *Aspergillus nidulans*, forward mutation	–	0	990.0000	Crebelli *et al.* (1986)
NCF, *Neurospora crassa*, forward mutation	–	0	7500.0000	Clark (1974)
*, Wasp, recessive/dominant lethal mutation	–	0	10.0000[e]	Grosch & Valcovic (1967)
DMX, *Drosophila melanogaster*, sex-linked recessive lethal mutation	–	0	20.0000	Pielou (1952)
DMX, *Drosophila melanogaster*, sex-linked recessive lethal mutation	–	0	0.0000	Clark (1974)
DML, *Drosophila melanogaster*, dominant lethal mutation	+	0	0.0000	Clark (1974)
DMN, *Drosophila melanogaster*, aneuploidy	+	0	0.0000	Clark (1974)
DMC, *Drosophila melanogaster*, chromosome loss	–	0	25.0000	Woodruff *et al.* (1983)
DIA, DNA damage, Chinese hamster V79 cells	–	–	354.0000	Swenberg *et al.* (1976)
DIA, DNA damage, Chinese hamster V79 cells	–	–	1060.0000	Swenberg (1981)
DIA, DNA damage, rat hepatocytes	–	0	106.0000	Sina *et al.* (1983)
URP, Unscheduled DNA synthesis, rat hepatocytes	–	0	35.0000	Maslansky & Williams (1981)
URP, Unscheduled DNA synthesis, rat hepatocytes	–	0	35.0000	Probst *et al.* (1981)
UIA, Unscheduled DNA synthesis, mouse hepatocytes	–	0	35.0000	Klaunig *et al.* (1984)
UIA, Unscheduled DNA synthesis, mouse hepatocytes	–	0	35.0000	Maslansky & Williams (1981)
UIA, Unscheduled DNA synthesis, hamster hepatocytes	–	0	35.0000	Maslansky & Williams (1981)
G9H, Gene mutation, Chinese V79 hamster cells, *hprt* locus	–	0	35.0000	Kelly-Garvert & Legator (1973)
G9H, Gene mutation, Chinese V79 hamster cells, *hprt* locus	–	0	14.2000	Tsushimoto *et al.* (1983)

Table 14 (contd)

Test system	Result[a] Without exogenous metabolic system	Result[a] With exogenous metabolic system	Dose[b] LED/HID	Reference
CIC, Chromosomal aberrations, Chinese hamster V79 cells	−	0	45.0000	Kelly-Garvert & Legator (1973)
CIC, Chromosomal aberrations, Chinese hamster B14F28 cells	+	0	49.0000	Mahr & Miltenburger (1976)
TBM, Cell transformation, BALB/c 3T3 mouse fibroblast cells	+	+	10.0000	Fitzgerald et al. (1989)
TCL, Cell transformation, mouse embryo cells	−	0	15.0000	Langenbach & Gingell (1975)
UHT, Unscheduled DNA synthesis, HeLa cells	−	0	18.0000	Brandt et al. (1972)
UHT, Unscheduled DNA synthesis, human fibroblasts	−	−	354.0000	Ahmed et al. (1977)
UHT, Unscheduled DNA synthesis, human lymphocytes	−	0	500.0000	Rocchi et al. (1980)
GIH, Gene mutation, human fibroblasts	−	−	35.0000	Tong et al. (1981)
CHL, Chromosomal aberrations, human lymphocytes in vitro	−	0	0.2000	Lessa et al. (1976)
HMM, Host-mediated assay, Neurospora crassa	−	0	150.0000 × 2 p.o.	Clark (1974)
HMM, Host-mediated assay, Salmonella typhimurium his G46	−	0	500.0000	Buselmaier et al. (1972)
MST, Mouse spot test in vivo	−	0	250.0000	Wallace et al. (1976)
CBA, Chromosomal aberrations, mouse bone-marrow cells	+	0	100.0000 × 1 i.p.	Johnson & Jalal (1973)
CBA, Chromosomal aberrations, rat bone marrow in vivo	−	0	200.0000 × 1 i.p.	Legator et al. (1973)
CBA, Chromosomal aberrations, rat bone marrow in vivo	−	0	100.0000 × 5 i.p.	Legator et al. (1973)
CBA, Chromosomal aberrations, rat bone marrow in vivo	−	0	100.0000 × 1 p.o.	Legator et al. (1973)
CBA, Chromosomal aberrations, rat bone marrow in vivo	−	0	80.0000 × 5 p.o.	Legator et al. (1973)
CGC, Chromosomal aberrations, mouse spermatocytes in vivo	(+)	0	150.0000	Clark (1974)
DLM, Dominant lethal test, mice	−	0	130.0000 × 1 i.p.	Epstein et al. (1972)
DLM, Dominant lethal test, mice	−	0	1200.0000 × 1 i.p.	Buselmaier et al. (1972)
DLM, Dominant lethal test, mice	(+)	0	150.0000 × 2 p.o.	Clark (1974)
DLR, Dominant lethal test, rats	(+)	0	50.0000	Palmer et al. (1973)
DLM, Dominant lethal test, mice	−	0	105.0000	Epstein & Shafner (1968)
CLH, Chromosomal aberrations, human lymphocytes in vivo	(+)	0	1.0000	Nazareth Rabello et al. (1975)

Table 14 (contd)

Test system	Result[a] Without exogenous metabolic system	With exogenous metabolic system	Dose[b] LED/HID	Reference
ICR, Inhibition of metabolic cooperation, rat liver epithelial cells	+	0	0.3500	Williams et al. (1981)
ICR, Inhibition of metabolic cooperation, Chinese hamster V79 cells	+	0	2.0000	Kurata et al. (1982)
ICR, Inhibition of metabolic cooperation, Chinese hamster V79 cells	+	0	3.6000	Tsushimoto et al. (1983)
ICR, Inhibition of metabolic cooperation, Chinese hamster V79 cells	+	0	6.0000	Wärngård et al. (1985)
ICR, Inhibition of metabolic cooperation, Chinese hamster V79 cells	+	0	10.0000	Zeilmaker & Yamasaki (1986)
ICR, Inhibition of metabolic cooperation, Chinese hamster V79 cells	+	0	0.5000	Aylsworth et al. (1989)
ICR, Inhibition of metabolic cooperation, Chinese hamster V79 cells	+	0	7.0000	Wärngård et al. (1989)
ICR, Inhibition of metabolic cooperation, mouse hepatocytes	+	0	1.0000	Klaunig & Ruch (1987)
ICR, Inhibition of metabolic cooperation, mouse hepatocytes	+	0	9.0000	Klaunig et al. (1990)
ICR, Inhibition of metabolic cooperation, Chinese hamster V79 cells	+	0	3.5000	Flodström et al. (1990)
ICR, Inhibition of metabolic cooperation, rat liver WB-F344 cells	+	0	3.5000	Flodström et al. (1990)
ICR, Inhibition of metabolic cooperation, Djungarian hamster fibroblasts, SV40 transformed	+	0	100.0000	Budunova et al. (1989)
ICH, Inhibition of metabolic cooperation, human skin fibroblasts	+	0	5.0000	Davidson et al. (1985)
ICH, Inhibition of metabolic cooperation, teratocarcinoma cells	+	0	5.0000	Zhong-Xiang et al. (1986)
* Reduction of gap junctions, rat liver cells in vivo	+	0	500.0000	Sugie et al. (1987)
SPM, Sperm morphology, mice	-	0	50.0000	Wyrobek & Bruce (1975)
SPM, Sperm morphology, mice	-	0	125.0000	Bruce & Heddle (1979)
SPM, Sperm morphology, mice	-	0	100.0000	Topham (1980)
SPR, Sperm morphology, rats	+	0	200.0000	Krause et al. (1975)

*Not displayed on profile

[a] +, positive; (+), weakly positive; -, negative; 0, not tested; ?, inconclusive (variable response in several experiments within an adequate study)

[b] In-vitro tests, μg/ml; in-vivo tests, mg/kg bw

[c] With S9 but no cofactors

[d] Also tested with 1,1,1-trichloropropene-2,3-oxide (microsomal epoxide hydrolase inhibitor)

[e] 10 μg per wasp

Table 15. Genetic and related effects of *para,para'*-TDE

Test system	Result[a] Without exogenous metabolic system	With exogenous metabolic system	Dose[b] LED/HID	Reference
SA0, *Salmonella typhimurium* TA100, reverse mutation	–	–	2500.0000	Moriya *et al.* (1983)
SA0, *Salmonella typhimurium* TA100, reverse mutation	–	–	500.0000	Glatt & Oesch (1987)
SA5, *Salmonella typhimurium* TA1535, reverse mutation	–	–	2500.0000	Moriya *et al.* (1983)
SA5, *Salmonella typhimurium* TA1535, reverse mutation	–	–	500.0000	Glatt & Oesch (1987)
SA7, *Salmonella typhimurium* TA1537, reverse mutation	–	–	2500.0000	Moriya *et al.* (1983)
SA7, *Salmonella typhimurium* TA1537, reverse mutation	–	–	500.0000	Glatt & Oesch (1987)
SA8, *Salmonella typhimurium* TA1538, reverse mutation	–	–	2500.0000	Moriya *et al.* (1983)
SA8, *Salmonella typhimurium* TA1538, reverse mutation	–	–	500.0000	Glatt & Oesch (1987)
SA9, *Salmonella typhimurium* TA98, reverse mutation	–	–	2500.0000	Moriya *et al.* (1983)
SA9, *Salmonella typhimurium* TA98, reverse mutation	–	–	500.0000	Glatt & Oesch (1987)
SAS, *Salmonella typhimurium* TA92, reverse mutation	–	–	500.0000	Glatt & Oesch (1987)
ECW, *Escherichia coli* WP2, *uvrA*, reverse mutation	–	–	500.0000	Glatt & Oesch (1987)
EC2, *Escherichia coli* WP2 *hcr*, reverse mutation	–	–	2500.0000	Moriya *et al.* (1983)
URP, Unscheduled DNA synthesis, rat hepatocytes	–	0	32.0000[c]	Maslansky & Williams (1981)
UIA, Unscheduled DNA synthesis, mouse hepatocytes	–	0	32.0000[c]	Maslansky & Williams (1981)
UIA, Unscheduled DNA synthesis, hamster hepatocytes	–	0	32.0000[c]	Maslansky & Williams (1981)
CIC, Chromosomal aberrations, Chinese hamster B14F28 cells	(+)	0	45.0000	Mahr & Miltenburger (1976)
CIA, Chromosomal aberrations, other animals cells *in vitro*	(+)	0	10.0000	Palmer *et al.* (1972)
TCL, Cell transformation, mouse embryo cells	–	0	15.0000[c]	Langenbach & Gingell (1975)
HMM, Host-mediated assay, *Salmonella typhimurium his* G46	–	0	500.0000[c]	Buselmaier *et al.* (1972)
ICR, Inhibition of metabolic cooperation, animal cells *in vitro*	+	0	5.0000	Kurata *et al.* (1982)

[a]+, positive; (+), weakly positive; –, negative; 0, not tested; ?, inconclusive (variable response in several experiments within an adequate study)
[b]In-vitro tests, μg/ml; in-vivo tests, mg/kg bw
[c]Isomer not specified

Table 16. Genetic and related effects of *ortho,para'*-TDE

Test system	Result[a] Without exogenous metabolic system	With exogenous metabolic system	Dose[b] LED/HID	Reference
SA0, *Salmonella typhimurium* TA100, reverse mutation	–	–	50.0000	Mortelmans et al. (1986)
SA5, *Salmonella typhimurium* TA1535, reverse mutation	–	–	50.0000	Mortelmans et al. (1986)
SA7, *Salmonella typhimurium* TA1537, reverse mutation	–	–	50.0000	Mortelmans et al. (1986)
SA9, *Salmonella typhimurium* TA98, reverse mutation	–	–	166.0000	Mortelmans et al. (1986)
URP, Unscheduled DNA synthesis, rat hepatocytes	–	0	32.0000[c]	Maslansky & Williams (1981)
UIA, Unscheduled DNA synthesis, mouse hepatocytes	–	0	32.0000[c]	Maslansky & Williams (1981)
UIA, Unscheduled DNA synthesis, hamster hepatocytes	–	0	32.0000[c]	Maslansky & Williams (1981)
SIC, Sister chromatid exchange, Chinese hamster cells *in vitro*	–	–	16.0000	Galloway et al. (1987)
CIC, Chromosomal aberrations, Chinese hamster CHO cells	–	–	50.0000	Galloway et al. (1987)
CIA, Chromosomal aberrations, other animals cells *in vitro*	(+)	0	10.0000	Palmer et al. (1972)
HMM, Host-mediated assay, *Salmonella typhimurium his* G46	–	0	500.0000[c]	Buselmaier et al. (1972)
TCL, Cell transformation, mouse embryo cells	–	0	15.0000[c]	Langenbach & Gingell (1975)

[a] +, positive; (+), weakly positive; –, negative; 0, not tested; ?, inconclusive (variable response in several experiments within an adequate study)

[b] In-vitro tests, μg/ml; in-vivo tests, mg/kg bw

[c] Isomer not specified

Table 17. Genetic and related effects of *para,para'*-DDE

Test system	Result[a] Without exogenous metabolic system	With exogenous metabolic system	Dose[b] LED/HID	Reference
PRB, Breakage in plasmid DNA *in vitro*	0	–	100.0000	Mamber *et al.* (1984)
PRB, Breakage in plasmid DNA *in vitro*	–	–	3180.0000	Brams *et al.* (1987)
ERD, *Escherichia coli*, WP2, differential toxicity	0	–	1000.0000	Mamber *et al.* (1984)
SA0, *Salmonella typhimurium* TA100, reverse mutation	0	–	2500.0000	McCann *et al.* (1975)
SA0, *Salmonella typhimurium* TA100, reverse mutation	–	–	370.0000	Van Dijck & Van de Voorde (1976)
SA0, *Salmonella typhimurium* TA100, reverse mutation	–	–	500.0000	Simmon & Kauhanen (1978)
SA0, *Salmonella typhimurium* TA100, reverse mutation	–	–	860.0000	Bartsch *et al.* (1980)
SA0, *Salmonella typhimurium* TA100, reverse mutation	–	–	5000.0000	De Flora (1981)
SA0, *Salmonella typhimurium* TA100, reverse mutation	–	–	2500.0000	Moriya *et al.* (1983)
SA0, *Salmonella typhimurium* TA100, reverse mutation	–	–	500.0000	Mortelmans *et al.* (1986)
SA0, *Salmonella typhimurium* TA100, reverse mutation	–	–	2500.0000	Brams *et al.* (1987)
SA0, *Salmonella typhimurium* TA100, reverse mutation	0	–	500.0000	Glatt & Oesch (1987)
SA0, *Salmonella typhimurium* TA100, reverse mutation	–	–	500.0000	De Flora *et al.* (1989)
SA0, *Salmonella typhimurium* TA100, reverse mutation	0	–	2500.0000	McCann *et al.* (1975)
SA5, *Salmonella typhimurium* TA1535, reverse mutation	–	–	500.0000	Marshall *et al.* (1976)
SA5, *Salmonella typhimurium* TA1535, reverse mutation	–	–	370.0000	Van Dijck & Van de Voorde (1976)
SA5, *Salmonella typhimurium* TA1535, reverse mutation	–	–	500.0000	Simmon & Kauhanen (1978)
SA5, *Salmonella typhimurium* TA1535, reverse mutation	–	–	5000.0000	De Flora (1981)
SA5, *Salmonella typhimurium* TA1535, reverse mutation	–	–	2500.0000	Moriya *et al.* (1983)
SA5, *Salmonella typhimurium* TA1535, reverse mutation	–	–	500.0000	Mortelmans *et al.* (1986)
SA5, *Salmonella typhimurium* TA1535, reverse mutation	0	–	500.0000	Glatt & Oesch (1987)
SA7, *Salmonella typhimurium* TA1537, reverse mutation	0	–	2500.0000	McCann *et al.* (1975)
SA7, *Salmonella typhimurium* TA1537, reverse mutation	–	–	500.0000	Marshall *et al.* (1976)
SA7, *Salmonella typhimurium* TA1537, reverse mutation	–	–	370.0000	Van Dijck & Van de Voorde (1976)
SA7, *Salmonella typhimurium* TA1537, reverse mutation	–	–	500.0000	Simmon & Kauhanen (1978)

Table 17 (contd)

Test system	Result[a]		Dose[b] LED/HID	Reference
	Without exogenous metabolic system	With exogenous metabolic system		
SA7, *Salmonella typhimurium* TA1537, reverse mutation	–	–	5000.0000	De Flora (1981)
SA7, *Salmonella typhimurium* TA1537, reverse mutation	–	–	2500.0000	Moriya *et al.* (1983)
SA7, *Salmonella typhimurium* TA1537, reverse mutation	–	–	500.0000	Mortelmans *et al.* (1986)
SA7, *Salmonella typhimurium* TA1537, reverse mutation	–	–	2500.0000	Brams *et al.* (1987)
SA7, *Salmonella typhimurium* TA1537, reverse mutation	0	–	500.0000	Glatt & Oesch (1987)
SA8, *Salmonella typhimurium* TA1538, reverse mutation	–	–	500.0000	Marshall *et al.* (1976)
SA8, *Salmonella typhimurium* TA1538, reverse mutation	–	–	370.0000	Van Dijck & Van de Voorde (1976)
SA8, *Salmonella typhimurium* TA1538, reverse mutation	–	–	500.0000	Simmon & Kauhanen (1978)
SA8, *Salmonella typhimurium* TA1538, reverse mutation	–	–	5000.0000	De Flora (1981)
SA8, *Salmonella typhimurium* TA1538, reverse mutation	–	–	2500.0000	Moriya *et al.* (1983)
SA8, *Salmonella typhimurium* TA1538, reverse mutation	–	–	2500.0000	Brams *et al.* (1987)
SA8, *Salmonella typhimurium*, TA1538, reverse mutation	0	–	500.0000	Glatt & Oesch (1987)
SA9, *Salmonella typhimurium* TA98, reverse mutation	0	–	2500.0000	McCann *et al.* (1975)
SA9, *Salmonella typhimurium* TA98, reverse mutation	–	–	370.0000	Van Dijck & Van de Voorde (1976)
SA9, *Salmonella typhimurium* TA98, reverse mutation	–	–	500.0000	Simmon & Kauhanen (1978)
SA9, *Salmonella typhimurium* TA98, reverse mutation	–	–	860.0000	Bartsch *et al.* (1980)
SA9, *Salmonella typhimurium* TA98, reverse mutation	–	–	5000.0000	De Flora (1981)
SA9, *Salmonella typhimurium* TA98, reverse mutation	–	–	2500.0000	Moriya *et al.* (1983)
SA9, *Salmonella typhimurium* TA98, reverse mutation	–	–	500.0000	Mortelmans *et al.* (1986)
SA9, *Salmonella typhimurium* TA98, reverse mutation	0	–	500.0000	Glatt & Oesch (1987)
SA9, *Salmonella typhimurium* TA98, reverse mutation	–	–	500.0000	De Flora *et al.* (1989)
SAS, *Salmonella typhimurium* TA1536, reverse mutation	–	–	500.0000	Marshall *et al.* (1976)
SAS, *Salmonella typhimurium* TA1978, reverse mutation	–	–	370.0000	Van Dijck & Van de Voorde (1976)
SAS, *Salmonella typhimurium* TA1950, reverse mutation	–	–	370.0000	Van Dijck & Van de Voorde (1976)
SAS, *Salmonella typhimurium* TA92, reverse mutation	0	–	500.0000	Glatt & Oesch (1987)
ECW, *Escherichia coli* WP2 *uvrA*, reverse mutation	–	–	500.0000	Glatt & Oesch (1987)
EC2, *Escherichia coli* WP2 *hcr*, reverse mutation	–	–	2500.0000	Moriya *et al.* (1983)
EC2, *Escherichia coli* WP2, reverse mutation	0	–	1000.0000	Mamber *et al.* (1984)

Table 17 (contd)

Test system	Result[a] Without exogenous metabolic system	With exogenous metabolic system	Dose[b] LED/HID	Reference
*, *Saccharomyces cerevisiae*, intrachromosomal recombination	+	0	100.0000	Schiestl et al. (1989)
*, *Saccharomyces cerevisiae*, intrachromosomal recombination	+	0	100.0000	Schiestl (1989)
SCH, *Saccharomyces cerevisiae*, homozygosis	−	−	25000.0000	Simmon & Kauhanen (1978)
DMX, *Drosophila melanogaster*, sex-linked recessive lethal mutations	+	0	10000.0000	Valencia et al. (1985)
DMH, *Drosophila melanogaster*, heritable translocation test	−	0	10000.0000	Valencia et al. (1985)
DIA, DNA damage, rat hepatocytes [?]	+	0	95.0000	Sina et al. (1983)
URP, Unscheduled DNA synthesis, rat hepatocytes	−	0	31.0000	Maslansky & Williams (1981)
URP, Unscheduled DNA synthesis, rat hepatocytes	−	0	2000.0000	Williams et al. (1982)
UIA, Unscheduled DNA synthesis, mouse hepatocytes	−	0	31.0000	Maslansky & Williams (1981)
URP, Unscheduled DNA synthesis hamster hepatocytes	−	0	31.0000	Maslansky & Williams (1981)
GCO, Gene mutation, Chinese hamster ovary cells *in vitro*	+	0	16.0000	Amacher & Zelljadt (1984)
GST, Gene mutation, mouse lymphoma L5178Y cells, *tk* locus	+	−	40.0000	Clive et al. (1979)
SIC, Sister chromatid exchange, Chinese hamster cells *in vitro*	−	(+)	5.0000	Galloway et al. (1987)
CIC, Chromosomal aberrations, Chinese hamster V79 cells	(+)	0	35.0000	Kelly–Garvert & Legator (1973)
CIC, Chromosomal aberrations, Chinese hamster B14F28 cells	(+)	0	44.0000	Mahr & Miltenburger (1976)
CIC, Chromosomal aberrations, Chinese hamster CHO cells	−	−	60.0000	Galloway et al. (1987)
CIA, Chromosomal aberrations, other animals cells *in vitro*	(+)	0	10.0000	Palmer et al. (1972)
HMM, Host-mediated assay, *Salmonella typhimurium hisG46*	−	0	500.0000	Buselmaier et al. (1972)
TCL, Cell transformation, mouse embryo cells	−	0	15.0000	Langenbach & Gingell (1975)
ICR, Inhibition of metabolic cooperation, animal cells *in vitro*	+	0	10.0000	Kurata et al. (1982)

*Not displayed on profile

[a]+, positive; (+), weakly positive; −, negative; 0, not tested; ?, inconclusive (variable response in several experiments within an adequate study)

[b]In-vitro tests, μg/ml; in-vivo tests, mg/kg bw

5. Summary of Data Reported and Evaluation

5.1 Exposure data

Technical-grade DDT is a complex mixture of *para,para'*-DDT, its isomers and related compounds. It has been used since 1943 as a nonsystemic insecticide with a broad spectrum of activities. DDT has been used extensively for the control of vectors of malaria, typhus, yellow fever and sleeping sickness, and also on food crops. Its use is banned in some countries and has been restricted since the 1970s in many others to the control of vector-borne diseases.

DDT has been formulated in almost every conceivable form, including granules and powders, solutions, concentrates, aerosols and others, alone and in combination with other insecticides.

DDT is ubiquitous in the environment. It is highly persistent and has been found extensively in foods, soils and sediments. Residual levels in human tissues have been declining slowly with the decreasing use of DDT worldwide.

Exposure may occur during its production and application and as a result of persistent residual levels in surface water and sediments, and in foods.

5.2 Carcinogenicity in humans

Slight excess risks for lung cancer were observed among workers at two DDT producing facilities in the USA. A nested case-control study in one of these investigations found a slight deficit of respiratory cancer. No other cancer occurred in sufficient numbers for analysis. In a prospective cohort study in which exposures were estimated on the basis of serum levels of DDT, the risk for lung cancer rose with increasing concentration but was based on small numbers.

Several investigators have compared serum or tissue levels of DDT and/or DDE among individuals with and without cancer, with inconsistent results.

Results from case-control studies of soft-tissue sarcoma do not point to an association.

An elevated risk for non-Hodgkin's lymphoma in relation to potential exposure to DDT was found in a study from Washington State in the USA, but not for other agricultural exposures. An elevated risk for malignant lymphomas was also found in a case-control study in northern Sweden, with adjustment for exposure to herbicides. The only study available found no association between exposure to DDT and primary liver cancer. In the USA, a slight increase in the risk for leukaemia occurred among farmers who reported use of DDT and many other agricultural exposures. The relative risks for leukaemia rose with frequency of use of DDT on animals.

Epidemiological data on cancer risks associated with exposure to DDT are suggestive, but limitations in the assessments of exposure in the studies and the finding of small and inconsistent excesses complicate an evaluation. The slight excesses of respiratory cancer seen among cohorts exposed to DDT are based on differences of five or fewer cases between exposed and unexposed groups. In case-control studies of lymphatic and haematopoietic cancers, exposure to agricultural pesticides other than DDT resulted in excesses as large as or larger than those associated with exposure to DDT. In most of the case-control studies, adjustment was not made for the potential influence of other exposures.

The cohort and case-control studies that have become available since the last evaluation was made in 1987 (see IARC, 1987) add to some extent to the concern about DDT. Most of these investigations were not specifically designed to evaluate the effects of DDT; consequently, the findings for DDT were not reported as fully as would have been desirable.

5.3 Carcinogenicity in experimental animals

DDT has been tested adequately for carcinogenicity by oral administration in mice, rats and hamsters, and by subcutaneous administration in mice. Following oral administration to mice, it caused liver-cell tumours, including carcinomas, in animals of each sex and hepatoblastomas in males. In one study, the incidence of lung carcinomas was increased, and in three studies the incidence of malignant lymphomas was increased; the incidence of lymphoma was decreased in two studies (see also General Remarks). The incidence of liver tumours was increased in mice following subcutaneous injection of DDT. Oral administration of DDT to rats increased the incidence of liver tumours in female rats in one study and in male rats in two studies. In two studies in which DDT was administered orally to hamsters at concentrations similar to or higher than those found to cause liver tumours in mice and rats, some increase in the incidence of adrenocortical adenomas was observed.

A metabolite of DDT, *para,para'*-DDE, has been tested for carcinogenicity by oral administration in mice and hamsters. A second metabolite, TDE, was tested by oral administration in mice and rats. TDE increased the incidence of liver tumours in male mice and of lung tumours in animals of each sex in one of the two studies in mice. An increase in the number of thyroid tumours was observed in one study in male rats. DDE produced a high incidence of liver tumours in male and female mice in two studies. An increased incidence of neoplastic liver nodules was observed in one study in male and female hamsters.

5.4 Other relevant data

The liver is the target organ for the chronic toxicity of DDT. This compound induced liver microsomal enzymes in rodents and primates and increased the frequency of enzyme-positive foci in rat liver.

DDT impaired reproduction and/or development in mice, rats, rabbits, dogs and avian species.

In one study, higher DDT levels were noted in the serum of women who had delivered prematurely than in those who had had a normal delivery. Studies of spontaneous abortion, gestational period and newborn status showed no clear association with body levels of DDT.

In one study, increased frequencies of chromatid-type but not chromosome-type aberrations were observed in peripheral lymphocytes of workers with increased plasma levels of DDT. No data were available on the genetic and related effects of metabolites of DDT in humans.

DDT reduced gap-junctional areas in rat liver cells *in vivo* and inhibited gap-junctional intercellular communication in rodent and human cell systems. Conflicting data were obtained with regard to some genetic endpoints. In most studies, DDT did not induce genotoxic effects in rodent or human cell systems nor was it mutagenic to fungi or bacteria.

para,para'-DDE weakly induced chromosomal aberrations in cultured rodent cells and caused mutation in mammalian cells and insects, but not bacteria. *para,para'*-DDE inhibited gap-junctional intercellular communication in cultured rodent cells.

In most studies, *para,para'*-TDE did not induce genetic effects in short-term tests *in vitro*. It inhibited gap-junctional intercellular communication in cultured rodent cells.

There is no evidence that *ortho,para'*-TDE induced genetic effects in short-term tests *in vitro* on the basis of the few studies available.

5.5 Evaluation[1]

There is *inadequate evidence* in humans for the carcinogenicity of DDT.

There is *sufficient evidence* in experimental animals for the carcinogenicity of DDT.

Overall evaluation

DDT *is possibly carcinogenic to humans (Group 2B).*

6. References

Adeshina, F. & Todd, E.L. (1990) Organochlorine compounds in human adipose tissue from North Texas. *J. Toxicol. environ. Health*, *29*, 147-156

Agarwal, H.C., Pillai, M.K.K., Yadav, D.V., Menon, K.B. & Gupta, R.K. (1976) Residues of DDT and its metabolites in human blood samples in Delhi, India. *Bull. World Health Organ.*, *54*, 349-351

Agency for Toxic Substances and Disease Registry (1989) *Toxicological Profile for p,p'-DDT, p,p'-DDE, and p,p'-DDD*, Springfield, VA, National Technical Information Service

Agthe, C., Garcia, H., Shubik, P., Tomatis, L. & Wenyon, E. (1970) Study of the potential carcinogenicity of DDT in Syrian golden hamsters. *Proc. Soc. exp. Med. (N.Y.)*, *134*, 113-116

Ahmed, F.E., Hart, R.W. & Lewis, N.J. (1977) Pesticide induced DNA damage and its repair in cultured human cells. *Mutat. Res.*, *42*, 161-174

Albone, E.S., Eglinton, G., Evans, N.C., Hunter, J.M. & Rhead, M.M. (1972) Fate of DDT in Severn estuary sediments. *Environ. Sci. Technol.*, *6*, 914-919

Al-Omar, M.A., Tameesh, A.H. & Al-Ogaily, N.H. (1985) Dairy product contamination with organochlorine insecticide residues in Baghdad district. *J. biol. Sci. Res.*, *16*, 133-144

Amacher, D.E. & Zelljadt, I. (1984) Mutagenic activity of some clastogenic chemicals at the hypoxanthine guanine phosphoribosyl transferase locus of Chinese hamster ovary cells. *Mutat. Res.*, *136*, 137-145

American Conference of Governmental Industrial Hygienists (1989) *Threshold Limit Values and Biological Exposure Indices for 1989-1990*, Cincinnati, OH, p. 19

Arbeidsinspectie (Labour Inspection) (1986) *De Nationale MAC-Lijst 1986* [National MAC List 1986], Voorburg, p. 10 (in Dutch)

Arbejdstilsynet (Labour Inspection) (1988) *Graensevaezdier for Staffe og Materialen* [Limit Values for Compounds and Materials] (No. 3.1.0.2), Copenhagen, p. 15 (in Danish)

Austin, H., Keil, J.E. & Cole, P. (1989) A prospective follow-up study of cancer mortality in relation to serum DDT. *Am. J. public Health*, *79*, 43-46

---

[1]For definition of the italicized terms, see Preamble, pp. 26-28.

Aylsworth, C.F., Trosko, J.E., Chang, C.C., Benjamin, K. & Lockwood, E. (1989) Synergistic inhibition of metabolic cooperation by oleic acid or 12-O-tetradecanoylphorbol-13-acetate and dichlorodiphenyltrichloroethane (DDT) in Chinese hamster V79 cells: implication of a role for protein kinase C in the regulation of gap junctional intercellular communication. *Cell Biol. Toxicol.*, 5, 27-37

Baker, M.T. & Van Dyke, R.A. (1984) Metabolism-dependent binding of the chlorinated insecticide DDT and its metabolite DDD, to microsomal protein lipids. *Biochem. Pharmacol.*, 33, 255-260

Baloch, U.K. (1985) Problems associated with the use of chemicals by agricultural workers. *Basic Life Sci.*, 34, 63-78

Banerjee, B.D. (1987) Effects of sub-chronic DDT exposure on humoral and cell-mediated immune responses in albino rats. *Bull. environ. Contam. Toxicol.*, 39, 827-834

Bang, Y.H., Arwati, S. & Gandahusada, S. (1982) A review of insecticide use for malaria control in central Java, Indonesia. *Malays. appl. Biol.*, 11, 85-96

Bartsch, H., Malaveille, C., Camus, A.-M., Martel-Planche, G., Brun, G., Hautefeuille, A., Sabadie, N., Barbin, A., Kuroki, T., Drevon, C., Piccoli, C. & Montesano, R. (1980) Validation and comparative studies on 180 chemicals with *S. typhimurium* strains and V79 Chinese hamster cells in the presence of various metabolizing systems. *Mutat. Res.*, 76, 1-50

Bennison, B.E. & Mostofi, F.K. (1950) Observations on inbred mice exposed to DDT. *J. natl Cancer Inst.*, 10, 989-992

Bergenstal, D.M., Hertz, R., Lipsett, M.B. & Moy, R.H. (1960) Chemotherapy of adrenocortical cancer with o,p'-DDD. *Ann. intern. Med.*, 53, 672-682

Bhuiya, Z.H. & Rothwell, D.F. (1969) Gas chromatographic analysis of technical DDT. *Pak. J. Sci. Res.*, 21, 94-96

Bitman, J. & Cecil, H.C. (1970) Estrogenic activity of DDT analogs and polychlorinated biphenyls. *J. agric. Food Chem.*, 18, 1108-1112

Bitman, J., Cecil, H.C., Harris, S.J. & Fries, G.F. (1969) DDT induces a decrease in eggshell calcium. *Nature*, 224, 44-46

Bledsoe, T., Island, D.P., Ney, R.L. & Liddle, G.W. (1964) An effect of o,p'-DDD on the extra-adrenal metabolism of cortisol in man. *J. clin. Endocrinol.*, 24, 1303-1311

Boyle, E., Jr (1970) Biological patterns in hypertension by race, sex, body weight and skin color. *J. Am. med. Assoc.*, 213, 1637-1643

Brams, A., Buchet, J.P., Crutzen-Fayt, M.C., De Meester, C., Lauwerys, R. & Léonard, A. (1987) A comparative study, with 40 chemicals, of the efficiency of the *Salmonella* assay and the SOS chromotest (kit procedure). *Toxicol. Lett.*, 38, 123-133

Brandt, V.N., Flamm, W.G. & Bernheim, N.J. (1972) The value of hydroxyurea in assessing repair synthesis of DNA in HeLa cells. *Chem.-biol. Interactions*, 5, 327-339

Brooks, G.T. (1974) *Chlorinated Insecticides*, Vol. 1, *Technology and Application*, Cleveland, OH, CRC Press, pp. 7-83

Brown, L.M., Blair, A., Gibson, R., Everett, G.D., Cantor, K.P., Schuman, L.M., Burmeister, L.F., Van Lier, S.F. & Dick, F. (1990) Pesticide exposures and other agricultural risk factors for leukemia among men in Iowa and Minnesota. *Cancer*, 50, 1685-1691

Bruce, W.R. & Heddle, J.A. (1979) The mutagenic activity of 61 agents as determined by the micronucleus, *Salmonella*, and sperm abnormality assays. *Can. J. Genet. Cytol.*, 21, 319-334

Bryan, T.E., Gildersleeve, R.P. & Wiard, R.P. (1989) Exposure of Japanese quail embryos to o,p'-DDT has long-term effects on reproductive behaviors, hematology, and feather morphology. *Teratology*, 39, 525-535

Budavari, S., ed. (1989) *The Merck Index*, 4th ed., Rahway, NJ, Merck & Co., p. 446

Budunova, I.V., Mittelman, L.A. & Belitsky, G.A. (1989) Identification of tumor promoters by their inhibitory effect on intercellular transfer of Lucifer yellow. *Cell Biol. Toxicol.*, *5*, 77-89

Buselmaier, W., Röhrborn, G. & Propping, P. (1972) Mutagenicity investigations with pesticides in the host-mediated assay and the dominant lethal test in mice (Ger.). *Biol. Zbl.*, *91*, 310-325

Bustos, S., Denegri, J.C., Diaz, F. & Tchernitchin, A.N. (1988) p,p'-DDT is an estrogenic compound. *Bull. environ. Contam. Toxicol.*, *41*, 496-501

Byeon, W.-H., Hyun, H.H. & Lee, S.Y. (1976) Mutagenicity of pesticides in the *Salmonella*/microsome system (Korean). *Korean J. Microbiol.*, *14*, 128-134

Cabral, J.R.P. (1985) DDT: laboratory evidence. In: Wald, N.J. & Doll, R., eds, *Interpretation of Negative Epidemiological Evidence for Carcinogenicity* (IARC Scientific Publications No. 65), Lyon, IARC, pp. 101-105

Cabral, J.R.P., Hall, R.K., Rossi, L., Bronczyk, S.A. & Shubik, P. (1982a) Effects of long-term intake of DDT on rats. *Tumori*, *68*, 11-17

Cabral, J.R.P., Hall, R.K., Rossi, L., Bronczyk, S.A. & Shubik, P. (1982b) Lack of carcinogenicity of DDT in hamsters. *Tumori*, *68*, 5-10

Caldwell, G.G., Cannon, S.B., Pratt, C.B. & Arthur, R.D. (1981) Serum pesticide levels in patients with childhood colorectal carcinoma. *Cancer*, *48*, 774-778

Campbell, M.A., Gyorkos, J., Leece, B., Homonko, K. & Safe, S. (1983) The effects of twenty-two organochlorine pesticides as inducers of the hepatic drug-metabolizing enzymes. *Gen. Pharmacol.*, *14*, 445-454

Chhabra, R.S. & Fouts, J.R. (1973) Stimulation of hepatic microsomal drug-metabolizing enzymes in mice by 1,1,1-trichloro-2,2-bis(*p*-chlorophenyl)ethane (DDT) and 3,4-benzpyrene. *Toxicol. appl. Pharmacol.*, *25*, 60-70

Clark, J.M. (1974) Mutagenicity of DDT in mice, *Drosophila melanogaster* and *Neurospora crassa*. *Aust. J. biol. Sci.*, *27*, 427-440

Clive, D., Johnson, K.O., Spector, J.F.S., Batson, A.G. & Brown, M.M.M. (1979) Validation and characterization of the L5178Y/TK$^{+/-}$ mouse lymphoma mutagen assay system. *Mutat. Res.*, *59*, 61-108

Codex Committee on Pesticide Residues (1989) *Codex Alimentarius* (Room Document 14), Geneva

Codex Committee on Pesticide Residues (1990) *Guide to Codex Maximum Limits for Pesticide Residues*, Part 2 (CAC/PR2-1990; CCPR Pesticide Classification No. 021), The Hague

Cook, W.A., ed. (1987) *Occupational Exposure Limits—Worldwide*, Washington DC, American Industrial Hygiene Association, pp. 119, 135, 177

County Natwest WoodMac (1990) *Agrochemical Services*, London, Wood Mackenzie & Co., p. 41

Crebelli, R., Bellincampi, D., Conti, G., Conti, L., Morpurgo, G. & Carere, A. (1986) A comparative study on selected chemical carcinogens for chromosome malsegregation, mitotic crossing-over and forward mutation induction in *Aspergillus nidulans*. *Mutat. Res.*, *172*, 139-149

Datta, P.R. & Nelson, M.J. (1968) Enhanced metabolism of methyprylon, meprobamate and chlordiazepoxide hydrochloride after chronic feeding of low dietary level of DDT to male and female rats. *Toxicol. appl. Pharmacol.*, *13*, 346-352

David, D. (1977) Influence of DDT on the germinal gonadal population of quail embryos throughout five successive generations (Fr.). *C.R. Acad. Sci. Paris*, *284*, 949-952

Davidson, J.S., Baumgarten, I. & Harley, E.H. (1985) Use of a new citrulline incorporation assay to investigate inhibition of intercellular communication by 1,1,1-trichloro-2,2-bis(*p*-chloro-phenyl)ethane in human fibroblasts. *Cancer Res.*, *45*, 515-519

Dean, M.E., Smeaton, T.C. & Stock, B.H. (1980) The influence of fetal and neonatal exposure to dichlorodiphenyltrichloroethane (DDT) on the testosterone status of neonatal male rat. *Toxicol. appl. Pharmacol.*, *53*, 315-322

De Flora, S. (1981) Study of 106 organic and inorganic compounds in the *Salmonella*/microsome test. *Carcinogenesis*, *2*, 283-298

De Flora, S., Zanacchi, P., Camoirano, A., Bennicelli, C. & Badolati, G.S. (1984) Genotoxic activity and potency of 135 compounds in the Ames reversion test and in a bacterial DNA-repair test. *Mutat. Res.*, *133*, 161-198

De Flora, S., Camoirano, A., Izzotti, A., D'Agostini, F. & Bennicelli, C. (1989) Photoactivation of mutagens. *Carcinogenesis*, *10*, 1089-1097

Deichmann, W.B. & Keplinger, M.L. (1966) Effect of combinations of pesticides and reproduction of mice (Abstract No. 11). *Toxicol. appl. Pharmacol.*, *8*, 337-338

Deichmann, W.B., Keplinger, M., Sala, F. & Glass, E. (1967) Synergism among oral carcingoens. IV. Simultaneous feeding of four tumorigens to rats. *Toxicol. appl. Pharmacol.*, *11*, 88-103

Deichmann, W.B., Keplinger, M., Dressler, I. & Sala, F. (1969) Retention of dieldrin and DDT in the tissue of dogs fed aldrin and DDT individually and as a mixture. *Toxicol. appl. Pharmacol.*, *14*, 205-213

Deichmann, W.B., MacDonald, W.E., Beasley, A.G. & Cubit, D. (1971) Subnormal reproduction in beagle dogs induced by DDT and aldrin. *Ind. Med.*, *38*, 10-20

Del Pup, J.A., Pasternack, B.S., Harley, N.H., Kane, P.B. & Palmes, E.D. (1978) Effects of DDT on stable laboratory mouse populations. *J. Toxicol. environ. Health*, *4*, 671-687

Deutsche Forschungsgemeinschaft (1989) *Maximum Concentrations at the Workplace and Biological Tolerance Values for Working Materials 1989* (Report No. 25), Weinheim, VCH Verlagsgessellschaft, p. 29

Ditraglia, D., Brown, D.P., Namekata, T. & Iverson, N. (1981) Mortality study of workers employed at organochlorine pesticide manufacturing plants. *Scand. J. Work Environ. Health*, *7* (Suppl. 4), 140-146

Durham, W.F., Ortega, P. & Hayes, W.J. (1963) The effect of various dietary levels of DDT on liver function, cell morphology and DDT storage in the rhesus monkey. *Arch. int. Pharmacodyn.*, *141*, 111-129

Eden, W.G. & Arthur, B.W. (1965) Translocation of DDT and heptachlor in soybeans. *J. econ. Entomol.*, *58*, 161-162

Epstein, S.S. & Shafner, H. (1968) Chemical mutagens in the human environment. *Nature*, *219*, 385-387

Epstein, S.S., Arnold, E., Andrea, J., Bass, W. & Bishop, Y. (1972) Detection of chemical mutagens by the dominant lethal assay in the mouse. *Toxicol. appl. Pharmacol.*, *23*, 288-325

Eriksson, M., Hardell, L., Berg, N.O., Moller, T. & Axelson, O. (1981) Soft-tissue sarcomas and exposure to chemical substances: a case-referent study. *Br. J. ind. Med.*, *38*, 27-33

Eriksson, M., Hardell, L. & Adami, H. (1990a) Exposure to dioxins as a risk factor for soft tissue sarcoma: a population-based case-control study. *J. natl Cancer Inst.*, *82*, 486-490

Eriksson, P., Nilsson-Håkansson, L., Nordberg, A., Aspberg, A. & Fredriksson, A. (1990b) Neonatal exposure to DDT and its fatty acid conjugate: effects on cholinergic and behavioural variables in the adult mouse. *Neurotoxicology*, *11*, 345-354

Fabro, S., McLachlan, J.A. & Dames, N.M. (1984) Chemical exposure of embryos during the preimplantation stages of pregnancy: mortality rate and intrauterine development. *Am. J. Obstet. Gynecol.*, *148*, 929-938

Fahmy, M.A.H., Fukudo, T.R., Metcalf, R.L. & Holmstead, R.L. (1973) Structure-activity correlations in DDT analogs. *J. agric. Food Chem.*, *21*, 585-591

FAO/WHO (1964) *Evaluation of the Toxicity of Pesticide Residues in Food: Report of a Joint Meeting of the FAO Committee on Pesticides in Agriculture and the WHO Expert Committee on Pesticide Residues* (FAO Meeting Report No. PL/1963/13: WHO/Food Add. 23), Rome

FAO/WHO (1965) *Evaluation of the Toxicity of Pesticide Residues in Food: Deliberations of the Joint Meeting of the FAO Committee on Pesticides in Agriculture and the WHO Expert Committee on Pesticide Residues* (FAO Meeting Report No. PL/1965/10/1; WHO/Food Add./27.65), Rome

FAO/WHO (1967a) *Pesticide Residues in Food. Joint Report of the FAO Working Party on Pesticide Residues and the WHO Expert Committee on Pesticide Residues* (FAO Agricultural Studies, No. 73; WHO Technical Report Series, No. 370), Rome

FAO/WHO (1967b) *Evaluation of Some Pesticide Residues in Food: Deliberations of the Joint Meeting of the FAO Committee on Pesticides in Agriculture and the WHO Expert Committee on Pesticide Residues* (FAO/PL:CP/15; WHO/Food Add./67.32), Rome

FAO/WHO (1968a) *Pesticide Residues. Report of the 1967 Joint Meeting of the FAO Working Party and the WHO Expert Committee* (FAO Meeting Report, No. PL:1967/M/11; WHO Technical Report Series, No. 391), Geneva

FAO/WHO (1968b) *1967 Evaluations of Some Pesticide Residues in Food: Deliberations of the Joint Meeting of the FAO Committee on Pesticides in Agriculture and the WHO Expert Committee on Pesticide Residues* (FAO/PL:1967/M/11/1; WHO/Food Add./68.30), Rome

FAO/WHO (1969) *1968 Evaluations of Some Pesticide Residues in Food* (FAO/PL:1968/M/9/1; WHO/Food Add./69.35), Geneva

FAO/WHO (1970a) *Pesticide Residues in Food. Report of the 1969 Joint Meeting of the FAO Working Party of Experts on Pesticide Residues and the WHO Expert Group on Pesticide Residues* (FAO Agricultural Studies. No. 84; WHO Technical Report Series, No. 458), Geneva

FAO/WHO (1970b) *1969 Evaluations of Some Pesticide Residues in Food: Deliberations of the Joint Meeting of the FAO Committee on Pesticides in Agriculture and the WHO Expert Committee on Pesticide Residues* (FAO/PL:1969/M/17/1; WHO/Food Add./70.38), Rome

FAO/WHO (1978) *Pesticide Residues in Food—1977. Report of the Joint Meeting of the FAO Panel of Experts on Pesticide Residues and Environment and the WHO Expert Group on Pesticide Residues* (FAO Plant Production and Protection Paper 10 Rev.), Rome

FAO/WHO (1980a) *Pesticide Residues in Food—1979. Report of the Joint Meeting of the FAO Panel of Experts on Pesticide Residues in Food and the Environment and the WHO Expert Group on Pesticide Residues* (FAO Plant Production and Protection Paper 20), Rome

FAO/WHO (1980b) *Pesticide Residues in Food: 1979 Evaluations. Data and Recommendations of the Joint Meeting of the FAO Committee on Pesticides in Agriculture and the WHO Expert Committee on Pesticide Residues* (FAO Plant Production and Protection Paper 20), Rome

FAO/WHO (1981) *Pesticide Residues in Food: 1980 Evaluations. Data and Recommendations of the Joint Meeting of the FAO Committee on Pesticides in Agriculture and the WHO Expert Committee on Pesticide Residues* (FAO Plant Production and Protection Paper 26 Sup.), Rome

FAO/WHO (1984) *Pesticide Residues in Food—1983. Report of the Joint Meeting of the FAO Panel of Experts on Pesticide Residues in Food and the Environment and the WHO Expert Group on Pesticide Residues* (FAO Plant Production and Protection Paper 56), Rome

FAO/WHO (1985) *Pesticide Residues in Food—1984. Report of the Joint Meeting on Pesticide Residues* (FAO Plant Production and Protection Paper 67), Rome

Fawcett, S.S., King, L.J., Bunyan, P.J. & Stanley, P.I. (1987) The metabolism of ^{14}C-DDT, ^{14}C-DDD, ^{14}C-DDE and ^{14}C-DDMU in rats and Japanese quail. *Xenobiotica, 17*, 525-538

Fitzgerald, D.J., Piccoli, C. & Yamasaki, H. (1989) Detection of non-genotoxic carcinogens in the BALB/c 3T3 cell transformation/mutation assay system. *Mutagenesis, 4*, 286-291

Fitzhugh, G.O. & Nelson, A.A. (1947) The chronic oral toxicity of DDT (2,2-bis(p-chlorophenyl)-1,1-trichloroethane. *J. Pharmacol. exp. Ther., 39*, 18-30

Flodin, U., Fredriksson, M., Persson, B. & Axelson, O. (1988) Chronic lymphatic leukaemia and engine exhausts, fresh wood, and DDT: a case-referent study. *Br. J. ind. Med., 45*, 33-38

Flodström, S., Hemming, H., Wärngard, L. & Ahlborg, U.G. (1990) Promotion of altered hepatic foci development in rat liver, cytochrome P450 enzyme induction and inhibition of cell-cell communication by DDT and some structurally related organohalogen pesticides. *Carcinogenesis, 11*, 1413-1417

Foxall, C.D. & Maroko, J.B.M. (1984) Persistence of DDT in soil and on foliage following its application to cotton crops in Kenya. *Environ. Contam.*, 91-95

Fransson, R., Nicotera, P., Wärngård, L. & Ahlborg, U.G. (1990) Changes in cytosolic Ca^{2+} are not involved in DDT-induced loss of gap junctional communication in WB-F344 cells. *Cell Biol. Toxicol., 6*, 235-244

Fry, D.M. & Toone, C.K. (1981) DDT-induced feminization of gull embryos. *Science, 213*, 922-924

Fuhremann, T.W. & Lichtenstein, E.P. (1980) A comparative study of the persistence, movement, and metabolism of six carbon-14 insecticides in soils and plants. *J. agric. Food Chem., 28*, 446-452

Galloway, S.M., Armstrong, M.J., Reuben, C., Colman, S., Brown, B., Cannon, C., Bloom, A.D., Nakamura, F., Ahmed, M., Duk, S., Rimpo, J., Margolin, B.H., Resnick, M.A., Anderson, B. & Zeiger, E. (1987) Chromosome aberrations and sister chromatid exchanges in Chinese hamster ovary cells: evaluations of 108 chemicals. *Environ. mol. Mutagenesis, 10* (Suppl. 10), 1-175

Gargus, J.L., Paynter, O.E. & Reese, W.H., Jr (1969) Utilization of newborn mice in the bioassay of chemical carcinogens. *Toxicol. appl. Pharmacol., 15*, 552-559

Gellert, R. & Heinrichs, W. (1975) Effects of DDT homologs administered to female rats during the perinatal period. *Biol. Neonate, 26*, 283-290

Gellert, R., Heinrichs, W. & Swerdloff, R. (1974) Effects of neonatally administered DDT homologs on reproductive function in male and female rats. *Neuroendocrinology, 16*, 84-94

Gingell, R. (1976) Metabolism of ^{14}C-DDT in the mouse and hamster. *Xenobiotica, 6*, 15-20

Gingell, R. & Wallcave, L. (1974) Species differences in the acute toxicity and tissue distribution of DDT in mice and hamsters. *Toxicol. appl. Pharmacol., 28*, 385-394

Glatt, H.R. & Oesch, F. (1987) Species differences in enzymes controlling reactive epoxides. *Arch. Toxicol., Suppl. 10*, 111-124

Gold, B. & Brunk, G. (1982) Metabolism of 1,1,1-trichloro-2,2-bis(p-chlorophenyl)ethane in the mouse. *Chem.-biol. Interactions, 41*, 327-339

Gold, B. & Brunk, G. (1984) A mechanistic study of the metabolism of 1,1-dichloro-2,2-bis(*p*-chlorophenyl)ethane (DDD) to 2,2-bis(p-chlorophenyl)acetic acid (DDA). *Biochem. Pharmacol., 33*, 979-982

Gold, B. & Brunk, G. (1986) The effect of subchronic feeding of 1,1-dichloro-2,2-bis(4'-chlorophenyl)ethene (DDE) on its metabolism in mice. *Carcinogenesis, 7*, 1149-1153

Gold, B., Leuschen, T., Brunk, G. & Gingell, R. (1981) Metabolism of a DDT metabolite via a chloroepoxide. *Chem.-biol. Interactions, 35*, 159-176

Government of Canada (1990) *Report on National Surveillance Data from 1984/85 to 1988/89*, Ottawa

Graillot, C., Gak, J.C., Lancret, C. & Truhaut, R. (1975) On the modes and mechanisms of toxic activity of organochlorine insecticides. II. Study in hamster of long-term toxicity of DDT (Fr.). *Eur. J. Toxicol.*, *8*, 353-359

Griffin, D.E., III & Hill, W.E. (1978) In vitro breakage of plasmid DNA by mutagens and pesticides. *Mutat. Res.*, *52*, 161-169

Grosch, D.S. & Valcovic, L.R. (1967) Chlorinated hydrocarbon insecticides are not mutagenic in *Bracon hebetor* tests. *J. econ. Entomol.*, *60*, 1177-1179

Halver, J.E. (1967) Crystalline aflatoxin and other vectors for trout hepatoma. In: Halver, J.E. & Mitchell, I.A., eds, *Trout Hepatoma Research Conference Papers* (Bureau of Sport Fisheries and Wild Life Research Rep. No. 70), Washington DC, Department of the Interior, pp. 78-102

Hardell, L. (1981) Relation of soft-tissue sarcoma, malignant lymphoma and colon cancer to phenoxy acids, chlorophenols and other agents. *Scand. J. Work Environ. Health*, *7*, 119-130

Hardell, L. & Eriksson, M. (1988) The association between soft tissue sarcomas and exposure to phenoxyacetic acids. *Cancer*, *62*, 652-656

Hardell, L. & Sandström, A. (1979) Case-control study: soft-tissue sarcomas and exposure to phenoxyacetic acids or chlorophenols. *Br. J. Cancer*, *39*, 711-717

Hardell, L., Eriksson, M., Lenner, P. & Lundgren, E. (1981) Malignant lymphoma and exposure to chemicals, especially organic solvents, chlorophenols and phenoxy acids: a case-control study. *Br. J. Cancer*, *43*, 169-176

Hardell, L., Johansson, B. & Axelson, O. (1982) Epidemiological study of nasal and nasopharyngeal cancer and their relation to phenoxy acid or chlorophenol exposure. *Am. J. ind. Med.*, *3*, 247-257

Hardell, L., Bengtsson, N.O., Jonsson, U., Eriksson, S. & Larsson, L.G. (1984) Aetiological aspects on primary liver cancer with special regard to alcohol, organic solvents and acute intermittent porphyria—an epidemiological investigation. *Br. J. Cancer*, *50*, 389-397

Harris, C.R. & Sans, W.W. (1967) Absorption of organochlorine insecticide residues from agricultural soils by root crops. *J. agric. Food Chem.*, *15*, 861-863

Hayes, W.J. (1982) *Pesticides Studied in Man*, Baltimore, MD, Williams & Wilkins, pp. 180-208

Health and Safety Executive (1987) *Occupational Exposure Limits 1987* (Guidance Note EH 40/87), London, Her Majesty's Stationery Office, p. 21

Health and Welfare Canada (1990) *National Pesticide Residue Limits in Foods*, Ottawa, Bureau of Chemical Safety, Food Directorate, Health Protection Branch

Hoar Zahm, S., Blair, A., Holmes, F.F., Boysen, C.D. & Robel, R.J. (1988) A case-referent study of soft-tissue sarcoma and Hodgkin's disease. *Scand. J. Work Environ. Health*, *14*, 224-230

Hoffman, D.L. & Mattox, V.R. (1972) Treatment of adrenocortical carcinoma with *o,p'*-DDD. *Med. Clin. N. Am.*, *56*, 999-1012

Hofvander, Y., Hagman, U., Linder, C.-E., Vaz, R. & Slorach, S.A. (1981) WHO Collaborative Breast Feeding Study: I. Organochlorine contaminants in individual samples of Swedish human milk, 1978-1979. *Acta paediatr. scand.*, *70*, 3-8

Horwitz, W., ed. (1975a) *Official Methods of Analysis of the Association of Official Analytical Chemists*, 12th ed., Washington DC, Association of Official Analytical Chemists, pp. 81-82

Horwitz, W., ed. (1975b) *Official Methods of Analysis of the Association of Official Analytical Chemists*, 12th ed., Washington DC, Association of Official Analytical Chemists, pp. 107-109

Horwitz, W., ed. (1975c) *Official Methods of Analysis of the Association of Official Analytical Chemists*, 12th ed., Washington DC, Association of Official Analytical Chemists, pp. 518-528

Horwitz, W., ed. (1975d) *Official Methods of Analysis of the Association of Official Analytical Chemists*, 12th ed., Washington DC, Association of Official Analytical Chemists, pp. 540-542

Hrdina, P.D., Singhal, R.L. & Ling, G.M. (1975) DDT and related chlorinated hydrocarbon insecticides: pharmacological basis of their toxicity in mammals. *Adv. Pharmacol. Chemother.*, *12*, 31-88

IARC (1974) *IARC Monographs on the Evaluation of Carcinogenic Risk of Chemicals to Man*, Vol. 5, *Some Organochlorine Pesticides*, Lyon, pp. 83-124

IARC (1987a) *IARC Monographs on the Evaluation of Carcinogenic Risks to Humans*, Suppl. 7, *Overall Evaluations of Carcinogenicity: An Updating of* IARC Monographs *Volumes 1 to 42*, Lyon, pp. 186-189

IARC (1987b) *IARC Monographs on the Evaluation of Carcinogenic Risks to Humans*, Suppl. 7, *Overall Evaluations of Carcinogenicity: An Updating of* IARC Monographs *Volumes 1 to 42*, Lyon, pp. 192-193

IARC (1989a) *IARC Monographs on the Evaluation of Carcinogenic Risks to Humans*, Vol. 47, *Some Organic Solvents, Resin Monomers and Related Compounds, Pigments and Occupational Exposures in Paint Manufacture and Painting*, Lyon, pp. 125-156

IARC (1989b) *IARC Monographs on the Evaluation of Carcinogenic Risks to Humans*, Vol. 45, *Occupational Exposures in Petroleum Refining; Crude Oil and Major Petroleum Fuels*, Lyon, pp. 39-117

Innes, J.R.M., Ulland, B.M., Valerio, M.G., Petrucelli, L., Fishbein, L., Hart, E.R., Pallotta, A.J., Bates, R.R., Falk, H.L., Gart, J.J., Klein, M., Mitchell, I. & Peters, J. (1969) Bioassay of pesticides and industrial chemicals for tumorigenicity in mice. A preliminary note. *J. natl Cancer Inst.*, *42*, 1101-1114

Ioannides, C., Lum, P.Y. & Parke, D.V. (1984) Cytochrome P-448 and the activation of toxic chemicals and carcinogens. *Xenobiotica*, *14*, 119-137

Ito, N., Tsuda, H., Hasegawa, R. & Imaida, K. (1983) Comparison of the promoting effect of various agents in induction of preneoplastic lesions in rat liver. *Environ. Health Perspect.*, *50*, 131-138

Izmerov, N.F., ed. (1983) *International Register of Potentially Toxic Chemicals. Scientific Reviews of Soviet Literature on Toxicity and Hazards of Chemicals: DDT* (Issue 39), Moscow, Centre of International Projects, United Nations Environment Programme

Jelinek, R., Peterka, M. & Rychter, Z. (1985) Chick embryotoxicity screening test—130 substances tested. *Indian J. exp. Biol.*, *23*, 588-595

Jensen, S. & Jansson, B. (1976) Anthropogenic substances in seal from the Baltic. Methyl sulfone metabolites of PCB and DDE. *Ambio*, *5*, 257-260

Johnson, G.A. & Jalal, S.M. (1973) DDT-induced chromosomal damage in mice. *J. Hered.*, *64*, 7-8

Kashyap, S.K., Nigam, S.K., Karnik, A.B., Gupta, R.C. & Chatterjee, S.K. (1977) Carcinogenicity of DDT (dichlorodiphenyl trichloroethane) in pure inbred Swiss mice. *Int. J. Cancer*, *19*, 725-729

Keil, J.E., Loadholt, C.D., Weinrich, M.C., Sandifer, S.H. & Boyle, E., Jr (1984) Incidence of coronary heart disease in blacks in Charleston, South Carolina. *Am. Heart J.*, *108*, 779-786

Kelly-Garvert, F. & Legator, M.S. (1973) Cytogenetic and mutagenic effects of DDT and DDE in a Chinese hamster cell line. *Mutat. Res.*, *17*, 223-229

Klaunig, J.E. & Ruch, R.J. (1987) Strain and species effects on the inhibition of hepatocyte intercellular communication by liver tumor promoters. *Cancer Lett.*, *36*, 161-168

Klaunig, J.E., Goldblatt, P.J., Hinton, D.E., Lipsky, M.M. & Trump, B.F. (1984) Carcinogen induced unscheduled DNA synthesis in mouse hepatocytes. *Toxicol. Pathol.*, *12*, 119-125

Klaunig, J.E., Ruch, R.J. & Weghorst, C.M. (1990) Comparative effects of phenobarbital, DDT, and lindane on mouse hepatocyte gap junctional intercellular communication. *Toxicol. appl. Pharmacol.*, *102*, 553-563

Klein, D., Dillon, J.C., Jirou-Najou, J.L., Gagey, M.J. & Debry, G. (1986) The elimination kinetics of organochlorine compounds during the first week of maternal breast feeding (Fr.). *Food chem. Toxicol.*, *24*, 869-873

Krause, W., Hamm, K. & Weissmüller, J. (1975) The effect of DDT on spermatogenesis of the juvenile rat. *Bull. environ. Contam. Toxicol.*, *14*, 171-179

Kreiss, K., Zack, M.M. & Kimbrough, R.D. (1981) Cross-sectional study of a community with exceptional exposure to DDT. *J. Am. med. Assoc.*, *245*, 1926-1930

Kurata, M., Hirose, K. & Umeda, M. (1982) Inhibition of metabolic cooperation in Chinese hamster cells by organochlorine pesticides. *Gann*, *73*, 217-221

Lacassagne, A. & Hurst, L. (1965) Experimental tumours of the interstitial gland of rats during oncogenesis by o,p-dichlorodiphenyldichloroethane in the testicle (Fr.). *Bull. Cancer*, *52*, 89-104

Langenbach, R. & Gingell, R. (1975) Cytotoxic and oncogenic activities of 1,1,1-trichloro-2,2-bis(*p*-chlorophenyl)ethane and metabolites to mouse embryo cells in culture. *J. natl Cancer Inst.*, *54*, 981-983

Larsen, K.D. & Jalal, S.M. (1974) DDT induced chromosome mutation in mice—further testing. *Can. J. Genet. Cytol.*, *16*, 491-497

Legator, M.S., Palmer, K.A. & Adler, I.-D. (1973) A collaborative study of in vivo cytogenetic analysis. I. Interpretation of slide preparations. *Toxicol. appl. Pharmacol.*, *24*, 337-350

Lessa, J.M.M., Beçak, W., Nazareth Rabello, M., Pereira, C.A.B. & Ungaro, M.T. (1976) Cytogenetic study of DDT on human lymphocytes *in vitro. Mutat. Res.*, *40*, 131-138

Lillard, D.A. & Noles, R.K. (1973) Effect of force molting and induced hyperthyroidism on the depletion of DDT residues from the laying hen. *Poultry Sci.*, *52*, 222-228

Lipsky, M.M., Trump, B.F. & Hinton, D.E. (1989) Histogenesis of dieldrin and DDT-induced hepatocellular carcinoma in BALB/c mice. *J. environ. Pathol. Toxicol. Oncol.*, *9*, 79-93

Luke, M.A., Masumoto, H.T., Cairns, T. & Hundley, H.K. (1988) Levels and incidences of pesticide residues in various foods and animal feeds analyzed by the Luke multiresidue methodology for fiscal years 1982-1986. *J. Assoc. off. anal. Chem.*, *71*, 415-433

Lund, B.-O. (1989) *Formation and Toxicity of Reactive Intermediates in the Metabolism of DDT in Mice* (Thesis), Uppsala, Swedish University of Agricultural Sciences

Lund, B.-O., Klasson-Wehler, E. & Brandt, I. (1986) o,p'-DDD in the mouse lung: selective uptake, covalent binding and effect on drug metabolism. *Chem.-biol. Interactions*, *60*, 129-141

Lund, B.-O., Bergman, Å. & Brandt, I. (1988) Metabolic activation and toxicity of a DDT-metabolite, 3-methylsulphonyl-DDE in the adrenal *zona fasciculata* in mice. *Chem.-biol. Interactions*, *65*, 25-40

Luquet, F.-M., Goursaud, J. & Casalis, J. (1974) Pollution of French human milk by organochlorine pesticide residues (Fr.). *Aliment. Vie*, *62*, 40-69

Luton, J.P., Mahoudeau, J.A., Bouchard, P., Thieblot, P., Hautecouverture, M., Simon, D., Laudat, M.H., Touitou, Y. & Bricaire, H. (1979) Treatment of Cushing's disease by o,p'-DDD. Survey of 62 cases. *New Engl. J. Med.*, *300*, 459-464

Mahr, U. & Miltenburger, H.G. (1976) The effect of insecticides on Chinese hamster cell cultures. *Mutat. Res.*, *40*, 107-118

Mamber, S.W., Bryson, V. & Katz, S.E. (1984) Evaluation of *Escherichia coli* K12 inductest for detection of potential chemical carcinogens. *Mutat. Res.*, *130*, 141-151

Marshall, T.C., Dorough, H.W. & Swim, H.E. (1976) Screening of pesticides for mutagenic potential using *Salmonella typhimurium* mutants. *J. agric. Food Chem.*, *24*, 560-563

Maslansky, C.J. & Williams, G.M. (1981) Evidence for an epigenetic mode of action in organochlorine pesticide hepatocarcinogenicity: a lack of genotoxicity in rat, mouse and hamster hepatocytes. *J. Toxicol. environ. Health*, 8, 121-130

Mason, R.R. & Schulte, G.J. (1981) Interaction of o,p'-DDT with the estrogen-binding protein (EBP) of DMBA-induced rat mammary tumors. *Res. Commun. chem. Pathol. Pharmacol.*, 33, 119-128

Matsui, S., Yamamoto, R. & Yamada, H. (1989) The *Bacillus subtilis*/microsome rec-assay for the detection of DNA damaging substances which may occur in chlorinated and ozonated waters. *Water Sci. Technol.*, 21, 875-887

McCann, J., Choi, E., Yamasaki, E. & Ames, B.N. (1975) Detection of carcinogens as mutagens in the *Salmonella*/microsome test: assay of 300 chemicals. *Proc. natl Acad. Sci. USA*, 72, 5135-5139

Mehrotra, K.M. (1985) Use of DDT and its environmental effects in India. *Proc. Indian natl Sci. Acad.*, B51, 169-184

Meister, R.T., ed. (1990) *Farm Chemicals Handbook 90*, Willoughby, OH, Meister Publishing Co., p. C91

Mellanby, K. (1989) DDT in perspective. In: *Progress and Prospects in Insect Control* (BCPC Monograph 43), Thornton Heath, British Crop Protection Council, pp. 3-20

Mes, J., Doyle, J.A., Adams, B.R., Davies, D.J. & Turton, D. (1984) Polychlorinated biphenyls and organochlorine pesticides in milk and blood of Canadian women during lactation. *Arch. environ. Contam. Toxicol.*, 13, 217-223

Milham, S.Y. (1983) *Occupational Mortality in Washington State 1950-1979* (DHHS No. 83-116), Cincinnati, OH, National Institute for Occupational Safety and Health

Mitjavila, S., Carrera, G. & Fernandez, Y. (1981) II. Evaluation of the toxic risk of accumulated DDT in the rat: during fat mobilization. *Arch. environ. Contam. Toxicol.*, 10, 471-481

Morgan, D.P. & Roan, C.C. (1971) Absorption, storage and metabolic conversion of ingested DDT and DDT metabolites in man. *Arch. environ. Health*, 22, 301-308

Morgan, D.P., Lin, L.I. & Saikaly, H.H. (1980) Morbidity and mortality in workers occupationally exposed to pesticides. *Arch. environ. Contam. Toxicol.*, 9, 349-382

Moriya, M., Ohta, T., Watanabe, K., Miyazawa, T., Kato, K. & Shirasu, Y. (1983) Further mutagenicity studies on pesticides in bacterial reversion assay systems. *Mutat. Res.*, 116, 185-216

Mortelmans, K., Haworth, S., Lawlor, T., Speck, W., Tainer, B. & Zeiger, E. (1986) *Salmonella* mutagenicity tests: II. Results from the testing of 270 chemicals. *Environ. Mutagenesis*, 8 (*Suppl. 7*), 1-119

Moser, G.J. & Smart, R.C. (1989) Hepatic tumor-promoting chlorinated hydrocarbons stimulate protein kinase C activity. *Carcinogenesis*, 10, 851-856

Murphy, P.G. (1971) The effect of size on the uptake of DDT from water by fish. *Bull. environ. Contam. Toxicol.*, 6, 20-23

Nazareth Rabello, M., Beçak, W., de Almeida, W.F., Pigati, P., Ungaro, M.T., Murata, T. & Pereira, C.A.B. (1975) Cytogenetic study on individuals occupationally exposed to DDT. *Mutat. Res.*, 28, 449-454

Nishimura, N., Nishimura, H. & Oshima, H. (1982) Survey on mutagenicity of pesticides by the *Salmonella*-microsome test. *J. Aichi med. Univ. Assoc.*, 10, 305-312

O'Leary, J.A., Davies, J.E. & Feldman, M. (1970) Spontaneous abortion and human pesticide residues of DDT and DDE. *Am. J. Obstet. Gynecol.*, 108, 1291-1291

Ottoboni, A. (1969) Effect of DDT on reproduction in the rat. *Toxicol. appl. Pharmacol.*, 14, 74-81

Ottoboni, A., Bissell, G. & Hexter, A. (1977) Effects of DDT on reproduction in multiple generations of beagle dogs. *Arch. environ. Contam. Toxicol.*, 6, 83-101

Palmer, K.A., Green, S. & Legator, M.S. (1972) Cytogenetic effects of DDT and derivatives of DDT in a cultured mammalian cell line. *Toxicol. appl. Pharmacol.*, *22*, 355-364

Palmer, K.A., Green, S. & Legator, M.S. (1973) Dominant lethal study of *p,p'*-DDT in rats. *Food Cosmet. Toxicol.*, *11*, 53-62

Peraino, C., Fry, R.J.M., Staffeldt, E. & Christopher, J.P. (1975) Comparative enhancing effects of phenobarbital, amobarbital, diphenylhydantoin and dichlorodiphenyltrichloroethane on 2-acetylaminofluorene-induced hepatic tumorigenesis in the rat. *Cancer Res.*, *35*, 2884-2890

Perini, G. & Ghezzo, F. (1970) Urinary dichlorodiphenylacetic acid (DDA) levels in the rural population of Ferrara (Ital.). *Arcisp. S. Anna di Ferrara*, *23*, 549-558

Persson, B., Dahlander, A.-M., Fredriksson, M., Brage, H.N., Ohlson, C.G. & Axelson, O. (1989) Malignant lymphomas and occupational exposures. *Br. J. ind. Med.*, *46*, 516-520

Pielou, D.P. (1952) The nonmutagenic action of *p,p'*-DDT and γ-hexachlorocyclohexane in *Drosophila melanogaster* Meig. (diptera: drosophilidae). *Can. J. Zool.*, *30*, 375-377

Planche, G., Croisy, A., Malaveille, C., Tomatis, L. & Bartsch, H. (1979) Metabolic and mutagenicity studies on DDT and 15 derivatives. Detection of 1,1-bis(*p*-chlorophenyl)-2,2-dichloroethane and 1,1,-bis(*p*-chlorophenyl)-2,2,2-trichloroethyl acetate (kelthane acetate) as mutagens in *Salmonella typhimurium* and of 1,1-bis(*p*-chlorophenyl) ethylene oxide, a likely metabolite, as an alkylating agent. *Chem.-biol. Interactions*, *25*, 157-175

Probst, G.S., McMahon, R.E., Hill, L.E., Thompson, C.Z., Epp, J.K. & Neal, S.B. (1981) Chemically-induced unscheduled DNA synthesis in primary rat hepatocyte cultures: a comparison with bacterial mutagenicity using 218 compounds. *Environ. Mutagenesis*, *3*, 11-32

Procianoy, R.S. & Schvartsman, S. (1981) Blood pesticide concentration in mothers and their newborn infants. Relation to prematurity. *Acta paediatr. scand.*, *70*, 925-928

Radomski, J.L., Deichmann, W.B., MacDonald, W.E. & Glass, E.M. (1965) Synergism among oral carcinogens. I. Results of simultaneous feeding of four tumorigens to rats. *Toxicol. appl. Pharmacol.*, *7*, 652-656

Rashid, K.A. & Mumma, R.O. (1986) Screening pesticides for their ability to damage bacterial DNA. *J. environ. Sci. Health*, *B21*, 319-334

Reif, V.D. & Sinsheimer, J.E. (1975) Metabolism of 1-(*o*-chlorophenyl)-1-(*p*-chlorophenyl)-2,2-dichloroethane (o,p'-DDD) in rats. *Drug Metab. Dispos.*, *3*, 15-25

Reuber, M.D. (1978) Carcinomas of the liver in Osborne-Mendel rats ingesting DDT. *Tumori*, *64*, 571-577

Reuber, M.D. (1979) Interstitial cell carcinomas of the testis in BALB/c male mice ingesting methoxychlor. *J. Cancer Res. clin. Oncol.*, *93*, 173-179

Ritter, L. & Wood, G. (1989) Evaluation and regulation of pesticides in drinking water. A Canadian approach. *Food Addit. Contam.*, *6* (Suppl. 1), S87-S94

Roan, C.C. (1970) They're eating DDT! *Farm Chem.*, *133*, 44, 46

Roan, C., Morgan, D. & Paschal, E.H. (1971) Urinary excretion of DDA following ingestion of DDA and DDT metabolites in man. *Arch. environ. Health*, *22*, 309-315

Robison, A.K., Schmidt, W.A. & Stancel, G.M. (1985a) Estrogenic activity of DDT: estrogen-receptor profiles and the responses of individual uterine cell types following o,p'-DDT administration. *J. Toxicol. environ. Health*, *16*, 493-508

Robison, A.K., Sirbasku, D.A. & Stancel, G.M. (1985b) DDT supports the growth of an estrogen-responsive tumor. *Toxicol. Lett.*, *27*, 109-113

Rocchi, P., Perocco, P., Alberghini, W., Fini, A. & Prodi, G. (1980) Effect of pesticides on scheduled and unscheduled DNA synthesis of rat thymocytes and human lymphocytes. *Arch. Toxicol.*, *45*, 101-108

Rogan, W.J., Gladen, B.C., McKinney, J.D., Carreras, N., Hardy, P., Thullen, J., Tingelstad, J. & Tully, M. (1986) Neonatal effects of transplacental exposure to PCBs and DDE. *J. Pediatr.*, *109*, 335-341

Rossi, L., Ravera, M., Repetti, G. & Santi, L. (1977) Long-term administration of DDT or phenobarbital-Na in Wistar rats. *Int. J. Cancer*, *19*, 179-185

Rossi, L., Barbieri, O., Sanguineti, M., Cabral, J.R.P., Bruzzi, P. & Santi, L. (1983) Carcinogenicity study with technical-grade dichlorodiphenyltrichloroethane and 1,1-dichloro-2,2,-bis(p-chloro-phenyl)ethylene in hamsters. *Cancer Res.*, *43*, 776-781

Rovinsky, F.Y., Afanasyev, M.I., Burtseva, L.V. & Yushkan, E.I. (1988) Methods of background environmental pollution monitoring applied in CMEA member countries. *Int. J. environ. anal. Chem.*, *32*, 167-176

Sadtler Research Laboratories (1980) *The Sadtler Standard Spectra, 1980 Cumulative Index*, Philadelphia, PA

Sadtler Research Laboratories (1990) *The Sadtler Standard Spectra, 1990 Cumulative Index*, Philadelphia, PA

Saxena, M.C., Siddiqui, M.K.J., Agarwal, V. & Kuuty, D. (1983) A comparison of organochlorine insecticide contents in specimens of maternal blood, placenta, and umbilical-cord blood from stillborn and live-born cases. *J. Toxicol. environ. Health*, *11*, 71-79

Schiestl, R.H. (1989) Nonmutagenic carcinogens induce intrachromosomal recombination in yeast. *Nature*, *337*, 285-288

Schiestl, R.H., Gietz, R.D., Mehta, R.D. & Hastings, P.J. (1989) Carcinogens induce intrachromosomal recombination in yeast. *Carcinogenesis*, *10*, 1445-1455

Scribner, J.D. & Mottet, N.K. (1981) DDT acceleration of mammary gland tumors induced in the male Sprague-Dawley rat by 2-acetamidophenanthrene. *Carcinogenesis*, *2*, 1235-1239

Shabad, L.M., Kolesnichenko, T.S. & Nikonova, T.V. (1973) Transplacental and combined long-term effect of DDT in five generations of A-strain mice. *Int. J. Cancer*, *11*, 688-693

Shellenberger, T.E. (1978) A multi-generation toxicity evaluation of p,p′-DDT and dieldrin with Japanese quail. I. Effects on growth and reproduction. *Drug chem. Toxicol.*, *1*, 137-146

Shivapurkar, N., Hoover, K.L. & Poirier, L.A. (1986) Effect of methionine and choline on liver tumor promotion by phenobarbital and DDT in diethylnitrosamine-initiated rats. *Carcinogenesis*, *7*, 547-550

Simmon, V.F. & Kauhanen, K. (1978) *In Vitro Microbiological Mutagenicity Assays of 1,3-Dichloropropene* (SRI International Report Project Lsu-5612), Washington DC, US Environmental Protection Agency

Simmon, V.F., Kauhanen, K. & Tardiff, R.G. (1977) Mutagenic activity of chemicals identified in drinking water. *Dev. Toxicol. environ. Sci.*, *2*, 249-258

Sina, J.F., Bean, C.L., Dysart, G.R., Taylor, V.I. & Bradley, M.O. (1983) Evaluation of the alkaline elution/rat hepatocyte assay as a predictor of carcinogen/mutagenic potential. *Mutat. Res.*, *113*, 357-391

Southern, A.L., Tochimoto, S., Strom, L., Ratuschni, A., Ross, H. & Gordon, G. (1966) Remission in Cushing's syndrome with o,p′-DDD. *J. clin. Endocrinol.*, *26*, 268-278

Sugie, S., Mori, H. & Takahashi, M. (1987) Effect of in vivo exposure to the liver tumor promoters phenobarbital or DDT on the gap junctions of rat hepatocytes: a quantitative freeze-fracture analysis. *Carcinogenesis*, *8*, 45-51

Swartz, W.J. (1984) Effects of 1,1-bis(p-chlorophenyl)-2,2,2-trichloroethane (DDT) on gonadal development in the chick embryo: a histological and histochemical study. *Environ. Res., 35,* 333-345

Swenberg, J.A. (1981) Utilization of the alkaline elution assay as a short-term test for chemical carcinogens. In: Stich, H.F. & San, R.H.C., eds, *Short-term Tests for Chemical Carcinogens,* New York, Springer-Verlag, pp. 48-58

Swenberg, J.A., Petzold, G.L. & Harbach, P.R. (1976) In vitro DNA damage/alkaline elution assay for predicting carcinogenic potential. *Biochem. biophys. Res. Commun., 72,* 732-738

Tarján, R. & Kemény, T. (1969) Multigeneration studies on DDT in mice. *Food Cosmet. Toxicol., 7,* 215-222

Taylor, D.G. (1977) *NIOSH Manual of Analytical Methods,* 2nd ed., Vol. 3 (DHEW (NIOSH) Publ. No. 77/157-C; US NTIS PB-276838), Cincinnati, OH, National Institute for Occupational Safety and Health, pp. S274-1—S274-7

Terracini, B., Testa, M.C., Cabral, J.R. & Day, N. (1973a) The effects of long-term feeding of DDT to BALB/c mice. *Int. J. Cancer, 11,* 747-764

Terracini, B., Cabral, R.J. & Testa, M.C. (1973b) A multigeneration study on the effect of continuous administration of DDT to BALB/c mice. In: Deichmann, W.B., ed., *Proceedings of the 8th Inter-American Conference on Toxicology: Pesticides and the Environment, A Continuing Controversy. Miami, Florida, 1973,* New York, Intercontinental Medical Book Corp., pp. 77-85

Thorpe, E. & Walker, A.I.T. (1973) The toxicology of dieldrin (HEOD). II. Comparative long-term oral toxicity studies in mice with dieldrin, DDT, phenobarbitone, β-BHC and γ-BHC. *Food Cosmet. Toxicol., 11,* 433-442

Tomatis, L., Turusov, V., Day, N. & Charles, R.T. (1972) The effect of long-term exposure to DDT on CF-1 mice. *Int. J. Cancer, 10,* 489-506

Tomatis, L., Turusov, V., Charles, R.T. & Boicchi, M. (1974) Effect of long-term exposure to 1,1-dichloro-2,2-bis(p-chlorophenyl)ethylene, to 1,1-dichloro-2,2-bis(p-chlorophenyl)ethane, and to the two chemicals combined on CF-1 mice. *J. natl Cancer Inst., 52,* 883-891

Tong, C., Fazio, M. & Williams, G.M. (1981) Rat hepatocyte-mediated mutagenesis of human cells by carcinogenic polycyclic aromatic hydrocarbons but not organochlorine pesticides. *Proc. Soc. exp. Biol. Med., 167,* 572-575

Topham, J.C. (1980) Do induced sperm-head abnormalities in mice specifically identify mammalian mutagens rather than carcinogens? *Mutat. Res., 74,* 379-387

Tsushimoto, G., Chang, C.C., Trosko, J.E. & Matsumura, F. (1983) Cytotoxic, mutagenic and cell-cell communication inhibitory properties of DDT, lindane and chlordane on Chinese hamster cells *in vitro. Arch. environ. Contam. Toxicol., 12,* 721-730

Turusov, V.S., Day, N.E., Tomatis, L., Gati, E. & Charles, R.T. (1973) Tumors in CF-1 mice exposed for six consecutive generations to DDT. *J. natl Cancer Inst., 51,* 983-997

Työsuojeluhallitus (National Finnish Board of Occupational Safety and Health) (1987) *HTP-Azvot 1987* [TLV Values 1987] (Safety Bull. 25), Helsinki, p. 12 (in Finnish)

Unger, M. & Olsen, J. (1980) Organochlorine compounds in the adipose tissue of deceased people with and without cancer. *Environ. Res., 23,* 257-263

Unger, M., Olsen, J. & Clausen, J. (1982) Organochlorine compounds in the adipose tissue of deceased persons with and without cancer: a statistical survey of some potential confounders. *Environ. Res., 29,* 371-376

Unger, M., Kiaer, H., Blichert-Toft, M., Olsen, J. & Clausen, J. (1984) Organochlorine compounds in human breast fat from deceased with and without breast cancer and in a biopsy material from newly diagnosed patients undergoing breast surgery. *Environ. Res.*, *34*, 24-28

Uphouse, L. & Williams, J. (1989) Sexual behavior of intact female rats after treatment with *o,p'*-DDT or *p,p'*-DDT. *Reprod. Toxicol.*, *3*, 33-41

US Environmental Protection Agency (1980) *Ambient Water Quality Criteria for DDT* (US EPA Report EPA 440/5-80-038; US NTIS PB81-117491), Washington DC, Office of Water Regulations and Standards

US Environmental Protection Agency (1986a) Method 8080. Organochlorine pesticides and PCBs. In: *Test Methods for Evaluating Solid Waste—Physical/Chemical Methods*, 3rd ed. (US EPA No. SW-846), Washington DC, Office of Solid Waste and Emergency Response

US Environmental Protection Agency (1986b) Method 8250. Gas chromatography/mass spectrometry for semivolatile organics: packed column technique. In: *Test Methods for Evaluating Solid Waste—Physical/Chemical Methods*, 3rd ed. (US EPA No. SW-846), Washington DC, Office of Solid Waste and Emergency Response

US Environmental Protection Agency (1986c) Method 8270. Gas chromatography/mass spectrometry for semivolatile organics: capillary column technique. In: *Test Methods for Evaluating Solid Waste—Physical/Chemical Methods*, 3rd ed. (US EPA No. SW-846), Washington DC, Office of Solid Waste and Emergency Response

US Environmental Protection Agency (1988a) Method TO-4. Method for the determination of organochlorine pesticides and polychlorinated biphenyls in ambient air. In: *Compendium of Methods for the Determination of Toxic Organic Compounds in Ambient Air* (US EPA Report No. EPA-600/4-89-017; US NTIS PB90-116989), Research Triangle Park, NC, Atmospheric Research and Exposure Assessment Laboratory

US Environmental Protection Agency (1988b) Method TO-10. Method for the determination of organochlorine pesticides in ambient air using low volume polyurethane foam (PUF) sampling with gas chromatography/electron capture detector (GC/ECD). In: *Compendium of Methods for the Determination of Toxic Organic Compounds in Ambient Air* (US EPA Report No. EPA-600/4-89-017; US NTIS PB90-116989), Research Triangle Park, NC, Atmospheric Research and Exposure Assessment Laboratory

US Environmental Protection Agency (1988c) Method 508. Determination of chlorinated pesticides in water by gas chromatography with an electron capture detector. In: *Methods for the Determination of Organic Compounds in Drinking Water* (EPA Report No. EPA-600/4-88-039; US NTIS PB89-220461), Cincinnati, OH, Environmental Monitoring Systems Laboratory

US Environmental Protection Agency (1989a) Method 608—organochlorine pesticides and PCBs. *US Code fed. Regul.*, *Title 40*, Part 136, Appendix A, pp. 354-374

US Environmental Protection Agency (1989b) Method 625—base/neutrals and acids. *US Code fed. Regul.*, *Title 40*, Part 136, Appendix A, pp. 447-474

US Food and Drug Administration (1990) Action levels for residues of certain pesticides in food and feed. *Fed. Reg.*, *55*, 14359-14363

US National Cancer Institute (1978) *Bioassays of DDT, TDE, and p,p'-DDE for Possible Carcinogenicity* (Technical Report No. 131; PB-286 367), Bethesda, MD

US National Technical Information Service (1968) *Evaluation of Carcinogenic, Teratogenic and Mutagenic Activities of Selected Pesticides and Industrial Chemicals*, Vol. 1, *Carcinogenic Study*, Washington DC

US Occupational Safety and Health Administration (1989) Air contaminants—permissible exposure limits. *US Code fed. Regul.*, *Title 29*, Part 1910.1000

Vainio, H. (1974) Enhancement of hepatic microsomal drug oxidation and glucuronidation in rat by 1,1,1-trichloro-2,2-bis(p-chlorophenyl)ethane (DDT) *Chem.-biol. Interactions, 9*, 7-14

Vainio, H. (1975) Stimulation of microsomal drug-metabolizing enzymes in rat liver by 1,1,1-trichloro-2,2-bis(p-chlorophenyl)ethane (DDT), pregnenolone-16α-carbonitrile (PCN) and polychlorinated biphenyls (PCB's). *Environ. Qual. Saf., Suppl. 3*, 486-490

Valencia, R., Mason, J.M., Woodruff, R.C. & Zimmering, S. (1985) Chemical mutagenesis testing in *Drosophila*. III. Results of 48 coded compounds tested for the National Toxicology Program. *Environ. Mutagenesis, 7*, 325-348

Van Dijck, P. & Van de Voorde, H. (1976) Mutagenicity *versus* carcinogenicity of organochlorine insecticides. *Med. Fac. Landbouau. Rijksuniv. Gent, 41*, 1491-1498

Walker, A.I.T., Thorpe, E. & Stevenson, D.E. (1973) The toxicology of dieldrin (HEOD). I. Long-term oral toxicity studies in mice. *Food Cosmet. Toxicol., 11*, 415-432

Wallace, E.Z., Silverstein, J.N., Villadolid, L.S. & Weisenfeld, S. (1961) Cushing's syndrome due to adrenocortical hyperplasia. *New Engl. J. Med., 265*, 1088-1093

Wallace, M.E., Knights, P. & Dye, A.O. (1976) Pilot study of the mutagenicity of DDT in mice. *Environ. Pollut., 11*, 217-222

Ware, G.W. (1975) Effects of DDT on reproduction in higher animals. *Residue Rev., 59*, 119-140

Ware, G.W., Estesen, B.J. & Cahill, W.P. (1970) Uptake of C^{14}-DDT from soil by alfalfa. *Bull. environ. Contam. Toxicol., 5*, 85-86

Wärngård, L., Flodström, S., Ljungquist, S. & Ahlborg, U.G. (1985) Inhibition of metabolic cooperation in Chinese hamster lung fibroblast cells (V79) in culture by various DDT-analogs. *Arch. environ. Contam. Toxicol., 14*, 541-546

Wärngård, L., Hemming, H., Flodström, S., Duddy, S.K. & Kass, G.E.N. (1989) Mechanistic studies on the DDT-induced inhibition of intercellular communication. *Carcinogenesis, 10*, 471-476

Wassermann, M., Ron, M., Bercovici, B., Wassermann, D., Cucos, S. & Pines, A. (1982) Premature delivery and organochlorine compounds: polychlorinated biphenyls and some organochlorine insecticides. *Environ. Res., 28*, 106-112

Weisburger, J.H. & Weisburger, E.K. (1968) Food additives and chemical carcinogens: on the concept of zero tolerance. *Food Cosmet. Toxicol., 6*, 235-242

Welch, R.M., Lewin, W. & Conney, A.H. (1969) Estrogenic action of DDT and its analogs. *Toxicol. appl. Pharmacol., 14*, 358-367

Wheatley, G.A. (1965) The assessment and persistence of residues of organochlorine insecticides in soils and their uptake by crops. *Ann. appl. Biol., 55*, 325-329

White, W.C. & Sweeney, T.R. (1945) The metabolism of 2,2-bis(p-chlorophenyl)-1,1,1-trichlorethane (DDT). I. A metabolite from rabbit urine, di(p-chlorophenyl)acetic acid; its isolation, identification and synthesis. *Public Health Rep., 60*, 66-71

WHO (1979) *DDT and its Derivatives* (Environmental Health Criteria 9), Geneva

WHO (1984) *Guidelines for Drinking Water Quality*, Vol. 1, *Recommendations*, Geneva, p. 69

WHO (1985) *Specifications for Pesticides Used in Public Health*, 6th ed., Geneva

WHO (1989) *DDT and its Derivatives—Environmental Aspects* (Environmental Health Criteria 83), Geneva,

Wicklund, K.G., Daling, J.R., Allard, J. & Weiss, N.S. (1988) Respiratory cancer among orchardists in Washington state, 1968 to 1980. *J. occup. Med., 30*, 561-564

Williams, G.M., Telang, S. & Tong, C. (1981) Inhibition of intercellular communication between liver cells by the liver tumor promoter 1,1,1-trichloro-2,2-bis(p-chlorophenyl)ethane. *Cancer Lett., 11*, 339-344

Williams, G.M., Laspia, M.F. & Dunkel, V.C. (1982) Reliability of the hepatocyte primary culture/DNA repair test in testing of coded carcinogens and noncarcinogens. *Mutat. Res.*, *97*, 359-370

Williams, S., ed. (1984a) *Official Methods of Analysis of the Association of Official Analytical Chemists*, 14th ed., Washington DC, Association of Official Analytical Chemists, pp. 533-543

Williams, S., ed. (1984b) *Official Methods of Analysis of the Association of Official Analytical Chemists*, 14th ed., Washington DC, Association of Official Analytical Chemists, p. 116

Williams, S., ed. (1985) *Official Methods of Analysis of the Association of Official Analytical Chemists*, 14th ed., Washington DC, Association of Official Analytical Chemists, pp. 385-386

Wolfe, H.R. & Armstrong, J.F. (1971) Exposure of formulating plant workers to DDT. *Arch. environ. Health*, *23*, 169-176

Wong, O., Brocker, W., Davis, H.V. & Nagle, G.S. (1984) Mortality of workers potentially exposed to organic and inorganic brominated chemicals, DBCP, Tris, PBB and DDT. *Br. J. ind. Med.*, *41*, 15-24

Woodruff, R.C., Phillips, J.P. & Irwin, D. (1983) Pesticide-induced complete and partial chromosome loss in screens with repair-defective females of *Drosophila melanogaster*. *Environ. Mutagenesis, 5*, 835-846

Woods, J.S. & Polissar, L. (1989) Non-Hodgkin's lymphoma among phenoxy herbicide-exposed farm workers in western Washington State. *Chemosphere*, *18*, 401-406

Woods, J.S., Polissar, L., Severson, R.K., Heuser, L.S. & Kulander, B.G. (1987) Soft tissue sarcoma and non-Hodgkin's lymphoma in relation to phenoxyherbicide and chlorinated phenol exposure in western Washington. *J. natl Cancer Inst.*, *78*, 899-910

Worthing, C.R. & Walker, S.B., eds (1987) *The Pesticide Manual—A World Compendium*, 8th ed., Thornton Heath, British Crop Protection Council, pp. 231-232

Wyrobek, A.J. & Bruce, W.R. (1975) Chemical induction of sperm abnormalities in mice. *Proc. natl Acad. Sci. USA*, *72*, 4425-4429

Zeilmaker, M.J. & Yamasaki, H. (1986) Inhibition of junctional intercellular communication as a possible short-term test to detect tumor-promoting agents: results with nine chemicals tested by dye transfer assay in Chinese hamster V79 cells. *Cancer Res.*, *46*, 6180-6186

Zhong-Xiang, L., Kavanagh, T., Trosko, J.E. & Chang, C.C. (1986) Inhibition of gap junctional intercellular communication in human teratocarcinoma cells by organochlorine pesticides. *Toxicol. appl. Pharmacol.*, *83*, 10-19

DELTAMETHRIN

1. Exposure Data

1.1 Chemical and physical data

Prior to 1980, deltamethrin was known as decamethrin. Of the eight possible stereoisomers with the general structure shown below (three asymmetric centres), only two isomers, 1R,3R,S(benzyl) and 1R,3S,S(benzyl) have insecticidal activity. The commercial product, deltamethrin, contains only the former (*cis*) isomer; products containing the latter are known as *trans*-deltamethrin. Deltamethrin has an α-cyanogroup on the 3-phenoxybenzyl alcohol and is a type II pyrethroid.

1.1.1 *Synonyms, structural and molecular data*

Deltamethrin

Chem. Abstr. Serv. Reg. No.: 52918-63-5
Replaced CAS Reg. Nos.: 55700-96-4; 62229-77-0
Chem. Abstr. Name: (1R-(1α(S*),3α))-3-(2,2-Dibromoethenyl)-2,2-dimethylcyclopropanecarboxylic acid, cyano(3-phenoxyphenyl)methyl ester
IUPAC Systematic Name: (S)-α-Cyano-3-phenoxybenzyl, (1R,3R)-3-(2,2-dibromovinyl)-2,2-dimethylcyclopropanecarboxylate
Synonyms: Decamethrin; Decamethrine; FMC 45498; NRDC 161; OMS 1998; RU 22974; RUP 987; *cis*-deltamethrin

trans-Deltamethrin

Chem. Abstr. Serv. Reg. No.: 64363-96-8
Chem. Abstr. Name: (1R-(1α(S*),3β))-3-(2,2-Dibromoethenyl)-2,2-dimethylcyclopropanecarboxylic acid, cyano(3-phenoxyphenyl)methyl ester
IUPAC Systematic Name: (S)-α-Cyano-3-phenoxybenzyl, (1R,3S)-3-(2,2-dibromovinyl)-2,2-dimethylcyclopropanecarboxylate
Synonym: RU 26979

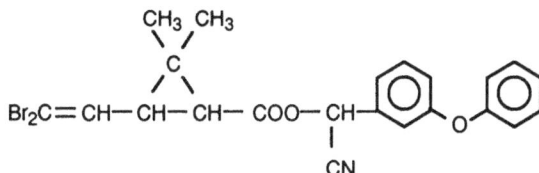

$C_{22}H_{19}Br_2NO_3$ Mol. wt: 505.2

1.1.2 *Chemical and physical properties of deltamethrin*

  (*a*) *Description*: White, odourless orthorhombic needles (Roussel-Uclaf, 1982; WHO, 1990)

  (*b*) *Boiling-point*: Decomposes above 300°C (WHO, 1990)

  (*c*) *Melting-point*: 101-102°C (Roussel-Uclaf, 1982); 98-101°C (Vaysse *et al.*, 1984; WHO, 1990)

  (*d*) *Spectroscopy data*: Infrared, nuclear magnetic resonance, ultraviolet and mass spectral data have been reported (Roussel-Uclaf, 1982).

  (*e*) *Solubility* at 20°C: Slightly soluble in water (< 0.002 mg/l); ethylene glycol, glycerol and isopropanol (< 0.01 g/100 ml); acetonitrile, cyclohexane and ethanol (0.01-0.1 g/100 ml); acetone, benzene, dimethyl sulfoxide, toluene and xylene (0.1-0.5 g/100 ml); cyclohexanone, dimethylformamide and tetrahydrofuran (> 0.5 g/100 ml) (Roussel-Uclaf, 1982; Vaysse *et al.*, 1984; WHO, 1990)

  (*f*) *Volatility*: Vapour pressure, 1.5×10^{-8} mm Hg [0.2×10^{-8} kPa] at 25°C (WHO, 1990)

  (*g*) *Stability*: Gradually undergoes photoisomerization to *trans*-deltamethrin and the 1S,3R stereoisomer; photodegrades on exposure to sunlight (Roussel-Uclaf, 1982); stable to heat (for six months at 40°C) and air but unstable in alkaline media (WHO, 1990)

  (*h*) *Octanol/water partition coefficient (P)*: log P, 5.43 (WHO, 1990)

  (*i*) *Conversion factor for airborne concentrations*[1]: $mg/m^3 = 20.66 \times ppm$

1.1.3 *Trade names, technical products and impurities*

Some common trade names for deltamethrin are Butox, Butoflin, Cislin, Crackdown, Decis and K-Othrine.

Technical-grade deltamethrin has a purity greater than 98% (WHO, 1990). The WHO (1985) specification for technical-grade deltamethrin intended for use in public health programmes requires that it contain a minimum of 98% deltamethrin and a maximum of 1% *trans*-deltamethrin.

Deltamethrin is formulated as solutions, emulsifiable concentrates, flowable powders, wettable powders, ultra-low volume concentrates, dusts, aerosols, granules and concentrated suspensions (Roussel-Uclaf, 1982; WHO, 1985; Royal Society of Chemistry, 1986; Collaborative International Pesticides Analytical Council Ltd, 1988). Deltamethrin is also registered in combination with dimethoate, heptenophos and sulfur (Royal Society of Chemistry, 1986).

1.1.4 *Analysis*

Selected methods for the analysis of deltamethrin in various matrices are given in Table 1. Several analytical methods have been developed for the qualitative determination of deltamethrin residues and formulations, including thin-layer chromatography, gas chromatography and high-performance liquid chromatography (Baker & Bottomley, 1982;

---

[1]Calculated from: mg/m^3 = (molecular weight/24.45) $\times$ ppm, assuming standard temperature (25°C) and pressure (760 mm Hg [101.3 kPa])

Papadopoulou-Mourkidou, 1983; Vaysse *et al.*, 1984; Meinard *et al.*, 1985; Izmerov, 1986; Worthing & Walker, 1987; Martijn & Dobrat, 1988; WHO, 1990).

Table 1. Methods for the analysis of deltamethrin[a]

Sample matrix	Sample preparation	Assay procedure[b]	Reference
Crops (non oily)	Extract with acetonitrile; wash with petroleum ether; extract with petroleum ether/ethyl ether; clean-up on Florisil	GC/ECD	Vaysse *et al.* (1984)
Crops (oily and moist)	Extract with petroleum ether/ethyl ether; concentrate; dissolve extract in dimethyl sulfoxide (DMSO); wash with petroleum ether; partition between DMSO/water and ethyl acetate; clean-up on Florisil	GC/ECD	Vaysse *et al.* (1984)
Formulations	Extract with isooctane/dioxane (80:20); filter	HPLC/UV	Vaysse *et al.* (1984)
Fruit (low fat content)	Extract with acetonitrile or hexane; filter; rewash filter; rewash; purify by liquid-liquid separation	GC/ECD	Roussel-Uclaf (1982)
Fruit (high fat content), milk	Extract with petroleum ether:ethyl ether (50:50); filter; rewash; filter; rewash; purify by liquid-liquid separation	GC/ECD	Roussel-Uclaf (1982)
Meat	Extract; purify by liquid-liquid separation	LG/GP-ECD	Roussel-Uclaf (1982)
Milk	Extract with hexane; partition with acetonitrile; clean-up on Florisil	GC/ECD	Vaysse *et al.* (1984)
Soil	Extract with acetone/hexane; partition extracts between water and hexane; clean-up on acid alumina column	GC/ECD	Vaysse *et al.* (1984)
Tissue	Extract with petroleum ether/ethyl ether; take up in acetonitrile; wash with petroleum ether; clean-up by gel permeation chromatography	GC/ECD	Vaysse *et al.* (1984)

[a]No limit of detection reported
[b]Abbreviations: GC/ECD, gas chromatography/electron capture detection; HPLC/UV, high performance liquid chromatography/ultraviolet detection; LC/GP-ECD, liquid chromatography/gel permeation-electron capture detection

1.2 Production and use

1.2.1 *Production*

Deltamethrin was first synthesized in 1974 and first marketed in 1977 (Vaysse *et al.*, 1984). Chemically, it is the [1R,3R (or *cis*); αS]-isomer of eight stereoisomeric esters of the dibromo analogue of chrysanthemic acid, 2,2-dimethyl-3-(2,2-dibromovinyl)cyclopropane-carboxylic acid, with α-cyano-3-phenoxybenzyl alcohol (WHO, 1990).

In 1987, worldwide production was about 250 tonnes. Production of deltamethrin increased steadily to this level from 75 tonnes in 1979 (WHO, 1990).

1.2.2 *Use*

Deltamethrin is a synthetic pyrethroid insecticide which possesses an extremely high level of activity against a wide range of insects (Worthing & Walker, 1987), including *Lepidoptera*, *Hemiptera*, *Diptera* and *Coleoptera* (Roussel-Uclaf, 1982). It acts by both direct contact and ingestion (Worthing & Walker, 1987).

It is used mostly for crop protection (85% of total production), of which 45% is used on cotton, 25% on fruit and vegetable crops, 20% on cereals, maize and soya beans and the remaining 10% on miscellaneous crops (WHO, 1990), such as coffee, maize (Health and Welfare Canada, 1990) and hops (Codex Committee on Pesticide Residues, 1990). It is also used in public health programmes (against Chagas' disease and malaria) and to protect stored crops, primarily cereal grains, coffee beans and dry beans. It can be used in animal facilities (WHO, 1990).

Deltamethrin is recommended for crop use at 10-15 g/ha (Roussel-Uclaf, 1982).

In the USSR, deltamethrin is approved for commercial application on sunflowers, cotton, potatoes and sugar beets (Izmerov, 1986).

1.3 Occurrence

1.3.1 *Soil*

When deltamethrin was applied to a sandy clay loam soil at 17.5 g/ha in an indoor incubation study and in two field experiments, its half-times were 4.9 and 6.9 weeks, respectively (Hill, 1983).

Chapman *et al.* (1981) examined the relative persistence of five pyrethroids, including deltamethrin, in sand and organic soil under laboratory conditions. All the insecticides (1 mg/kg) were degraded more rapidly in natural soils than in sterilized soils, suggesting the importance of microbial degradation. About 52% of the deltamethrin applied was recovered from sand and 74% from organic soil eight weeks after treatment of natural soil.

The degradation of deltamethrin was investigated by Zhang *et al.* (1984) in an organic soil over a 180-day period. The half-time was found to be 72 days, indicating that delta-methrin is likely to be less susceptible to degradation in organic soils than in mineral soils. The degradation of deltamethrin was also studied in two German soils: the half-times for sandy soil and sandy loam soil were reported to be 35 and 60 days, respectively (WHO, 1990).

1.3.2 *Food*

Some 598 samples of food were analysed as part of the Canadian national surveillence programme in 1984-89. Three samples contained residues (2/25 samples of apples and 1/21 of strawberries) at levels of 0.004-0.006 mg/kg (Government of Canada, 1990).

A trial in Tunisia in 1987 involving one application at a rate of 50 g active ingredient/ha of formulated product (0.1% concentrate) on pears resulted in average residue of 0.04 mg/kg after 14 days. When stored potatoes were dusted with one application of a dust powder formulation of deltamethrin at a rate of 100 g/100 kg potatoes, samples collected at 113 days showed residue levels averaging 0.07 mg/kg (FAO/WHO, 1988).

The level in wheat grain treated with deltamethrin at the rate of 2 mg/kg was 1.08 mg/kg after storage for 9 months. When the wheat was milled and baked, the residue level in white bread was 0.11 mg/kg (as reported by WHO, 1990).

1.3.3 *Occupational exposure*

Workers packaging deltamethrin in a small importing factory in China were reported to have been exposed to airborne levels of 0.5-12 $\mu g/m^3$, with resulting skin contact (He *et al.*, 1988).

1.4 Regulations and guidelines

The FAO/WHO Joint Meeting on Pesticide Residues evaluated deltamethrin at its meetings in 1980, 1981, 1982, 1984, 1985, 1986 and 1987 (FAO/WHO, 1981, 1982, 1983a,b, 1985, 1986a,b, 1987, 1988). In 1982, an acceptable daily intake of 0.01 mg/kg bw was established (Codex Committee on Pesticide Residues, 1990; WHO, 1990).

Maximum residue levels have been established by the Codex Alimentarius Commission for deltamethrin in or on the following agricultural commodities (in mg/kg): tea (black, green), 10; hops (dry) and wheat bran (unprocessed), 5; coffee beans, 2; beans (dry), cereal grains, field peas (dry), lentils (dry) and wheat wholemeal, 1; leafy vegetables, legume animal feeds (dry) and straw and fodder (dry) of cereal grains, 0.5; *Brassica* vegetables (head cabbages, flowerhead brassicas), fruiting vegetables (cucurbits) and fruiting vegetables (except cucurbits), 0.2; bulb vegetables (except fennel (bulb)), legume vegetables, oilseed, oilseed (except peanut), olives, pome fruit and wheat flour, 0.1; artichokes (globe), bananas, cocoa beans, grapes, kiwifruit, mandarins, oranges (sweet, sour), stone fruit and strawberries, 0.05; figs, legume oilseeds, melons (except watermelon), milks, mushrooms, peanuts, pineapples and vegetables (root, tuber), 0.01 (Codex Committee on Pesticide Residues, 1990).

The US Environmental Protection Agency (1987) proposed that a tolerance of 0.2 ppm (mg/kg) be established for the combined residues of deltamethrin and a tolerance of 1.0 ppm for its *trans*-isomer in or on imported tomatoes and concentrated tomato products.

National and regional pesticide residue limits for deltamethrin in foods are present in Table 2.

Table 2. National and regional pesticide residue limits for deltamethrin in foods[a]

Country or region	Residue limit (mg/kg)	Commodities
Argentina	1	Stored cereal grains in general
	0.1	Apples, beans, cabbage, cauliflower, maize, cotton, eggplant, flax, peaches, peanuts, pears, peas, peppers, sorghum, soya, sunflower, sweet corn, Swiss chard, tomatoes
	0.05	Artichokes
	0.01	Potatoes
Australia	10 (provisional)	Wheat bran, wheat pollard
	2	Cereal grains (whole grain)
	0.2	Milk (fat basis)
	0.1	Berry vegetables, meat fat (cattle, goats, sheep), oilseeds, sweet maize, vegetables (pod, seed)
	0.05[b]	Cole crops

Table 2 (contd)

Country or region	Residue limit (mg/kg)	Commodities
Austria	5.0	Hops
	0.5	Artichokes, asparagus, beans (broad, green), bulb vegetables, cabbage, cardoon, cereals, chard, cucumber, eggplant, fennel, fruit used as vegetables, garden celery, kitchen herbs, lettuce, melons, mushrooms, parsley (without root), peas (green), pepper cress, peppers, potatoes, pumpkin, rapeseed, rhubarb stalks, spinach, squash, sweet maize, tomatoes, zucchini
	0.2	Fruit, other vegetables
Belgium	0.2	Pome fruit, vegetables
	0.1	Other fruit
	0.05	Potatoes, strawberries
	0 (0.05)^c	Other foodstuffs of vegetable origin
Brazil	1.0	Coffee, maize (stored in bulk, on cob, in sacks), rice (stored in sacks), wheat
	0.1	Kale
	0.05	Broccoli, citrus fruit (peel), rice, sorghum
	0.04	Peaches
	0.03	Cauliflower, cucumbers, eggplant, garlic, onions, tomatoes
	0.02	Apples, cottonseed, plums
	0.01	Peppers, wheat
	0.005	Cabbage, maize, peanuts, potatoes
	0.002	Figs, honeydew melons, soya beans
	0.001	Citrus fruit (edible parts), string beans, watermelons
Canada	Negligible	Apples, asparagus, barley, blueberries, broccoli, Brussels' sprouts, cabbages, cauliflower, cucumbers, flax, lentils, mustard, oats, pears, peaches, peppers, potatoes, rapeseed (canola oil), Saskatoon berries, sunflowers, strawberries, wheat
Denmark	0.5	Leafy vegetables
	0.1	Fruit (pome, stone)
Finland	0.5	Food products
France	1	Cereal grains
	0.5	Vegetable greens (salad)
	0.2	Fruit, other vegetables
Germany	10	Hops, tea
	2	Raw coffee
	0.5	Green cabbage, legumes
	0.2	Fruit used as vegetables (except mushrooms), pome fruit, vegetables (leaf, sprout (except green cabbage, onions, shallots)), wheat bran
	0.1	Berries (except strawberries), cereals, cereal products (except wheat bran), grapes, oilseeds, olives, onions, shallots, stone fruit
	0.05	Spices, tea-like products, other foods of plant origin
Hungary	0.1	Crops and food

Table 2 (contd)

Country or region	Residue limit (mg/kg)	Commodities
Italy	0.5	Broad beans, cabbages, carrots, citrus fruit, maize, cucumbers, drupes, eggplants, figs, grapes, kidney beans, lettuce, olives, peas, pomes, potatoes, strawberries, sugar beets, tobacco, tomatoes, wheat
Netherlands	0.2	Leafy vegetables
	0.1	Other fruit
	0.05[d]	Meat, milk, other vegetables, potatoes, strawberries
	0 (0.05)[e]	Other foodstuffs
South Africa	1.0	Oats, rye, wheat
	0.1	Apples, beans, cruciferae, grapes, lucerne, mealies (green), peaches, pears, plums
	0.05	Groundnuts, peas, prickly pears, sorghum, sweet potatoes, tomatoes
Spain	2	Hops (dried)
	0.5	Grains (cereal, legume), leafy vegetables
	0.2	Other vegetables (except bulbs, roots, tubers)
	0.05	Fruit
	0.01	Vegetables (bulb, root, tuber), other plant products
Sweden	0.05[b]	Potatoes
Switzerland	0.1	Fruit (except grapes)
	0.05	Cereal, grapes, mushrooms, rapeseed, vegetables (except potatoes)
	0.03	Milk
	0.01	Maize, potatoes
Taiwan	1.0	Tea leaves
	0.5	Leafy vegetables with large wrapper leaves, leafy vegetables with small leaves
	0.2	Berries, fruit vegetables
	0.1	Melons
	0.05	Rice
	0.01	Tropical fruit
Yugoslavia	0.2	Cabbage, cabbage-like plants
	0.1	Fruit, vegetables (except cabbage)

[a]From Health and Welfare Canada (1990)

[b]The maximum residue limit has been set at or about the limit of analytical determination.

[c]The figure in parentheses is the lower limit for determining residues in the corresponding product according to the standard method of analysis.

[d]A pesticide may be used on an eating or drinking ware or raw material without a demonstrable residue remaining; the value listed is considered the highest concentration at which this requirement is deemed to have been met.

[e]Residues shall be absent; the value in parentheses is the highest concentration at which this requirement is still deemed to have been met.

2. Studies of Cancer in Humans

No data were available to the Working Group.

3. Studies of Cancer in Experimental Animals

Oral administration

Mouse: Groups of 30 male and 30 female C57Bl/6 mice, six weeks of age, were given 1 or 4 mg/kg bw deltamethrin (99.5% pure) dissolved in arachis oil by gavage daily on five days a week for 104 weeks. Further groups of 50 males and 50 females received 8 mg/kg bw deltamethrin daily for 104 weeks. Control groups of 50 males and 50 females were given arachis oil or left untreated. The experiment was terminated when the mice were 120 weeks of age. The survival rate was similar in treated and control groups (40-64%), except in high-dose females, of which only 32% were alive at 120 weeks. There was no increase in the incidence of tumours at any site in experimental groups (Cabral *et al.*, 1990).

Rat: Groups of 50 male and 50 female BD VI rats, six weeks of age, were given 0, 3 or 6 mg/kg bw deltamethrin (99.5% pure) in arachis oil by gavage daily on five days a week for 104 weeks. Control rats received arachis oil alone. The experiment was terminated when the rats were 120 weeks of age. The survival pattern was comparable in all groups; 60% or more rats were alive at 120 weeks. The incidence of thyroid adenomas in males (19/50) that received 3 mg/kg bw and in females (14/49) that received 6 mg/kg bw was significantly higher than that in controls (6/48 males, $p = 0.003$; 4/47 females, $p = 0.011$) (Cabral *et al.*, 1990). [The Working Group noted that the type of thyroid adenoma was not specified.]

4. Other Relevant Data

The toxicity of deltamethrin has been reviewed (FAO/WHO, 1981, 1982, 1983a,b; WHO, 1990). For a general introduction to the toxicokinetics of pyrethroids, see the monograph on permethrin.

4.1 Absorption, distribution, metabolism and excretion

4.1.1 *Humans*

The cutaneous and gastrointestinal absorption of deltamethrin in humans has been demonstrated after acute poisonings due to occupational overexposure or ingestion of deltamethrin products. The presence of a deltamethrin metabolite (3-(2,2-dibromovinyl)-2,2-dimethylcyclopropane carboxylic acid) (see Fig. 1) has been reported in the urine of people with acute deltamethrin intoxication (He *et al.*, 1989), confirming the absorption and metabolic degradation of this insecticide in the human body.

4.1.2 *Experimental systems*

The metabolic pathways of deltamethrin in mammals are shown in Figure 1. The metabolism of this compound has been studied in rats *in vivo* (Ruzo *et al.*, 1978, 1979) and

Fig. 1. Metabolic pathways of deltamethrin in mammals[a]

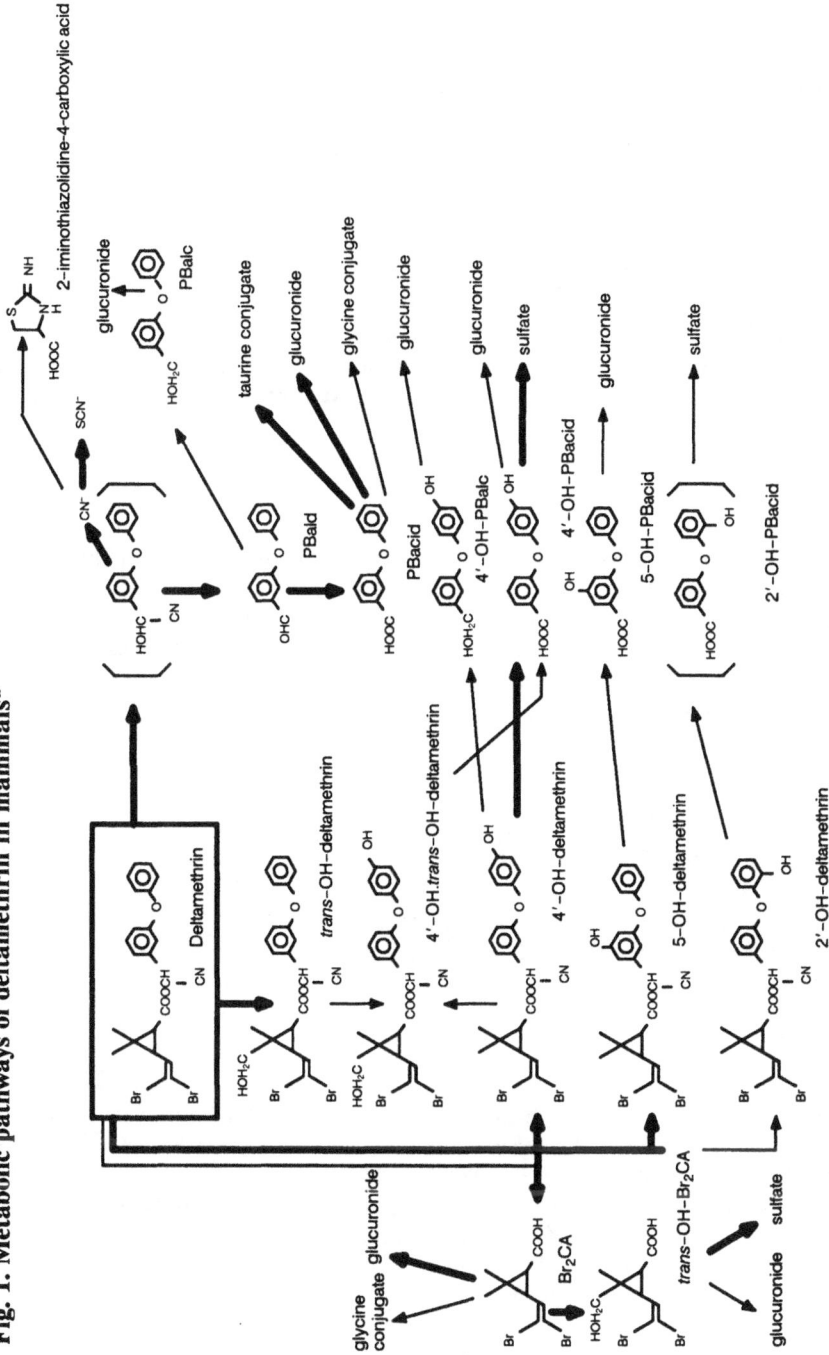

[a]From WHO (1990); Br$_2$CA, 3-(2,2-dibromovinyl)-2,2-dimethylcyclopropane carboxylic acid; PBacid, 3-phenoxybenzoic acid; PBald, 3-phenoxy-benzaldehyde; PBalc, 3-phenoxybenzyl alcohol

in vitro (Soderlund & Casida, 1977; Shono *et al.*, 1979) and shown to occur *via* ester hydrolysis, oxidation, hydroxylation and conjugation.

Deltamethrin was labelled with ^{14}C in the dibromovinyl substituent or in the benzylic carbon and administered orally to rats and mice. Eight days later, the highest concentrations were retained in fat tissue, regardless of the labelling position, suggesting that unmetabolized deltamethrin is retained in fat. When the ^{14}C-label was in the cyano group, the greatest radiocarbon activity was found in skin and stomach and, in the rat, also in the intestines and blood, due to remaining thiocyanate. In rats, 80-90 % of the radiolabel was eliminated within 24 h. When the ^{14}C-label was in the cyano group, elimination was slower, owing to retention of thiocyanate. In general, unmetabolized deltamethrin and hydroxylated metabolites were excreted in the faeces, while more polar hydrolysis products and conjugates were eliminated in the urine. Mice had a somewhat slower rate of elimination than rats (48-60% within 24 h) (Ruzo *et al.*, 1978, 1979).

4.2 Toxic effects

4.2.1 *Humans*

He *et al.* (1989) reviewed 325 cases of deltamethrin intoxication from the Chinese medical literature. Common findings included paraesthesia, particularly involving the face, dizziness, headache, nausea, anorexia and fatigue. Less common findings included chest tightness, palpitations, blurred vision, increased sweating and low-grade fever. Muscular fasciculations, convulsions and coma were reported in some of the more severely poisoned cases. Two deaths from convulsions were reported.

4.2.2 *Experimental systems*

The acute toxicity of deltamethrin is high, with an oral LD_{50} (in an oily vehicle) of approximately 50 mg/kg bw for adult male and 30 mg/kg bw for adult female rats (Kavlock *et al.*, 1979; Gaines & Linder, 1986). A suspension of deltametrin in 10% gum-arabic solution reduced the oral toxicity in rats by more than 100-fold (Pham *et al.*, 1984).

Signs of acute intoxication in rats and mice included salivation, ataxia and choreoathetotic movements (Kavlock *et al.*, 1979; Pham *et al.*, 1984).

Deltamethrin has been demonstrated to bind covalently to mammalian hepatic proteins *in vitro*, although the binding was less pronounced than that of cismethrin (Catinot *et al.*, 1989).

The following studies were reported in a review (WHO, 1990). In Sprague-Dawley rats given up to 10 mg/kg bw deltamethrin by gavage daily for 13 weeks, slight hyperexcitability was noted in some animals at the highest dose. Lower body weight gain was noted in males at 2.5 and 10 mg/kg. No other treatment-related effect was reported. In dogs treated at similar doses (by gelatin capsule) over 13 weeks, dilated pupils were seen at doses of 2.5 and 10 mg/kg bw per day. The incidence of vomiting increased dose-dependently at doses from 1 mg/kg bw. The central nervous system was the main target of toxicity, with various neurological symptoms at the higher doses. No histopathological lesion was found, neither was any other toxic effect found.

In 24-month studies, no treatment-related non-neoplastic effect was found in mice fed dietary levels of up to 100 mg/kg (CD-1 mice) or in mice given up to 8 mg/kg bw by gavage on five days a week (C57Bl/6 mice). In Charles River CD rats fed up to 50 mg/kg of diet deltamethrin for 24 months, no significant treatment-related non-neoplastic effect was noted, except for slightly less weight gain at the 50 mg/kg dose level. In dogs given up to 40 mg/kg deltamethrin in the diet for 24 months, no treatment-related non-neoplastic effect was noted.

4.3 Reproductive and developmental effects

4.3.1 *Humans*

No data were available to the Working Group.

4.3.2 *Experimental systems*

Deltamethrin dissolved in corn oil was given to CD-1 mice at 0, 3, 6 or 12 mg/kg by gavage on days 7-16 of gestation and to Sprague-Dawley rats at 0, 1.25, 2.5 or 5.0 mg/kg by gavage on days 7-20 of gestation. Mice and rats were sacrificed on day 18 or 20 of gestation, respectively. In mice, there was a dose-dependent decrease in maternal weight and an increase in supernumary ribs; however, there was no effect on number of implantation sites, perinatal mortality, fetal weight, ossification centres or visceral abnormalities. In rats, there was a dose-dependent decrease in maternal body weight with no effect on fetal parameters (Kavlock *et al.*, 1979).

In a screening study for developmental toxicity, 25 CD-1 mice were treated with deltamethrin at 10 mg/kg [dose reported correctly in follow-up study] in corn oil by gavage on days 8-12 of gestation, and 24 controls were treated with corn oil. There was no effect on the number of pregnancies, maternal weight gain during pregnancy, number of pups born alive or pup weights on postnatal days 1 or 3 (Chernoff & Kavlock, 1982). An extension of the experiment up to 250 days of life to assess growth, viability, morphology and reproductive function of the offspring showed no effect of deltamethrin on these parameters (Gray & Kavlock, 1984).

In a similar screening test in ICR/SIM mice, animals were treated with a minimally toxic maternal dose (14 mg/kg bw per day) by oral intubation (in corn oil) on days 8-12 of gestation. Although maternal weight gain was decreased, there was no effect on neonatal survival or weight gain (Seidenberg *et al.*, 1986). A repetition using similar procedures with deltamethrin at 10 mg/kg bw per day suggested an effect on neonatal survival (Kavlock *et al.*, 1987).

Quail embryos received an intravitelline injection of purified technical-grade or a commercial preparation of deltamethrin (25 g deltamethrin/litre excipient, essentially xylene). The number of germ cells was decreased by both preparations, but the commercial preparation was more potent than the purified deltamethrin, being active independently of the route of treatment (injection, spraying, treatment of parents *via* feed). Both xylene and deltamethrin appeared to be responsible for the decrease in germ cell number (David, 1982).

Treatment of quail eggs with deltamethrin by immersion in aqueous emulsions (equivalent to 0-1.5 g active ingredient in 110 litres applied per hectare) on days 0, 4 or 14 of incubation had no effect on hatchability or developmental malformation. An effect on incubation time was seen at the highest concentration when given at the preincubation stage (Martin, 1990).

4.4 Genetic and related effects (see also Table 3 and Appendices 1 and 2)

4.4.1 *Humans*

No data were available to the Working Group.

4.4.2 *Experimental systems*

Deltamethrin did not induce point mutation in bacteria or cultured mammalian cells or DNA damage in yeast, but it induced chromosomal aberrations in root meristem cells of *Allium cepa*.

In vivo, deltamethrin induced chromosomal aberrations and micronucleus formation in bone-marrow cells of mice. In a study by oral administration, no chromosomal aberration was observed in mouse bone marrow, but morphological sperm abnormalities were induced in mice. [The Working Group noted that the studies by Páldy (1981) and Hoellinger *et al.* (1987) could not be evaluated because of inadequacies of experimental design and reporting.]

5. Summary of Data Reported and Evaluation

5.1 Exposure data

Deltamethrin is a highly active contact insecticide. It was first marketed in 1977 and is used mostly on cotton and on crops such as coffee, maize, cereals, fruit, vegetables and hops. It is also used in public health programmes and for the protection of stored crops.

Deltamethrin has been formulated as solutions, concentrates, granules, powders and aerosols, alone and in combination with other pesticides.

Exposure can occur during its production and application and, at much lower levels, from the consumption of food containing residues.

5.2 Carcinogenicity in humans

No data were available to the Working Group.

5.3 Carcinogenicity in experimental animals

Deltamethrin was tested for carcinogenicity in one experiment in mice and in one experiment in rats by oral administration. In mice, no increase in tumour incidence was seen. In rats, a statistically significant increase in the incidence of unspecified thyroid adenomas was observed in low-dose males and high-dose females.

5.4 Other relevant data

No data were available on the genetic and related effects of deltamethrin in humans.

Deltamethrin induced micronucleus formation and chromosomal aberrations in bone marrow and abnormal sperm morphology in mice treated *in vivo*. The only other indication of genotoxic potential was induction of chromosomal aberrations in plants.

Table 3. Genetic and related effects of deltamethrin

Test system	Result[a] Without exogenous metabolic system	Result[a] With exogenous metabolic system	Dose[b] LED/HID	Reference
SA0, Salmonella typhimurium TA100, reverse mutation	–	–	2500.0000	Kavlock et al. (1979)
SA0, Salmonella typhimurium TA100, reverse mutation (plate incorporation)	–	–	300.0000	Pluijmen et al. (1984)
SA0, Salmonella typhimurium TA100, reverse mutation (fluctuation test)*	–	–	10.0000	Pluijmen et al. (1984)
SA5, Salmonella typhimurium TA1535, reverse mutation	–	–	2500.0000	Kavlock et al. (1979)
SA7, Salmonella typhimurium TA1537, reverse mutation	–	–	2500.0000	Kavlock et al. (1979)
SA8, Salmonella typhimurium TA1538, reverse mutation	–	–	2500.0000	Kavlock et al. (1979)
SA9, Salmonella typhimurium TA98, reverse mutation	–	–	2500.0000	Kavlock et al. (1979)
SA9, Salmonella typhimurium TA98, reverse mutation (plate incorporation)	–	–	300.0000	Pluijmen et al. (1984)
SA9, Salmonella typhimurium TA98, reverse mutation (fluctuation test)*	–	–	10.0000	Pluijmen et al. (1984)
EC2, Escherichia coli WP2, reverse mutation	–	–	500.0000	Kavlock et al. (1979)
SSB, Saccharomyces cerevisiae D3, DNA damage	–	–	50000.0000	Kavlock et al. (1979)
ACC, Allium cepa, chromosomal aberrations	+	0	0.5000 (6–8 h)	Chauhan et al. (1986)
G9O, Gene mutation, Chinese hamster V79 cells, ouabain resistance	–	–	40.0000	Pluijmen et al. (1984)
G9H, Gene mutation, Chinese hamster V79 cells, hprt locus	+	0	40.0000	Pluijmen et al. (1984)
CBA, Chromosomal aberrations, Swiss albino mouse bone marrow	+	0	10.0000 × 1, i.p.	Bhunya & Pati (1990)
CBA, Chromosomal aberrations, Swiss albino mouse bone marrow	+	0	20.0000 × 1, p.o.	Bhunya & Pati (1990)
CBA, Chromosomal aberrations, Swiss albino mouse bone marrow	+	0	20.0000 × 1, s.c.	Bhunya & Pati (1990)
CBA, Chromosomal aberrations, Swiss albino mouse bone marrow	–	0	6.8000 × 5, p.o.	Poláková & Vargová (1983)
MVM, Micronucleus test, Swiss albino mouse bone marrow	+	0	10.0000 × 2, i.p.	Bhunya & Pati (1990)
SPM, Sperm morphology, Swiss albino mouse	+	0	10.0000 × 5, i.p.	Bhunya & Pati (1990)
ICR, Inhibition of intercellular communication, V79 cells	–	0	8.0000	Flodström et al. (1988)

*Not displayed on profile

[a] +, positive; (+), weakly positive; –, negative; 0, not tested; ?, inconclusive (variable response in several experiments within an adequate study)

[b] In-vitro tests, μg/ml; in-vivo tests, mg/kg bw

5.5 Evaluation[1]

No data were available from studies in humans.

There is *inadequate evidence* for the carcinogenicity of deltamethrin in experimental animals.

Overall evaluation

Deltamethrin *is not classifiable as to its carcinogenicity to humans (Group 3).*

6. References

Baker, P.G. & Bottomley, P. (1982) Determination of residues of synthetic pyrethroids in fruit and vegetables by gas-liquid and high-performance liquid chromatography. *Analyst, 107,* 206-212

Bhunya, S.P. & Pati, P.C. (1990) Effect of deltamethrin, a synthetic pyrethroid, on the induction of chromosome aberrations, micronuclei and sperm abnormalities in mice. *Mutagenesis, 5,* 229-232

Cabral, J.R.P., Galendo, D., Laval, M. & Lyandrat, N. (1990) Carcinogenicity studies with deltamethrin in mice and rats. *Cancer Lett., 49,* 147-152

Catinot, R., Hoellinger, H., Sonnier, M., Do, C.-T., Pichon, J. & Nguyen, H.N. (1989) In vitro covalent binding of the pyrethroids cismethrin, cypermethrin and deltamethrin to rat liver homogenate and microsomes. *Arch. Toxicol., 63,* 214-220

Chapman, R.A., Tu, C.M., Harris, C.R. & Cole, C. (1981) Persistence of five pyrethroid insecticides in sterile and natural, mineral and organic soil. *Bull. environ. Contam. Toxicol., 26,* 513-519

Chauhan, L.K.S., Dikshith, T.S.S. & Sundararaman, V. (1986) Effect of deltamethrin on plant cells. I. Cytological effects on the root meristems of *Allium cepa. Mutat. Res., 171,* 25-30

Chernoff, N. & Kavlock, R.J. (1982) An *in vivo* teratology screen utilizing pregnant mice. *J. Toxicol. environ. Health, 10,* 541-550

Codex Committee on Pesticide Residues (1990) *Guide to Codex Maximum Limits for Pesticide Residues,* Part 2 (CAC/PR 2—1990; CCPR Pesticide Classification No. 135), The Hague

David, D. (1982) Influence of technical and commercial decamethrin, a new synthetic pyrethroid, on the gonadic germ population in quail embryos. *Arch. Anat. Hist. Embr. norm. exp., 65,* 99-110

FAO/WHO (1981) *Pesticide Residues in Food: 1980 Evaluations* (FAO Plant Production and Protection Paper 26 Sup.), Rome

FAO/WHO (1982) *Pesticide Residues in Food: 1981 Evaluations* (FAO Plant Production and Protection Paper 42), Rome

FAO/WHO (1983a) *Pesticide Residues in Food—1982. Report of the Joint Meeting of the FAO Panel of Experts on Pesticide Residues in Food and the Environment and the WHO Expert Group on Pesticide Residues* (FAO Plant Production and Protection Paper 46), Rome

FAO/WHO (1983b) *Pesticide Residues in Food: 1982 Evaluations* (FAO Plant Production and Protection Paper 49), Rome

FAO/WHO (1985) *Pesticide Residues in Food in 1984* (Plant Production and Protection Paper 67), Rome

FAO/WHO (1986a) *Pesticide Residues in Food in 1985* (FAO Plant Production and Protection Paper 68), Rome

---

[1]For definition of the italicized terms, see Preamble, pp. 26-28.

FAO/WHO (1986b) *Pesticide Residues in Food in 1986* (FAO Plant Production and Protection Paper 77), Rome

FAO/WHO (1987) *Pesticide Residues in Food in 1987* (FAO Plant Production and Protection Paper 84), Rome

FAO/WHO (1988) *Pesticide Residues in Food in 1988. Evaluations. Part 1—Residues*, Rome, pp. 61-66

Flodström, S., Wärngård, L., Ljungquist, S. & Ahlborg, U.G. (1988) Inhibition of metabolic cooperation in vitro and enhancement of enzyme altered foci incidence in rat liver by the pyrethroid insecticide fenvalerate. *Arch. Toxicol.*, *61*, 218-223

Gaines, T.B. & Linder, R.E. (1986) Acute toxicity of pesticides in adult and weanling rats. *Fundam. appl. Toxicol.*, *7*, 299-308

Government of Canada (1990) *Report on National Surveillance Data from 1984/85 to 1988/89*, Ottawa

Gray, L.E., Jr & Kavlock, R.J. (1984) An extended evaluation of an in vivo teratology screen utilizing postnatal growth and viability in the mouse. *Teratog. Carcinog. Mutagenesis*, *4*, 403-426

He, F., Shun, J., Han, K., Wu, Y., Yao, P., Wang, S. & Liu, L. (1988) Effects of pyrethroid insecticides on subjects engaged in packaging pyrethroids. *Br. J. ind. Med.*, *45*, 548-551

He, F., Wang, S., Liu, L., Chen, S., Zhang, Z. & Sun, J. (1989) Clinical manifestations and diagnosis of acute pyrethroid poisoning. *Arch. Toxicol.*, *63*, 54-58

Health and Welfare Canada (1990) *National Pesticide Residue Limits in Foods*, Ottawa, Bureau of Chemical Safety, Food Directorate, Health Protection Branch

Hill, B.D. (1983) Persistence of deltamethrin in a Lethbridge sandy clay loam. *J. environ. Sci. Health*, *B18*, 691-703

Hoellinger, H., Lecorsier, A., Sonnier, M., Leger, C., Do, C.-T. & Nguyen, H.-N. (1987) Cytotoxicity, cytogenotoxicity and allergenicity tests on certain pyrethroids. *Drug chem. Toxicol.*, *10*, 291-310

Izmerov, N.F., ed. (1986) *International Register of Potentially Toxic Chemicals. Scientific Reviews of Soviet Literature on Toxicity and Hazards of Chemicals: Decamethrin* (Issue 102), Moscow, Centre of International Projects, United Nations Environment Programme

Kavlock, R., Chernoff, N., Baron, R., Linder, R., Rogers, E., Carver, B., Dilley, J. & Simmon, V. (1979) Toxicity studies with decamethrin, a synthetic pyrethroid insecticide. *J. environ. Pathol. Toxicol.*, *2*, 751-765

Kavlock, R.J., Short, R.D., Jr & Chernoff, N. (1987) Further evaluation of an in vivo teratology screen. *Teratog. Carcinog. Mutagenesis*, *7*, 7-16

Martijn, A. & Dobrat, W., eds (1988) *CIPAC Handbook*, Vol. D, *Analysis of Technical and Formulated Pesticides*, Cambridge, Collaborative International Pesticides Analytical Council Ltd, pp. 57-66

Martin, P.A. (1990) Effects of carbofuran, chloropyrifos and deltamethrin on hatchability, deformity, chick size and incubation time of Japanese quail (*Coturnix japonica*) eggs. *Environ. Toxicol. Chem.*, *9*, 529-534

Meinard, C., Bruneau, P. & Perronnet, J. (1985) High-performance liquid chromatograph coupled with two detectors: a UV spectrometer and a polarimeter. Example in the field of pyrethroids: identification of enantiomers. *J. Chromatogr.*, *349*, 109-116

Páldy, A. (1981) Examination of the mutagenic effect of synthetic pyrethroids on mouse bone-marrow cells. In: *Proceedings of the 21st Hungarian Annual Meeting on Biochemistry*, Veszprém, Budapest, National Institute of Public Health, pp. 227-228

Papadopoulou-Mourkidou, E. (1983) Analysis of established pyrethroid insecticides. *Res. Rev.*, *89*, 179-208

Pham, H.C., Navarro-Delmasure, C., Pham, H.C.A., Clavel, P., Van Haverbeke, G. & Cheav, S.L. (1984) Toxicological studies of deltamethrin. *Int. J. Tissue React.*, *6*, 127-133

Pluijmen, M., Drevon, C., Montesano, R., Malaveille, C., Hautefeuille, A. & Bartsch, H. (1984) Lack of mutagenicity of synthetic pyrethroids in *Salmonella typhimurium* strains and in V79 Chinese hamster cells. *Mutat. Res.*, *137*, 7-15

Poláková, H. & Vargová, M. (1983) Evaluation of the mutagenic effects of decamethrin: cytogenetic analysis of bone marrow. *Mutat. Res.*, *120*, 167-171

Roussel-Uclaf (1982) *Deltamethrin Monograph*, Paris

Royal Society of Chemistry (1986) *European Directory of Agrochemical Products*, Vol. 3, *Insecticides, Acaricides, Nematicides*, Cambridge, pp. 166-175

Ruzo, L.O., Unai, T. & Casida, J.E. (1978) Decamethrin metabolism in rats. *J. agric. Food Chem.*, *26*, 918-925

Ruzo, L.O., Engel, J.L. & Casida, J.E. (1979) Decamethrin metabolites from oxidative, hydrolytic and conjugative reactions in mice. *J. agric. Food Chem.*, *27*, 725-731

Seidenberg, J.M., Anderson, D.G. & Becker, R.A. (1986) Validation of an in vivo developmental toxicity screen in the mouse. *Teratog. Carcinog. Mutagenesis*, *6*, 361-374

Shono, T., Ohsawa, K. & Casida, J.E. (1979) Metabolism of *trans*- and *cis*-permethrin, *trans*- and *cis*-cypermethrin, and decamethrin by microsomal enzymes. *J. agric. Food Chem.*, *27*, 316-325

Soderlund, D.M. & Casida, J.E. (1977) Effect of pyrethroid structure on rates of hydrolysis and oxidation by mouse liver microsomal enzymes. *Pestic. Biochem. Physiol.*, *7*, 391-401

US Environmental Protection Agency (1987) Pesticide tolerance for deltamethrin. *Fed. Reg.*, *52*, 49171-49172, 49177-49178

Vaysse, M., Giudicelli, J.C., Devaux, P. & L'Hotellier, M. (1984) Decis. In: Zweig, G. & Sherma, J., eds, *Analytical Methods for Pesticides and Plant Growth Regulators*, Vol. XIII, *Synthetic Pyrethroids and Other Pesticides*, New York, Academic Press, pp. 53-68

WHO (1985) *Specifications for Pesticides Used in Public Health: Insecticides—Molluscicides—Repellents Methods*, 6th ed., Geneva, pp. 270-296

WHO (1990) *Deltamethrin* (Environmental Health Criteria 97), Geneva

Worthing, C.R. & Walker, S.B., eds (1987) *The Pesticide Manual—A World Compendium*, 8th ed., Thornton Heath, British Crop Protection Council, pp. 234-235

Zhang, L.-Z., Khan, S.U., Akhtar, M.H. & Ivarson, K.C. (1984) Persistence, degradation and distribution of deltamethrin in an organic soil under laboratory conditions. *J. agric. Food Chem.*, *32*, 1207-1211

DICHLORVOS

This substance was considered by a previous Working Group in 1978 (IARC, 1979a). Since that time, new data have become available, and these have been incorporated into the monograph and taken into consideration in the present evaluation.

1. Exposure Data

1.1 Chemical and physical data

1.1.1 *Synonyms, structural and molecular data*

Chem. Abstr. Serv. Reg. No.: 62-73-7
Replaced CAS Reg. Nos.: 8023-22-1; 8072-21-7; 8072-39-7; 8076-16-2; 11095-17-3; 11096-21-2; 11111-31-2; 11126-72-0; 12772-40-6; 55819-32-4; 62139-95-1; 62655-59-8; 95828-55-0; 116788-91-1
Chem. Abstr. Name: Phosphoric acid, 2,2-dichloroethenyl dimethyl ester
IUPAC Systematic Name: 2,2-Dichlorovinyl dimethyl phosphate
Synonyms: 2,2-Dichloroethenol, dimethyl phosphate; dimethyl dichlorovinyl phosphate; dimethyl 2,2-dichloroethenyl phosphate; dimethyl 2,2-dichlorovinyl phosphate; *O,O*-dimethyl 2,2-dichlorovinyl phosphate; 2,2-dichloroethenyl dimethyl phosphate; phosphoric acid, 2,2-dichlorovinyl dimethyl ester

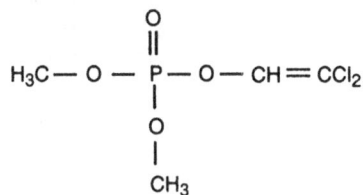

$$H_3C - O - \overset{\displaystyle O}{\underset{\displaystyle \underset{\displaystyle CH_3}{|}}{\overset{\displaystyle ||}{P}}} - O - CH = CCl_2$$

C$_4$H$_7$Cl$_2$O$_4$P   Mol. wt: 221.0

1.1.2 *Chemical and physical properties*

From AMVAC Chemical Corp. (1986), otherwise specified
(a) *Description*: Clear, colourless to pale yellow, almost odourless liquid
(b) *Boiling-point*: 117°C at 10 mm Hg [1.33 kPa]
(c) *Melting-point*: < -60°C (AMVAC Chemical Corp., 1990)
(d) *Density*: 1.422 at 25°C/4°C
(e) *Spectroscopy data*: Infrared (prism [7721]; grating [44551P]) spectroscopy data have been reported (Sadtler Research Laboratories, 1980).

(f) *Solubility*: Completely miscible with aromatic hydrocarbons, chlorinated hydro-carbons, alcohols, ketones and esters; slightly soluble in water (approx. 1%) and glycerine (approx. 0.5%); insoluble in kerosene and aliphatic hydrocarbons

(g) *Volatility*: Vapour pressure, 0.012 mm Hg [1.6×10^{-3} kPa] at 20°C

(h) *Stability*: Hydrolysed by water and readily decomposed by strong acids and bases; breaks down on standing in the presence of traces of moisture, with the formation of acidic products that catalyse further decomposition; corrosive to black iron and mild steel (WHO, 1989)

(i) *Octanol/water partition coefficient (P)*: log P, 1.47 (WHO, 1989)

(j) *Half-time in water*: 301 min at pH 8; 462 min at pH 7; 2100 min at pH 6; 4620 min at pH 5.4 (Latif *et al.*, 1984)

(k) *Conversion factor for airborne concentrations*[1]: mg/m^3 = 9.04 $\times$ ppm

1.1.3 *Trade names, technical products and impurities*

Some examples of trade names are: Atgard; Bibesol; Brevinyl; Canogard; Chlorvinphos; DDVP; Dedevap; Des; Dichlofos; Dichlorman; Dichlorovos; Divipan; ENT 20738; Equigard; Equigel; Estrosel; Estrosol; Fecama; Fekama; Insectigas D; Mopari; Nefrafos; Nerkol; Nogos; Novotox; Nuan; Nuvan; OKO; OMS 14; Panaplate; Phosvit; Prima U; SD 1750; Szklarniak; TAP 9VP; Task; Unifos; Unitox; Vapona; Vapona Insecticide; Vaponite; Vinylofos; Vinylophos; Winylophos

WHO (1985, 1989) specifications for technical-grade dichlorvos for public health use require a minimum purity of 97%; the value was previously 93% (WHO, 1967).

Dichlorvos is available in the USA as a technical-grade product with a minimal purity of 93 or 96% (AMVAC Chemical Corp., 1986, 1990). In the past, 2-4% epichlorohydrin (see IARC, 1987a) was added to stabilize the technical-grade product; other stabilizers may now be used in some products, but improved technology and purity has largely eliminated the need for them (WHO, 1989). Analysis of a sample of commercial-grade dichlorvos (produced in about 1970) showed the following constituents (%): dichlorvos, 95-97; dipterex (trichlorfon; *0,0*-dimethyl 2,2,2-trichloro-1-hydroxyethylphosphonate) (see IARC, 1983a, 1987b), 1.5-3; *O,O*-dimethyl 2-chlorovinyl phosphate, 0.4-0.7; *O,O*-dimethyl methyl-phosphate, trace-0.1; *O,O,O*-trimethyl phosphate, 0.3-0.8; and chloral (trichloro-acetaldehyde), 0.1-0.5 (Santodonato *et al.*, 1985).

In the USA and Europe, registered formulations include dusts, granules, pellets/tablets, impregnated resin strips, emulsifiable concentrates, soluble concentrates, wettable powders and pressurized formulations (Royal Society of Chemistry, 1986; US Environmental Protection Agency, 1987). In the USSR, dichlorvos is formulated as emulsion concentrates, pellets and aerosols (Izmerov, 1984). Dichlorvos is also formulated in combination with dimethoate, dinocap, fenchlorphos, fenitrothion, iodofenphos, lindane (see IARC, 1987c), malathion (see IARC, 1983b, 1987d), methoxychlor (see IARC, 1979b, 1987e), phosalone,

---

[1]Calculated from: mg/m^3 = (molecular weight/24.45) $\times$ ppm, assuming standard temperature (25°C) and pressure (760 mm Hg [101.3 kPa])

piperonyl butoxide (see IARC, 1983c, 1987f), pirimiphos-methyl, propoxur, tetrasul, pyrethrins and trichlorfon (Royal Society of Chemistry, 1986).

1.1.4 *Analysis*

Selected methods for the analysis of dichlorvos in various matrices are given in Table 1. Dichlorvos residues can be determined by gas chromatography; the same method can be used for product analysis. Alternative methods include infrared spectrometry and reaction with excess iodine, with estimation by titration (WHO, 1989). Several other methods in various media have been reviewed (Porter, 1964; Anon., 1972; Vevai, 1974; Worthing & Walker, 1987; WHO, 1989).

Table 1. Methods for the analysis of dichlorvos

Sample matrix	Sample preparation	Assay procedure[a]	Limit of detection	Reference
Air	Collect vapours on polyurethane foam; extract with 5% diethyl ether in hexane	GC/ECD	Not reported	US Environmental Protection Agency (1988a)
	Adsorb on XAD-2; desorb with toluene	GC/FPD	0.2 µg/sample	US National Institute for Occupational Safety and Health (1979)
Water	Extract with dichloromethane; isolate extract; dry; concentrate with methyl *tert*-butyl ether	GC/NPD	2.5 µg/l	US Environmental Protection Agency (1988b)
Groundwater, soil, wastes	Extract with dichloromethane; dry; concentrate; clean-up using Florisil column or gel permeation; exchange into hexane	GC/MS	0.1 µg/l	US Environmental Protection Agency (1986)
Formulations	Dissolve in chloroform; concentrate using evaporation (baits & emulsifiable concentrate forms)	IR	Not reported	Williams (1984)
	Extract with sodium hydroxide; dry using anhydrous sodium sulfate (spray solutions & sprays in hydrocarbon solvents)	IR	Not reported	Williams (1984)
Fruits and vegetables	Acidify with hydrochloric acid; extract with hexane; clean-up on silicic acid column	GC/MCD	0.05 ppm (mg/kg)	US Food and Drug Administration (1989a)
Animal tissues, crops, milk	Acidify with hydrochloric acid; extract with hexane; clean-up with anhydrous sodium sulfate	GC/TD or GC/ECD[b]	0.01-0.02 ppm (mg/l or mg/kg) (milk & tissues)	US Food and Drug Administration (1989a)

Table 1 (contd)

Sample matrix	Sample preparation	Assay procedure[a]	Limit of detection	Reference
Animal tissues, crops, eggs, milk	Extract into hexane; clean-up on silicic acid column with dichloro-methane:hexane (3:2) eluant	GC/FPD	0.002 ppm (mg/l milk)	US Food and Drug Administration (1989b)

[a]Abbreviations: GC/ECD, gas chromatography/electron capture detection; GC/FPD, gas chromatography/ flame photometric detection; GC/MS, gas chromatography/mass spectrometry; GC/NPD, gas chromatography/nitrogen-phosphorus detection; GC/MCD, gas chromatography/microcoulometric detection; GC/TD, gas chromatography/thermionic detection; IR, infrared spectrophotometry
[b]Used if interfering organophosphorus or organochlorine pesticides are present

1.2 Production and use

1.2.1 *Production*

Dichlorvos was first synthesized in the late 1940s (Tinker, 1972). It has been commercially manufactured and used throughout the world since 1961 (WHO, 1989). It was first found as a highly insecticidal impurity of trichlorfon (chlorophos) in 1955; trichlorfon is rapidly converted to dichlorvos at above pH 6 (Eto, 1974). Dichlorvos is manufactured by the dehydrochlorination of trichlorfon in aqueous alkali at 40-50 °C or by the reaction between chloral and trimethyl phosphite (WHO, 1989).

Dichlorvos is produced currently in Argentina, Brazil, Germany, India, Israel, Japan, the Republic of Korea, Mexico, the Netherlands, Spain, Sweden, Switzerland and the USA (Meister, 1990). The present worldwide production of dichlorvos is about 4000 tonnes per year (WHO, 1989). Worldwide production figures for 1984 were as follows (tonnes): eastern Europe, 220; western Europe, 300; Latin America, 400; south-east Asia, 500; USA, 500; Japan, 1100; Middle East, India and Pakistan, 1200 (WHO, 1989).

1.2.2 *Use*

Dichlorvos is a contact and stomach insecticide with fumigant and penetrant action. It is used as granules or impregnated resin to control internal and external parasites (especially fleas and ticks) in livestock and as aerosols or liquid sprays or as impregnated cellulose, ceramic or resin strips to control insects in houses, buildings and outdoor areas (especially flies and mosquitos). It is also used to protect certain crops (and other plants) from insects in the field and in storage. Dichlorvos is not generally applied directly to soil, but it is added to water to control parasites in the case of intensive fish farming (WHO, 1989). It is used as an antihelminthic by incorporation in animal feeds (Worthing & Walker, 1987).

Worldwide, it is estimated that 60% is used in plant protection, 30% for public health and vector control and 10% to protect stored products (WHO, 1989).

In the USA, in 1971, 16 tonnes of dichlorvos were used on crops (mainly tobacco) and 1100 tonnes were used on livestock and livestock buildings; in 1976, 50 tonnes were used on crops and 390 on livestock. In 1975, 80% of the dichlorvos produced in the USA was formulated into polyvinyl chloride resin strips containing 20% by weight of dichlorvos, which were used primarily in households. These strips were first marketed in 1967 to control flies and mosquitoes in the home; they were introduced earlier in dairy and poultry operations. Flea collars containing dichlorvos, for dogs and cats, have also been commercially marketed (Santodonato et al., 1985).

In the USA in 1980, the yearly agricultural usage of dichlorvos (active ingredient) was estimated as follows (tonnes): dairy cattle, 340; beef cattle, 30; hogs, 6; poultry, 2; and other livestock, 14; about 50 tonnes were used for treatment of tobacco. Overall, 680-1200 tonnes of dichlorvos were used for agricultural uses, 450 tonnes for public health and about 450 tonnes for household use (US Environmental Protection Agency, 1980). Less than 450 tonnes of dichlorvos (active ingredient) are believed to have been used in the USA in 1989.

In Finland, about 1500 kg (active ingredient) of dichlorvos were sold in 1988 (Agrochemical Producers' Association of Finland, 1989).

1.3 Occurrence

1.3.1 Air

Dichlorvos is degraded rapidly in air, the rate depending on humidity. The method of application is an important factor in determining its concentration in air (Gillett et al., 1972a).

Examples of indoor air concentrations resulting from household and public health use are shown in Table 2 (WHO, 1989).

The highest exposure recorded in a vaporizer production plant and its packaging rooms was 3 mg/m^3, with an average value of 0.7 mg/m^3 (Menz et al., 1974). The mean concentration of dichlorvos in air did not exceed 0.5 ppb (0.005 mg/m^3) in the office and insecticide storage rooms of commercial pest control buildings and 0.1 ppb (0.001 mg/m^3) in vehicles (Wright & Leidy, 1980).

Dichlorvos was sprayed at 8 ml active ingredient/100 m^3 in a unit used for mushroom cultures, and kept closed for 24 h. The air concentration decreased from 3.3 to 0.006 mg/m^3 in 24 h. The unit was also treated with paper strips drenched in 50% dichlorvos formulations (40 ml/100 m^3), which gave air concentrations of 0.38 and 0.024 mg/m^3 at 3 and 24 h, respectively (Grübner, 1972).

Following weekly 6-h applications, the maximum concentrations of dichlorvos observed in a large warehouse ranged from 2.4 to 7 mg/m^3. The amount of dichlorvos dispensed per application was 25-59 mg/m^3, which resulted in average air concentrations after eight applications of 4 mg/m^3 (Gillenwater et al., 1971).

The work place concentration resulting from hot spraying of dichlorvos in six greenhouses at 0.4 ml/m^3 was 7-24 mg/m^3 (average, 16 mg/m^3) (Wagner & Hoyer, 1975). Spraying of 12 glass and plastic greenhouses gave concentrations between 0.7 and 2.7 mg/m^3 (average, 1.3 mg/m^3). Field application by spraying resulted in air concentrations of 0.01-0.26 mg/m^3 (average, 0.08 mg/m^3) (as reported by WHO, 1989). The air concentration of dichlorvos in greenhouses immediately after spraying with 0.2-0.3% dichlorvos solutions was 1.2 mg/m^3, which decreased to 0.01 mg/m^3 within 24 h. Disturbing the plants resulted in an increase of 10-26% in the dichlorvos concentration in air (Zotov et al., 1977).

In a study designed to test the aeration period needed for safe reentry into a room following dichlorvos treatment with a pressurized home-fogger, the air levels after 30 min

Table 2. Indoor air concentrations of dichlorvos following various applications[a]

Location	Application	Dose[b]	Temperature (°)	RH[c] (%)	Ventilation	Time after application	Concentration (mg/m³)
Food shops	Resin strips	1 strip/30 m³			Normal	First week	0.03
						4 weeks	0.02
						10 weeks	0.01
Houses	Resin strips	1 strip/30 m³	18–35	20–60	Normal	First week	0.06–0.17
						2–3 weeks	0.01
Hospital wards	Resin strips	1 strip/30 m³	20–27	35–70	Varied	Several days	0.10–0.28
						20–30 days	0.02
Hospital wards	Strips of paper drenched in 50% dichlorvos solution hanging in rooms for 24–36 h	0.2 ml ai/m³	–	–	2 h	3 days	0.06
		0.2 ml ai/m³	17	–	2 h	66 h	0.1–0.3
		0.2 ml ai/m³	17	–	2 h	90 h	0.3
		0.8 ml ai/m³	30	High	2 h	3 h	3.7
						46 h	0.6
Houses	0.5% solution according to typical pest control practice	225 or 1200 ml	26	47–60	None	0	0.4
						8 h	0.2
						24 h	<0.1
Bathroom (sealed)	0.5% solution wall spray	25 ml	26	60	None	0	1.1
						4 h	0.3
						24 h	<0.1
Living room (experimental)	Spray cans	2.3 mg ai/m³	20–22		30 min	0	0.24
					1 h	0	0.13
	Fogging	240 mg ai/m³	20–22		None	1 h	37
					None	24 h	5.5
					1 h	1 h	2.5
					120 h	1 h	<0.2
Apartments[d]	0.5% solution	190 mg ai/m³	26	82	–	0–2 h	0.5
						2–24 h	0.2

[a]Reviewed by WHO (1989)
[b]ai, active ingredient
[c]RH, relative humidity
[d]From Gold et al. (1984)
–, not stated

were below the industrial workplace permissible exposure level of 1 mg/m^3. Without ventilation, 18 h were required to reach an acceptable level. Because of concern for the health of infants and elderly persons, the acceptable level for homes was established at 1/40 of the permissible exposure level. Rooms treated with this type of applicator and ventilated after treatment were considered safe for reentry after 10 h (as reported by WHO, 1989).

Monitoring of mushroom-growing houses in the USA gave air concentrations of 0.1 mg/m^3; swabs of exposed surfaces revealed maximal residues of 0.026 μg/cm^2 (as reported by WHO, 1989).

In houses treated for pest control with 230-330 g dichlorvos as an aerosol and 40-50 g as emulsion spray, the mean dichlorvos residue on surfaces was 0.24 μg/cm^2 at the end of day 1 and decreased to 0.06 μg/cm^2 by day 5 (Das et al., (1983).

1.3.2 Water

In water, dichlorvos is hydrolysed into dimethyl phosphoric acid and dichloroacetic acid (WHO, 1989).

1.3.3 Soil

Dichlorvos vaporized in a mushroom house to give 0.2-0.4 mg/m^3 degraded rapidly in the moist loam soil, with only 37% remaining after 3 days. The amount of free dichloroacetaldehyde at that time was 4% (Hussey & Hughes, 1964).

Dichlorvos is degraded by microorganisms. Bacillus cereus utilizes it as a single carbon source. In soil columns perfused with an aqueous solution containing dichlorvos at 1 kg/litre, 30% of the loss of the compound was attributed to microbial action (Lamoreaux & Newland, 1978). Species of Pseudomonas derived from sewage converted dichlorvos to dichloro-ethanol, dichloroacetic acid and ethyl dichloroacetate (Lieberman & Alexander, 1983). Fungi, such as Trichoderma viride, also degrade dichlorvos into water-soluble metabolites (Matsumura & Boush, 1968).

1.3.4 Plants

Dichlorvos is rapidly lost from leaf surfaces by volatilization and hydrolysis, with a half-time of only a few hours. A small amount penetrates the waxy layers of plant tissues, where it may persist for longer (FAO/WHO, 1971).

In California, the estimated safe level of dislodgeable foliar dichlorvos from turf is 0.06 μg/cm^2 (WHO, 1989). Studies by Goh et al. (1986a,b) found that dislodgeable foliar dichlorvos residues decreased rapidly after 2-6 h and were not detectable after 24-48 h.

1.3.5 Food

Data on residues in food commodities resulting from pre- and post-harvest treatment and from use on animals were summarized by FAO/WHO (1967, 1968, 1971, 1975).

In Canada, of 262 bovine and porcine fat samples analysed between 1973 and 1981, only one was contaminated with dichlorvos (Frank et al., 1983). In a national surveillence programme in Canada, 1984-85 to 1988-89, no residue was found in 898 samples of fruit, vegetables, meat or wine (Government of Canada, 1990).

Normally, dichlorvos residues present in food are destroyed by washing and cooking. Abbott et al. (1970) confirmed the absence of residues in a total-diet study in the United

Kingdom, 1966-67, finding no dichlorvos in 462 samples. A total-diet study carried out in the USA from 1975 to 1976 gave similar results (Johnson *et al.*, 1981).

Food, meals and unwrapped ready-to-eat foodstuffs exposed to dichlorvos from resin strips had mean residue levels of < 0.05 mg/kg (range, < 0.01-0.1 mg/kg) (Elgar *et al.*, 1972a,b) and < 0.02 mg/kg (Collins & deVries, 1973). No residue of dichloroacetaldehyde (< 0.03 mg/kg) was detected in the ready-to-eat foodstuffs (Elgar *et al.*, 1972b). Food and beverages exposed to air concentrations of 0.04-0.58 mg/m^3 for 30 min contained dichlorvos residues of 0.005-0.5 mg/kg, except for margarine which had up to 1.7 mg/kg (Dale *et al.*, 1973).

1.3.6 *Occupational exposure*

Mixed dermal and inhalation exposures were assessed for 13 professional pesticide applicators after a day's work spraying dichlorvos preparations. Absorbent pads recorded average exposures of 0.08 µg/cm^2 on the back and 0.04 µg/cm^2 on the chest. Levels found in respirator filters were 1.1 µg/cm^2, in contrast to surface residues of 0.04-0.5 µg/cm^2 measured at various sites around the treated houses. Although the men wore protective equipment, some absorption of dichlorvos occurred, as shown by the recovery of 0.32-1.4 µg dimethylphosphate from their urine (Das *et al.*, 1983).

1.4 Regulations and guidelines

The FAO/WHO Joint Meeting on Pesticide Residues evaluated dichlorvos at its meetings in 1965, 1966, 1967, 1969, 1970, 1974 and 1977 (FAO/WHO, 1965, 1967, 1968, 1970, 1971, 1975, 1978). In 1966, the Meeting established an acceptable daily intake for humans of 0.004 mg/kg bw (FAO/WHO, 1967).

Maximum residue levels have been established by the Codex Alimentarius Commission for dichlorvos in or on the following agricultural commodities (in mg/kg): fruit (e.g., apples, peaches, pears, strawberries), 0.1; mushrooms and vegetables (except lettuce), 0.5; head lettuce, 1; cereal grains, coffee beans, dried lentils, dried soya beans and peanuts, 2; and cacao beans, 5. As such residues decline rapidly during storage and shipment, these limits are based on residues likely to be found at harvest (Codex Committee on Pesticide Residues, 1990).

Maximum residue limits have also been established by the Codex Alimentarius Commission for dichlorvos in or on the following animal commodities (in mg/kg): milk, 0.02; eggs, goat meat, meat of cattle, pigs, sheep and poultry, 0.05, based on residues likely to be found at slaughter (Codex Committee on Pesticide Residues, 1990).

In the USSR, dichlorvos residues are not allowed in fishing areas; however, a level of 0.1 mg/l was established for other surface waters (Izmerov, 1984).

National and regional pesticide residue limits for dichlorvos in foods are presented in Table 3.

Table 3. National and regional pesticide residue limits for dichlorvos in foods[a]

Country or region	Residue limit (mg/kg)	Commodities
Argentina	2	Stored cereals in general
Australia	5	Cocoa beans
	2	Cereal grains, coffee beans (green), lentils, nuts, peanuts, soya beans
	1	Lettuce
	0.5	Mushrooms, tomatoes, vegetables (except lettuce)
	0.1	All foods for which no other maximum residue limit is specified (e.g., bread, cakes, cooked meats), fruit
	0.05	Eggs, meat, poultry
	0.02	Whole milk
Austria	2.0	Cereals
	0.1	Other foods of vegetable origin
	0.05	Eggs (without shell), meat, milk
Belgium	5	Cocoa beans
	2	Coffee beans, grains, leguminous vegetables (dried)
	0.5	Flour
	0.1	Fruit, vegetables
	0.05	Animal fats, fowl, game, hare, meat, meat products, poultry
	0.02	Milk and dairy products
	0 (0.02)[b]	Other foodstuffs of animal and vegetable origin
Brazil	5.0	Cocoa
	2.0	Barley, maize, coffee, cottonseed, peanuts, rice, rye, soya beans, wheat
	1.0	Lettuce, ornamental plants, tobacco
	0.5	Chick peas, eggs (without shell), field beans, onions, potatoes, vegetables (except lettuce)
	0.1	Apples, bran, Brazil nuts, cakes, citrus fruits, flour, mushrooms, piñon seed, strawberries, watermelon
	0.05	Meat and meat products, poultry
	0.02	Milk
Canada	2.0	Non-perishable packaged foods of high fat content (> 6%)
	0.5	Non-perishable packaged foods of low fat content (< 6%)
	0.25	Tomatoes
	Negligible	Beef and dairy cattle (meat and milk), foods exposed in food storage areas, homes and restaurants to dichlorvos generated from 20% resin strips
Chile	2.0	Lentils, raw cereals
	1.0	Lettuce
	0.5	Cereal products, garden vegetables (except lettuce)
	0.1	Fruits
	0.05	Eggs, carcasses, poultry
	0.02	Whole milk
China	0.2	Vegetables
	0.1	Grain
	None	Vegetable oils

Table 3 (contd)

Country or region	Residue limit (mg/kg)	Commodities
Czechoslovakia	2.0	Imported lentils, peanuts, raw cereals, soya beans, unroasted coffee
	1.0	Imported head lettuce
	0.5	Imported mill products, mushrooms, tomatoes
	0.2	Dried medicinal herbs (for preservation)
	0.1	Foodstuffs in general (for preservation), fruits, vegetables
	0.1	Imported fruits, various foodstuffs
	0.02	Imported eggs (without shell), milk
Denmark	2	Cereals
	1	Leafy vegetables
	0.5	Mushrooms
	0.1	Berries and small fruits, citrus fruits, other fruits, pome and stone fruits
European Community	2.0	Barley, buckwheat, grain sorghum, maize, millet, oats, other cereals, paddy rice, rye, triticale, wheat
	0.1	Other products
Finland	1.0	Cereal grains
	0.2	Flour
	0.1	Fruit, vegetables
France	2	Wheat
	0.1	Fruits, vegetables
Germany	2.0	Cereals
	0.5	Cereal products
	0.1	Other foods of plant origin
Hungary	2.0	Barley grain, maize, oat grain, rice (brown, polished), rye, sorghum, triticale, wheat grain
	1.0	Greenhouse lettuce, lettuce
	0.5	Beetroot, Brussels' sprouts, cabbage, carrots, cauliflower, celery, celery leaf, garlic, green beans, greenhouse cucumber, greenhouse green paprika, greenhouse tomatoes, horseradish, kohlrabi, mushrooms, paprika, peas, parsley, parsley root, radishes, red onion, savoy, sorrel, spinach
	0.2	Apples, apricots, cherries, grapes, greengages, peaches, pears, plums, quince, sour cherries, wine grapes
India	1.0	Food grains
	0.25	Milled food grains
	0.15	Vegetables
	0.1	Fruit
Ireland	1.0	Lettuce
	0.5	Mushrooms, other vegetables
	0.1	Other products

Table 3 (contd)

Country or region	Residue limit (mg/kg)	Commodities
Israel	5.0	Cocoa beans
	2.0	Coffee beans, raw cereals (e.g., barley, maize, oats, rice, sorghum, wheat), lentils, peanuts, soya beans
	1.0	Lettuce
	0.5	Milled products from raw grain, mushrooms, vegetables (except lettuce), tomatoes
	0.1	Fruit (e.g., apples, peaches, pears, strawberries), miscellaneous food items not otherwise specified that were treated with dichlorvos in warehouses, shops, etc. (e.g., bread, cakes, cheese, cooked meat)
	0.05	Eggs (without shell), meat of cattle, goats, sheep, pigs and poultry
	0.02	Milk
Italy	2.0	Cereals in bulk
	0.5	Milled products (from treated cereals)
	0.1	Fruits, garden vegetables, sugar beets
Japan	0.3[c]	Strawberries
	0.1	Asparagus, celery, eggplants, garden radishes, garden radish leaves, grapes, Japanese pears, Spanish paprika, spinach, stone leeks
	0.1[c]	Fruit (except strawberries); rice, oats and other minor cereals; potatoes, tea, vegetables
Kenya	5.0	Cocoa beans
	2.0	Coffee beans, lentils, peanuts, raw grain (e.g., barley, maize, oats, rice, rye, sorghum, wheat), soya beans
	1.0	Lettuce
	0.5	Fresh vegetables (except lettuce), milled products from raw grain, mushrooms, tomatoes
	0.1	
	0.05	Fresh fruit (e.g., apples, peaches, pears, strawberries), miscellaneous food items not otherwise specified
	0.02	Eggs (without shell), meat of cattle, goats, pigs, poultry and sheep Milk (whole)
Netherlands	5	Cocoa beans
	2	Buckwheat cereal, coffee beans, peanuts, pod vegetables, pulses
	0.5	Whole meal flour
	0.1	Fruit, other vegetables
	0.05	Eggs, meat, poultry meat
	0.02[d]	Milk
	0 (0.02)[e]	Other crops and foodstuffs
New Zealand	2.0	Cereals, fruit, vegetables
Peru	5.0	Cocoa beans
	2.0	Coffee beans, grain cereals, grain lentils, grain soya, peanuts
	1.0	Lettuce
	0.5	Edible mushrooms, tomatoes, vegetables (except lettuce)
	0.3	Cereal products (ground, for human consumption)
	0.1	Bread, cakes, cheese, cooked meat, fruits (except citrus)
	0.05	Eggs (without shell), meat of cattle, goats, hogs, poultry, sheep
	0.02	Whole milk
Romania	0.05	Eggs (without shell), meat
	0.02	Whole milk

Table 3 (contd)

Country or region	Residue limit (mg/kg)	Commodities
Singapore	0.5	Fruit, grains, vegetables
South Africa	0.1	Bananas, beans, cherries, cruciferae, grapes, lettuce, tomatoes, wheat
	0.05	Carcass meat (on the rendered or extracted carcass fat), eggs (without shell)
	0.02	Milk (on a fat basis)
Spain	2.0	Cereal grains
	0.1	Other plant products
Sweden	2.0	Cereals
	0.5[f]	Flakes and flour made from cereals, hulled grain
	0.1[f]	Fruit (fresh and dried, fresh and deep-frozen berries), vegetables (green and root)
	0.1	Butter, cheese
	0.05	Raw meat, eggs
	0.02	Milk
Switzerland	2.0	Cereals, cocoa beans
	0.3	Cereal products, vegetables (canned, fresh, frozen)
	0.1	Citrus fruit, fruit, other foodstuffs
	0.01	Milk
Taiwan	0.5	Fruit, vegetables, leafy vegetables with large wrapper leaves, leafy vegetables with small leaves, melon, mushrooms, peas, snap beans
	0.1	Root vegetables
United Kingdom	2	Barley, maize, oats, other cereals, paddy rice, rye, wheat
	1	Lettuce
	0.5	Beans, Brussels' sprouts, cabbage, carrots, cauliflower, celery, cucumbers, leeks, lettuce, mushrooms, onions, peas, potatoes, swedes, tomatoes, turnips
	0.1	Apples, bananas, blackcurrants, citrus, grapes, nectarines, peaches, pears, plums, raspberries, strawberries
	0.05	Eggs (birds' eggs in shell (other than eggs for hatching) and whole egg products and egg yolk products (whether fresh, dried or otherwise prepared)), meat, fat and preparations of meat, milk
	0.02	Milk (fresh raw cows' milk and fresh whole-cream cows' milk expressed as whole milk)
USA[g]	2.0	Raw agricultural commodities (nonperishable, packaged or bagged, containing more than 6% fat (post-harvest))
	1.0	Lettuce[h]
	0.5	Cucumbers[h], dried figs, mushrooms[h] and tomatoes (pre- and post-harvest)[h]; radishes, raw agricultural commodities (nonperishable, bulk stored regardless of fat content (post-harvest)); raw agricultural commodities (nonperishable, packaged or bagged, containing 6% fat or less (post-harvest))
	0.1	Figs
	0.1 (negligible)	Edible tissue of swine
	0.05 (negligible)	Eggs and poultry (fat, meat, and meat by-products)
	0.02 (negligible)	Cattle, goats, horses, sheep (fat, meat and meat by-products), milk

Table 3 (contd)

Country or region	Residue limit (mg/kg)	Commodities
USSR	0.3	Bran, grain
	0.05	Apples, grapes
	Not permitted	Flour, grouts
Yugoslavia	2.0	Cereals
	0.3	Processed cereals, vegetables
	0.1	Other foodstuffs

[a]From Health and Welfare Canada (1990)
[b]Residues should not be present; the value in parentheses indicates the lower limit for residue determination according to the standard method of analysis, this limit having been used to reach the no-residue conclusion.
[c]Standard for withholding registration of agricultural chemicals
[d]A pesticide may be used on an eating or drinking ware or raw material without a demonstrable residue remaining; the value listed is considered the highest concentration at which this requirement is deemed to have been met.
[e]Residues shall be absent; the value in parentheses is the highest concentration at which this requirement is still deemed to have been met.
[f]If analysis shows that two or more of certain substances are present in the same sample, in addition to the limit which applies for each substance, a maximum level of 1.0 mg/kg applies to the sum of the residues of these substances.
[g]From US Environmental Protection Agency (1989a,b)
[h]Residues expressed as naled

Occupational exposure limits and guidelines for dichlorvos in some countries and regions are given in Table 4.

Table 4. Occupational exposure limits and guidelines for dichlorvos[a]

Country or region	Year	Concentration[b] (mg/m^3)	Interpretation[c]
Austria	1987	1	TWA
Belgium	1987	1	TWA
China	1987	0.3	TWA
Denmark	1987	1	TWA
Finland	1987	1	TWA
		3	STEL
Germany	1989	1	TWA
Hungary	1987	0.2	TWA
		0.2	STEL
India	1987	1	TWA
		3	STEL
Indonesia	1987	1	TWA
Mexico	1987	1.5	TWA
Netherlands	1987	1	TWA

Table 4 (contd)

Country or region	Year	Concentration[b] (mg/m³)	Interpretation[c]
Romania	1987	0.5	TWA
		1.5	STEL
Switzerland	1987	1	TWA
Taiwan	1987	1	TWA
United Kingdom	1987	1	TWA
		3	STEL
URSS	1987	0.2	TWA
USA			
ACGIH		0.9	Guideline
OSHA		1	TWA
Venezuela	1987	1	TWA
		3	Ceiling
Yugoslavia	1987	0.1	TWA

[a]From Izmerov (1984); Cook (1987); American Conference of Governmental Industrial Hygienists (ACGIH) (1989); Deutsche Forschungsgemeinschaft (1989); US Occupational Safety and Health Administration (OSHA) (1989)
[b]All values given are with skin notation
[c]TWA, time-weighted average; STEL, short-term exposure limit

2. Studies of Cancer in Humans

2.1 Case reports

In a case series, four children with aplastic anaemia and one with acute lymphoblastic leukaemia were reported by their parents to have been exposed at home to dichlorvos and propoxur (Reeves *et al.*, 1981).

2.2 Case-control studies

In a case-control study of leukaemia in the USA (Brown *et al.*, 1990), described in detail in the monograph on occupational exposure in spraying and application of insecticides (p. 68), significant excesses of leukaemia were noted among farmers who reported use of dichlorvos on animals (odds ratio, 2.0; 95% confidence interval [CI], 1.2-3.5). Risks were greater among those who had first used dichlorvos 20 or more years before diagnosis of leukaemia (odds ratio, 2.4; 95% CI, 1.1-5.4). The risks were greatest among farmers who used dichlorvos on animals on 10 or more days per year (odds ratio, 3.8; 95% CI, 1.0-14.8). The risk for leukaemia in this study was also associated with use of other agricultural pesticides, including crotoxyphos, famphur, pyrethrins, methoxychlor, nicotine and DDT, and it was not possible to evaluate exposure to dichlorvos in the absence of these other pesticides.

3. Studies of Cancer in Experimental Animals

The Working Group was aware of a study by Horn *et al.* (1987), which was of short duration and not considered informative for an evaluation.

3.1 Oral administration

3.1.1 *Mouse*

Groups of 50 male and 50 female B6C3F$_1$ hybrid mice, five to seven weeks of age, were fed technical-grade dichlorvos (minimum purity, 94%) in the diet at initial doses of 1000 and 2000 mg/kg. After two weeks, the doses were reduced to 300 and 600 mg/kg of diet, respectively, due to severe toxicity, and treated animals were maintained at these dietary levels for 78 weeks followed by 12-14 weeks on dichlorvos-free diets, after which time (92-94 weeks) the animals were killed and necropsied. The measured time-weighted average doses were 318 and 635 mg/kg of diet, respectively. Groups of 10 male and 10 female mice that served as matched controls were maintained on dichlorvos-free diets for 92 weeks; further control data were obtained from pooled control animals (100 males and 80 females). In females, 13/50 low-dose animals died before week 90; survival to 90 weeks was greater than 84% in all other groups. Average weights of high-dose males and females were generally lower than those of the low-dose and control groups, but the differences did not exceed 10%. The only findings of note were two squamous-cell carcinomas of the oesophagus (in one low-dose male and one high-dose female), one papilloma of the oesophagus (in a high-dose female) and three cases of focal hyperplasia of the oesophageal epithelium (in three low-dose males) (US National Cancer Institute, 1977). [The Working Group noted the short duration of treatment.]

Groups of 50 male and 50 female B6C3F$_1$ mice, eight weeks of age, were administered 0, 10 or 20 (males) and 0, 20 or 40 mg/kg bw (females) dichlorvos (99% pure) in corn oil by gavage per day on five days per week for 103 weeks. Survival was not affected by treatment. The incidence of squamous-cell papillomas of the forestomach was increased in males and females. A significant dose-response trend for the incidence of squamous-cell papillomas was seen in males (1/50 control, 1/50 low-dose, 5/50 high-dose; $p = 0.032$) and in females (5/49 control, 6/49 low-dose, 18/50 high-dose; $p = 0.002$). In females, the incidence in the high-dose group was significantly greater than that in controls ($p = 0.004$). Two of 50 high-dose females also had squamous-cell carcinomas (US National Toxicology Program, 1989).

3.1.2 *Rat*

Groups of 50 male and 50 female Osborne-Mendel rats, five to seven weeks of age, were fed diets containing 150 or 1000 mg/kg of diet technical-grade dichlorvos (minimum purity, 94%); due to severe toxicity, the high-dose was reduced to 300 mg/kg of diet after three weeks. Both groups were treated for 80 weeks and were maintained for a further 30 weeks on a dichlorvos-free diet. Time-weighted average doses were 150 and 326 mg/kg of diet, respectively. Groups of 10 males and 10 females served as matched controls and groups of 60 animals of each sex as pooled controls. Weight gain was consistently lower in high-dose groups than in low-dose and control groups. No significant difference in survival was observed between treated and control groups at 105 weeks. The incidence of malignant fibrous histiocytomas in male rats showed a statistically significant trend (pooled control, 2/58; low-dose, 4/48; high-dose, 8/50; $p = 0.018$); a histiocytoma occurred in 1/10 matched male controls (US National Cancer Institute, 1977). [The Working Group noted the short duration of treatment].

Technical-grade dichlorvos (97% purity) was administered by gavage in water to 70 male and 70 female rats (inbred strain BD IX/Bln), six to eight weeks of age, at a dose of 0.1 mg per animal twice a week; or to 99 male and 99 female rats at a dose of 0.1 mg per animal three times a week for 60 weeks. Groups of 59 male and 60 female rats served as vehicle controls. Animals were killed 111 weeks after the beginning of treatment. There was no difference in median survival times between treated and control animals. Forestomach papillomas were observed in two males and in one female that received 0.3 mg dichlorvos. One male and one female rat receiving 0.3 mg had two and five papillomas of the urinary bladder, respectively (Horn et al., 1988). [The Working Group noted the short duration of exposure.]

Groups of 50 male and 50 female Fischer 344/N rats, seven weeks of age, were administered 0, 4 or 8 mg/kg bw dichlorvos (99% pure) per day in corn oil by gavage on five days per week for 103 weeks. Survival was 31/50 control, 25/50 low-dose and 24/50 high-dose males and 31/50 control, 26/50 low-dose and 24/50 high-dose females; body weight gain was not affected by administration of dichlorvos. The incidence of acinar-cell adenomas of the pancreas was increased in treated males (16/50 control, 25/49 low-dose and 30/50 high-dose; $p < 0.001$ for trend). Further examination of horizontal sections of all pancreases revealed increases of reduced statistical significance (25/50, 30/50 and 33/50; [p for trend = < 0.05]). There were also more male rats with multiple adenomas in the treated groups than among controls (2/50, 7/49 and 13/50). Mononuclear-cell leukaemia occurred with a significant dose-response trend in male rats ($p = 0.011$), and the incidence in each of the treated groups was significantly greater than that in controls (11/50 control, 20/50 low-dose and 21/50 high-dose males). In females, fibroadenomas and adenomas of the mammary gland occurred with a significant dose-response trend ($p = 0.028$), and the incidence in both treated groups was significantly greater than that in controls (9/50 control, 19/50 low-dose and 17/50 high-dose females). Two female rats in the control group and two in the low-dose group had carcinomas of the mammary gland (US National Toxicology Program, 1989).

3.2 Inhalation and/or intratracheal administration

Rat: Groups of 50 male and 50 female Carworth Farm E strain rats, five weeks of age, were exposed continuously to atmospheres containing 0 (control), 0.05, 0.5 or 5 mg/m^3 technical-grade dichlorvos (purity, > 97%) for 104 weeks. The mean values for the entire test period were 0.05, 0.48 and 4.7 mg/m^3 [range ± 20%]. All treated groups showed decreased weight gain compared with controls, especially in the high-dose group. The numbers of males surviving at 99-102 weeks were 11/50 control, 21/50 low-dose, 15/50 mid-dose and 32/50 high-dose; survival in females at 104 weeks was 22/47 control, 27/47 low-dose, 26/47 mid-dose and 34/47 high-dose. Complete necropsy and histopathology were performed on 20-32% of males and 22-38% of females, reducing the effective numbers of animals per group to between 10 and 18. No significant increase in tumour incidence could be attributed to treatment (Blair *et al.*, 1976). [The Working Group noted the small numbers of animals submitted for complete necropsy.]

Studies of cancer in experimental animals are summarized in Table 5.

4. Other Relevant Data

The toxicity of dichlorvos has been reviewed (FAO/WHO, 1965, 1967, 1968, 1971; Anon., 1974; FAO/WHO, 1978; WHO, 1989).

4.1 Absorption, distribution, metabolism and excretion

4.1.1 *Humans*

Dichlorvos is rapidly hydrolysed in human blood (half-time, 7-11 min), and no unchanged dichlorvos was found (detection limit, 0.1 µg/g) in blood samples taken 1 min after cessation of inhalation by two male volunteers exposed to 0.25 mg/m3 for 10 h or to 0.7 mg/m^3 for 20 h (Blair *et al.*, 1975).

A human volunteer who ingested 5 mg [^{14}C-vinyl]-dichlorvos excreted radiolabel at a rate similar to that seen after comparable oral dosing of rats, mice and hamsters, except that the output of ^{14}CO$_2$ was somewhat greater. The urinary metabolites were tentatively identified as demethyldichlorvos, urea and hippuric acid (Hutson & Hoadley, 1972a).

More recently, it was established that dimethylphosphate is a metabolite in the urine of workers occupationally exposed to dichlorvos (Das *et al.*, 1983).

4.1.2 *Experimental systems*

The metabolism and disposition of dichlorvos have been reviewed (Wright *et al.*, 1979).

Metabolic disposition studies using radiolabelled dichlorvos have been reported in rats, mice, hamsters, pigs and humans. Labelling at different sites (e.g., ^{14}C-methyl, ^{14}C-vinyl, ^{36}Cl-chlorovinyl, ^{32}P-phosphate) has enabled specific pathways to be traced (Hutson *et al.*, 1971; Hutson & Hoadley, 1972a,b; Page *et al.*, 1972; Potter *et al.*,, 1973; Blair *et al.*, 1975). Furthermore, metabolic disposition has been determined after both inhalation exposure and oral administration (including slow-release polyvinyl chloride-pelleted dose forms).

There are two main metabolic pathways for dichlorvos: (1) ester hydrolysis of the *PO*-vinyl group to yield dimethylphosphate and dichloroacetaldehyde and (2) oxidative *O*-demethylation to demethyldichlorvos and formaldehyde. An alternative pathway for *O*-demethylation involves conjugation with glutathione (Dicowsky & Morello, 1971; Hutson *et al.*, 1971; Hutson & Hoadley, 1972a,b; Page *et al.*, 1972; Potter *et al.*,, 1973; Blair *et al.*, 1975). Hydrolysis of the *O*-demethylated metabolite yields methylphosphate and, eventually, phosphoric acid and methanol (WHO, 1989). Radiolabel from [^{14}C-methyl]- and [^{14}C-vinyl]-dichlorvos is ultimately incorporated into CO$_2$ (e.g., 39% of an oral dose of [^{14}C-vinyl]-dichlorvos over four days in rats) and enters the 1 and 2-carbon metabolic pools, resulting in the labelling of amino acids, proteins and purines. This labelling may confound the interpretation of studies of tissue disposition and urinary excretion if the chemical specificity and source of the radiolabel are not determined.

Patterns of urinary metabolites indicate that metabolic clearance varies very little by species or route. The hydrolysis pathway generally predominates over the *O*-demethylation pathway, although the latter is more prominent in mice.

Table 5. Studies of cancer in experimental animals

Reference	Species/strain	Sex	Dose schedule	Experimental parameter/observation	0	1	2	3	Statistical conclusion	Comment
US National Cancer Institute (1977)	Mouse B6C3F1	M	In diet for 80 weeks	Dose (mg/kg of diet)[a]	0	0	318	635		
				Oesophageal carcinoma				1/50		
		F	In diet for 80 weeks	Dose (mg/kg of diet)	0	0	318	635		No significant increase in tumours
				Oesophageal carcinoma				1/50		
				Oesophageal papilloma				1/50		
US National Toxicology Program (1989)	Mouse B6C3F1	M	Gavage, 5 days/week for 103 weeks	Dose (mg/kg bw)	0	10	20	–		
				Forestomach papilloma	1/50	1/50	5/50		$p = 0.032$ trend	
		F	Gavage, 5 days/week for 103 weeks	Dose (mg/kg bw)	0	20	40	–		
				Forestomach papilloma	5/49	6/49	18/50		$p = 0.002$ trend	
				Forestomach carcinoma	0/49	0/49	2/50			
US National Cancer Institute (1977)	Rat Osborne-Mendel	M	In diet for 80 weeks	Dose (mg/kg of diet)[a]	0	0	150	326		
				Malignant fibrous histiocytomas	1/10	2/58	4/48	8/50	$p = 0.018$ trend	
		F	In diet for 80 weeks	Dose (mg/kg of diet)	0	0	150	326		No significant increase in tumours
Horn et al. (1988)	Rat BDIX/Bln	M	Gavage, 2 or 3 per week for 60 weeks	Dose (mg/animal) per week	0	0.1 × 2	0.1 × 3			
				Forestomach papillomas	0/10	0/13	2/26		NS	Number of animals with papillomas
				Urinary bladder papillomas	0/55	0/65	1/95		NS	
		F	Gavage 2 or 3 per week for 60 weeks	Dose (mg/animal) per week	0	0.1 × 2	0.1 × 3			
				Forestomach papillomas	0/22	0/20	1/38		NS	Number of animals with papillomas
				Urinary bladder papillomas	0/6	0/7	1/10		NS	
US National Toxicology Program (1989)	Rat Fischer 344/N	M	Gavage, 5 days/weeks for 103 weeks	Dose (mg/kg bw)	0	4	8			
				Pancreatic acinar-cell adenomas	25/50	30/50	33/50		$p < 0.05$ trend	
				Mononuclear-cell leukaemia	11/50	20/50	21/50		$p = 0.011$ trend	
		F	Gavage, 5 days/weeks for 103 weeks	Dose (mg/kg bw)	0	4	8	–		
				Pancreatic acinar-cell adenomas	2/50	3/50	6/50		NS	
				Mammary fibroadenomas/adenomas	9/50	19/50	17/50		$p = 0.028$ trend	

[a]Groups: 0, matched controls; 1, pooled controls

Hydrolytic metabolism of dichlorvos to dimethylphosphate and dichloroacetaldehyde, which in turn is rapidly reduced to dichloroethanol and conjugated with glucuronic acid, is so rapid that the half-time for the reaction *in vivo* has not been determined with any accuracy. *In vitro*, the half-time for blood-catalysed hydrolysis ranges from 2 min in rabbits to 30 min in rats. In human blood, the half-time is approximately 10 min, and the K_m for the reaction has been estimated to be approximately 3 μM. For this reason, unchanged dichlorvos is detected in blood only at relatively high dose rates (Blair *et al.*, 1975).

4.2 Toxic effects

4.2.1 *Humans*

The adverse effects of dichlorvos in humans have been reviewed (Cavagna & Vigliani, 1970; Gillett *et al.*, 1972a,b; Hayes, 1982). Depression of plasma cholinesterase is the most sensitive indicator of exposure to dichlorvos but is not necessarily an indicator of toxicity. At higher dose levels, red blood cell cholinesterase may also be affected.

Dichlorvos was administered in the form of slow-release polyvinyl resin formulation pellets as single doses (1-32 mg/kg bw) to 107 men and as repeated doses (1-32 mg/kg bw per day for 2-7 days; 1-16 mg/kg bw per day for up to three weeks) to 38 men. Maximal plasma cholinesterase depression occurred at approximately 6 mg/kg bw (single dose) and 1 mg/kg bw per day (repeated dose over three weeks). The single-dose threshold for plasma cholinesterase depression was approximately 1-3 mg/kg bw. Red blood cell cholinesterase activity was depressed at doses approximately four-fold higher. While the incidence of transient gastrointestinal and central nervous system-related subjective effects which accompanied the cholinesterase depression was relatively low at the lowest dose rates, they were sufficiently adverse to cause subjects given repeated doses of 8-32 mg/kg bw per day to withdraw from the study (Slomka & Hine, 1981).

Airborne levels of dichlorvos which cause slight to moderate cholinesterase depression have been reported to be 0.7 mg/m³ average over one year in factory workers producing dichlorvos vaporizers (Menz *et al.*, 1974) and 0.1 mg/m³ for 24 h per day in children and adults hospitalized for various periods in wards provided with dichlorvos-impregnated plastic strips. Plasma (but not red blood cell) cholinesterase levels were slightly depressed in 11 hospitalized babies exposed to air levels of over 0.1 mg/m³ for 24 h per day, but children of 2-7 years were not affected at the same exposure level for 16 h per day (Cavagna *et al.*, 1969). As reported in an abstract, neither plasma nor red blood cell cholinesterase depression was found in 22 newborn babies when the average air levels of dichlorvos were reported to be up to 0.159 mg/m³ (Vigliani, 1971).

Lethal exposures to dichlorvos have been reported in connection with accidental splashing of a concentrated formulation, coupled with failure to wash the material off (Hayes, 1982). A case of systemic poisoning resulted from an accident in which dichlorvos spray leaked down a man's back (Bisby & Simpson, 1975). Another accidental incident of skin contact resulted in symptomatic effects followed by the development of a persistent contact dermatitis (Mathias, 1983).

4.2.2 *Experimental systems*

The toxicology of dichlorvos in experimental animals has been reviewed (Attfield & Webster, 1966; Gillett *et al.*, 1972a,b; Anon., 1974; Wright *et al.*, 1979).

Dichlorvos is acutely neurotoxic by virtue of its ability to inhibit brain cholinesterase. The acute oral LD_{50} in rats was cited as 56-80 (Durham *et al.*, 1957) and 25-30 mg/kg bw (Ben-Dyke *et al.*, 1970) and that in mice as 140-275 mg/kg bw (Anon., 1974; Holmstedt *et al.*, 1978). The oral LD_{50} of dichlorvos in young pigs was 157 mg/kg bw; no death occurred in animals administered up to 100 mg/kg of a polyvinyl chloride formulation of dichlorvos (Stanton *et al.*, 1979). The large range cited for the dermal LD_{50} (75-900 mg/kg bw) in rats suggests that skin absorption is vehicle-dependent (Jones *et al.*, 1968).

Exposures after which cholinesterase depression was the only discernible toxic effect include two-year inhalation exposure of rats to 0.5-5 mg/m^3 (Blair *et al.*, 1976), 90-day feeding of 0.4-70 mg/kg bw per day to rats (effects observed at 3.5 mg/kg per day and above; Durham *et al.*, 1957), administration for 30 days of 1-16 mg/kg bw per day in polyvinyl chloride pellets to pigs (Stanton *et al.*, 1979) and administration for 10-21 days of 10-80 mg/kg bw per day in polyvinyl chloride pellets to rhesus monkeys (Hass *et al.*, 1972).

Dichlorvos has been ascribed only a slight risk of causing delayed neuropathy, because doses that inhibit neuropathy target esterase and result in ataxia in hens exceed the LD_{50} by several fold; protection with atropine is required if the test is to be completed (Johnson, 1978; Caroldi & Lotti, 1981; Johnson, 1981).

Both humoral immune response and cell-mediated immunity were inhibited in rabbits treated orally with dichlorvos for five days a week for up to five to six weeks at high dose rates (0.31-2.5 mg/kg bw: 2.5-20% of the LD_{50}; Dési *et al.*, 1978, 1980). Immunosuppression was also observed in mice given 120 mg/kg bw orally, but the authors commented that this phenomenon, seen with other organophosphonates and the cholinomimetic compound, arecoline, may be secondary to a profound cholinergic stimulation (Casale *et al.*, 1983).

The diurnal rhythm of the pituitary/adrenal axis was altered in rats given 2 ppm (mg/l) dichlorvos in the drinking-water for two weeks (approximate intake, 0.3 mg/kg bw per day), causing changes in plasma adrenocorticotrophic hormone levels and adrenal cholesterol ester concentrations. While adrenocorticotrophic hormone secretion is believed to be acetylcholine-sensitive, there was no detectable change in cholinesterase activity (Civen *et al.*, 1980).

Reactions with macromolecules: Dichlorvos is a phosphorylating and alkylating agent (Wright *et al.*, 1979). 4-Nitrobenzylpyridine is alkylated by dichlorvos (half-time, 28 min) more slowly than methyl methanesulfonate (half-time, 9.6 min). Metabolites of dichlorvos did not react with 4-nitrobenzylpyridine in this system (Bedford & Robinson, 1972). The relative reactivity of dichlorvos toward 4-nitrobenzylpyridine and acetylcholinesterase was greatly in favour of esterase phosphorylation (WHO, 1989), indicating that dichlorvos-associated methylation of DNA purines may not be as important *in vivo* as the esterase phosphorylation reaction (Wright *et al.*, 1979; Wooder *et al.*, 1977).

There may appear to be some conflict between this conclusion and the detection of radiolabelled N-7-methylated guanine in mouse urine following administration of [^{14}C-methyl]- or [^{3}H-methyl]-dichlorvos (24-90 µCi intraperitoneally or an estimated

8.5-11 μCi by inhalation) (Wennerberg & Löfroth, 1974). Since, however, methylated purines occur naturally in urine and [^{14}C-methyl]-dichlorvos metabolites enter the 1- and 2-carbon metabolic pool, it has been suggested that the mechanism of methylation may be indirect (Wooder & Wright, 1981). No N-7-guanine methylation was found in the DNA of lung, liver, heart, brain, testes or spleen of 20 rats exposed to [^{14}C-methyl]-dichlorvos by inhalation at 0.064 μg/l for 12 h (estimated total dose, 6 μg; specific activity, 113 μCi/mmol; resulting in a DNA detection limit of 0.000001% of the dose) (Wooder et al., 1977).

Segerbäck and Ehrenberg (1981) also concluded that the likelihood of DNA methylation after dosing with dichlorvos in vivo is extremely small. Their estimate of the amount of DNA methylation in mice after intraperitoneal dosing with 1.9 μmol/kg bw [0.42 mg/kg] is of the order of 8×10^{-13} mol methyl per gram of DNA.

4.3 Reproductive and developmental effects

4.3.1 Humans

No data were available to the Working Group.

4.3.2 Experimental systems

Female Sherman rats were treated intraperitoneally with dichlorvos at 15 mg/kg bw in peanut oil on day 11 of gestation. No difference was noted in weight gain, number of fetuses per litter, number of resorptions per pregnant rat or weight of the fetuses or placentae on day 20 of gestation. Three omphalocoeles occurred among 41 offspring in the treated group, but no malformation was noted among controls (Kimbrough & Gaines, 1968).

No adverse developmental effect was observed in CF-1 mice administered the maximal tolerated dose by gavage on days 6-15 of gestation or in New Zealand rabbits administered 60 and 5 mg/kg bw per day on days 6-18 of gestation or by inhalation at 4 mg/m^3 for 7 h per day (Schwetz et al., 1979).

Pregnant rabbits were treated [route not given] with dichlorvos at a dose of 6 mg/kg bw per day for the last 10 days of gestation. Light-microscopic examination of the brains of six pups from treated and six from untreated dams sacrificed at birth revealed no alteration in brain morphology; electron microscopic examination suggested 'immaturity' or delay in brain development in the treated animals. Synaptic junctions quantified in the motor cortex using electron microscopy were considered to be immature (Dambska et al., 1979). [The Working Group noted the lack of adequate controls and the poor description of the study.]

Carworth E rats and Dutch rabbits were exposed to dichlorvos in air at concentrations of up to 6.25 mg/m^3 and 4 mg/m^3, respectively, for 23 h per day on seven days per week from the day of mating until the end of gestation. These treatments produced a dose-dependent decrease in plasma, red cell and brain cholinesterase activity in both species but had no effect on the number of pregnancies, the number of resorptions, the number of fetal deaths, litter size or fetal weight in rats or rabbits (Thorpe et al., 1972).

In pregnant sows fed a polyvinyl chloride formulation of dichlorvos at doses of 5 or 25 mg/kg bw per day for the last 30 days of gestation, no alteration in reproductive performance was observed. Plasma and red cell cholinesterase activities and, at the high dose, myometrial acetylcholinesterase activity were decreased in the sows; the rhomb-encephalic acetylcholinesterase level was increased in fetuses (Stanton et al., 1979).

A series of early studies reported in abstracts also examined reproductive and developmental effects. No effect on reproduction or development was seen in more than 6000 offspring of male and female rats treated for three generations with dichlorvos in feed at doses of up to 500 ppm [mg/kg] (Witherup *et al.*, 1971). In rabbits treated orally with a polyvinyl chloride formulation of dichlorvos, maternal toxicity was seen at 34 mg/kg; no alteration was observed in reproductive or developmental parameters at doses not associated with maternal toxicity (Vogin *et al.*, 1971). No effect on reproduction or development was seen over two generations in male and female swine treated for 37 months at doses in the feed of up to 500 ppm [mg/kg] (Collins *et al.*, 1971).

4.4 Genetic and related effects (see also Table 6 and Appendices 1 and 2)

4.4.1 *Humans*

No data were available to the Working Group.

4.4.2 *Experimental systems*

The genetic activity of dichlorvos has been reviewed (Ramel *et al.*, 1980).

In bacteria, dichlorvos bound covalently to DNA, RNA and protein and caused DNA damage and point mutations. Bacterial mutagenicity was reduced in the presence of liver preparations. Dichlorvos induced gene conversion, mutation and aneuploidy in yeast and fungi, and mutation, chromosomal aberrations and micronucleus formation in plants. In *Drosophila melanogaster*, chromosomal aberrations but not sex-linked recessive lethal mutation were induced. Autosomal lethal and polygenic viability mutations were induced in *D. melanogaster* by treatment over multiple generations. [The Working Group considered that these tests are not well validated.] In mammalian cells *in vitro*, dichlorvos caused DNA strand breaks, mutation, sister chromatid exchange, chromosomal aberrations and cell transformation. In human cells *in vitro*, it induced unscheduled DNA synthesis but neither chromosomal aberrations nor sister chromatid exchange.

No significant response was observed *in vivo* in any of the mammalian tests used for the induction of unscheduled DNA synthesis, sister chromatid exchange, micronucleus formation, chromosomal aberrations or dominant lethal mutation.

5. Summary of Data Reported and Evaluation

5.1 Exposure data

Dichlorvos has been used widely as an insecticide since 1961 to control internal and external parasites in livestock and domestic animals, to control insects in houses, and in crop protection.

Dichlorvos has been formulated for use as dusts, granules, pellets/tablets, impregnated resin strips and concentrates.

Household and public health uses represent the main sources of human exposure to dichlorvos. Exposure may also occur during its production and application.

Table 6. Genetic and related effects of dichlorvos

Test system	Result[a] Without exogenous metabolic system	With exogenous metabolic system	Dose[b] LED/HID	Reference
PRB, Prophage induction	+	+	60.0000	Houk & DeMarini (1987)
ECB, *Escherichia coli* WP2, DNA strand breaks	+	0	2000.0000	Green et al. (1974)
ECB, *Escherichia coli* WP67, DNA strand breaks	+	0	500.0000	Green et al. (1974)
ECB, *Escherichia coli* ColE1 plasmid, DNA strand breaks	+	0	1000.0000	Griffin & Hill (1978)
ECD, *Escherichia coli pol A*, differential toxicity (spot test)	+	0	13.0000	Rosenkranz (1973)
ECD, *Escherichia coli pol A*, differential toxicity (liquid)	+	0	1400.0000	Rosenkranz (1973)
BSD, *Bacillus subtilis rec*, differential toxicity	+	0	2000.0000	Shirasu et al. (1976)
BSD, *Bacillus subtilis rec*, differential toxicity	+	0	0.0000	Kawachi et al. (1980)
BRD, Bacteria (other), differential toxicity	(+)	0	50000.0000	Adler et al. (1976)
BRD, Bacteria (other), differential toxicity	+	0	2.0000	Braun et al. (1982)
SA0, *Salmonella typhimurium* TA100, reverse mutation	+	+	300.0000	Byeon et al. (1976)
SA0, *Salmonella typhimurium* TA100, reverse mutation	+	+	275.0000	Löfroth (1978)
SA0, *Salmonella typhimurium* TA100, reverse mutation	+	+	0.0000	Kawachi et al. (1980)
SA0, *Salmonella typhimurium* TA100, reverse mutation	+	0	0.0000	Ishidate et al. (1981)
SA0, *Salmonella typhimurium* TA100, reverse mutation	+	(+)	1.0000	Braun et al. (1982)
SA0, *Salmonella typhimurium* TA100, reverse mutation	+	+	375.0000	Moriya et al. (1983)
SA0, *Salmonella typhimurium* TA100, reverse mutation	(+)	+	250.0000	Breau et al. (1985)
SA0, *Salmonella typhimurium* TA100, reverse mutation	+	-	250.0000	Choi et al. (1985)
SA0, *Salmonella typhimurium* TA100, reverse mutation	+	+	167.0000	Zeiger et al. (1988)
SA0, *Salmonella typhimurium* TA100, reverse mutation	+	+	500.0000	US National Toxicology Program (1989)
SA2, *Salmonella typhimurium* TA102, reverse mutation	-	-	0.0000	Choi et al. (1985)
SA3, *Salmonella typhimurium* TA1530, reverse mutation	+	0	0.0000	Hanna & Dyer (1975)
SA5, *Salmonella typhimurium* TA1535, reverse mutation	+	0	0.0000	Hanna & Dyer (1975)
SA5, *Salmonella typhimurium* TA1535, reverse mutation	(+)	(+)	1500.0000	Byeon et al. (1976)
SA5, *Salmonella typhimurium* TA1535, reverse mutation	+	0	2500.0000	Shirasu et al. (1976)
SA5, *Salmonella typhimurium* TA1535, reverse mutation	+	0	1500.0000	Carere et al. (1978)
SA5, *Salmonella typhimurium* TA1535, reverse mutation	-	-	2500.0000	Moriya et al. (1978)

Table 6 (contd)

Test system	Result[a] Without exogenous metabolic sytem	Result[a] With exogenous metabolic system	Dose[b] LED/HID	Reference
SA5, *Salmonella typhimurium* TA1535, reverse mutation	+	0	0.0000	Choi et al. (1985)
SA7, *Salmonella typhimurium* TA1537, reverse mutation	−	0	0.0000	Hanna & Dyer (1975)
SA7, *Salmonella typhimurium* TA1537, reverse mutation	−	0	2500.0000	Shirasu et al. (1976)
SA7, *Salmonella typhimurium* TA1537, reverse mutation	−	0	2800.0000	Carere et al. (1978)
SA7, *Salmonella typhimurium* TA1537, reverse mutation	−	−	2500.0000	Moriya et al. (1983)
SA8, *Salmonella typhimurium* TA1538, reverse mutation	−	0	0.0000	Hanna & Dyer (1975)
SA8, *Salmonella typhimurium* TA1538, reverse mutation	−	0	2500.0000	Shirasu et al. (1976)
SA8, *Salmonella typhimurium* TA1538, reverse mutation	−	−	1500.0000	Byeon et al. (1976)
SA8, *Salmonella typhimurium* TA1538, reverse mutation	−	0	2800.0000	Carere et al. (1978)
SA8, *Salmonella typhimurium* TA1538, reverse mutation	−	−	2500.0000	Moriya et al. (1983)
SA8, *Salmonella typhimurium* TA1538, reverse mutation	−	−	0.0000	Choi et al. (1985)
SA9, *Salmonella typhimurium* TA98, reverse mutation	−	−	1500.0000	Byeon et al. (1976)
SA9, *Salmonella typhimurium* TA98, reverse mutation	−	0	0.0000	Kawachi et al. (1980)
SA9, *Salmonella typhimurium* TA98, reverse mutation	−	−	2500.0000	Moriya et al. (1983)
SA9, *Salmonella typhimurium* TA98, reverse mutation	−	−	0.0000	Breau et al. (1985)
SA9, *Salmonella typhimurium* TA98, reverse mutation	−	−	0.0000	Choi et al. (1985)
SA9, *Salmonella typhimurium* TA98, reverse mutation	−	−	500.0000	Zeiger et al. (1988)
SA9, *Salmonella typhimurium* TA98, reverse mutation	−	−	500.0000	US National Toxicology Program (1989)
SAS, *Salmonella typhimurium* 64–320, reverse mutation	+	0	500.0000	Voogd et al. (1972)
SAS, *Salmonella typhimurium* C117, reverse mutation	(+)	0	6630.0000	Dyer & Hanna (1973)
SAS, *Salmonella typhimurium* C117, reverse mutation	−	0	0.0000	Hanna & Dyer (1975)
SAS, *Salmonella typhimurium* G46, reverse mutation	−	0	0.0000	Hanna & Dyer (1975)
SAS, *Salmonella typhimurium* TA1536, reverse mutation	−	0	2500.0000	Shirasu et al. (1976)
SAS, *Salmonella typhimurium* TA1536, reverse mutation	−	0	2800.0000	Carere et al. (1978)
ECF, *Escherichia coli* B, forward mutation	+	0	1100.0000	Wild (1973)
ECK, *Escherichia coli* K12, forward or reverse mutation	+	0	145.0000	Mohn (1973)
ECW, *Escherichia coli* WP2 *uvrA*, reverse mutation	+	0	2000.0000	Bridges et al. (1973)

Table 6 (contd)

Test system	Result[a]		Dose[b] LED/HID	Reference
	Without exogenous metabolic sytem	With exogenous metabolic system		
ECW, *Escherichia coli* WP2 *uvrA*, reverse mutation	+	0	0.0000	Hanna & Dyer (1975)
ECW, *Escherichia coli* WP2 *uvrA*, reverse mutation	+	0	0.0000	Nagy et al. (1975)
ECW, *Escherichia coli* WP2 *uvrA*, reverse mutation	+	0	2000.0000	Bridges (1978)
EC2, *Escherichia coli* WP2, reverse mutation	–	0	0.0000	Dean (1972a)
EC2, *Escherichia coli* WP2, reverse mutation	+	0	2000.0000	Bridges et al. (1973)
EC2, *Escherichia coli* WP2, reverse mutation	+	0	0.0000	Hanna & Dyer (1975)
EC2, *Escherichia coli* WP2, reverse mutation	(+)	0	0.0000	Nagy et al. (1975)
EC2, *Escherichia coli* WP2, reverse mutation	+	0	5.0000	Green et al. (1976)
EC2, *Escherichia coli* WP2, reverse mutation	+	0	2500.0000	Shirasu et al. (1976)
EC2, *Escherichia coli* WP2, reverse mutation	+	0	5.0000	Bridges (1978)
EC2, *Escherichia coli* WP2, reverse mutation	+	0	2500.0000	Moriya et al. (1983)
ECR, *Escherichia coli* B(sd–4), reverse mutation	+	0	220.0000	Löfroth et al. (1969)
ECR, *Escherichia coli* K12 HfrH, reverse mutation	+	0	1000.0000	Voogd et al. (1972)
EC2, *Escherichia coli* WP67, reverse mutation	+	0	1000.0000	Bridges et al. (1973)
EC2, *Escherichia coli* WP67, reverse mutation	+	0	0.0000	Hanna & Dyer (1975)
EC2, *Escherichia coli* CM561, reverse mutation	–	0	2000.0000	Bridges et al. (1973)
EC2, *Escherichia coli* CM561, reverse mutation	–	0	0.0000	Hanna & Dyer (1975)
EC2, *Escherichia coli* CM571, reverse mutation	–	0	2000.0000	Bridges et al. (1973)
EC2, *Escherichia coli* CM571, reverse mutation	–	0	0.0000	Hanna & Dyer (1975)
EC2, *Escherichia coli* CM611, reverse mutation	–	0	2000.0000	Bridges et al. (1973)
EC2, *Escherichia coli* CM611, reverse mutation	–	0	0.0000	Hanna & Dyer (1975)
ECR, *Escherichia coli* CM881, reverse mutation	+	0	0.1000	Bridges (1978)
ECR, *Escherichia coli* B/r WP2, reverse mutation	+	+	2500.0000	Moriya et al. (1978)
KPF, *Klebsiella pneumoniae*, forward mutation	+	0	500.0000	Voogd et al. (1972)
SCG, *Saccharomyces cerevisiae*, gene conversion	+	0	4000.0000	Dean et al. (1972)
SCG, *Saccharomyces cerevisiae*, gene conversion	+	0	1326.0000	Fahrig (1973)
SCG, *Saccharomyces cerevisiae*, gene conversion	+	0	1770.0000	Fahrig (1976)
SCH, *Saccharomyces cerevisiae*, homozygosis by gene conversion	+	0	5000.0000	Choi et al. (1985)

Table 6 (contd)

Test system	Result[a]		Dose[b] LED/HID	Reference
	Without exogenous metabolic sytem	With exogenous metabolic system		
ANG, *Aspergillus nidulans*, genetic crossing-over	+	0	2800.0000	Morpurgo *et al.* (1977)
SZF, *Schizosaccharomyces pombe*, forward mutation	+	(+)	330.0000	Gilot–Delhalle *et al.* (1983)
ANR, *Aspergillus nidulans*, reverse mutation	+	0	14000.0000	Morpurgo *et al.* (1977)
ANN, *Aspergillus nidulans*, aneuploidy	+	0	800.0000	Morpurgo *et al.* (1979)
HSM, *Hordeum* species, mutation	–	0	166.0000	Bhan & Kaul (1975)
HSM, *Hordeum* species, mutation	+	0	1500.0000	Panda & Sharma (1979)
HSM, *Hordeum* species, mutation	+	0	5000.0000	Singh *et al.* (1980)
HSM, *Hordeum* species, mutation	+	0	0.0000	Sharma *et al.* (1983)
TSM, *Tradescantia paludosa*, mutation	–	0	0.0000	Schairer *et al.* (1978)
TSI, *Tradescantia paludosa*, micronuclei	+	0	0.0000	Ma *et al.* (1984)
ACC, *Allium cepa*, chromosomal aberrations	+	0	50.0000	Rao *et al.* (1987)
HSC, *Hordeum* species, chromosomal aberrations	+	0	55.0000	Bhan & Kaul (1975)
HSC, *Hordeum* species, chromosomal aberrations	+	0	100.0000	Panda & Sharma (1979)
HSC, *Hordeum* species, chromosomal aberrations	+	0	0.0000	Sharma *et al.* (1983)
VFC, *Vicia faba*, chromosomal aberrations	+	0	125.0000	Amer & Ali (1986)
PLC, *Capsicum annuum*, chromosomal aberrations	+	0	5000.0000	Devadas *et al.* (1986)
DMG, *Drosophila melanogaster*, crossing–over/recombination	–	0	350.0000	Jayasuriya & Ratnayake (1973)
DMX, *Drosophila melanogaster*, sex–linked recessive lethal mutations	–	0	350.0000	Jayasuriya & Ratnayake (1973)
DMX, *Drosophila melanogaster*, sex–linked recessive lethal mutations	–	0	0.0900	Kramers & Knaap (1978)
DMX, *Drosophila melanogaster*, sex–linked recessive lethal mutations	–	0	0.0700	Sobels & Todd (1979)
*, *Drosophila melanogaster*, polygenic viability mutations	+	0	4.0000	Marcos *et al.* (1989)
*, *Drosophila melanogaster*, autosomal recessive lethal mutations	+	0	0.7500	Hanna & Dyer (1975)

Table 6 (contd)

Test system	Result[a] Without exogenous metabolic sytem	Result[a] With exogenous metabolic system	Dose[b] LED/HID	Reference
DMC, *Drosophila melanogaster*, chromosomal aberrations	+	0	1.0000	Gupta & Singh (1974)
DIA, DNA strand breaks, Chinese hamster V–79–4 cells *in vitro*	(+)	0	2000.0000	Green et al. (1974)
G9O, Gene mutation, Chinese hamster V79 lung cells (ouabain)	–	0	1100.0000	Aquilina et al. (1984)
GST, Gene mutation, mouse lymphoma L5178Y cells *in vitro*, *tk* locus	+	0	25.0000	US National Toxicology Program (1989)
SIC, Sister chromatid exchange, Chinese hamster cells *in vitro*	+	0	20.0000	Tezuka et al. (1980)
SIC, Sister chromatid exchange, Chinese hamster cells *in vitro*	+	0	7.0000	Nishio & Uyeki (1981)
SIC, Sister chromatid exchange, Chinese hamster cells *in vitro*	+	0	22.0000	Shirasu et al. (1984)
SIC, Sister chromatid exchange, Chinese hamster cells *in vitro*	+	+	25.0000	US National Toxicology Program (1989)
SIR, Sister chromatid exchange, rat cells *in vitro*	+	0	10.0000	Lin et al. (1988)
CIC, Chromosomal aberrations, Chinese hamster cells *in vitro*	–	0	1000.0000	Sasaki et al. (1980)
CIC, Chromosomal aberrations, Chinese hamster cells *in vitro*	+	0	110.0000	Tezuka et al. (1980)
CIC, Chromosomal aberrations, Chinese hamster cells *in vitro*	+	0	130.0000	Ishidate et al. (1981)
CIR, Chromosomal aberrations, rat cells *in vitro*	+	0	80.0000	Lin et al. (1988)
TCS, Cell transformation, Syrian hamster embryo cells *in vitro*	+	0	0.0000	Tu et al. (1986)
TCL, Cell transformation, rat tracheal epithelial cells *in vitro*	+	0	40.0000	Lin et al. (1988)
UHL, Unscheduled DNA synthesis, human lymphocytes *in vitro*	+	0	5.0000	Perocco & Fini (1980)
UIH, Unscheduled DNA synthesis, EUE human cells *in vitro*	+	0	14365.0000	Aquilina et al. (1984)
SHF, Sister chromatid exchange, human fibroblasts *in vitro*	–	0	10.0000	Nicholas et al. (1978)
SHL, Sister chromatid exchange, human lymphocytes *in vitro*	–	0	10.0000	Nicholas et al. (1978)
CHL, Chromosomal aberrations, human lymphocytes *in vitro*	–	0	40.0000	Dean (1972b)
HMM, Host–mediated assay, *Salmonella typhimurium* in mice	–	0	25.000	Buselmaier et al. (1972)
HMM, Host–mediated assay, *Salmonella typhimurium* in mice	–	0	8.0000	Voogd et al. (1972)
HMM, Host–mediated assay, *Saccharomyces cerevisiae* in mice	–	0	100.0000	Dean et al. (1972)
UPR, Unscheduled DNA synthesis, rat hepatocytes *in vivo*	–	0	35.0000	Mirsalis et al. (1989)
SVA, Sister chromatid exchange, mouse lymphocytes *in vivo*	–	0	25.0000	Kligerman t al. (1985)

Table 6 (contd)

Test system	Result[a]		Dose[b] LED/HID	Reference
	Without exogenous metabolic sytem	With exogenous metabolic system		
MVM, Micronucleus test, mouse bone-marrow cells *in vivo*	–	0	0.0150	Paik & Lee (1977)
CBA, Chromosomal aberrations, mouse bone-marrow cells *in vivo*	–	0	15.0000 (16-h inhal.)	Dean & Thorpe (1972a)
CBA, Chromosomal aberrations, Chinese hamster bone marrow *in vivo*	–	0	15.0000	Dean & Thorpe (1972a)
CBA, Chromosomal aberrations, mouse bone-marrow cells *in vivo*	–	0	100.0000	Kurinnyi (1975)
CBA, Chromosomal aberrations, mouse bone-marrow cells *in vivo*	–	0	10.0000	Moutschen–Dahmen et al. (1981)
CBA, Chromosomal aberrations, mouse bone-marrow cells *in vivo*	–	0	0.3300[c]	Degraeve et al. (1984a)
CBA, Chromosomal aberrations, Syrian hamster bone marrow *in vivo*	(+)	0	15.0000	Dzwonkowska & Hübner (1986)
CCC, Chromosomal aberrations, mouse spermatocytes *in vivo*	–	0	0.3300[c]	Degraeve et al. (1984a)
CCC, Chromosomal aberrations, mouse spermatocytes *in vivo*	–	0	10.0000	Degraeve et al. (1984b)
CGC, Chromosomal aberrations, mouse spermatogonia *in vivo*	–	0	0.3300[c]	Degraeve et al. (1984a)
CGC, Chromosomal aberrations, mouse spermatogonia *in vivo*	–	0	10.0000	Degraeve et al. (1984b)
DLM, Dominant lethal test, mice	–	0	53.0000 (16-h inhal.)	Dean & Thorpe (1972b)
DLM, Dominant lethal test, mice	–	0	16.5000	Epstein et al. (1972)
DLM, Dominant lethal test, mice	–	0	50.0000	Dean & Blair (1976)
DLM, Dominant lethal test, mice	–	0	10.0000	Moutschen–Dahmen et al. (1981)
DLM, Dominant lethal test, mice	–	0	0.3300[c]	Degraeve et al. (1984a)
BID, Binding to calf thymus DNA *in vitro*	+	0	20000.0000	Löfroth (1970)
BID, Binding to DNA, *Escherichia coli* WP2 *uvrA in vitro*	+	0	300.0000	Lawley et al. (1974)
BID, Binding to DNA, HeLa cells *in vitro*	+	0	215.0000	Lawley et al. (1974)
BID, Binding to DNA, *Escherichia coli* B *in vitro*	+	0	155.0000	Wennerberg & Löfroth (1974)
BID, Binding to calf thymus DNA *in vitro*	+	0	3.7500	Segerbäck (1981)

Table 6 (contd)

Test system	Result[a] Without exogenous metabolic sytem	With exogenous metabolic system	Dose[b] LED/HID	Reference
BIP, Binding to RNA/protein, *Escherichia coli* WP2 *uvrA in vitro*	+	0	215.0000	Lawley *et al.* (1974)
BIP, Binding to RNA/protein, HeLa cells *in vitro*	+	0	215.0000	Lawley *et al.* (1974)
BIP, Binding to RNA/protein, *Escherichia coli* B *in vitro*	+	0	155.0000	Wennerberg & Löfroth (1974)
BVD, Binding to DNA, rats *in vivo*	–	0	0.0150 (12-h inhal.)	Wooder *et al.* (1977)
BVD, Binding to DNA, mice *in vivo*	–	0	0.4000	Segerbäck (1981)
BVP, Binding to RNA/protein, rats *in vivo*	–	0	0.0150 (12-h inhal.)	Wooder *et al.* (1977)
SPF, Sperm morphology, F1 mice *in vivo*	(+)	0	12.0000	Wyrobeck & Bruce (1975)

*Not displayed on profile

[a] +, positive; (+), weakly positive; –, negative; 0, not tested; ?, inconclusive (variable response in several experiments within an adequate study)

[b] In-vitro tests, µg/ml; in-vivo tests, mg/kg bw

[c] In drinking-water

5.2 Carcinogenicity in humans

One case-control study of leukaemia in the USA found an association with use of dichlorvos on animals; there were few exposed subjects, and they had potential exposure to many pesticides.

5.3 Carcinogenicity in experimental animals

Dichlorvos was tested for carcinogenicity by oral administration in two experiments in mice and in three experiments in rats. A few rare oesophageal squamous-cell tumours were found in mice treated with dichlorvos in the diet. A dose-related increase in the incidence of squamous-cell tumours (mainly papillomas) was noted in the forestomachs of mice that received dichlorvos in corn oil by gavage. In rats that received dichlorvos in water by gavage, a few squamous-cell papillomas of the forestomach were seen. In rats that received dichlorvos in corn oil by gavage, a dose-related increase in the incidence of mononuclear-cell leukaemia and an increased incidence of pancreatic acinar-cell adenomas were observed in males.

5.4 Other relevant data

A variety of studies in several species did not demonstrate developmental toxicity due to dichlorvos.

In vitro, dichlorvos phosphorylates esterases to a greater extent than it methylates nucleophiles; the likelihood of DNA methylation *in vivo* is extremely small.

Immunosuppression has been noted after short-term administration of high doses of dichlorvos which are associated with profound cholinergic hyperstimulation.

No data were available on the genetic and related effects of dichlorvos in humans.

Dichlorvos was not shown to have genetic activity in various assays in mammals *in vivo*. It induced gene mutation and chromosomal damage in cultured mammalian cells ·and in insects, plants, fungi, yeast and bacteria.

5.5 Evaluation[1]

There is *inadequate evidence* in humans for the carcinogenicity of dichlorvos.

There is *sufficient evidence* in experimental animals for the carcinogenicity of dichlorvos.

Overall evaluation

Dichlorvos *is possibly carcinogenic to humans (Group 2B).*

6. References

Abbott, D.C., Crisp, S., Tarrant, K.R. & Tatton, J.O'G. (1970) Pesticide residues in the total diet in England and Wales, 1966-1967. III. Organophosphorus pesticide residues in the total diet. *Pestic. Sci., 1*, 10-13

---

[1]For definition of the italicized terms, see Preamble, pp. 26-28.

Adler, B., Braun, R., Schöneich, J. & Böhme, H. (1976) Repair-defective mutants of *Proteus mirabilis* as a prescreening system for the detection of potential carcinogens. *Biol. Zbl.*, *95*, 463-469

Agrochemical Producers' Association of Finland (1989) 1988 Finnish pesticide sales. *AGROW*, *97*, 11-12

Amer, S.M. & Ali, E.M. (1986) Cytological effects of pesticides. XVII. Effect of the insecticide dichlorvos on root-mitosis of *Vicia faba*. *Cytologia*, *51*, 21-25

American Conference of Governmental Industrial Hygienists (1989) *Threshold Limit Values and Biological Exposure Indices for 1989-1990*, Cincinnati, OH, p. 20

AMVAC Chemical Corp. (1986) *Product Data Sheet: DDVP Technical*, Los Angeles, CA

AMVAC Chemical Corp. (1990) *Material Safety Data Sheet: DDVP Technical Grade*, Los Angeles, CA

Anon. (1972) Vapona® insecticide. *Anal. Methods pestic. plant growth Regul.*, *6*, 529-533

Anon. (1974) Studies on dichlorvos. *Food Cosmet. Toxicol.*, *28*, 765-772

Aquilina, G., Benigni, R., Bignami, M., Calcagnile, A., Dogliotti, E., Falcone, E. & Carere, A. (1984) Genotoxic activity of dichlorvos, trichlorfon and dichloroacetaldehyde. *Pestic. Sci.*, *15*, 439-442

Attfield, J.G. & Webster, D.A. (1966) Dichlorvos. *Chem. Ind.*, 12 February, pp. 272-278

Bedford, C.T. & Robinson, J. (1972) The alkylating properties of organophosphates. *Xenobiotica*, *2*, 307-337

Ben-Dyke, R., Sanderson, D.M. & Noakes, D.N. (1970) Acute toxicity data for pesticides. *World Rev. Pest Control*, *9*, 119-127

Bhan, A.K. & Kaul, B.L. (1975) Cytotoxic activity of dichlorvos in barley. *Indian J. exp. Biol.*, *13*, 403-405

Bisby, J.A. & Simpson, G.R. (1975) An unusual presentation of systemic organophosphate poisoning. *Med. J. Aust.*, *2*, 394-395

Blair, D., Hoadley, E.C. & Hutson, D.H. (1975) The distribution of dichlorvos in the tissues of mammals after its inhalation or intravenous administration. *Toxicol. appl. Pharmacol.*, *31*, 243-253

Blair, D., Dix, K.M., Hunt, P.F., Thorpe, E., Stevenson, D.E. & Walker, A.I.T. (1976) Dichlorvos—a 2-year inhalation carcinogenesis study in rats. *Arch. Toxicol.*, *35*, 281-294

Braun, R., Schöneich, J., Weissflog, L. & Dedek, W. (1982) Activity of organophosphorus insecticides in bacterial tests for mutagenicity and DNA repair—direct alkylation *vs* metabolic activation and breakdown. I. Butonate, vinylbutonate, trichlorfon, dichlorvos, dimethyl dichlorvos and dimethyl vinylbutonate. *Chem.-biol. Interactions*, *39*, 339-350

Breau, A.P., Mitchell, W.M., Swinson, J. & Field, L. (1985) Mutagenic and cell transformation activities of representative phosphorothioate esters *in vitro*. *J. Toxicol. environ. Health*, *16*, 403-413

Bridges, B.A. (1978) On the detection of volatile liquid mutagens with bacteria: experiments with dichlorvos and epichlorhydrin. *Mutat. Res.*, *54*, 367-371

Bridges, B.A., Mottershead, R.P., Green, M.H.L. & Gray, W.J.H. (1973) Mutagenicity of dichlorvos and methyl methanesulfonate for *Escherichia coli* WP2 and some derivatives deficient in DNA repair. *Mutat. Res.*, *19*, 295-303

Brown, L.M., Blair, A., Gibson, R., Everett, G.D., Cantor, K.P., Schuman, L.M., Burmeister, L.F., Van Lier, S.F. & Dick, F. (1990) Pesticide exposures and other agricultural risk factors for leukemia among men in Iowa and Minnesota. *Cancer*, *50*, 6585-6591

Buselmaier, W., Röhrborn, G. & Propping, P. (1972) Mutagenicity investigations with pesticides in the host-mediated assay and dominant lethal test in the mouse (Ger.). *Biol. Zbl.*, *91*, 311-325

Byeon, W.-H., Hyun, H.H. & Lee, S.Y. (1976) Mutagenicity of pesticides in the *Salmonella*/microsome system (Korean). *Korean J. Microbiol.*, *14*, 128-134

Carere, A., Ortali, V.A., Cardamone, G. & Morpurgo, G. (1978) Mutagenicity of dichlorvos and other structurally related pesticides in *Salmonella* and *Streptomyces*. *Chem.-biol. Interactions*, *22*, 297-308

Caroldi, S. & Lotti, M. (1981) Delayed neurotoxicity caused by a single massive dose of dichlorvos to adult hens. *Toxicol. Lett.*, *9*, 157-159

Casale, G.P., Cohen, S.D. & DiCapua, R.A. (1983) The effects of organophosphate-induced cholinergic stimulation on the antibody response to sheep erythrocytes in inbred mice. *Toxicol. appl. Pharmacol.*, *68*, 198-205

Cavagna, G. & Vigliani, E.C. (1970) Problems of health and safety when using Vapona as an insecticide in domestic quarters (Fr.). *Med. Lav.*, *61*, 409-423

Cavagna, G., Locati, G. & Vigliani, E.C. (1969) Clinical effects of exposure to DDVP (Vapona) insecticide in hospital wards. *Arch. environ. Health*, *19*, 112-123

Choi, E.U., Kim, Y.K. & Roh, J.K. (1985) Genetic toxicity of pesticides used in Korea on *Salmonella typhimurium* and *Saccharomyces cerevisiae*. *Environ. Mutagen. Carcinogens*, *5*, 11-18

Civen, M., Leeb, J.E., Wishnow, R.M., Wolfsen, A. & Morin, R.J. (1980) Effects of low level administration of dichlorvos on adrenocorticotrophic hormone secretion, adrenal cholesteryl ester and steroid metabolism. *Biochem. Pharmacol.*, *29*, 635-641

Codex Committee on Pesticide Residues (1990) *Guide to Codex Maximum Limits for Pesticide Residues*, Part 2 (CAC/PR 2—1990; CCPR Pesticide Classification No. 120), The Hague

Collins, R.D. & deVries, D.M. (1973) Air concentrations and food residues from use of Shell's No-Pest® insecticide strip. *Bull. environ. Contam. Toxicol.*, *9*, 227-233

Collins, J.A., Schooley, M.A. & Singh, V.K. (1971) The effect of dietary dichlorvos on swine reproduction and viability of their offspring (Abstract No. 41). *Toxicol. appl. Pharmacol.*, *19*, 377

Cook, W.A., ed. (1987) *Occupational Exposure Limits—Worldwide*, Washington DC, American Industrial Hygiene Association, pp. 120, 136, 181

Dale, W.E., Miles, J.W. & Weathers, D.B. (1973) Measurements of residues of dichlorvos absorbed by food exposed during disinfection of aircraft. *J. agric. Food Chem.*, *21*, 858-860

Dambska, M., Iwanowski, L. & Kozłowski, P. (1979) The effect of transplacental intoxication with dichlorvos on the development of cerebral cortex in newborn rabbits. *Neuropathol. Pol.*, *17*, 571-576

Das, Y.T., Taskar, P.K., Brown, H.D. & Chattopadhyay, S.K. (1983) Exposure of professional pest control operator to dichlorvos (DDVP) and residue on house structures. *Toxicol. Lett.*, *17*, 95-99

Dean, B.J. (1972a) The mutagenic effects of organophosphorus pesticides on microorganisms. *Arch. Toxicol.*, *30*, 67-74

Dean, B.J. (1972b) The effect of dichlorvos on cultured human lymphocytes. *Arch. Toxicol.*, *30*, 75-78

Dean, B.J. & Blair, D. (1976) Dominant lethal assay in female mice after oral dosing with dichlorvos or exposure to atmospheres containing dichlorvos. *Mutat. Res.*, *40*, 67-72

Dean, B.J. & Thorpe, E. (1972a) Cytogenetic studies with dichlorvos in mice and Chinese hamsters. *Arch. Toxicol.*, *30*, 39-49

Dean, B.J. & Thorpe, E. (1972b) Studies with dichlorvos vapour in dominant lethal mutation tests in mice. *Arch. Toxicol.*, *30*, 51-59

Dean, B.J., Doak, S.M.A. & Funnell, J. (1972) Genetic studies with dichlorvos in the host-mediated assay and in liquid medium using *Saccharomyces cerevisiae*. *Arch. Toxicol.*, *30*, 61-66

Degraeve, N., Chollet, M.-C. & Moutschen, J. (1984a) Cytogenetic and genetic effects of subchronic treatments with organophosphorus insecticides. *Arch. Toxicol.*, *56*, 66-67

Degraeve, N., Chollet, M.-C. & Moutschen, J. (1984b) Cytogenetic effects induced by organophosphorus pesticides in mouse spermatocytes. *Toxicol. Lett.*, *21*, 315-319

Dési, I., Varga, L. & Farkas, I. (1978) Studies on the immunosuppressive effect of organochlorine and organophosphoric pesticides in subacute experiments. *J. Hyg. Epidemiol. Microbiol. Immunol.*, *22*, 115-122

Dési, I., Varga, L. & Farkas, I. (1980) The effect of DDVP, an organophosphorus pesticide on the humoral and cell-mediated immunity of rabbits. *Arch. Toxicol.*, *Suppl. 4*, 171-174

Deutsche Forschungsgemeinschaft (1989) *Maximum Concentrations at the Workplace and Biological Tolerance Values for Working Materials. 1989* (Report No. XXV), Weinheim, VCH Verlagsgesellschaft, p. 32 (in German)

Devadas, N., Rajam, M.V. & Subhash, K. (1986) Comparative mutagenicity of four organophosphorus insecticides in meiotic system of red pepper. *Cytologia*, *51*, 645-653

Dicowsky, L. & Morello, A. (1971) Glutathione-dependent degradation of 2,2-dichlorovinyl dimethyl phosphate (DDVP) by the rat. *Life Sci.*, *10*, 1031-1037

Durham, W.F., Gaines, T.B., McCauley, R.H., Jr, Sedlak, V.A., Mattson, A.M. & Hayes, W.J., Jr (1957) Studies on the toxicity of O,O-dimethyl-2,2-dichlorovinyl phosphate (DDVP). *Arch. ind. Health*, *15*, 340-349

Dyer, K.F. & Hanna, P.J. (1973) Comparative mutagenic activity and toxicity of triethylphosphate and dichlorvos in bacteria and *Drosophila*. *Mutat. Res.*, *21*, 175-177

Dzwonkowska, A. & Hübner, H. (1986) Induction of chromosomal aberrations in the Syrian hamster by insecticides tested *in vivo*. *Arch. Toxicol.*, *58*, 152-156

Elgar, K.E., Mathews, B.L. & Bosio, P. (1972a) Dichlorvos residues in food arising from the domestic use of dichlorvos PVC strips. *Pestic. Sci.*, *3*, 601-607

Elgar, K.E., Mathews, B.L. & Bosio, P. (1972b) Vapona strips in shops: residues in foodstuffs. *Environ. Qual. Saf.*, *1*, 217-221

Epstein, S.S., Arnold, E., Andrea, J., Bass, W. & Bishop, Y. (1972) Detection of chemical mutagens by the dominant lethal assay in the mouse. *Toxicol. appl. Pharmacol.*, *23*, 288-325

Eto, M. (1974) *Organophosphorus Pesticides: Organic and Biological Chemistry*, Cleveland, OH, CRC Press, Inc., p. 235

Fahrig, R. (1973) Evidence of a genetic action of organophosphorus insecticides (Ger.). *Naturwissenschaften*, *60*, 50-51

Fahrig, R. (1976) The effect of dose and time on the induction of genetic alterations in *Saccharomyces cerevisiae* by aminoacridines in the presence and absence of visible light irradiation in comparison with the dose-effect-curves of mutagens with other type of action. *Mol. gen. Genet.*, *144*, 131-140

FAO/WHO (1965) *Evaluation of the Toxicity of Pesticide Residues in Food* (FAO Meeting Report, No. PL/1965/10/1; WHO/Food Add./27.65), Rome

FAO/WHO (1967) *Evaluation of Some Pesticide Residues in Food* (FAO/PL:CP/15; WHO/Food Add./67.32), Rome

FAO/WHO (1968) *1967 Evaluations of Some Pesticide Residues in Food* (FAO/PL:1967/M/11/1; WHO/Food Add./68.30), Rome

FAO/WHO (1970) *1969 Evaluations of Some Pesticide Residues in Food* (FAO/PL/1969/M/17/1; WHO/Food Add./70.38), Rome

FAO/WHO (1971) *1970 Evaluations of Some Pesticide Residues in Food* (AGP: 1970/M/12/1; WHO/Food Add./71.42), Rome

FAO/WHO (1975) *1974 Evaluations of Some Pesticide Residues in Food* (WHO Pesticide Residues Series No. 4), Geneva

FAO/WHO (1978) *Pesticide Residues in Food: 1977 Evaluations* (FAO Plant Production and Protection Paper 10 Sup.), Rome

Frank, R., Braun, H.E. & Fleming, G. (1983) Organochlorine and organophosphorus residues in fat of bovine and porcine carcasses marketed in Ontario, Canada from 1969 to 1981. *J. Food Prot.*, *46*, 893-900

Gillenwater, H.B., Harein, P.K., Loy, E.W., Jr, Thompson, J.F., Laudani, H. & Eason, G. (1971) Dichlorvos applied as a vapor in a warehouse containing packaged foods. *J. stored Prod. Res.*, *7*, 45-56

Gillett, J.W., Harr, J.R., Lindstrom, F.T., Mount, D.A., St Clair, A.D. & Weber, L.J. (1972a) Evaluation of human health hazards on use of dichlorvos (DDVP), especially in resin strips. *Residue Rev.*, *44*, 115-159

Gillett, J.W., Harr, J.R., St Clair, A.D. & Weber, L.J. (1972b) Comment on the distinction between hazard and safety in evaluation of human health hazards on use of dichlorvos, especially in resin strips. *Residue Rev.*, *44*, 161-184

Gilot-Delhalle, J., Colizzi, A., Moutschen, J. & Moutschen-Dahmen, M. (1983) Mutagenicity of some organophosphorus compounds at the *ade*6 locus of *Schizosaccharomyces pombe*. *Mutat. Res.*, *117*, 139-148

Goh, K.S., Edmiston, S., Maddy, K.T. & Margetich, S. (1986a) Dissipation of dislodgeable foliar residue for chlorpyrifos and dichlorvos treated lawn: implication for safe entry. *Bull. environ. Contam. Toxicol.*, *37*, 33-40

Goh, K.S., Edmiston, S., Maddy, K.T., Meinders, D.D. & Margetich, S. (1986b) Dissipation of dislodgeable foliar residue of chlorpyrifos and dichlorvos on turf. *Bull. environ. Contam. Toxicol.*, *37*, 27-32

Gold, R.E., Holcslaw, T., Tupy, D. & Ballard, J.B. (1984) Dermal and respiratory exposure to applicators and occupants of residences treated with dichlorvos (DDVP). *J. econ. Entomol.*, *77*, 430-436

Government of Canada (1990) *Report on National Surveillance Data from 1984/85 to 1988/89*, Ottawa

Green, M.H.L., Medcalf, A.S.C., Arlett, C.F., Harcourt, S.A. & Lehmann, A.R. (1974) DNA strand breakage caused by dichlorvos, methyl methanesulfonate and iodoacetamide in *Escherichia coli* and cultured Chinese hamster cells. *Mutat. Res.*, *24*, 365-378

Green, M.H.L., Muriel, W.J. & Bridges, B.A. (1976) Use of a simplified fluctuation test to detect low levels of mutagens. *Mutat. Res.*, *38*, 33-42

Griffin, D.E., III & Hill, W.E. (1978) In vitro breakage of plasmid DNA by mutagens and pesticides. *Mutat. Res.*, *52*, 161-169

Grübner, P. (1972) Residue problems in the use of phosphoric acid ester insecticides in mushroom cultures (Ger.). *Nachrichtenbl. Pflanzenshutzdienst*, *26*, 245-247

Gupta, A.K. & Singh, J. (1974) Dichlorvos (DDVP) induced breaks in the salivary gland chromosomes of *Drosophila melanogaster*. *Curr. Sci.*, *43*, 661-662

Hanna, P.J. & Dyer, K.F. (1975) Mutagenicity of organophosphorus compounds in bacteria and *Drosophila*. *Mutat. Res.*, *28*, 405-420

Hass, D.K., Collins, J.A. & Kodama, J.K. (1972) Effects of orally administered dichlorvos in rhesus monkeys. *J. Am. vet. Med. Assoc.*, *161*, 714-719

Hayes, W.J. (1982) *Pesticides Studied in Man*, Baltimore, MD, Williams & Wilkins, pp. 348-351

Health and Welfare Canada (1990) *National Pesticide Residue Limits in Foods*, Ottawa, Bureau of Chemical Safety, Food Directorate, Health Protection Branch

Holmstedt, B., Nordgren, I., Sandoz, M. & Sundwall, A. (1978) Metrifonate. Summary of toxicological and pharmacological information available. *Arch. Toxicol.*, *41*, 3-29

Horn, K.-H., Teichmann, B. & Schramm, T. (1987) Investigation of dichlorvos (DDVP). I. Testing of dichlorvos for carcinogenic activity in mice (Ger.). *Arch. Geschwulstforsch.*, *57*, 353-360

Horn, K.-H., Teichmann, B., Schramm, T. & Nischan, P. (1988) Investigation of dichlorvos (DDVP). II. Testing of dichlorvos for carcinogenic activity in rats (Ger.). *Arch. Geschwulstforsch.*, *58*, 1-9

Houk, V.S. & DeMarini, D.M. (1987) Induction of prophage lambda by chlorinated pesticides. *Mutat. Res.*, *182*, 193-201

Hussey, N.W. & Hughes, J.T. (1964) Investigations on the use of dichlorvos in the control of the mushroom phorid, *Megaselia halterata* (Wood). *Ann. appl. Biol.*, *54*, 129-139

Hutson, D.H & Hoadley, E.C. (1972a) The comparative metabolism of [^{14}C-vinyl]dichlorvos in animals and man. *Arch. Toxikol.*, *30*, 9-18

Hutson, D.H. & Hoadley, E.C (1972b) The metabolism of [^{14}C-methyl]dichlorvos in the rat and the mouse. *Xenobiotica*, *2*, 107-116

Hutson, D.H., Hoadley, E.C. & Pickering, B.A. (1971) The metabolic fate of [vinyl-1-^{14}C]dichlorvos in the rat after oral and inhalational exposure. *Xenobiotica*, *6*, 593-611

IARC (1979a) *IARC Monographs on the Evaluation of the Carcinogenic Risk of Chemicals to Humans*, Vol. 20, *Some Halogenated Hydrocarbons*, Lyon, pp. 97-127

IARC (1979b) *IARC Monographs on the Evaluation of the Carcinogenic Risk of Chemicals to Humans*, Vol. 20, *Some Halogenated Hydrocarbons*, Lyon, pp. 259-281

IARC (1983a) *IARC Monographs on the Evaluation of the Carcinogenic Risk of Chemicals to Humans*, Vol. 30, *Miscellaneous Pesticides*, Lyon, pp. 207-231

IARC (1983b) *IARC Monographs on the Evaluation of the Carcinogenic Risk of Chemicals to Humans*, Vol. 30, *Miscellaneous Pesticides*, Lyon, pp. 103-129

IARC (1983c) *IARC Monographs on the Evaluation of the Carcinogenic Risk of Chemicals to Humans*, Vol. 30, *Miscellaneous Pesticides*, Lyon, pp. 183-195

IARC (1987a) *IARC Monographs on the Evaluation of Carcinogenic Risks to Humans*, Suppl. 7, *Overall Evaluations of Carcinogenicity: An Updating of* IARC Monographs *Volumes 1 to 42*, Lyon, pp. 202-203

IARC (1987b) *IARC Monographs on the Evaluation of Carcinogenic Risks to Humans*, Suppl. 7, *Overall Evaluations of Carcinogenicity: An Updating of* IARC Monographs *Volumes 1 to 42*, Lyon, p. 73

IARC (1987c) *IARC Monographs on the Evaluation of Carcinogenic Risks to Humans*, Suppl. 7, *Overall Evaluations of Carcinogenicity: An Updating of* IARC Monographs *Volumes 1 to 42*, Lyon, pp. 220-222

IARC (1987d) *IARC Monographs on the Evaluation of Carcinogenic Risks to Humans*, Suppl. 7, *Overall Evaluations of Carcinogenicity: An Updating of* IARC Monographs *Volumes 1 to 42*, Lyon, p. 65

IARC (1987e) *IARC Monographs on the Evaluation of Carcinogenic Risks to Humans*, Suppl. 7, *Overall Evaluations of Carcinogenicity: An Updating of* IARC Monographs *Volumes 1 to 42*, Lyon, p. 66

IARC (1987f) *IARC Monographs on the Evaluation of Carcinogenic Risks to Humans*, Suppl. 7, *Overall Evaluations of Carcinogenicity: An Updating of* IARC Monographs *Volumes 1 to 42*, Lyon, p. 70

Ishidate, M., Jr, Sofuni, T. & Yoshikawa, K. (1981) Chromosomal aberration tests *in vitro* as a primary screening tool for environmental mutagens and/or carcinogens. *Gann Monogr. Cancer Res.*, *27*, 95-108

Izmerov, N.P., ed. (1984) *International Register of Potentially Toxic Chemicals, Scientific Reviews of Soviet Literature on Toxicity and Hazards of Chemicals: DDVP* (Issue 79), Moscow, Centre of International Projects, United Nations Environment Programme

Jayasuriya, V.U. de S. & Ratnayake, W.E. (1973) Screening of some pesticides on *Drosophila melanogaster* for toxic and genetic effects. *Drosophila Inf. Serv., 50*, 184-186

Johnson, M.K. (1978) The anomalous behaviour of dimethyl phosphates in the biochemical test for delayed neurotoxicity. *Arch. Toxicol., 41*, 107-110

Johnson, M.K. (1981) Delayed neurotoxicity—do trichlorphon and/or dichlorvos cause delayed neuropathy in man or in test animals? *Acta pharmacol. toxicol., 49* (Suppl. V), 87-98

Johnson, R.D., Manske, D.D. & Podrebarac, D.S. (1981) Pesticide, metal and other chemical residues in adult total diet samples. XII. August 1975-July 1976. *Pestic. Monit. J., 15*, 54-69

Jones, K.H., Sanderson, D.M. & Noakes, D.N. (1968) Acute toxicity data for pesticides (1968). *World Rev. Pest. Control, 7*, 135-143

Kawachi, T., Komatsu, T., Kada, T., Ishidate, M., Sasaki, M., Sugiyama, T. & Tazima, Y. (1980) Results of recent studies on the relevance of various short-term screening tests in Japan. In: Williams, G.M., Kroes, R., Waaijers, H.W. & van de Poll, K.W., eds, *The Predictive Value of Short-term Screening Tests in Carcinogenicity Evaluation*, Amsterdam, Elsevier/North-Holland Biomedical Press, pp. 253-267

Kimbrough, R.D. & Gaines, T.B. (1968) Effect of organic phosphorus compounds and alkylating agents on the rat fetus. *Arch. environ. Health, 16*, 805-808

Kligerman, A.D., Erexson, G.L. & Wilmer, J.L. (1985) Induction of sister-chromatid exchange (SCE) and cell-cycle inhibition in mouse peripheral blood B lymphocytes exposed to mutagenic carcinogens *in vivo. Mutat. Res., 157*, 181-187

Kramers, P.G.N. & Knaap, A.G.A.C. (1978) Absence of a mutagenic effect after feeding dichlorvos to larvae of *Drosophila melanogaster. Mutat. Res., 57*, 103-105

Kurinnyi, A.I. (1975) Comparative study of the cytogenetic effect of certain organophosphorus pesticides (Russ.). *Genetika, 11*, 64-69

Lamoreaux, R.J. & Newland, L.W. (1978) The fate of dichlorvos in soil. *Chemosphere, 10*, 807-814

Latif, S., Haken, J.K. & Wainwright, M.S. (1984) Gas chromatographic analysis of insecticidal preparations using carbon dioxide propellants. *J. Chromatogr., 287*, 77-84

Lawley, P.D., Shah, S.A. & Orr, D.J. (1974) Methylation of nucleic acids by 2,2-dichlorovinyl dimethyl phosphate (dichlorvos, DDVP). *Chem.-biol. Interactions, 8*, 171-182

Lieberman, M.T. & Alexander, M. (1983) Microbial and nonenzymatic steps in the decomposition of dichlorvos. *J. agric. Food Chem., 31*, 265-167

Lin, S.Y., Lee, T.C., Cheng, C.S. & Wang, T.C. (1988) Cytotoxicity, sister-chromatid exchange, chromosome aberration and transformation induced by 2,2-dichlorovinyl-*O,O*-dimethyl phosphate. *Mutat. Res., 206*, 439-445

Löfroth, G. (1970) Alkylation of DNA by dichlorvos. *Naturwissenschaften, 57*, 393-394

Löfroth, G. (1978) The mutagenicity of dichloroacetaldehyde. *Z. Naturforsch., 33*, 783-785

Löfroth, G., Kim, C. & Hussain, S. (1969) Alkylating property of 2,2-dichlorovinyl dimethyl phosphate: a disregarded hazard. *EMS News Lett., 2*, 21-26

Ma, T.-H., Harris, M.M., Anderson, V.A., Ahmed, I., Mohammad, K., Bare, J.L. & Lin, G. (1984) *Tradescantia*-micronucleus (Trad-MCN) tests on 140 health-related agents. *Mutat. Res., 138*, 157-167

Marcos, R., Andreu, H., Velásquez, A., Xamena, N. & Creus, A. (1989) Induction of polygenic mutations affecting viability in *Drosophila* after dichlorvos and malathion treatments. *Genét. Ibér.*, *41*, 147-159

Mathias, C.G.T. (1983) Persistent contact dermatitis from the insecticide dichlorvos. *Contact Derm.*, *9*, 217-218

Matsumura, F. & Boush, G.M. (1968) Degradation of insecticides by a soil fungus *Trichoderma viride*. *J. econ. Entomol.*, *61*, 610-612

Meister, R.T., ed. (1990) *Farm Chemicals Handbook '90*, Willoughby, OH, Meister Publishing Co., pp. C91-C92

Menz, M., Luetkemeier, H. & Sachsse, K. (1974) Long-term exposure of factory workers to dichlorvos (DDVP) insecticide. *Arch. environ. Health*, *28*, 72-76

Mirsalis, J.C., Tyson, C.K., Steinmetz, K.L., Loh, E.K., Hamilton, C.M., Bakke, J.P. & Spalding, J.W. (1989) Measurement of unscheduled DNA synthesis and S-phase synthesis in rodent hepatocytes following in vivo treatment: testing of 24 compounds. *Environ. mol. Mutagenesis*, *14*, 155-164

Mohn, G. (1973) 5-Methyltryptophan resistance mutations in *Escherichia coli* K-12. Mutagenic activity of monofunctional alkylating agents including organophosphorus insecticides. *Mutat. Res.*, *20*, 7-15

Moriya, M., Kato, K. & Shirasu, Y. (1978) Effects of cysteine and a liver metabolic activation system on the activities of mutagenic pesticides. *Mutat. Res.*, *57*, 259-263

Moriya, M., Ohta, T., Watanabe, K., Miyazawa, T., Kato, K. & Shirasu, Y. (1983) Further mutagenicity studies on pesticides in bacterial reversion assay systems. *Mutat. Res.*, *116*, 185-216

Morpurgo, G., Aulicino, F., Bignami, M., Conti, L., Velcich, A. & Montalenti, S.G. (1977) Relationship between structure and mutagenicity of dichlorvos and other pesticides. *Accad. naz. Lincei Rend. Cl. Sci. fis. mat. nat.*, *62*, 692-701

Morpurgo, G., Bellincampi, D., Gualandi, G., Baldinelli, L. & Crescenzi, O.S. (1979) Analysis of mitotic nondisjunction with *Aspergillus nidulans*. *Environ. Health Perspect.*, *31*, 81-95

Moutschen-Dahmen, J., Moutschen-Dahmen, M. & Degraeve, N. (1981) Metrifonate and dichlorvos: cytogenetic investigations. *Acta pharmacol. toxicol.*, *49*, 29-39

Nagy, Z., Mile, I. & Antoni, F. (1975) The mutagenic effect of pesticides on *Escherichia coli* WP2 try⁻. *Acta microbiol. acad. sci. hung.*, *22*, 309-314

Nicholas, A.H., Vienne, M. & Van den Berghe, H. (1978) Sister chromatid exchange frequencies in cultured human cells exposed to an organophosphorus insecticide: dichlorvos. *Toxicol. Lett.*, 2, 271-275

Nishio, A. & Uyeki, E.M. (1981) Induction of sister chromatid exchanges in Chinese hamster ovary cells by organophosphate insecticides and their oxygen analogs. *J. Toxicol. environ. Health*, *8*, 939-946

Page, A.C., Loeffler, J.E., Hendrickson, H.R., Huston, C.K & DeVries, D.M. (1972) Metabolic fate of dichlorvos in swine. *Arch. Toxikol.*, *30*, 19-27

Paik, S.G. & Lee, S.Y. (1977) Genetic effects of pesticides in the mammalian cells. I. Induction of micronucleus. *Korean J. Zool.*, *20*, 19-28

Panda, B.B. & Sharma, C.B.S.R. (1979) Organophosphate induced chlorophyl mutations in *Hordeum vulgare*. *Theor. appl. Genet.*, *55*, 253-255

Perocco, P. & Fini, A. (1980) Damage by dichlorvos of human lymphocyte DNA. *Tumori*, *66*, 425-430

Porter, P.E. (1964) Vapona insecticide (DDVP). In: Zweig, G., ed., *Analytical Methods for Pesticides, Plant Growth Regulators, and Food Additives*, Vol. II, *Insecticides*, New York, Academic Press, pp. 561-579

Potter, J.C., Boyer, A.C., Marxmiller, R.L., Young, R. & Loeffler, J.E. (1973) Radioisotopic residues and residues of dichlorvos and its metabolites in pregnant sows and their progeny dosed with dichlorvos-^{14}C or dichlovos-^{36}Cl formulated as PVC pellets. *J. agric. Food Chem.*, 21, 734-738

Ramel, C., Drake, J. & Sugimura, T. (1980) ICPEMC Publication No. 5. An evaluation of the genetic toxicity of dichlorvos. *Mutat. Res.*, 76, 297-309

Rao, B.V., Sharma, C.B.S.R. & Rao, B.G.S. (1987) Cytological effects of organophosphorus insecticides on *Allium cepa* root-meristems. *Cytologia*, 52, 365-371

Reeves, J.D., Driggers, D.A. & Kiley, V.A. (1981) Household insecticide associated aplastic anaemia and acute leukaemia in children. *Lancet*, ii, 300-301

Rosenkranz, H.S. (1973) Preferential effect of dichlorvos (Vapona) on bacteria deficient in DNA polymerase. *Cancer Res.*, 33, 458-459

Royal Society of Chemistry (1986) *European Directory of Agrochemical Products*, Vol. 3, *Insecticides, Acaricides, Nematicides*, Cambridge, pp. 198-212

Sadtler Research Laboratories (1980) *The Sadtler Standard Spectra, 1980, Cumulative Index*, Philadelphia, PA

Santodonato, J., Bosch, S., Meylan, W., Becker, J. & Neal, M. (1985) *Monograph on Human Exposure to Chemicals in the Workplace: Dichlorvos* (US NTIS PB86-148343), Washington DC, US National Technical Information Service

Sasaki, M., Sugimura, K., Yoshida, M.A. & Abe, S. (1980) Cytogenetic effects of 60 chemicals on cultured human and Chinese hamster cells. *Kromosomo II*, 20, 574-584

Schairer, L.A., Van't Hof, J., Hayes, C.G., Burton, R.M. & de Serres, F.J. (1978) Measurement of biological activity of ambient air mixtures using a mobile laboratory for *in situ* exposures: preliminary results from the *Tradescantia* plant test system. In: Waters, M.D., Nesnow, S., Huisingh, J.L., Sandhu, S.S. & Claxton, L., eds, *Application of Short-term Bioassays in the Fractionation and Analysis of Complex Environmental Mixtures* (EPA-600/9-78-027), Research Triangle Park, NC, US Environmental Protection Agency, pp. 421-440

Schwetz, B.A., Ioset, H.D., Leong, B.K.J. & Staples, R.E. (1979) Teratogenic potential of dichlorvos given by inhalation and gavage to mice and rabbits. *Teratology*, 20, 383-388

Segerbäck, D. (1981) Estimation of genetic risks of alkylating agents. V. Methylation of DNA in the mouse by DDVP (2,2-dichlorovinyl dimethyl phosphate). *Hereditas*, 94, 73-76

Segerbäck, D. & Ehrenberg, L. (1981) Alkylating properties of dichlorvos (DDVP). *Acta pharmacol. toxicol.*, 49 (Suppl. V), 56-66

Sharma, C.B.S.R., Panda, B.B., Behera, B.N. & Rao, R.N. (1983) Progeny testing in barley for monitoring environmental mutagens. In: Sinha, R.P. & Sinha, U., eds, *Current Approaches in Cytogenetics*, Patna, Delhi, Spectrum Publishing, pp. 245-255

Shirasu, Y., Moriya, M., Kato, K., Furuhashi, A. & Kada, T. (1976) Mutagenicity screening of pesticides in the microbial system. *Mutat. Res.*, 40, 19-30

Shirasu, Y., Moriya, M., Tezuka, H., Teramoto, S., Ohta, T. & Inoue, T. (1984) Mutagenicity of pesticides. *Environ. Sci. Res.*, 31, 617-624

Singh, R.M., Singh, A.K., Singh, R.B., Singh, J. & Singh, B.D. (1980) Chlorophyll mutations induced by seed treatment with certain insecticides in barley *Hordeum vulgare*. *Indian J. exp. Biol.*, 18, 1396-1397

Slomka, M.B. & Hine, C.H. (1981) Clinical pharmacology of dichlorvos. *Acta pharmacol. toxicol.*, *49* (Suppl. V), 105-108

Sobels, F.H. & Todd, N.K. (1979) Absence of a mutagenic effect of dichlorvos in *Drosophila melanogaster*. *Mutat. Res.*, *67*, 89-92

Stanton, H.C., Albert, J.R. & Mersmann, H.J. (1979) Studies on the pharmacology and safety of dichlorvos in pigs and pregnant sows. *Am. J. vet. Res.*, *40*, 315-320

Tezuka, H., Ando, N., Suzuki, R., Terahata, M., Moriya, M. & Shirasu, Y. (1980) Sister-chromatid exchanges and chromosomal aberrations in cultured Chinese hamster cells treated with pesticides positive in microbial reversion assays. *Mutat. Res.*, *78*, 177-191

Thorpe, E., Wilson, A.B., Dix, K.M. & Blair, D. (1972) Teratological studies with dichlorvos vapour in rabbits and rats. *Arch. Toxicol.*, *30*, 29-38

Tinker, J. (1972) The Vapona dossier. *New Sci.*, *53*, 489-492

Tu, A., Hallowell, W., Pallotta, S., Sivak, A., Lubet, R.A., Curren, R.D., Avery, M.D., Jones, C., Sedita, B.A., Huberman, E., Tennant, R., Spalding, J. & Kouri, R.E. (1986) An interlaboratory comparison of transformation in Syrian hamster embryo cells with model and coded chemicals. *Environ. Mutagenesis*, *8*, 77-98

US Environmental Protection Agency (1980) *Preliminary Quantitative Usage Analysis of DDVP*, Washington DC, Office of Pesticide Programs

US Environmental Protection Agency (1986) Method 8140. Organophosphorus pesticides. In: *Test Methods for Evaluating Solid Waste—Physical/Chemical Methods*, 3rd ed. (US EPA Publ. No. SW-846), Washington DC, Office of Solid Waste and Emergency Response

US Environmental Protection Agency (1987) *Guidance for the Reregistration of Pesticide Products Containing DDVP as the Active Ingredient*, Washington DC, Office of Pesticide Programs, p. 132

US Environmental Protection Agency (1988a) Method TO-10. Method for the determination of organochlorine pesticides in ambient air using low volume polyurethane foam (PUF) sampling with gas chromatography/electron capture detector (GC/ECD). In: *Compendium of Methods for the Determination of Toxic Organic Compounds in Ambient Air* (US EPA Report No. EPA-600/4-89-017; US NTIS PB90-116989), Research Triangle Park, NC, Atmospheric Research and Exposure Assessment Laboratory

US Environmental Protection Agency (1988b) Method 507. Determination of nitrogen- and phosphorus-containing pesticides in water by gas chromatography with a nitrogen-phosphorus detector. In: *Methods for the Determination of Organic Compounds in Drinking Water* (USA EPA Report No. EPA-600/4-88-039; US NTIS PB89-220461), Cincinnati, OH, Environmental Monitoring Systems Laboratory, pp. 143-170

US Environmental Protection Agency (1989a) 2,2-Dichlorovinyl dimethyl phosphate; tolerances for residues. Part 180—Tolerances and exemptions from tolerances for pesticide chemicals in or on raw agricultural commodities. *US Code fed. Regul.*, *Title 40*, Part 180.235, pp. 370-371

US Environmental Protection Agency (1989b) 2,2-Dichlorovinyl dimethyl phosphate. Part 185—Tolerances for pesticides in food. *US Code fed. Regul.*, *Title 40*, Part 185.1900, p. 476

US Food and Drug Administration (1989a) Naled. In: *Pesticide Analytical Manual*, Vol. II, *Methods Which Detect Multiple Residues*, Washington DC, US Department of Health and Human Services

US Food and Drug Administration (1989b) 2,2-Dichlorovinyl dimethyl phosphate. In: *Pesticide Analytical Manual*, Vol. II, *Methods Which Detect Multiple Residues*, US Department of Health and Human Services

US National Cancer Institute (1977) *Bioassay of Dichlorvos for Possible Carcinogenicity* (Carcinogenesis Technical Report Series No. 10; DHEW Publ. No. (NIH) 77-810), Washington DC, US Government Printing Office

US National Institute for Occupational Safety and Health (1979) *NIOSH Manual of Analytical Methods*, Vol. 5, *Dichlorvos P&CAM 295* (DHEW (NIOSH) Publ. No. 79-141), 2nd ed., Cincinnati, OH, US Department of Health, Education, and Welfare, pp. 295-1–295-10

US National Toxicology Program (1989) *Toxicology and Carcinogenesis Studies of Dichlorvos (CAS No. 62-73-7) in F344/N Rats and B6C3F1 Mice (Gavage Studies)* (NTP Technical Report 342; NIH Publ. No. 89-2598), Research Triangle Park, NC

US Occupational Safety and Health Administration (1989) Air contaminants—permissible exposure limits. *US Code fed. Regul., Title 29*, Part 1910.1000

Vevai, E.J. (1974) Know your pesticide, its salient points and uses in pest control. 5. Dichlorvos. *Pesticides, 8* 15-23

Vigliani, E.C. (1971) Exposure of newborn babies to *Vapona®* insecticide (Abstract No. 48). *Toxicol. appl. Pharmacol., 19*, 379-380

Vogin, E.E., Carson, S. & Slomka, M.B. (1971) Teratology studies with dichlorvos in rabbits (Abstract No. 42). *Toxicol. appl. Pharmacol., 19*, 377-378

Voogd, C.E., Jacobs, J.J.J.A.A. & van der Stel, J.J. (1972) On the mutagenic action of dichlorvos. *Mutat. Res., 16*, 413-416

Wagner, R. & Hoyer, J. (1975) Methods employed in determining workplace concentrations and occupational hygienic conditions during and after hot spraying of pesticides in greenhouses (Ger.). *Z. ges. Hyg., 21*, 18-20

Wennerberg, R. & Löfroth, G. (1974) Formation of 7-methylguanine by dichlorvos in bacteria and mice. *Chem.-biol. Interactions, 8*, 339-348

WHO (1967) *Specifications for Pesticides Used in Public Health*, Geneva, pp. 69-75

WHO (1985) *Specifications for Pesticides Used in Public Health*, 6th ed., Geneva, pp. 163-168

WHO (1989) *Dichlorvos* (Environmental Health Criteria 79), Geneva

Wild, D. (1973) Chemical induction of streptomycin-resistant mutations in *Escherichia coli*: dose and mutagenic effects of dichlorvos and methyl methanesulfonate. *Mutat. Res., 19*, 33-41

Williams, S., ed. (1984) *Official Methods of Analysis of the Association of Official Analytical Chemists*, 14th ed., Washington DC, Association of Official Analytical Chemists, pp. 126-127

Witherup, S., Jolley, W.J., Stemmer, K. & Pfitzer, E.A. (1971) Chronic toxicity studies with 2,2-dichlorovinyl dimethyl phosphate (DDVP) in dogs and rats including observations on rat reproduction (Abstract No. 40). *Toxicol. appl. Pharmacol., 19*, 377

Wooder, M.F. & Wright, A.S. (1981) Alkylation of DNA by organophosphorus pesticides. *Acta pharmacol. toxicol., 49* (Suppl. V), 51-55

Wooder, M.F., Wright, A.S. & King, L.J. (1977) In vivo alkylation studies with dichlorvos at practical use concentrations. *Chem.-biol. Interactions, 19*, 25-46

Worthing, C.R. & Walker, S.B., eds (1987) *The Pesticide Manual—A World Compendium*, 8th ed., Thornton Heath, British Crop Protection Council, pp. 269-270

Wright, C.G. & Leidy, R.B. (1980) Air samples in vehicles and buildings turn up only very low levels of organic phosphate insecticides. *Pest Control, 48*, 22, 24, 26, 68

Wright, A.S., Hutson, D.H. & Wooder, M.F. (1979) The chemical and biochemical reactivity of dichlorvos. *Arch. Toxicol., 42*, 1-18

Wyrobek, A.J. & Bruce, W.R. (1975) Chemical induction of sperm abnormalities in mice. *Proc. natl Acad. Sci. USA, 72*, 4425-4429

Zeiger, E., Anderson, B., Haworth, S., Lawlor, T. & Mortelmans, K. (1988) *Salmonella* mutagenicity tests: IV. Results from the testing of 300 chemicals. *Environ. mol. Mutagenesis, 11* (Suppl. 12), 1-158

Zotov, V.M., Svirin, J.N. & Prucakova, R.M. (1977) The development of health regulations for occupational exposure in greenhouses treated with chemical pesticides (Russ.). *Gig. Tr. prof. Zabol., 3,* 49-50

FENVALERATE

1. Exposure Data

1.1 Chemical and physical data

Fenvalerate is a mixture of four stereoisomers (RR, RS, SR, SS) due to the two asymmetric carbon atoms in the molecule. It has an α-cyanogroup on the 3-phenoxybenzyl alcohol and is a type II pyrethroid. The SS stereoisomer is the most biologically active and is sold as esfenvalerate.

1.1.1 *Synonyms, structural and molecular data*

Fenvalerate

Chem. Abstr. Serv. Reg. No.: 51630-58-1
Chem. Abstr. Name: 4-Chloro-α-(1-methylethyl)benzeneacetic acid, cyano(3-phenoxyphenyl)methyl ester
IUPAC Systematic Name: (RS)-α-Cyano-3-phenoxybenzyl (RS)-2-(4-chlorophenyl)-3-methylbutyrate
Synonyms: α-Cyano-3-phenoxybenzyl 2-(4-chlorophenyl)isovalerate; α-cyano-3-phenoxybenzyl α-(4-chlorophenyl)isovalerate; α-cyano-3-phenoxybenzyl isopropyl-4-chlorophenylacetate; cyano(3-phenoxyphenyl)methyl 4-chloro-α-(1-methylethyl)benzeneacetate; OMS 2000

Fenvalerate β

Chem. Abstr. Serv. Reg. No.: 66267-77-4
Chem. Abstr. Name: (R-(R*,S*))-4-Chloro-α-(1-methylethyl) benzeneacetic acid, cyano(3-phenoxyphenyl)methyl ester
IUPAC Systematic Name: (R)-α-Cyano-3-phenoxybenzyl (S)-2-(4-chlorophenyl)-3-methylbutyrate
Synonyms: Fenvalerate β; Fenvalerate Aβ; S 5602Aβ

Esfenvalerate

Chem. Abstr. Serv. Reg. No.: 66230-04-4
Replaced CAS Reg. No.: 72650-28-3
Chem. Abstr. Name: (S-(R*,R*))-4-Chloro-α-(1-methylethyl) benzeneacetic acid, cyano(3-phenoxyphenyl)methyl ester
IUPAC Systematic Name: (S)-α-Cyano-3-phenoxybenzyl (S)-2-(4-chlorophenyl)-3-methylbutyrate

Synonyms: (S)-α-Cyano-3-phenoxybenzyl (S)-2-(4-chlorophenyl)isovalerate; fenvalerate α; fenvalerate Aα; OMS 3023

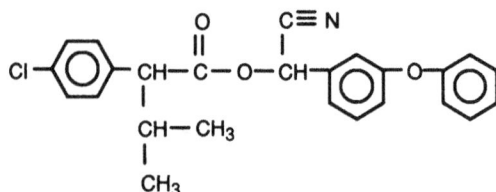

$$Cl-\langle\bigcirc\rangle-\underset{\underset{CH_3}{\overset{\displaystyle |}{CH-CH_3}}}{\overset{\displaystyle |}{CH}}-\overset{\overset{\displaystyle O}{||}}{C}-O-\underset{}{\overset{\overset{\displaystyle C\equiv N}{|}}{CH}}\langle\bigcirc\rangle-O-\langle\bigcirc\rangle$$

$C_{25}H_{22}ClNO_3$ Mol. wt: 419.91

1.1.2 *Chemical and physical properties*

Fenvalerate

(a) *Description*: Viscous yellow or brown liquid, sometimes partly crystalline at room temperature (Worthing & Walker, 1987; WHO, 1990)

(b) *Boiling-point*: 300°C at 37 mm Hg [4.9 kPa] (WHO, 1990)

(c) *Density*: 1.175 (25/25°C) (Worthing & Walker, 1987)

(d) *Solubility*: Slightly soluble in water (< 1 mg/l at 20°C); readily soluble in most organic solvents (acetone, chloroform, cyclohexanone, ethanol, xylene; all > 1 kg/kg at 23°C) (Worthing & Walker, 1987; Royal Society of Chemistry, 1989)

(e) *Volatility*: Vapour pressure, 2.8×10^{-7} mm Hg [0.37×10^{-7} kPa] at 25°C (Royal Society of Chemistry, 1989; WHO, 1990)

(f) *Stability*: Stable to light, heat and moisture; relatively stable in acidic media, but rapidly hydrolysed in alkaline media, with optimal stability at pH 4 (Worthing & Walker, 1987; Royal Society of Chemistry, 1989; WHO, 1990)

(g) *Octanol/water partition coefficient (P)*: log P, 6.2 (WHO, 1990)

(h) *Half-time*: Four to 15 days (natural water); eight to 14 days (on plants); one to 18 days (on soil); 15 days to three months (in soil) (WHO, 1990)

(i) *Conversion factor for airborne concentrations*[1]: mg/m^3 = 17.17 × ppm

Esfenvalerate

(a) *Description*: White crystalline solid (Budavari, 1989)

(b) *Melting-point*: 59-60.2°C (Budavari, 1989)

(c) *Solubility*: Practically insoluble in water; soluble in most organic solvents (acetone, acetonitrile, chloroform, dimethyl formamide, dimethyl sulfoxide, ethyl acetate, ethyl cellosolve, α-methylnaphthalene, xylene); slightly soluble in n-hexane, kerosene and methanol (Budavari, 1989; Royal Society of Chemistry, 1989)

(d) *Volatility*: Vapour pressure, 5×10^{-7} mm Hg [0.67×10^{-7} kPa] at 25°C (Budavari, 1989)

---

[1]Calculated from: mg/m^3 = (molecular weight/24.45) × ppm, assuming standard temperature (25°C) and pressure (760 mm Hg [101.3 kPa])

(e) *Stability*: Stable at normal temperatures; incompatible with alkaline substances such as soda ash and lye (Du Pont, 1988a)

(f) *Octanol/water partition coefficient (P)*: log P, 4.42 (Verschueren, 1983)

1.1.3 *Trade names, technical products and impurities*

Some trade names include:

Fenvalerate: Aqmatrine; Belmark; Ectrin; Evercide 2362; Fenkill; Fenval; Phenvalerate; Pydrin®; S-5602; Sanmarton; SD 43775; Sumibac; Sumicidin; Sumifleece; Sumifly; Sumipower; Sumitick; Sumitox; WL 43775

Esfenvalerate: Asana; Halmark; S-1844; S 5602Aα; Sumi-alfa; Sumi-alpha; Sumicidin Aα

Fenvalerate is a synthetic pyrethroid with no cyclopropane ring in the molecule. Technical-grade fenvalerate is 90-94% pure and consists of equal portions of the four stereoisomers (RR, RS, SR, SS). It may be formulated as emulsifiable concentrates, ultra-low volume concentrates, dusts or wettable powders (WHO, 1990).

Fenvalerate formulations currently registered in the USA, Europe and India are emulsifiable concentrates (Royal Society of Chemistry, 1986; Du Pont, 1988b; E.I. duPont de Nemours & Co., 1988a, 1989a; Roussel Bio Corp., 1989; All India Medical Corp., undated). Xylene (see IARC, 1989) may be present in the concentrates (E.I. duPont de Nemours & Co., 1988a).

Esfenvalerate is available in the USA as a technical-grade product with a purity of 75%. It is formulated in the USA as an emulsifiable concentrate (Du Pont, 1988a; E.I. duPont de Nemours & Co., Inc., 1988b,c, 1989b,c; Du Pont, 1990). The concentrate may contain xylene (E.I. duPont de Nemours & Co., Inc., 1988b,c, 1989b,c) or ethylbenzene (DuPont, 1990).

Fenvalerate is also formulated in combination with oxydemeton-methyl (Royal Society of Chemistry, 1986).

1.1.4 *Analysis*

Selected methods for the analysis of fenvalerate in various matrices are given in Table 1. Residues and environmental samples of fenvalerate can be analysed by gas chromatography with electron capture detection, with a minimum detection level of 0.005 mg/kg; products can be analysed by gas chromatography with flame ionization detection (WHO, 1990). Additional methods for formulation and residue analysis have been reviewed (Baker & Bottomley, 1982; Papadopoulou-Mourkidou, 1983; Shell Development Co., 1984).

A method has been described that allows detection of the presence of fenvalerate (as its separate diastereoisomers) in commercially available insecticidal preparations using high-pressure liquid chromatography with a normal-phase system (Mourot *et al.*, 1979). A gas chromatographic method is available for determination of the chemical purity and diastereoisomers of fenvalerate (Horiba *et al.*, 1980), and a gas chromatographic method for the determination of esfenvalerate in technical preparations has been described (Sakaue *et al.*, 1987).

Table 1. Methods for the analysis of fenvalerate

Sample matrix	Sample preparation	Assay procedure[a]	Limit of detection	Reference
Animal tissues, crops (oily)	Extract with hexane:isopropanol (3:1); remove isopropanol by water partitioning; partition with acetonitrile; exchange to hexane; clean-up on Florisil column	GC/ECD	0.01 ppm (mg/kg)	US Food and Drug Administration (1989)
Cream, milk, milk fat	Extract with dichloromethane; extract solids with acetone; exchange to hexane; combine hexane and dichloromethane extracts; remove solvent; solubilize fat with hexane and partition with acetonitrile; wash with hexane; backwash with acetonitrile; combine acetonitrile extracts and dilute with sodium chloride; extract with hexane; concentrate; clean-up on Florisil column	GC/ECD	Not reported	US Food and Drug Administration (1989)
Crops (non-oily)	Extract with hexane:isopropanol (3:1); remove isopropanol by water partitioning; exchange to hexane; clean-up on Florisil column	GC/ECD	0.01 ppm (mg/kg)	US Food and Drug Administration (1989)
Eggs	Extract with hexane:acetonitrile; wash acetonitrile phase with hexane; backwash with acetonitrile; combine acetonitrile extracts and dilute with sodium chloride; extract with hexane; concentrate; clean-up on Florisil column	GC/ECD	Not reported	US Food and Drug Administration (1989)
Formulations	Dissolve in hexane; filter; analyse directly	HPLC/UV	Not reported	Papadopoulou-Mourkidou (1985)
Gauze patches	Extract with acetone:hexane (1:1); evaporate to dryness; dissolve residue in hexane; clean-up on Florisil column	GC/ECD	Not reported	US Food and Drug Administration (1989)
Hair	Extract with 5% (v/v) ethyl acetate in hexane; inject directly	GC/ECD	Not reported	US Food and Drug Administration (1989)
Soil	Extract by high frequency vibration in acetone:hexane (1:1); exchange to hexane; clean-up on Florisil column	GC/ECD	0.01 ppm (mg/kg)	US Food and Drug Administration (1989)
Water	Extract by partitioning with hexane; clean-up on Florisil column	GC/ECD	0.05 ppm (mg/l)	US Food and Drug Administration (1989)

[a]Abbreviations: GC/ECD, gas-liquid chromatography/electron capture detection; HPLC/UV, high performance liquid chromatography/ultraviolet detection

1.2 Production and use

1.2.1 *Production*

Fenvalerate was first marketed in 1976. Approximately 1000 tonnes were produced annually worldwide in 1979-83 (WHO, 1990); annual production is now believed to be about 2000 tonnes. The history of the development, manufacture and commercialization of fenvalerate has been reviewed in detail (Yoshioka, 1978; Rogosheske *et al.*, 1982; Yoshioka, 1985). It is produced currently in India, Japan, the United Kingdom and the USA (Meister, 1990).

Fenvalerate can be prepared by esterification of 3-phenoxybenzaldehyde cyanohydrin with 2-(4-chlorophenyl)isovaleroyl chloride, or by condensation of 3-phenoxy-α-halobenzyl cyanide with the isovaleric acid in the presence of a base such as potassium carbonate. More conveniently, fenvalerate can be provided by the Francis reaction using the isovaleroyl chloride, the aldehyde and sodium cyanide.

The most active isomer, esfenvalerate, can be derived from (S)-2-(4-chlorophenyl)-isovaleroyl chloride and (S)-3-phenoxymandelic acid. It can be prepared most efficiently, however, from the (R,S) alcohol ester of the (S) acid through preferential precipitation (Yoshioka, 1978).

1.2.2 *Use*

Fenvalerate is a highly active contact insecticide that is effective against a wide range of pests, including strains resistant to organochlorine, organophosphorus and carbamate insecticides (Worthing & Walker, 1987). It is used mainly in agriculture, with about 90% used on cotton. It is also used on other crops, such as vines, tomatoes, potatoes, pomes, other fruit and a wide variety of other crops (WHO, 1990). It is also used in public health and animal husbandry, e.g., for controlling flies in cattle sheds (Worthing & Walker, 1987).

It is used in homes and gardens for insect control and around the foundations of buildings to control termites and carpenter ants (Roussel Bio Corp., 1989; WHO, 1990).

1.3 Occurrence

1.3.1 *Food*

Of a total of 946 samples analysed in the 1984-89 Canadian national surveillance programme, seven were found to contain fenvalerate residues, at levels of 0.02-0.096 mg/kg. Most were in pears (6/114 samples) and one in lettuce (1/11 samples) (Government of Canada, 1990). In Sweden, 163 of 165 samples of imported fruit and vegetables contained residues up to 0.2 mg/kg; one had a residue of 0.54 mg/kg (FAO/WHO, 1985)

Of 19 851 food and feed samples analysed in the USA during 1982-86, only 25 had fenvalerate residues; one sample had a level of 1 mg/kg, and the rest were lower (Luke *et al.*, 1988).

In stored grain treated with 1 mg/kg, over 70% of an applied dose remained in wheat after 10 months. White bread contained the same residue levels as the white flour from which it was prepared (WHO, 1990).

When fenvalerate was applied to peanuts in the USA at rates up to 0.45 kg active ingredient/ha, the residues in whole nuts were < 0.1 mg/kg; those in nut meat did not exceed the detection limit of 0.01 mg/kg (FAO/WHO, 1982).

Trials in the USA and Canada on lettuce, spinach, celery and Brassica vegetables showed residue levels of less than 1 mg/kg seven days after treatment at rates of 0.05-0.45 kg/ha. In cabbage, the maximum residue seven days or more after application was 4.3 mg/kg for an application rate of 0.45 kg/ha. Treatments with 0.45 and 0.22 kg/ha fenvalerate gave residue levels of 4.3 and 1.7 mg/kg, respectively, in lettuce (FAO/WHO, 1982).

In apples, following application at rates up to 1.12 kg/ha, residues at day 0 or after were < 2.0 mg/kg. In another trial in the USA, residues of 2.2 mg/kg were found after 42 days following four treatments with 0.67 kg/ha. The residue found in pears in the USA was 4.3 mg/kg 20 days after a second treatment of 0.45 kg/ha. In other countries, residues in pears did not exceed 2 mg/kg 14 days after treatment (FAO/WHO, 1982).

Grapes treated in the USA, Canada and Japan at rates up to 0.22 kg/ha generally contained residues of less than 1 mg/kg 14 days after application; the maximum residue found was 3.8 mg/kg. Wine made from grapes containing up to 3.44 mg/kg fenvalerate contained no detectable residue seven days after treatment (FAO/WHO, 1982).

Apples treated with fenvalerate were processed into apple sauce, juice, pomace and peels plus cores. The sauce and juice contained essentially no residue; whole apples contained about 0.4 ppm (mg/kg), pomace contained about 2 ppm (mg/kg) and peels plus cores, 1.5 ppm (mg/kg) (Spittler et al., 1982).

Fenvalerate-treated tomatoes were processed into chopped fresh tomatoes, canned quarters, juice, paste and by-product skins and seeds. The fresh produce contained 0.26 ppm (mg/kg) and skins and seeds, 1.9 ppm (mg/kg). Residues averaged 0.12 ppm (mg/kg) in the paste but were barely detectable in other products (Spittler et al., 1984).

1.3.2 Occupational exposure

At a fenvalerate packing plant in China, workers were reported to be exposed to 12-55 $\mu g/m^3$ in the air, with resulting skin contact (He et al., 1988).

1.4 Regulations and guidelines

Maximum residue levels have been established by the Codex Alimentarius Commission for fenvalerate (fat-soluble residue) in or on the following agricultural commodities (in mg/kg): alfalfa fodder, 20; kale, 10; Brussels' sprouts, kiwifruit, peaches and wheat bran (unprocessed), 5; cabbages (head), 3; broccoli, cauliflower, celery, cereal grains, cherries, citrus fruit, lettuce (head), pome fruit and wheat wholemeal, 2; beans (except broad and soya beans), berries and other small fruit, Chinese cabbage (pak-choi), meat (fat) and tomatoes, 1; squash (summer, winter), sweet peppers and watermelon, 0.5; cotton seed, cucumbers, melons (except watermelon), tree nuts and wheat flour, 0.2; beans (shelled), cotton-seed oil (crude, edible), milks, peanuts (whole), peas (shelled), soya beans (dried), sunflower seeds and sweet maize (on-the-cob), 0.1; vegetables (root, tuber), 0.05; edible offal (mammalian), 0.02 (Codex Committee on Pesticide Residues, 1990).

Fenvalerate was evaluated by the Joint Meeting of the FAO/WHO Expert Committee on Pesticide Residues in 1979, 1981, 1982, 1984, 1985, 1986, 1987 and 1988 (FAO/WHO, 1980, 1982, 1983, 1985, 1986a,b, 1988a,b). In 1986, the Committee established an acceptable daily intake for humans of 0.02 mg/kg bw (Codex Committee on Pesticide Residues, 1990; WHO, 1990).

The US Environmental Protection Agency (1987) calculated an acceptable daily intake of 0.025 mg/kg per day for fenvalerate and a maximum permissible intake of 1.5 mg/kg per day for a 60-kg human.

National and regional pesticide residue limits for fenvalerate in foods are presented in Table 2. Additionally, the US Environmental Protection Agency (1989c) established a food additive tolerance of 0.05 ppm (mg/kg) for residues of fenvalerate in or on all food items (other than those already covered by a higher tolerance as a result of use on growing crops) in food handling establishments where food and food products are held, processed or prepared.

Table 2. National and regional pesticide residue limits for fenvalerate in foods[a]

Country or region	Residue limit (mg/kg)	Commodities
Argentina	2	Citrus fruit, peaches, sunflower seeds without husks
	1	Apples, flax, peas (fresh), soya beans, sunflowers
	0.5	Pears
	0.25	Peas (dried)
	0.2	Cotton, sorghum
	0.1	Sweet maize, tomatoes
	0.05	Soya seeds without husks
	0.02	Maize
Australia	5	Wheat bran
	2	Celery, cereal grains
	1	Cole crops, pome fruit, stone fruit, strawberries
	0.5	Fat of meat of goats and sheep, oilseeds, pod vegetables, seed vegetables
	0.2	Fat of meat of cattle, milk (fat basis), milk products (fat basis), tomatoes
	0.05	Sweet maize
Austria	2	Fruit, vegetables
	0.5	Other foodstuffs of vegetable origin
	0.05	Meat
Belgium	1	Cabbage and related plants, pome fruit
	0.5	Other fruit
	0.05	Potatoes
	0 (0.05)[b]	Other foodstuffs of vegetable origin
Brazil	1.0	Kale, rice
	0.2	Lard, meat (in fat), meats
	0.1	Coffee beans, cottonseed, soya beans, tomatoes
	0.04	Wheat
	0.01	Maize, field beans
Canada	Negligible	Apples, Brussels' sprouts, cabbages, cattle, cauliflower, pears, peanuts, potatoes
Chile	10	Cabbages, lettuce, peaches
	2	Apples, pears
	1.5	Sheep carcasses
	1.0	Beef carcasses, milk, tomatoes
	0.25	Dried beans
	0.05	Hog carcasses
	0.02	Goat carcasses, potatoes

Table 2 (contd)

Country or region	Residue limit (mg/kg)	Commodities
Denmark	2	Fruit (citrus, pome, stone), leafy vegetables
	1	Berries and small fruit, other vegetables
	0.05	Carrots, other root vegetables and onions, potatoes
Finland	2	Citrus fruit
	1.0	Grapes
	0.5	Other foodstuffs (excluding cereal grains)
France	0.5	Fruit (pome, stone), grapes
Germany	2	Berries, stone fruit (except plums)
	1.0	Cabbages, grapes, pome fruit
	0.5	Plums
	0.05	Maize, meat, meat products, potatoes, rape, sugar beets
	0.02	Other foodstuffs of plant origin
	0.01	Dairy products, milk
Hungary	1.0	Not specified
Italy	1.5[c]	Apples, grapes, oranges, peaches, pears
Japan	20	Exocarp of summer oranges
	1	Fruit (except exocarp of summer oranges)
	0.5	Sugar beets, vegetables
	0.1	Pulses
	0.05	Potatoes, etc.
Netherlands[c]	1	Cabbage species, leafy vegetables, pome fruit
	0.05[d]	Cereals, meat, milk, potatoes
	0 (0.05)[e]	Other foodstuffs
New Zealand[c]	5	*Brassica* vegetables
	3	Kiwifruit
	1.0	Legume vegetables, pome fruit
	0.2	Tomatoes
South Africa	0.5	Apples, cottonseed, mealies (green), pears
	0.3	Beans
	0.2	Sorghum, sunflower seeds
	0.1	Peas, potatoes, tomatoes
	0.05	Grapes, mangoes
Spain[c]	10	Alfalfa
	5	Beetroot tops, maize, sorghum
	2	Citrus fruit, drupes, pomes
	1.00	Grapes
	0.50	Straw of cereals
	0.20	Cucumbers
	0.05	Other plant products
Sweden[c]	1.0	Fruit, vegetables
	0.05[f]	Potatoes

Table 2 (contd)

Country or region	Residue limit (mg/kg)	Commodities
Switzerland	0.5	All foodstuffs (except fruit and milk)
	0.4	Fruit
	0.01	Milk
Taiwan	2	Leafy vegetables with small leaves
	1.0	Nut fruit
	0.5	Leafy vegetables with large wrapper leaves
	0.1	Rice, root vegetables
USA[g]	50	Maize (fodder, forage)
	20	Dried apple pomace (animal feed), sugar-cane bagasse (animal feed), turnip tops
	15	Almond hulls
	10	Cabbage, collards, dried tomato pomace (animal feed), stone fruit
	8	Radish tops
	7	Milk (fat)
	3	Blueberries, caneberries, currants, elderberries, gooseberries, huckleberries
	2	Apples, beans (snap), broccoli, pears, sugar-cane, sunflower hulls (animal feed)
	1.5	Cattle, goats, hogs, horses, sheep (fat, meat, meat by-products)
	1.0	Cantaloupes, eggplants, honeydew melons, muskmelons, peas, peppers, pumpkins, soya bean hulls (animal feed), sunflower seeds, tomatoes, water-melons, winter squash
	0.5	Carrots, cauliflower, cucumbers, summer squash, turnip roots
	0.3	Milk, radish roots
	0.25	Beans (dried), peas (dried)
	0.2	Almonds, artichokes, cottonseed, English walnuts, filberts, pecans
	0.1	Maize (sweet, kernels, cob), okra (Florida only), peanut hulls
	0.05	Soya beans
	0.02	Maize (grain), peanuts, potatoes
Yugoslavia	1.0	Fruit, grapes
	0.5	Other foodstuffs
	0.1	Rape

[a]From Health and Welfare Canada (1990)

[b]The figure in parentheses is the lower limit for determining residues in the corresponding product according to the standard method of analysis.

[c]Sum of steroisomers

[d]A pesticide may be used on an eating or drinking ware or raw material without a demonstrable residue remaining; the value listed is considered to be the highest concentration at which this requirement is deemed to have been met.

[e]Residues shall be absent; the value in parentheses is the highest concentration at which this requirement is still deemed to have been met.

[f]Limit of determination with current analytical methodology

[g]From US Environmental Protection Agency (1989a,b)

2. Studies of Cancer in Humans

No data were available to the Working Group.

3. Studies of Cancer in Experimental Animals

Oral administration

Mouse: Groups of 50 male and 50 female $B6C3F_1$ mice, 7-9 weeks old, were fed 10, 50, 250 or 1250 mg/kg of diet fenvalerate (95.8% pure) for two years. Two control groups of 50 males and 50 females were fed basal diet. The experiment was terminated after 104-105 weeks. There was a significant increase in mortality in male mice that received 10 and 1250 mg/kg and increased mortality in females that received the highest dose of fenvalerate. There was no significant increase in the incidence of tumours at any site in treated animals (Parker *et al.*, 1983).

Groups of 50 male and 50 female C57Bl/6 mice six weeks old were administered 40 or 80 mg/kg bw fenvalerate (99% pure) in arachis oil daily by gavage on five days a week for 104 weeks. Two groups of 50 males and 50 females were given arachis oil alone or were untreated. The experiment was terminated when the mice were 120 weeks of age, when the number of surviving high-dose females was slightly less (34%) than that among controls (40-44%). There was no significant increase in the incidence of tumours at any site in treated animals (Cabral & Galendo, 1990).

In a study designed to evaluate the effect of fenvalerate treatment on the onset of malignant lymphomas in female SJL/ola mice, groups of 24-26 females eight weeks of age, were given 0 or 80 mg/kg bw fenvalerate (92% pure) or 80 mg/kg bw fenvalerate (99% pure) in arachis oil by gavage once a week for 12 weeks and were observed for an additional 40 weeks, at which time the experiment was terminated. A slight increase in mortality was noted in the group that received 92% fenvalerate. Malignant lymphomas developed in all groups, and there was a shortening of the latent period in mice treated with 92% fenvalerate (Cabral & Galendo, 1990). [The Working Group noted that the statistical significance of the finding could not be determined.]

Rat: Groups of 93 male and 93 female Sprague-Dawley rats, 7-8 weeks of age, were fed 1, 5, 25 or 250 mg/kg of diet fenvalerate (95.8% pure) dissolved in hexane for up to 104 weeks. Control rats (183 males and 183 females) were maintained on a basal diet. Ten rats from each experimental group and 20 rats from each control group were killed at three, six, 12 and 18 months; the remaining rats were killed at 104 weeks. In a second study, groups of 50 males and 50 females were fed 0 or 1000 mg/kg of diet fenvalerate for 104 weeks. No significant difference in mortality was observed between experimental and control groups. In the first experiment, a significant [trend test: $p = 0.002$] increase in the incidence of benign mammary tumours was observed in females: 25/102 controls, 16/49 at 1 mg/kg, 18/51 at 5 mg/kg, 21/51 at 25 mg/kg and 20/48 at 250 mg/kg. No such increase was observed in the second experiment (20/49 and 16/50 in treated and control animals, respectively). Subcutaneous spindle-cell sarcomas developed in 5/51 males that received 1000 mg/kg fenvalerate; one intrathoracic spindle-cell sarcoma developed in 50 control males [$p > 0.05$]

(Parker *et al.*, 1984). [The Working Group noted the variable historical incidence of benign mammary tumours in this strain of rats.]

4. Other Relevant Data

4.1 Absorption, distribution, metabolism and excretion

4.1.1 *Humans*

No data were available to the Working Group.

4.1.2 *Experimental systems*

For a general introduction to the toxicokinetics of pyrethroids, see the monograph on permethrin. The metabolic pathways of fenvalerate in mammals are depicted in Figure 1 (WHO, 1990). These have mainly been studied using racemic fenvalerate.

Following its oral administration to rats and mice, fenvalerate is apparently rapidly absorbed. After a single oral administration of labelled fenvalerate to rats, excretion of radiolabel from the acid or benzoyl moieties was fairly rapid; the total recovery of radiolabel in the urine, faeces and expired air was 93-99% in six days. Excretion of radiolabel from the cyanogroup was relatively slower and the label was retained as thiocyanate, particularly in the hair, skin and stomach contents (Kaneko *et al.*, 1981).

A lipophilic metabolite, cholesteryl[2R]-2-(4-chlorophenyl)isovalerate (CPIA-cholesterol ester), has been detected in several tissues, notably the adrenal glands, liver and mesenteric lymph nodes, of rats and mice (Kaneko *et al.*, 1986). This metabolite has been indicated as the causative agent for microgranulomatous changes (see below) following administration of fenvalerate (Okuno *et al.*, 1986a). *In vitro* in homogenates from various tissues of mice, rats, dogs and monkeys, only the [2R, αS] isomer gave CPIA-cholesterol ester as a major metabolite. Mouse tissues were more efficient in producing the metabolite than those of other species (Miyamoto *et al.*, 1986), and microsomes from mouse liver produced less CPIA-cholesterol than did those from brain, kidney and spleen (Takamatsu *et al.*, 1987).

4.2 Toxic effects

The toxicity of fenvalerate has been reviewed (FAO/WHO, 1980, 1982, 1985; WHO, 1990).

4.2.1 *Humans*

Thirty-six adult volunteers received topical applications of fenvalerate on each ear lobe (0.081 mg/cm^2, approximately the field concentration of fenvalerate, in 0.05 ml of vehicle). Numbness, itching, burning, stinging, pricking and warmth were the most frequently reported sensations, and these occurred intermittently or continuously (Knox *et al.*, 1984). Similar results were obtained in another study (Flannigan *et al.*, 1985) and after occupational exposures (Tucker & Flannigan, 1983). Electrophysiological studies were performed on the arms and legs of subjects who had experienced paraesthesia after exposure to fenvalerate and other pyrethroids; there was no abnormal finding (Le Quesne *et al.*, 1980).

Fig. 1. Metabolic pathways of fenvalerate in mammals[a]

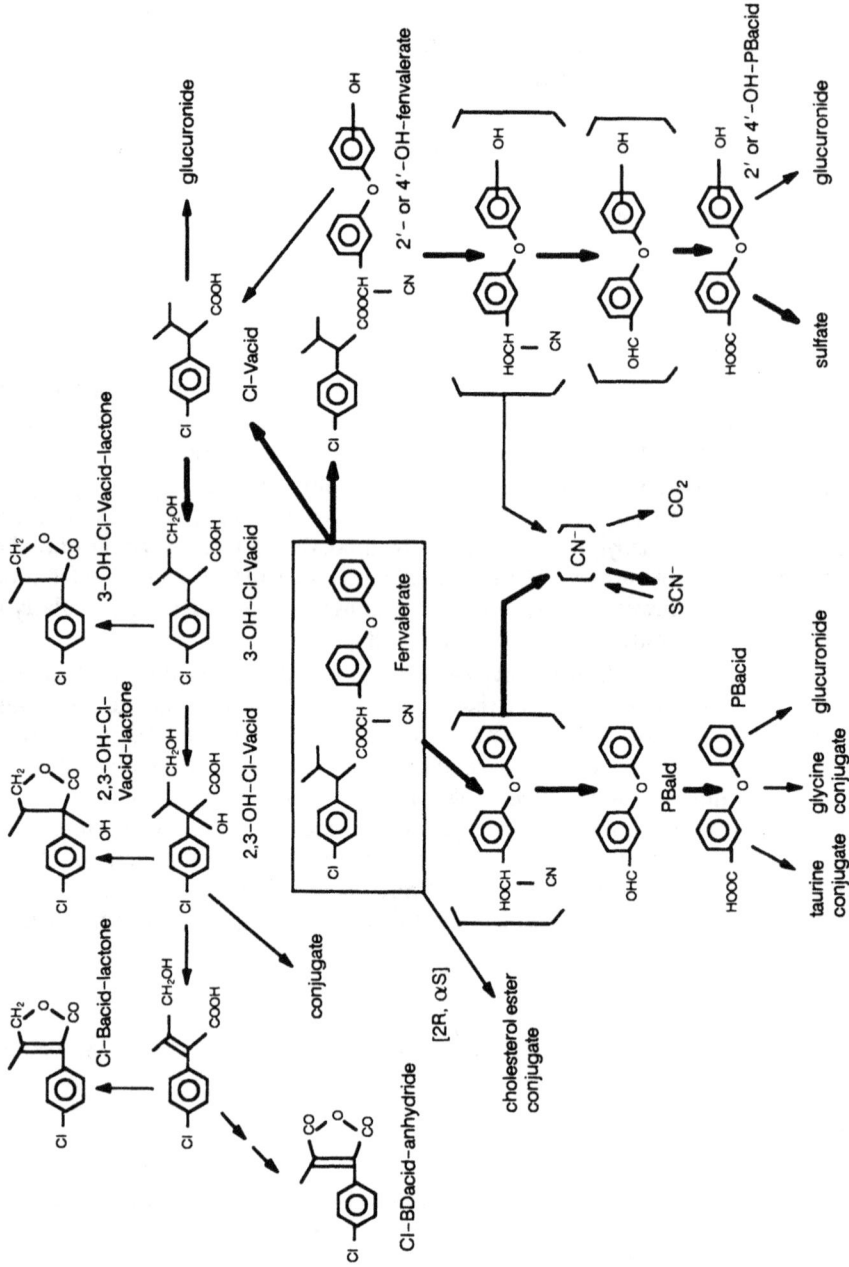

[a]From WHO (1990); Cl-Vacid, 2-(4-chlorophenyl)isovaleric acid; Cl-BDacid, 2-(4-chlorophenyl)-cis-2-butenedioic acid; Cl-Bacid-lactone, 2-(4-chlorophenyl)-3-methyl-2-butene-4-olide; PBacid, 3-phenoxybenzoic acid; PBald, 3-phenoxybenzaldehyde

He *et al.* (1989) reviewed 196 cases of fenvalerate intoxication from the Chinese medical literature. Common findings included paraesthesia, particularly involving the face, dizziness, headache, nausea, anorexia and fatigue. Less common findings included chest tightness, palpitations, blurred vision, increased sweating and low-grade fever. Muscular fasciculations, convulsions and coma were reported among some of the more severely poisoned cases. Five deaths (two from combined exposures) were reported.

4.2.2 *Experimental systems*

The oral LD_{50} of technical-grade fenvalerate was reported to be 451 mg/kg bw in rats and 100-300 mg/kg bw in mice, when given in dimethyl sulfoxide; when polyethylene glycol/water was used as the vehicle, the LD_{50}s were much higher. Signs of intoxication reported in rats were restlessness, tremors, piloerection, occasional diarrhoea and an abnormal gait following oral administration; surviving rats recovered rapidly and were asymptomatic after three to four days. It has been reported that comparative studies of the acute toxicity of several metabolites of fenvalerate in mice following intraperitoneal administration indicated a lower toxicity of the metabolites than that of the parent compound (WHO, 1990).

Absolute and relative increases in liver weight were noted in a 13-week study in Fischer 344 rats fed decarboxyfenvalerate (one major photodegradation product of fenvalerate) in the diet at 300, 3000 or 10 000 mg/kg diet. Hepatocellular hypertrophy and focal necrosis were found in animals fed 3000 or 10 000 mg/kg diet (Parker *et al.*, 1986). The incidence and severity of hepatic multifocal microgranulomas were increased in a dose-dependent way in male and female beagle dogs fed 250, 500 or 1000 mg/kg diet technical-grade fenvalerate for six months (Parker *et al.*, 1984). Multifocal microgranulomas were also observed in liver and spleen of mice fed technical-grade fenvalerate in the diet for two years at concentrations of 250-1250 mg/kg and in lymph nodes of mice fed 50-1250 mg/kg (Parker *et al.*, 1983). Microgranulomas were also observed in liver, spleen and lymph nodes of mice given 20-160 mg/kg bw fenvalerate for 10 weeks. Under similar conditions, hamsters showed slight hepatocyte hypertrophy at 80 and 160 mg/kg but no microgranulomas at any dose level (Cabral & Galendo, 1990). The causative agent of these changes has been reported to be the metabolite CPIA-cholesterol ester (Okuno *et al.*, 1986a).

The pathological changes were caused only by feeding the 2R,αS isomer of fenvalerate, i.e., the only isomer that can be metabolized to CPIA-cholesterol (Okuno *et al.*, 1986a). In another study, Wistar rats and ddY mice were fed diets containing 10-3000 ppm (mg/kg) technical-grade fenvalerate for 24-28 and 17-20 months, respectively. The no-observed-effect level for the development of microgranulomas was found to be 150 and 30 ppm (mg/kg) for rats and mice, respectively. A study in which ddY mice were exposed for six weeks to a diet containing 1000 or 3000 ppm (mg/kg) technical-grade fenvalerate and then to a control diet up to 12 months indicated that the microgranulomatous changes are reversible with time (Okuno *et al.*, 1986b).

It has been reported that, at very high doses of fenvalerate, surviving rats may show neuropathology of the sciatic nerve that might be reversible (WHO, 1990). In mice and rats given single oral doses of technical-grade fenvalerate, reversible ataxia and incoordination were observed at 56-320 mg/kg bw and sparse axonal damage in peripheral nerves at 180-1000 mg/kg bw (Parker *et al.*, 1985).

Technical-grade fenvalerate (in arachis oil) given by gavage (75 mg/kg bw per day, on five days a week for 10 weeks) induced significantly more γ-glutamyl transpeptidase-positive enzyme-altered foci per cubic centimetre and a larger percentage of liver tissue occupied by focus tissue in partially hepatectomized, *N*-nitrosodiethylamine-initiated male Sprague-Dawley rats than in a vehicle control group. Analysis of the size distribution of foci in fenvalerate- and vehicle-treated rats showed elevated incidences of foci in fenvalerate-treated rats at all focus sizes. Fenvalerate did not increase serum transaminase activities or cause other histopathological changes (Flodström *et al.*, 1988).

In contrast, fenvalerate given in the diet (at up to 1500 ppm [mg/kg]) for six weeks, two weeks after a single intraperitoneal dose of *N*-nitrosodiethylamine (200 mg/kg bw), to male Fischer rats that were also subjected to a two-thirds partial hepatectomy three weeks after the start of the study, did not increase the number or area of glutathione *S*-transferase (placental form)-positive liver-cell foci at eight weeks; positive controls treated with 2-acetylaminofluorene or sodium phenobarbital after *N*-nitrosodiethylamine initiation showed these changes. Neurological signs, including altered response to sensory stimuli, staggering gate and tremors, were observed in rats given 1500 mg/kg fenvalerate in the diet, and relative liver weights were increased in animals administered 500 mg/kg or more in the diet (Hagiwara *et al.*, 1990).

4.3 Reproductive and prenatal effects

4.3.1 *Humans*

No data were available to the Working Group.

4.3.2 *Experimental systems*

In a review of reproductive and developmental toxicology studies in mice, rats and rabbits, no adverse effect was reported (WHO, 1990).

4.4 Genetic and related effects (see also Table 3 and Appendices 1 and 2)

4.4.1 *Humans*

No data were available to the Working Group.

4.4.2 *Experimental systems*

Several unpublished reports are cited in a recent review (WHO, 1990).

Fenvalerate did not cause mutation in bacteria or in *Drosophila melanogaster*, but weak induction of aneuploidy was observed in *D. melanogaster*. A weak induction of sister chromatid exchange and induction of chromosomal aberrations were observed in cultured human lymphocytes.

In vivo, there was evidence of clastogenic effects of fenvalerate in mouse bone marrow; significant effects were reported following a single oral or intraperitoneal administration, yet a single subcutaneous administration had no significant effect. In mice, fenvalerate increased the frequency of micronucleated polychromatic erythrocytes in bone marrow and the frequency of sperm with abnormal morphology.

Table 3. Genetic and related effects of fenvalerate

Test system	Result[a] Without exogenous metabolic system	Result[a] With exogenous metabolic system	Dose[b] LED/HID	Reference
SA0, *Salmonella typhimurium* TA100, reverse mutation (fluct. test)	−	−	10.0000	Pluijmen *et al.* (1984)
SA0, *Salmonella typhimurium* TA100, reverse mutation	−	−	1750.0000	Herrera & Laborda (1988)
SA4, *Salmonella typhimurium* TA104, reverse mutation	−	−	1750.0000	Herrera & Laborda (1988)
SA5, *Salmonella typhimurium* TA1535, reverse mutation (spot test)	−	−	500.0000	Herrera & Laborda (1988)
SA7, *Salmonella typhimurium* TA1537, reverse mutation (spot test)	−	−	500.0000	Herrera & Laborda (1988)
SA8, *Salmonella typhimurium* TA1538, reverse mutation (spot test)	−	−	500.0000	Herrera & Laborda (1988)
SA9, *Salmonella typhimurium* TA98, reverse mutation (fluct. test)	−	−	10.0000	Pluijmen *et al.* (1984)
SA9, *Salmonella typhimurium* TA98, reverse mutation	−	−	1750.0000	Herrera & Laborda (1988)
SAS, *Salmonella typhimurium* TA97, reverse mutation	−	−	1750.0000	Herrera & Laborda (1988)
DMX, *Drosophila melanogaster*, sex-linked recessive lethal mutation	−	0	20.0000 adult feeding	Batiste–Alentorn *et al.* (1987)
DMX, *Drosophila melanogaster*, sex-linked recessive lethal mutation	−	0	25.0000 larval feeding	Batiste–Alentorn *et al.* (1987)
DMX, *Drosophila melanogaster*, sex-linked recessive lethal mutation	−	0	20.0000 adult injection	Batiste–Alentorn *et al.* (1987)
DMC, *Drosophila melanogaster*, chromosome breakage	−	0	10.0000 adult feeding	Batiste–Alentorn *et al.* (1987)
DMC, *Drosophila melanogaster*, chromosome breakage	−	0	50.0000 larval feeding	Batiste–Alentorn *et al.* (1987)
DMC, *Drosophila melanogaster*, chromosome breakage	−	0	20.0000 adult injection	Batiste–Alentorn *et al.* (1987)
DMN, *Drosophila melanogaster*, aneuploidy	(+)	0	5.0000 adult feeding	Batiste–Alentorn *et al.* (1987)
DMN, *Drosophila melanogaster*, aneuploidy	−	0	50.0000 larval feeding	Batiste–Alentorn *et al.* (1987)
DMN, *Drosophila melanogaster*, aneuploidy	−	0	20.0000 adult injection	Batiste–Alentorn *et al.* (1987)
SHL, Sister chromatid exchange, human lymphocytes *in vitro*	(+)	0	10.0000	Puig *et al.* (1989)
CHL, Chromosomal aberrations, human lymphocytes *in vitro*	+	0	4.0000	Puig *et al.* (1989)
MVM, Micronucleus test, mouse bone marrow *in vivo*	+	0	150.0000 × 2 i.p.	Pati & Bhunya (1989)
CBA, Chromosomal aberrations, mouse bone marrow *in vivo*	+	0	150.0000 × 1 i.p.	Pati & Bhunya (1989)
CBA, Chromosomal aberrations, mouse bone marrow *in vivo*	+	0	200.0000 × 1 p.o.	Pati & Bhunya (1989)
CBA, Chromosomal aberrations, mouse bone marrow *in vivo*	−	0	200.0000 × 1 s.c.	Pati & Bhunya (1989)
ICR, Inhibition of intercellular communication, V79 cells *in vitro*	+	0	4.0000	Flodström *et al.* (1988)
SPM, Sperm abnormalities, mice *in vivo*	+	0	20.0000 × 5 i.p.	Pati & Bhunya (1989)

[a] +, positive; (+), weakly positive; −, negative; 0, not tested; ?, inconclusive (variable response in several experiments within an adequate study)

[b] In-vitro tests, μg/ml; in-vivo tests, mg/kg bw

Fenvalerate and a major metabolite, 2-(4-chlorophenyl)isovaleric acid, inhibited gap-junctional intercellular communication in Chinese hamster V79 cells (Flodström *et al.*, 1988).

5. Summary of Data Reported and Evaluation

5.1 Exposure data

Fenvalerate is a highly active contact insecticide. It has been used since 1976, mostly in agriculture but also in public health programmes, in homes and gardens and on cattle, alone or in combination with other insecticides. It has been formulated as concentrates, dusts and wettable powders.

Exposure to fenvalerate can occur during its production and application and, at much lower levels, from consumption of foods containing residues.

5.2 Carcinogenicity data in humans

No data were available to the Working Group.

5.3 Carcinogenicity in experimental animals

Fenvalerate was tested for carcinogenicity in two experiments in mice and in two experiments in rats by oral administration. There was no increase in the incidence of tumours in mice. In rats, there was an increased incidence of benign mammary tumours in females in one study. In another study at a higher dose, no increase in tumour incidence was seen in animals of either sex.

5.4 Other relevant data

In one study, fenvalerate increased the frequency of enzyme-positive foci in rat liver.

Administration of fenvalerate to mice *in vivo* induced chromosomal aberrations and micronuclei in bone marrow and morphological abnormalities in sperm. Induction of chromosomal aberrations and sister chromatid exchange was observed in cultured human cells, and aneuploidy was seen in insects. Fenvalerate inhibited gap-junctional intercellular communication in cultured mammalian cells. It did not induce mutation in insects or bacteria.

5.5 Evaluation[1]

No data were available from studies in humans.

There is *inadequate evidence* for the carcinogenicity of fenvalerate in experimental animals.

Overall evaluation

Fenvalerate *is not classifiable as to its carcinogenicity to humans (Group 3).*

---

[1]For definition of the italicized terms, see Preample, pp. 26-28.

6. References

All India Medical Corp. (undated) *Data Sheet: Fenvalerate 20% E.C.—Sumitox 20% E.C.—Synthetic Pyrethroid Insecticide*, Bombay, AIMCO Pesticides

Baker, P.G. & Bottomley, P. (1982) Determination of residues of synthetic pyrethroids in fruit and vegetables by gas-liquid and high-performance liquid chromatography. *Analyst, 107*, 206-212

Batiste-Alentorn, M., Xamena, N., Velázquez, A., Creus, A. & Marcos, R. (1987) Non-mutagenicity of fenvalerate in *Drosophila. Mutagenesis, 2*, 7-10

Budavari, S., ed. (1989) *The Merck Index*, 11th ed., Rahway, NJ, Merck & Co., p. 629

Cabral, J.R.P. & Galendo, D. (1990) Carcinogenicity study of the pesticide fenvalerate in mice. *Cancer Lett., 49*, 13-18

Codex Committee on Pesticide Residues (1990) *Guide to Codex Maximum Limits for Pesticide Residues*, Part 2, (CAC/PR 2—1990; CCPR Pesticide Classification No. 119); The Hague

Du Pont (1988a) *Material Safety Data Sheet: Asana® Insecticide Technical*, Wilmington, DE

Du Pont (1988b) *Material Safety Data Sheet: Pydrin® Insecticide Technical*, Wilmington, DE

Du Pont (1990) *Material Safety Data Sheet: Asana® XL Insecticide*, Wilmington, DE

E.I. duPont de Nemours & Co. (1988a) Material safety data sheet: Pydrin insecticide 2.4 emulsifiable concentrate. In: *MSDS Reference for Crop Protection Chemicals*, New York, Chemical and Pharmaceutical Press, pp. 454-456

E.I. duPont de Nemours & Co. (1988b) Material safety data sheet: Asana insecticide 1.9 emulsifiable concentrate. In: *MSDS Reference for Crop Protection Chemicals*, New York, Chemical and Pharmaceutical Press, pp. 300-302

E.I. duPont de Nemours & Co. (1988c) Material safety data sheet: Asana XL insecticide 0.66 emulsifiable concentrate. In: *MSDS Reference for Crop Protection Chemicals*, New York, Chemical and Pharmaceutical Press, pp. 303-305

E.I. duPont de Nemours & Co. (1989a) Sample label: Pydrin® insecticide 2.4 emulsifiable concentrate. In: *Crop Protection Chemical Reference CPCR®*, 5th ed., New York, Chemical and Pharmaceutical Press, pp. 964-972

E.I. duPont de Nemours & Co. (1989b) Sample label: Asana® insecticide 1.9 emulsifiable concentrate. In: *Crop Protection Chemical Reference CPCR®*, 5th ed., New York, Chemical and Pharmaceutical Press, pp. 724-730

E.I. duPont de Nemours & Co. (1989c) Sample label: Asana® XL insecticide 0.66 emulsifiable concentrate. In: *Crop Protection Chemical Reference CPCR®*, 5th ed., New York, Chemical and Pharmaceutical Press, pp. 730-737

FAO/WHO (1980) *Pesticide Residues in Food: 1979 Evaluations* (FAO Plant Production and Protection Paper 20 Sup.), Rome

FAO/WHO (1982) *Pesticide Residues in Food—1981 Evaluations* (FAO Plant Production and Protection Paper 42), Rome

FAO/WHO (1983) *Pesticide Residues in Food—1982 Evaluations* (FAO Plant Production and Protection Paper 46), Rome

FAO/WHO (1985) *Pesticide Residues in Food—1984 Evaluations* (FAO Plant Production and Protection Paper 67), Rome

FAO/WHO (1986a) *Pesticide Residues in Food—1985 Evaluations* (FAO Plant Production and Protection Paper 68), Rome

FAO/WHO (1986b) *Pesticide Residues in Food—1986 Evaluations* (FAO Plant Production and Protection Paper 77), Rome

FAO/WHO (1988a) *Pesticide Residues in Food—1987 Evaluations* (FAO Plant Production and Protection Paper 86/1), Rome

FAO/WHO (1988b) *Pesticide Residues in Food—1987 Evaluations* (FAO Plant Production and Protection Paper 93/1), Rome

Flannigan, S.A., Tucker, S.B., Key, M.M., Ross, C.E., Fairchild, E.J., II, Grimes, B.A. & Harrist, R.B. (1985) Synthetic pyrethroid insecticides: a dermatological evaluation. *Br. J. ind. Med.*, *42*, 363-372

Flodström, S., Wärngård, L., Ljungquist, S. & Ahlborg, U.G. (1988) Inhibition of metabolic cooperation *in vitro* and enhancement of enzyme altered foci incidence in rat liver by the pyrethroid insecticide fenvalerate. *Arch. Toxicol.*, *61*, 218-223

Government of Canada (1990) *Report on National Surveillance Data from 1984/85 to 1988/89*, Ottawa

Hagiwara, A., Yamada, M., Hasegawa, R., Fukushima, S. & Ito, N. (1990) Lack of enhancing effects of fenvalerate and esfenvalerate on induction of preneoplastic glutathione S-transferase placental form positive liver cell foci in rats. *Cancer Lett.*, *54*, 67-73

He, F., Sun, J., Han, K., Wu, Y., Yao, P., Wang, S. & Liu, L. (1988) Effects of pyrethroid insecticides on subjects engaged in packaging pyrethroids. *Br. J. ind. Med.*, *45*, 548-551

He, F., Wang, S., Liu, L., Chen, S., Zhang, Z. & Sun, J. (1989) Clinical manifestations and diagnosis of acute pyrethroid poisoning. *Arch. Toxicol.*, *63*, 54-58

Health and Welfare Canada (1990) *National Pesticide Residue Limits in Foods*, Ottawa, Bureau of Chemical Safety, Food Directorate, Health Protection Branch

Herrera, A. & Laborda, E. (1988) Mutagenic activity of synthetic pyrethroids in *Salmonella typhimurium*. *Mutagenesis*, *3*, 509-514

Horiba, M., Kitahara, H., Takahashi, K., Yamamoto, S. & Murano, A. (1980) Gas chromatographic determination of fenvalerate (S-5602) in technical preparations. *Agric. biol. Chem.*, *44*, 1197-1199

IARC (1989) *IARC Monographs on the Evaluation of Carcinogenic Risks to Humans*, Vol. 47, *Some Organic Solvents, Resin Monomers and Related Compounds, Pigments and Occupational Exposures in Paint Manufacture and Painting*, Lyon, pp. 125-156

Kaneko, H., Ohkawa, H. & Miyamoto, J. (1981) Comparative metabolism of fenvalerate and the [2S,αS]-isomer in rats and mice. *J. Pestic. Sci.*, *6*, 317-326

Kaneko, H., Matsuo, M. & Miyamoto, J. (1986) Differential metabolism of fenvalerate and granuloma formation. I. Identification of cholesterol ester derived from a specific chiral isomer of fenvalerate. *Toxicol. appl. Pharmacol.*, *83*, 148-156

Knox, J.M., Tucker, S.B. & Flannigan, S.A. (1984) Parasthesia from cutaneous exposure to a synthetic pyrethroid insecticide. *Arch. Dermatol.*, *120*, 744-746

Le Quesne, P.M., Maxwell, I.C. & Butterworth, S.T.G. (1980) Transient facial sensory symptoms following exposure to synthetic pyrethroids: a clinical and electrophysiological assessment. *Neurotoxicology*, *2*, 1-11

Luke, M.A., Masumoto, H.T., Cairns, T. & Hundley, H.K. (1988) Levels and incidences of pesticide residues in various foods and animal feeds analyzed by the Luke multiresidue methodology for fiscal years 1982-1986. *J. Assoc. off. anal. Chem.*, *71*, 415-433

Meister, R.T., ed. (1990) *Farm Chemicals Handbook '90*, Willoughby, OH, Meister Publishing Co., pp. C25-C26, C131-C132, C273

Miyamoto, J., Kaneko, H. & Takamatsu, Y. (1986) Stereoselective formation of a cholesterol ester conjugate from fenvalerate by mouse microsomal carboxyesterase(s). *J. biochem. Toxicol.*, *1*, 79-94

Mourot, D., Delépine, B., Boisseau, J. & Gayot, G. (1979) High-pressure liquid chromatography of a new pyrethroid insecticide, sumicidin. *J. Chromatogr.*, *168*, 277-279

Okuno, Y., Seki, T., Ito, S., Kaneko, H., Watanabe, T., Yamada, T. & Miyamoto, J. (1986a) Differential metabolism of fenvalerate and granuloma formation. II. Toxicological significance of a lipophilic conjugate from fenvalerate. *Toxicol. appl. Pharmacol.*, *83*, 157-169

Okuno, Y., Ito, S., Seki, T., Hiromori, T., Murakami, M., Kadota, T. & Miyamoto, J. (1986b) Fenvalerate-induced granulomatous changes in rats and mice. *J. toxicol. Sci.*, *11*, 53-66

Papadopoulou-Mourkidou, E. (1983) Analysis of established pyrethroid insecticides. *Residue Rev.*, *89*, 179-208

Papadopoulou-Mourkidou, E. (1985) Direct analysis of fenvalerate isomers by liquid chromatography. Application to formulation and residue analysis of fenvalerate. *Chromatographia*, *20*, 376-378

Parker, C.M., McCullough, C.B., Gellatly, J.B.M. & Johnston, C.D. (1983) Toxicologic and carcinogenic evaluation of fenvalerate in the B6C3F$_1$ mouse. *Fundam. appl. Toxicol.*, *3*, 114-120

Parker, C.M., Piccirillo, V.J., Kurtz, S.L., Garner, F.M., Gardiner, T.H. & Van Gelder, G.A. (1984) Six-month feeding study of fenvalerate in dogs. *Fundam. appl. Toxicol.*, *4*, 577-586

Parker, C.M., Albert, J.R., Van Gelder, G.A., Patterson, D.R. & Taylor, J.L. (1985) Neuropharmacologic and neuropathologic effect of fenvalerate in mice and rats. *Fundam. appl. Toxicol.*, *5*, 278-286

Parker, C.M., Wimberley, H.C., Lam, A.S., Gardiner, T.H. & Van Gelder, G.A. (1986) Subchronic feeding study of decarboxyfenvalerate in rats. *J. Toxicol. environ. Health*, *18*, 77-90

Pati, P.C. & Bhunya, S.P. (1989) Cytogenetic effects of fenvalerate in mammalian in vivo test systems. *Mutat. Res.*, *222*, 149-154

Pluijmen, M., Drevon, C., Montesano, R., Malaveille, C., Hautefeuille, A. & Bartsch, H. (1984) Lack of mutagenicity of synthetic pyrethroids in *Salmonella typhimurium* strains and in V79 Chinese hamster cells. *Mutat. Res.*, *137*, 7-15

Puig, M., Carbonell, E., Xamena, N., Creus, A. & Marcos, R. (1989) Analysis of cytogenetic damage induced in cultured human lymphocytes by the pyrethroid insecticides cypermethrin and fenvalerate. *Mutagenesis*, *4*, 72-74

Rogosheske, S.E., Baker, G.J. & Preiss, F.J. (1982) Fenvalerate—its development and application for domestic and industrial use. *Chem. Times Trends*, *5*, 42-44, 64

Roussel Bio Corp. (1989) *Specimen Label: Gold Crest® Tribute® Termiticide/ Insecticide Concentrate*, Englewood Cliffs, NJ

Royal Society of Chemistry (1986) *European Directory of Agrochemical Products*, Vol. 3, *Insecticides, Acaricides, Nematicides*, Cambridge, pp. 4-10

Royal Society of Chemistry (1989) *The Agrochemicals Handbook* [Dialog Information Services (File 306)], Cambridge

Sakaue, S., Kida, S. & Doi, T. (1987) Gas chromatographic determination of esfenvalerate (Sumi-alpha®) in technical preparations. *Agric. Biol. Chem.*, *51*, 1671-1673

Shell Development Co. (1984) Pydrin®: insecticide. In: Zweig, G. & Sherma, J., eds, *Analytical Methods for Pesticides and Plant Growth Regulators*, Vol. XIII, *Synthetic Pyrethroids and Other Pesticides*, New York, Academic Press, pp. 121-131

Spittler, T.D., Argauer, R.J., Lisk, D.J., Mumma, R.O. & Winhett, G. (1982) Gas-liquid chromatographic determination of fenvalerate insecticide residues in processed apple products and by-products. *J. Assoc. off. anal. Chem.*, *65*, 1106-1111

Spittler, T.D., Argauer, R.J., Lisk, D.J., Mumma, R.O., Winnett, G. & Fen, D.N. (1984) Gas chromatographic determination of fenvalerate insecticide residues in processed tomato products and by-products. *J. Assoc. off. anal. Chem.*, *67*, 834-836

Takamatsu, Y., Kaneko, H., Abiko, J., Yoshitake, A. & Miyamoto, J. (1987) In vivo and in vitro stereoselective hydrolysis of four chiral isomers of fenvalerate. *J. Pestic. Sci.*, *12*, 397-404

Tucker, S.B. & Flannigan, S.A. (1983) Cutaneous effects from occupational exposure to fenvalerate. *Arch. Toxicol.*, *54*, 195-202

US Environmental Protection Agency (1987) *Pesticide Fact Sheet Number 145: Fenvalerate*, Washington DC, Office of Pesticide Programs

US Environmental Protection Agency (1989a) Cyano(3-phenoxphenyl)methyl 4-chloro-*alpha*-(methylethyl)benzeneacetate; tolerances for residues. Part 180—Tolerances and exemptions from tolerances for pesticide chemicals in or on raw agricultural commodities. *US Code fed. Regul.*, *Title 40*, Part 180.379, pp. 357-358

US Environmental Protection Agency (1989b) Cyano(3-phenoxphenyl)methyl 4-chloro-*alpha*-(methylethyl)benzeneacetate. Part 186—Tolerances for pesticides in animal feeds. *US Code fed. Regul.*, *Title 40*, Part 186.1300, p. 444

US Environmental Protection Agency (1989c) Cyano(3-phenoxphenyl)methyl 4-chloro-*alpha*-(methylethyl)benzeneacetate. Part 185—Tolerances for pesticides in food. *US Code fed. Regul.*, *Title 40*, Part 185.1300, p. 473

US Food and Drug Administration (1989) Cyano(3-phenoxyphenyl)methyl 4-chloro-*alpha*-(1-methyl-ethyl)benzeneacetate. In: *Pesticide Analytical Manual*, Vol. II, *Methods Which Detect Multiple Residues*, Washington DC, US Department of Health and Human Services

Verschueren, K. (1983) *Handbook of Environmental Data on Organic Chemicals*, 2nd ed., New York, Van Nostrand Reinhold Co., p. 670

WHO (1990) *Fenvalerate* (Environmental Health Criteria 95), Geneva

Worthing, C.R. & Walker, S.B., eds (1987) *The Pesticide Manual—A World Compendium*, 8th ed., Thornton Heath, British Crop Protection Council, pp. 395-396

Yoshioka, H. (1978) Development of fenvalerate, a new and unique synthetic pyrethroid containing the phenylisovaleric acid moiety. *Rev. plant Prot. Res.*, *11*, 39-52

Yoshioka, H. (1985) Development of fenvalerate. *Chemtech*, *15*, 482-486

PERMETHRIN

1. Exposure Data

1.1 Chemical and physical data

Permethrin is typically a mixture of (+) *cis* and (+) *trans* esters of the general structure shown below, in either a 40:60 or 25:75 ratio.

1.1.1 *Synonyms, structural and molecular data*

Table 1. Chemical Abstract Services Registry numbers, names and synonyms of permethrin

Name	CAS Reg. Nos[a]	Chem. Abstr. names[b] and synonyms
Permethrin	52645-53-1 (57608-04-5; 60018-94-2; 63364-00-1; 75497-64-2; 93388-66-0)	**3-(2,2-Dichloroethenyl)-2,2-dimethylcyclopropanecarboxylic acid, (3-phenoxyphenyl)methyl ester;** *meta*-phenoxybenzyl 3-(2,2-dichlorovinyl)-2,2-dimethylcyclopropanecarboxylate; 3-phenoxybenzyl (1RS)-*cis,trans*-3-(2,2-dichlorovinyl)-2,2-dimethylcyclopropanecarboxylate (IUPAC); 3-phenoxybenzyl (1RS,3RS;1RS,3SR)-3-(2,2-dichlorovinyl)-2,2-dimethylcyclopropanecarboxylate (IUPAC); 3-phenoxybenzyl-2,2-dimethyl-3-(2,2-dichlorovinyl)cyclopropanecarboxylate; FMC 33297; FMC 41655; ICI-PP 557; NRDC 143; OMS 1821; WL 43479
trans-Permethrin	61949-77-7	**trans-3-(2,2-Dichloroethenyl)-2,2-dimethylcyclopropanecarboxylic acid, (3-phenoxyphenyl)methyl ester;** *trans-meta*-phenoxybenzyl 3-(2,2-dichlorovinyl)-2,2-dimethylcyclopropanecarboxylate
cis-Permethrin	61949-76-6	**cis-3-(2,2-Dichloroethenyl)-2,2-dimethylcyclopropanecarboxylic acid, (3-phenoxyphenyl)methyl ester;** *cis-meta*-phenoxybenzyl 3-(2,2-dichlorovinyl)-2,2-dimethylcyclopropanecarboxylate; *cis*-permethrin
(-)-*trans*-Permethrin	54774-47-9	**(1S-trans)-3-(2,2-Dichloroethenyl)-2,2-dimethylcyclopropanecarboxylic acid, (3-phenoxyphenyl)methyl ester;** 1S-*trans*-permethrin
(-)-*cis*-Permethrin	54774-46-8	**(1S-cis)-3-(2,2-Dichloroethenyl)-2,2-dimethylcyclopropanecarboxylic acid, (3-phenoxyphenyl)methyl ester;** 1S-*cis*-permethrin
(+)-*cis*-Permethrin	54774-45-7	**(1R-cis)-3-(2,2-Dichloroethenyl)-2,2-dimethylcyclopropanecarboxylic acid, (3-phenoxyphenyl)methyl ester;** 1R-*cis*-permethrin; NRDC 167
(±)-*cis*-Permethrin	52341-33-0	**cis-(±)-3-(2,2-Dichloroethenyl)-2,2-dimethylcyclopropanecarboxylic acid, (3-phenoxyphenyl)methyl ester;** (±)-*cis*-FMC 33297; FMC 35171; NRDC 148; 1RS-*cis*-permethrin

Table 1 (contd)

Name	CAS Reg. Nos[a]	Chem. Abstr. names[b] and synonyms
(±)-*trans*-Permethrin	52341-32-9	*trans*-(±)-3-(2,2-Dichloroethenyl)-2,2-dimethylcyclopropane-carboxylic acid, (3-phenoxyphenyl)methyl ester; NRDC 146; 1RS-*trans*-permethrin
(+)-*trans*-Permethrin	51877-74-8	Biopermethrin; (1R-*trans*)-3-(2,2-dichloroethenyl)-2,2-dimethyl-cyclopropanecarboxylic acid, (3-phenoxyphenyl)methyl ester; NRDC 147; 1R-*trans*-permethrin; RU 22090

[a]Replaced CAS Registry number(s) in parentheses
[a]In bold

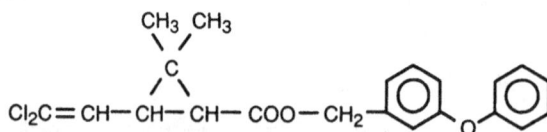

$C_{21}H_{20}Cl_2O_3$ Mol. wt: 391.3

1.1.2 *Chemical and physical properties*

(a) *Description*: Colourless to white, odourless crystalline solid (pure); viscous brown liquid or crystalline solid with a sweet odour (technical) (Swaine & Tandy, 1984; Roussel Bio Corp., undated)

(b) *Boiling-point*: 220°C at 0.05 mm Hg [6.7×10^{-3} kPa] (Roussel Bio Corp., undated);

(c) *Melting-point*: 34-39°C (technical), 63-65°C (*cis*-isomers), 44-47°C (*trans*-isomers) (Worthing & Walker, 1987; WHO, 1990)

(d) *Solubility*: Insoluble in water (0.2 mg/l at 30°C); soluble in or miscible with most organic solvents (acetone (450 g/l), chloroform, cyclohexanone, ethanol, ether, hexane (> 1 kg/kg at 25°C), methanol (258 g/kg at 25°C), dichloromethane, xylene (> 1 kg/kg at 25°C) (Swaine & Tandy, 1984; Worthing & Walker, 1987; The Royal Society of Chemistry, 1989; WHO, 1990; Roussel Bio Corp., undated)

(e) *Volatility*: Vapour pressure, 3.4×10^{-7} mm Hg [0.45×10^{-7} kPa] at 25°C (technical) (FMC Corp., 1984); 15×10^{-9} mm Hg [2.0×10^{-9} kPa] at 20°C (*cis*-isomer), 7.5×10^{-9} mm Hg [1.0×10^{-9} kPa] at 20°C (*trans*-isomer) (Swaine & Tandy, 1984)

(f) *Stability*: Stable in neutral and weak acidic media, but hydrolysis can occur under alkaline or strongly acidic conditions (Swaine & Tandy, 1984).

(g) *Half-time*: 10-25 days at 25°C in soil, depending on soil type (Roussel Bio Corp., undated)

(h) *Octanol/water partition coefficient (P)*: log P, 6.5 (WHO, 1990)

(i) *Conversion factor for airborne concentrations*[1]: mg/m^3 = 16.0 × ppm

1.1.3 *Trade names, technical products and impurities*

Some examples of trade names are: Adion; Ambush; Ambushfog; Anomethrin N; Antiborer 3768; Atroban; BW-21-Z; Cellutec; Chinetrin; Coopex; Corsair; Diffusil H; Dragon; Ecsumin; Ectiban; Efmethrin; Eksmin; Exmin; Imperator; Indothrin; Ipitox; Kafil; Kavil; Kestrel; LE 79-519; MP 79; NIA 33297; Outflank; Perigen; Permanone; Permasect; Permit; Perthrine; Picket; Pounce; PP 557; Pramex; Pynosect; Qamlin; S 3151; SBP 1513; SBP 15131TEC; Spartan; Stockade; Stomoxin; Talcord; Torpedo

Technical-grade permethrin contains from a minimum of 35% to a maximum of 55% (±)-*cis* isomer and from a minimum of 45% to a maximum of 65% (±)-*trans* isomer (Roussel Bio Corp., 1987; Anon., 1989). In the common technical-grade products, the *cis:trans* ratio is either 2:3 (WHO, 1990) or 1:3 (Worthing & Walker, 1987).

Permethrin is available in the USA as a technical-grade product containing 91.0-95.0% w/w of the pure chemical and 5.0-9.0% impurities (Fairfield American Corp., 1989; Roussel Bio Corp., 1989; ICI Americas, 1990).

Several of the minor components have been identified in technical permethrin. These were principally: ethyl (±)-*cis,trans*-3-(2,2-dichlorovinyl)-2,2-dimethylcyclopropane-1-carboxylate, 3-phenoxytoluene, 4-phenoxybenzyl (±)-*cis,trans*-3-(2,2-dichlorovinyl)-2,2-dimethylcyclopropane-1-carboxylate, and 6-bromo-3-phenoxybenzyl (±)-*cis,trans*-3-(2,2-dichlorovinyl)-2,2-dimethylcyclopropane-1-carboxylate. Other minor components were found to be xylene (see IARC, 1989), 3-phenoxybenzyl alcohol, *N,N*-diethyl-3-phenoxybenzylamine, 3-phenoxybenzaldehyde and 4-(2,2-dichlorovinyl)-5,5-dimethyloxacyclopentane-2-one (Horiba *et al.*, 1977).

Permethrin is formulated as granules, emulsifiable concentrates, wettable powders, dusts, smokes, ultra-low-volume sprays, fumigants, aerosols, fogging solutions and water-dispersible granules. In one European country, registered permethrin products also include capsule suspensions and lacquer formulations (Papadopoulou-Mourkidou, 1983; Swaine & Tandy, 1984; The Royal Society of Chemistry, 1986, 1989; Meister, 1990). In Europe, permethrin is also registered in combination with piperonyl butoxide (see IARC, 1983, 1987), tetramethrin, plifenate and other pyrethrins (Royal Society of Chemistry, 1986).

1.1.4 *Analysis*

Selected methods for the analysis of permethrin in various matrices are given in Table 2. Permethrin can be determined in pesticide formulations using gas chromatography with flame ionization detection (Association of Official Analytical Chemists, 1986; WHO, 1990).

Several other methods for the determination of permethrin (and its individual isomers) in various matrices, including high-performance liquid chromatography and gas chromatography, have been reviewed (Horiba *et al.*, 1977; Miyamoto *et al.*, 1981; Baker & Bottomley, 1982; Papadopoulou-Mourkidou, 1983; Nehmer & Dimov, 1984; Swaine & Tandy, 1984).

---

[1]Calculated from: mg/m^3 = (molecular weight/24.45) × ppm, assuming standard temperature (25°C) and pressure (760 mm Hg [101.3 kPa])

Table 2. Methods for the analysis of permethrin

Sample matrix	Sample preparation	Assay procedure[a]	Limit of detection	Reference
Water	Extract with dichloromethane; isolate extract; dry; concentrate with methyl *tert*-butyl ether	GC/ECD	0.5 µg/l (for isomers)	US Environmental Protection Agency (1989a)
Waste-water	Extract with dichloromethane; dry; exchange into hexane	GC/ECD	0.2 µg/l (for isomers)	US Environmental Protection Agency (undated)
Soil	Extract with methanol:water (9:1); partition into dichloromethane; clean-up on activated Florisil column	GC/CCD[b]	0.05 ppm (mg/kg)	US Food and Drug Administration (1989)
Crops	Extract with hexane; remove oil by gel permeation chromatography; clean-up on activated Florisil column	GC/CCD[b] GC/ECD[b]	0.05 ppm (mg/kg)	US Food and Drug Administration (1989)
Milk, animal tissue	Extract with acetone:hexane (1:1); partition into dimethylformamide (in 1% aqueous sodium sulfate solution); back-extract into hexane; clean-up on activated Florisil column	GC/ECD[b]	0.01 ppm (mg/l or mg/kg)	US Food and Drug Administration (1989)
Eggs	Extract with acetone/hexane (1:1); wash with 10% sodium chloride solution; partition into dimethylformamide (in 1% aqueous sodium sulfate solution); back-extract into hexane; clean-up on activated Florisil column plus Merckogel or Fractosil	GC/ECD[b]	0.02 ppm (mg/kg) (0.01 ppm for isomers)	US Food and Drug Administration (1989)

[a]Abbreviations: GC/CCD, gas chromatography/Coulson conductivity detection; GC/ECD, gas chromatography/electron capture detection
[b]Method is suitable for determining total permethrin or the individual *cis*- and *trans*-permethrin isomers

1.2 Production and use

1.2.1 *Production*

Permethrin was first synthesized in 1973 (Swaine & Tandy, 1984) and first marketed in 1977 (WHO, 1990).

The starting acid is prepared by a variation of the conventional chrysanthemic acid synthesis using ethyldiazoacetate in which 1,1-dichloro-4-methyl-1,3-pentadiene is reacted with ethyldiazoacetate in the presence of a copper catalyst and the resulting ethyl (±)-*cis*,*trans*-2,2-dimethyl-3-(2,2-dichlorovinyl)cyclopropanecarboxylate hydrolysed to the free acid. The *cis*- and *trans*-isomers can be separated from one another by selective crystallization from *n*-hexane in which the *cis*-isomer is more soluble. The starting acid is then reacted with 3-phenoxybenzyl alcohol to give permethrin (Sittig, 1980).

Permethrin is produced currently in Japan, the United Kingdom and the USA (Meister, 1990).

1.2.2 *Use*

Permethrin is a synthetic contact pyrethroid insecticide with a high level of activity against a wide range of insects, including *Lepidoptera*, *Hemiptera*, *Diptera* and *Coleoptera*. It is used mainly in agriculture, where it is fast acting and effective against all growth stages, particularly larvae. About 60% of the permethrin produced is used on cotton plants. Other crops to which permethrin is applied are maize, soya beans, coffee, tobacco, rape seed oil, wheat, barley, alfalfa, vegetables and fruit (WHO, 1990).

Permethrin is also used for control of insects in household and animal facilities and in forest pest control, as a fog in mushroom houses, and as a wood preservative. Other applications are in public health, particularly for insect control in buildings and in aircraft, treatment of mosquito nets and control of human lice (WHO, 1990). It is also used for termite control as a barrier treatment on building foundations (Anon., 1989).

Approximately 600 tonnes of permethrin are used annually worldwide. The major countries or regions that were using permethrin in 1980 were (tonnes): the USA (263), Brazil (38), Mexico (36) and Central America (27) (WHO, 1990). In Finland, about 3.5 tonnes (active ingredient) permethrin were used in 1988 (Agrochemical Producers' Association of Finland, 1989)

1.3 Occurrence

1.3.1 *Food*

Samples (1954) of fruits, vegetables, grains, meats, dairy products and wine were analysed as part of the Canadian national surveillance programme in 1984-89. A total of 29 samples contained permethrin residues; of these 25 of 118 were in lettuce, 2 of 100 in pears and 2 of 97 in tomatoes. The residue levels ranged from 0.01 to 1.67 mg/kg (Government of Canada, 1990).

Cows were fed *cis:trans* (40:60)-permethrin at rates of 0.2-150 mg/kg diet for 28-31 days. Residues plateaued in milk, with means of < 0.01 µg/g and 0.3 µg/g at dietary levels of 0.2 and 150 mg/kg, respectively. Milk levels declined to < 0.01 µg/g within five days after permethrin administration ceased. Residue levels of < 0.01-0.04 and 2.8-6.2 µg/g fat were found in perirenal fat of cows given dietary levels of 0.2 and 150 mg/kg, respectively (as reported by WHO, 1990). Levels of radioactivity retained in tissues and secreted in milk were appreciably higher in goats treated with *cis*-permethrin than with *trans*-permethrin (Hunt & Gilbert, 1977). In goats dosed orally with 40:60 *cis:trans* permethrin equivalent to 10 mg/kg in the diet for seven days, residues in milk also plateaud at 0.02-0.03 µg permethrin equivalents/g after five days (FAO/WHO, 1982).

In supervised trials in Spain and the USA with citrus fruits, permethrin residues in the edible parts did not exceed 0.01 mg/kg and 0.05 mg/kg, respectively, when applied at the recommended rates. The residues were found almost exclusively in the peel (FAO/WHO, 1982).

1.3.2 *Occupational exposure*

Four of five workers in Sweden who packed conifer seedlings for 6 h in a tunnel that had been sprayed 1 h earlier with a 2% aqueous solution of permethrin, resulting in atmospheric concentrations of permethrin of 0.011-0.085 mg/m^3 in the breathing zone, did not excrete detectable amounts of acid pyrethrin metabolites in the urine. One very short person whose face was close to the plants and who had the highest concentration of permethrin in the breathing zone excreted 0.26 µg/ml permethrin acid metabolites in the urine the following morning; in the afternoon, excretion was below the detection limit of the method. A group of five workers who planted the treated conifer seedlings were exposed to non-detectable to low permethrin levels in the breathing zone (mean, 0.002 mg/m^3; range, not detected-0.006 mg/m^3) and excreted no detectable amount of permethrin metabolites in the urine (Kolmodin-Hedman *et al.*, 1982).

1.4 Regulations and guidelines

The FAO/WHO Joint Meeting on Pesticide Residues evaluated permethrin at its meetings in 1979, 1980, 1981, 1982, 1983, 1984, 1985, 1987, 1988 and 1989 (FAO/WHO, 1980, 1981, 1982, 1983, 1985a,b, 1986, 1987, 1988, 1990). In 1987, an acceptable daily intake of 0.05 mg/kg bw was established (40% *cis*:60% *trans* and 25% *cis*:75% *trans* material) (FAO/WHO, 1987).

Maximum residue levels have been established by the Codex Alimentarius Commission for permethrin in or on the following agricultural commodities (in mg/kg): coffee beans, pistachio nuts, potatoes, rape seeds, soya beans and sugar beets, 0.05; almonds, carrots, crude soya bean oil, dried beans, edible cottonseed oil, eggs, Japanese radishes, kohlrabi, melons (except watermelon), milks (fat), mushrooms, peanuts, shelled peas and sweet corn, 0.1; cauliflower, citrus fruits, cottonseed, cucumbers, gherkins, horseradish, leeks, spring onions, summer squash, wheat flour (post-harvest treatment) and winter squash, 0.5; asparagus, blackberries, Brussels' sprouts, common beans, dewberries (boysenberries and loganberries), eggplants, olives, peppers, raspberries (red and black), strawberries, sunflower seeds, sunflower seed oil (crude and edible) and tomatoes, 1; broccoli, celery, cereal grains (post-harvest treatment), currants (black, red and white), gooseberries, grapes, head lettuce, kiwifruit, pome fruit, spinach, stone fruit and wholemeal wheat (post-harvest treatment), 2; cabbage (Chinese, head and savoy) and kale, 5; unprocessed wheat bran (post-harvest treatment), 10; dry sorghum straw and fodder and tea (green and black), 20; dried apple pomace, dried hops and soya bean fodder, 50; alfalfa and maize fodder, 100 (Codex Committee on Pesticide Residues, 1990).

Maximum residue levels have been established by the Codex Alimentarius Commission for permethrin in or on the following animal commodities (in mg/kg): edible offal (mammalian; accommodates veterinary uses) and poultry meat, 0.1; meat (fat; accommodates veterinary uses), 1 (Codex Committee on Pesticide Residues, 1990).

National and regional pesticide residue limits for permethrin in foods are presented in Table 3.

Table 3. National and regional pesticide residue limits for permethrin in foods[a]

Country or region	Residue limit (mg/kg)	Commodities
Australia	10	Bran
	5	Celery, lettuce
	2	Brussels' sprouts, cereal grains, kiwifruit, mushrooms
	1	Cole crops (except Brussels' sprouts)
	0.5	Edible offal of goat, green beans
	0.4	Tomatoes
	0.2	Cottonseed, rapeseed, sunflower seeds
	0.1	Beans (mung, navy), cattle, goats, pigs, poultry, and sheep (fat of meat), eggs, linseed, lupins, soya beans, sugar-cane
	0.05	Cattle and goat milk (in the fat), milk products (fat basis), potatoes, sweet corn
Austria[b]	50	Hops
	1.0	Meat, cereals, fruits, vegetables
	0.1	Eggs (without shell), milk
Belgium[b]	2	Grains, kiwi fruit
	1	Other fruit, other vegetables
	0.05	Animal fats, meat (poultry, hares, fowl, game), meat products, milk, milk products, mushrooms, potatoes
	0 (0.05)[c]	Other foodstuffs of vegetable origin
	0 (0.01)[c]	Other foodstuffs of animal origin
Brazil	0.5	Cottonseed, rice
	0.3	Tomatoes
	0.1	Cabbage, cauliflower, corn, kale
	0.02	Wheat
	0.01	Coffee (shelled), soya beans
Canada	2.0	Grapes
	1.0	Apples, lettuce, peaches, pears
	0.5	Beans, broccoli, Brussels sprouts, cabbage, celery, cucumbers, peppers, plums, tomatoes
	Negligible	Asparagus, cattle (meat and milk), beetroot, blueberries, cauliflower, corn, flax, horseradish, kiwi fruits, onion, potatoes, poultry (meat and eggs), radishes, rapeseed (canola oil), sugar beets (sugar), sunflowers, turnips, wheat
Chile	0.05	Carcasses, eggs, milk, poultry
Denmark[b]	5	Leafy vegetables
	2	Berries, fruit (pome, small, stone, other), other vegetables
	0.5	Citrus fruit
	0.1	Carrots
Finland[b]	2.0	Citrus fruit
	0.5	Other foodstuffs (except cereal grains)
France[b]	2.0	Kiwifruit
	1.0	Cabbage, fruit, vegetable greens (salad)
	0.5	Other vegetables
	0.1	Maize

Table 3 (contd)

Country or region	Residue limit (mg/kg)	Commodities
Germany	50	Hops
	10	Bran
	2	Cereals (except maize), cereal products (except bran), currants, kiwi-fruit, lettuce
	1.0	Other fruit, other leafy and sprout vegetables
	0.5	Fruit used as vegetables
	0.2	Maize, oilseed
	0.1	Root vegetables
	0.05	Citrus juices, kiwifruit (without peel), raw coffee, spices, tea, tea-like products, other foodstuffs of plant origin
Italy	1.0	Apples, cabbage, carrots, cereals, citrus fruit, cucurbitaceae, drupes, grapes, leeks, lettuce, mushrooms (cultivated), olives, pears, potatoes, solanaceae, spinach, sugar beets, tobacco, turnips
Japan[d]	20	Tea
	15	Exocarp of summer oranges
	5	Fruit (except exocarp of summer oranges)
	3	Vegetables
	0.5	Sugar beets
	0.2	Potatoes, etc.
Netherlands[b]	2	Kiwifruit, leafy vegetables
	1	Other fruit, other vegetables
	0.05[e]	Mushrooms, potatoes, animal products
	0 (0.05)[f]	Other foodstuffs
New Zealand	2.0	Kiwifruit
	1.0	*Brassica* vegetables, fruit (berry, pome)
	0.5	Fruiting vegetables, grapes, legumes
South Africa[b]	0.5	Apples, grapes, lucerne, mealies (green), pears, sorghum
	0.1	Beans, peas, tomatoes
	0.05	Cottonseed, groundnuts, potatoes
Spain[b]	20	Hops (dried)
	10	Alfalfa (dried)
	1.0	Fruit, fruit vegetables
	0.5	Cottonseed, sunflower seeds
	0.05	Beetroot, maize, potatoes, rapeseed, sorghum grains, soya beans
	0.01	Other plant products
Sweden[b]	2.0	Fruit, vegetables
	0.05	Potatoes
Switzerland	2.0[g]	Kiwifruit (whole)
	0.8	Cabbage
	0.5	Other foodstuffs
	0.4	Fruit (except grapes and kiwifruit), vegetables (except cabbage and potatoes)
	0.1[g]	Kiwifruit (pulp)
	0.05	Milk
	0.01	Potatoes

Table 3 (contd)

Country or region	Residue limit (mg/kg)	Commodities
Taiwan	2.0	Leafy vegetables with large wrapper leaves, leafy vegetables with small leaves
	1.0	Fruit vegetables
	0.5	Rice
USA[h]	60	Maize (fodder, forage)
	55	Alfalfa (hay)
	25	Alfalfa (fresh)
	20	Almond hulls, head lettuce, leafy vegetables (except *Brassica*), spinach, collards, turnip greens
	15	Range grasses
	10	Artichokes
	6.25	Milk fat (reflecting 0.25 ppm in whole milk)
	6	Cabbage, mushrooms
	5	Celery, peaches, watercress
	3	Cherries, pears, cucurbit vegetables, fat (cattle, goats, hogs, horses, sheep), meat by-products (hogs)
	2	Kiwifruit, tomatoes, meat by-products (cattle, goats, horses, sheep)
	1.0	Asparagus, avocados, bell peppers, broccoli, Brussels' sprouts, cauliflower, eggplant, eggs, horseradish, papayas (limited to Florida), turnip roots (regional registration)
	0.5	Cottonseed
	0.25	Meat (cattle, goats, hogs, horses, poultry, sheep)
	0.15	Fat (poultry)
	0.1	Garlic, onions (dry bulb), pistachios, sweet maize (kernel plus cob with husks removed)
	0.05	Almonds, apples, maize grain (field, pop), filberts, potatoes, soya beans, walnuts, meat (poultry)

[a]From Health and Welfare Canada

[b]Sum of isomers

[c]The figure in parentheses is the lower limit for determining residues in the corresponding product according to the standard method of analysis.

[d]Standard for withholding registration of agricultural chemicals

[e]A pesticide may be used on an eating or drinking ware or raw material without a demonstrable residue remaining; the value listed is considered the highest concentration at which this requirement is deemed to have been met.

[f]Residues shall be absent; the value in parentheses is the highest concentration at which this requirement is still deemed to have been met.

[g]These upper 'limit values' are maximum concentrations which, if exceeded, mean that the food is judged unfit for human consumption.

[h]From US Environmental Protection Agency (1989b); includes its metabolites, 3-(2,2-dichloro-ethenyl)-2,2-dimethylcyclopropane carboxylic acid and (3-phenoxybenzyl)methanol

2. Studies of Cancer in Humans

No data were available to the Working Group.

3. Studies of Cancer in Experimental Animals

Oral administration

Mouse: Four groups of 70 male and 70 female Swiss-derived mice, four to five weeks old, were fed 0, 250, 1000 or 2500 mg/kg of diet permethrin (*cis:trans* isomer, 40:60; > 93.9% pure) for 98 weeks. Survival in control and experimental groups was comparable; more than 75% of animals survived beyond 52 weeks and 20% or more survived until the termination of experiment. In male mice, there was a slight increase in the incidence of pulmonary adenomas: 11/70 control, 6/69 low dose, 13/70 mid dose and 17/70 high dose (p = 0.04 test for trend) (Ishmael & Litchfield, 1988).

Rat: Four groups of 60 male and 60 female pathogen-free Alpk:AP (Wistar-derived) rats, aged four to five weeks, were fed 0, 500, 1000 or 2500 mg/kg of diet permethrin (*cis:trans* isomer, 40:60; > 93.9% pure) for 104 weeks, at which time the experiment was terminated. Survival in control and experimental groups was similar; more than 92% survived beyond 52 weeks and 42% or more survived until termination of the experiment. There was no difference in the incidence of tumours between the control and experimental groups (Ishmael & Litchfield, 1988).

4. Other relevant data

The toxicity of permethrin has been reviewed (FAO/WHO, 1980, 1982, 1988; WHO, 1990).

4.1 Absorption, distribution, metabolism and excretion

4.1.1 *Humans*

Ten scabies patients (five men and five women) had about 25 g (range, 21-32 g) of a 5% permethrin cream applied to the skin of the whole body, with the exception of the head and neck. Dermal absorption of permethrin was calculated from the quantity of conjugated and nonconjugated *cis*- and *trans*-3-(2,2-dichlorovinyl)-2,2-dimethylcyclopropane carboxylic acid (CVA) metabolites of permethrin determined in the urine. In samples of urine collected by seven patients one and two days after application of the permethrin cream, 414 and 439 µg mean total CVA were found, respectively. The mean total CVA in the urine of three patients who collected their urine in the same container for two days was 1435 µg. The urinary concentration of *trans*-CVA varied during the first 48 h from 0.11 to 1.07 µg/ml and that of the *cis*-isomer from 0.02 to 0.21 µg/ml. CVA was still detectable in the urine of three patients after a week and in the urine of one patient, reported to be an alcoholic, after two weeks. The absorption of permethrin over the first 48 h after application was estimated from the urinary CVA excretion levels to be 6 mg (range, 3-11 mg), i.e., 0.5% of the dose applied (van der Rhee *et al.*, 1989).

Among approximately 350 people who were individually dusted against body lice with 30-50 g of powders containing 2.5 or 5.0 g/kg permethrin (*cis:trans*, 25:75), the mean amount of permethrin absorbed during the first 24 h after treatment was estimated to be 14 µg/kg bw among 19 of the subjects using the powder containing 2.5 g/kg permethrin and 39 µg/kg bw among 15 of the subjects using the 5 g/kg powder. No residue was found in samples of urine taken 30 and 60 days after treatment (Nassif *et al.*, 1980).

4.1.2 *Experimental systems*

Pyrethroids are absorbed through the skin and the respiratory and digestive tracts, although absorption from the gastrointestinal tract appears to be incomplete. Pyrethroids undergo metabolic degradation at numerous sites (Miyamoto, 1976). In mammals, they are generally metabolized through ester hydrolysis, oxidation and conjugation (WHO, 1990).

The metabolism of permethrin has been studied in great detail in various species of mammals using isomers labelled in the alcohol or acid moiety. The metabolic pathways of permethrin in mammals are given in Figure 1 (WHO, 1990). It is metabolized and almost completely eliminated from the body within approximately 12 days in rats, goats and cows following oral administration; *trans*-permethrin is eliminated more rapidly than is *cis*-permethrin, and trace tissue residue levels of the *cis* isomer were higher than those of the *trans* isomer in these species (Elliot *et al.*, 1976, Gaughan *et al.*, 1977, 1978; Ivie & Hunt, 1980). Absorption through the skin has been demonstrated in mice (Shah *et al.*, 1981), rats (Shah *et al.*, 1987; Sidon *et al.*, 1988) and monkeys (Sidon *et al.*, 1988). Dermal absorption was greater in rats than in monkeys (Sidon *et al.*, 1988). After an intramuscular injection of ^{14}C-labelled permethrin, the urinary half-time values were similar for the *cis* and *trans* isomers in rats and monkeys. Radiocarbon from *trans*-permethrin was excreted mostly in the urine, whereas that from the *cis*-permethrin was eliminated in both urine and faeces (Sidon *et al.*, 1988).

4.2 Toxic effects

4.2.1 *Humans*

Volunteers received applications to an area of 4 cm^2 on an ear lobe of 0.05 ml of a field-strength preparation of technical (94-96% active ingredients) or formulated (32-36%) permethrin (0.13 mg/cm^2) or of the inert ingredients; 0.05 ml of the vehicle (ethanol as the control for technical permethrin and water as the control for formulated permethrin) was applied to the other lobe. The intensity of paraesthesia induced by permethrin was four-fold stronger than that induced by a similar application of fenvalerate, permethrin being the least active compound for both the technical and formulated preparations. No cutaneous sensation was elicited by the inert ingredients. Paraesthesia appeared after a latent period of about 30 min, peaked between 8 and 12 h and disappeared after about 24 h. Further studies using a range of doses demonstrated that the response was dose-related (Flannigan *et al.*, 1985).

Workers who handled seedlings treated with permethrin (*cis:trans*, 25:75 wettable powder or *cis:trans*, 40:60) reported irritation on the skin (63% of subjects) and in the upper respiratory tract (33%) (Kolmodin-Hedman *et al.*, 1982).

A group of 435 patients, most of them children, were treated for pediculosis capitis; approximately half of the group were treated with a single, 10-min application of 25-50 ml of a permethrin (1%) and isopropanol (20%) cream rinse after towel drying of washed hair, and the remainder were treated with a liquid product containing pyrethrins (0.3%), piperonyl

Fig. 1. Metabolic pathways of permethrin in mammals[a]

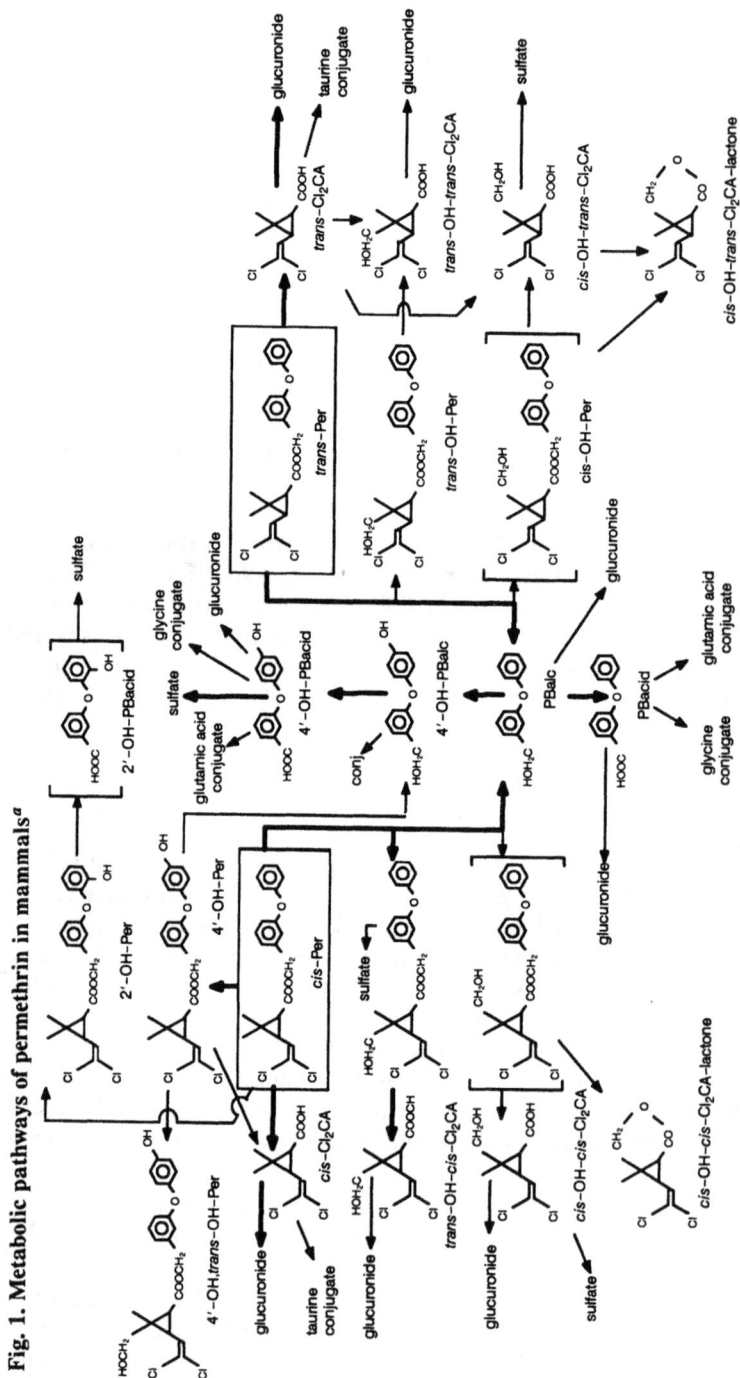

[a]From WHO (1990); Per, permethrin; Cl₂CA, chrysanthemic acid; PBacid, 3-phenoxybenzoic acid; PBalc, 3-phenoxybenzyl alcohol

butoxide (3%), petroleum distillate (1.2%) and benzyl alcohol (2.4%). Cutaneous side-effects (pruritus, mild transient skin burning, stinging sensations, skin tingling, erythema and scalp rash) were reported by 7% of the patients in the first group and by 16% of those in the second (DiNapoli *et al.*, 1988). Similar results and side-effects were reported by Brandenburg *et al.* (1986).

One of 28 subjects with pediculosis pubis treated with a 1% permethrin rinse developed mild scrotal erythema and irritation 12 h after application (Kalter *et al.*, 1987).

Of 10 scabies patients treated with one application of 25 g (range, 21-32 g) of a 5% permethrin cream, followed by a thorough washing approximately 8-20 h after treatment, six had limited, mild-to-moderate not pre-existing eczema on the scabies-affected skin at one or more examinations (van der Rhee *et al.*, 1989).

4.2.2 *Experimental systems*

Synthetic pyrethroids act on axons in the peripheral and central nervous system by interacting with sodium channels in mammals and/or insects. The mechanism of toxicity of synthetic pyrethroids and their classification into two types were reviewed by WHO (1990). Permethrin does not contain an α-cyano-group and is a type I pyrethroid.

Oral LD_{50}s in aqueous suspension generally ranged from approximately 3000 to > 4000 mg/kg bw, while the use of corn oil as the vehicle generally gave LD_{50} values of about 500 mg/kg bw (WHO, 1990). *cis*-Permethrin is considerably more toxic than *trans*-permethrin when given orally to rats (in WHO, 1990) or intraperitoneally or intravenously to mice (Glickman *et al.*, 1982). After oral administration of 40:60 *cis:trans* permethrin to rats, signs of poisoning became apparent after 2 h and persisted for up to three days; these included whole-body tremors, sometimes accompanied by salivation. Other signs were hyperactivity, hyperexcitability, urination, defaecation and ataxia (WHO, 1990).

In several subacute and subchronic studies by oral administration of permethrin to mice, rats and dogs, repeated findings were increases in absolute and relative liver weights, proliferation of smooth endoplasmic reticulum and increased activity of microsomal oxidative enzymes. In 90-day studies in rats, increased absolute and relative liver weights were reported to be evident with doses of 100 mg/kg of diet; in dogs, such effects were reported to be apparent with doses of 50 mg/kg bw and upwards for 90 days. In some but not all studies, high doses of permethrin were reported to damage peripheral nerves in rats (WHO, 1990). In rats fed diets of 20, 100 or 500 ppm (mg/kg) permethrin [isomeric composition unspecified] for two years or in rats from the third generation in a three-generation study with dietary exposure to 20 or 100 ppm, however, there was no evidence of morphological damage to nervous tissue when compared to control groups (Dyck *et al.*, 1984).

Long-term studies with rats and mice fed diets containing up to 2500 ppm (mg/kg) permethrin (40:60 *cis:trans*) indicated effects on the central nervous system, such as tremors and hypersensitivity to noise, in rats only and only during the first two weeks. Liver hypertrophy, increased microsomal enzyme activity and proliferation of smooth endoplasmic reticulum occurred in both species but was less pronounced in mice (Ishmael & Litchfield, 1988).

Permethrin (80:20 *cis:trans*) (50 mg/kg bw per day orally to rats) increased the levels of cytochrome P450 in liver after four, eight or 12 days of administration and NADPH cytochrome c reductase after eight or 12 days. A mixture containing less of the *cis* form (40:60 *cis:trans*) increased the levels of the two enzymes only after eight or 12 days of administration (Carlson & Schoenig, 1980). Treatment of rats with 190 mg/kg bw permethrin (25:75 *cis:trans* permethrin) intraperitoneally for three days decreased antipyrine half-time, and γ-glutamyl-transpeptidase activity in plasma was significantly increased within 21 and 14 days at doses of 95 and 190 mg/kg bw per day, respectively (Anadon *et al.*, 1988).

4.3 Reproductive and developmental effects

4.3.1 *Humans*

No data were available to the Working Group.

4.3.2 *Experimental systems*

Following immersion of fertile mallard eggs (30 per dose group) for 30 sec in an aqueous solution of permethrin, the LC_{50} for embryonic death was > 40 lb/acre at 100 gal/acre (> 45 kg/ha at 935 l/ha; more than 100 times the usual field application rate); no malformation was observed in mallard chicks (Hoffman & Albers, 1984).

Sprague-Dawley rats, weighing 180-200 g, were treated with permethrin in water at concentrations ranging from 500 to 4000 ppm (mg/l) or with drinking-water (control) on days 6-15 of gestation. At concentrations of 2500 ppm or more, the protein and glycogen content of the placenta was reduced (actual weight not given). The resorption index was increased at all doses, but there was no change in the number of live fetuses at day 20 of gestation in any treatment group (Spencer & Berhane, 1982).

4.4 Genetic and related effects (see also Table 5 and Appendices 1 and 2)

4.4.1 *Humans*

No data were available to the Working Group.

4.4.2 *Experimental systems*

Several unpublished studies were cited in a recent review (WHO, 1990).

Permethrin did not induce mutation in either bacteria or cultured Chinese hamster V79 cells. It did not induce mutation or aneuploidy in *Drosophila melanogaster*, nor did it inhibit gap-junctional intercellular communication in V79 cells.

[The Working Group noted that the studies by Páldy (1981) and by Hoellinger *et al.* (1987) on rodent bone marrow *in vivo* could not be evaluated because of inadequacies in the experimental design and reporting of the studies.]

5. Summary of Data Reported and Evaluation

5.1 Exposure

Permethrin is a highly active contact insecticide, which was first marketed in 1977. It is used mainly on cotton and food crops. Other uses are in forestry and for public health purposes, in public buildings, residences and aircraft.

Table 5. Genetic and related effects of permethrin

Test system	Result[a]		Dose[b]	Reference
	Without exogenous metabolic system	With exogenous metabolic system		
SA0, *Salmonella typhimurium* TA100, reverse mutation	–	–	490.0000	Bartsch *et al.* (1980)
SA0, *Salmonella typhimurium* TA100, reverse mutation	–	–	2500.0000	Moriya *et al.* (1983)
SA0, *Salmonella typhimurium* TA100, reverse mutation	–	–	150.0000	Pluijmen *et al.* (1984)
SA0, *Salmonella typhimurium* TA100, reverse mutation (fluct. test)	–	–	10.0000	Pluijmen *et al.* (1984)
SA0, *Salmonella typhimurium* TA100, reverse mutation	–	–	2730.0000	Pednekar *et al.* (1987)
SA0, *Salmonella typhimurium* TA100, reverse mutation	–	–	3000.0000	Herrera & Laborda (1988)
SA4, *Salmonella typhimurium* TA104, reverse mutation (spot test)	–	–	3000.0000	Herrera & Laborda (1988)
SA5, *Salmonella typhimurium* TA1535, reverse mutation	–	–	2500.0000	Moriya *et al.* (1983)
SA5, *Salmonella typhimurium* TA1535, reverse mutation (spot test)	–	–	500.0000	Herrera & Laborda (1988)
SA7, *Salmonella typhimurium* TA1537, reverse mutation	–	–	2500.0000	Moriya *et al.* (1983)
SA7, *Salmonella typhimurium* TA1537, reverse mutation (spot test)	–	–	500.0000	Herrera & Laborda (1988)
SA8, *Salmonella typhimurium* TA1538, reverse mutation	–	–	2500.0000	Moriya *et al.* (1983)
SA8, *Salmonella typhimurium* TA1538, reverse mutation (spot test)	–	–	500.0000	Herrera & Laborda (1988)
SA9, *Salmonella typhimurium* TA98, reverse mutation	–	–	490.0000	Bartsch *et al.* (1980)
SA9, *Salmonella typhimurium* TA98, reverse mutation	–	–	2500.0000	Moriya *et al.* (1983)
SA9, *Salmonella typhimurium* TA98, reverse mutation	–	–	150.0000	Pluijmen *et al.* (1984)
SA9, *Salmonella typhimurium* TA98, reverse mutation (fluct. test)	–	–	10.0000	Pluijmen *et al.* (1984)
SA9, *Salmonella typhimurium* TA98, reverse mutation	–	–	2730.0000	Pednekar *et al.* (1987)
SA9, *Salmonella typhimurium* TA98, reverse mutation	–	–	3000.0000	Herrera & Laborda (1988)
SAS, *Salmonella typhimurium* TA97a, reverse mutation	–	–	2730.0000	Pednekar *et al.* (1987)
SAS, *Salmonella typhimurium* TA97, reverse mutation	–	–	3000.0000	Herrera & Laborda (1988)
EC2, *Escherichia coli* WP2 *hcr*, reverse mutation	–	–	2500.0000	Moriya *et al.* (1983)

Table 5 (contd)

Test system	Result[a]		Dose[b]	Reference
	Without exogenous metabolic system	With exogenous metabolic system		
DMN, *Drosophila melanogaster*, chromosome loss	–	0	5.0000 (feeding solution)	Woodruff *et al.* (1983)
DMX, *Drosophila melanogaster*, sex-linked recessive lethal mutation	–	0	1.0000 (feeding solution)	Gupta et al (1990)
G9O, Gene mutation, Chinese hamster V79 cells, ouabain resistance	–	0[c]	40.0000	Pluijmen *et al.* (1984)
G9H, Gene mutation, Chinese hamster V79 cells, *hprt* locus	–	0[c]	40.0000	Pluijmen *et al.* (1984)
ICR, Inhibition of intercellular communication, V79 cells *in vitro*	–	0	8.0000	Flodström *et al.* (1988)

[a], negative; 0, not tested
[b]In-vitro tests, μg/ml; in-vivo tests, mg/kg bw
[c]Data obtained in the presence of an exogenous metabolic system were inadequate for an evaluation

Permethrin has been formulated as granules, powders, emulsifiable concentrates, aerosols and other forms.

Exposure can occur during its production and application and, at much lower levels, from consumption of food containing residues.

5.2 Carcinogenicity data in humans

No data were available to the Working Group.

5.3 Carcinogenicity in experimental animals

One preparation of permethrin (*cis:trans*, 40:60) was tested for carcinogenicity in one study in mice and in one study in rats by oral administration in the diet. In mice, a marginal increase in the incidence of pulmonary adenomas was observed in males. No increased tumour incidence was observed in treated rats.

5.4 Other relevant data

Permethrin has caused dermal irritation after topical exposure. It induced microsomal enzymes in rats and mice.

No data were available on the genetic and related effects of permethrin in humans. No effect was observed in the limited number of short-term tests available.

5.5 Evaluation[1]

No data were available from studies in humans.

There is *inadequate evidence* for the carcinogenicity of permethrin in experimental animals.

Overall evaluation

Permethrin *is not classifiable as to its carcinogenicity to humans (Group 3).*

6. References

Agrochemical Producers' Association of Finland (1989) 1988 Finnish pesticide sales. *AGROW*, 97, 11-12

Anadon, A., Diez, M.J., Sierra, M., Sanchez, J.A. & Teran, M.T. (1988) Microsomal enzyme induction by permethrin in rats. *Vet. hum. Toxicol.*, 30, 309-312

Anon. (1989) *CPCR® Crop Protection Chemicals Reference*, 5th ed., New York, Chemical and Pharmaceutical Press, pp. 1224-1234, 1268-1277, 1431-1434

Association of Official Analytical Chemists (1986) Permethrin in pesticide formulations. Gas chromatographic method. First action. CIPAC-AOAC method. In: *Changes in Official Methods of Analysis*, 14th ed., 2nd Suppl., Washington DC, pp. 351-352

---

[1]For definition of the italicized terms, see Preamble, pp. 26-28.

Baker, P.G. & Bottomley, P. (1982) Determination of residues of synthetic pyrethroids in fruit and vegetables by gas-liquid and high-performance liquid chromatography. *Analyst, 107,* 206-212

Bartsch, H., Malaveille, C., Camus, A.-M., Martel-Planche, G., Brun, G., Hautefeuille, A., Sabadie, N., Barbin, A., Kuroki, T., Drevon, C., Piccoli, C. & Montesano, R. (1980) Validation and comparative studies on 180 chemicals with *S. typhimurium* strains and V79 Chinese hamster cells in the presence of various metabolizing systems. *Mutat. Res., 76,* 1-50

Brandenburg, K., Deinard, A.S., DiNapoli, J., Englender, S.J., Orthoefer, J. & Wagner, D. (1986) 1% permethrin cream rinse vs 1% lindane shampoo in treating pediculosis capitis. *Am. J. Dis. Child., 140,* 894-896

Carlson, G.P. & Schoenig, G.P. (1980) Induction of liver microsomal NADPH cytochrome c reductase and cytochrome P-450 by some new synthetic pyrethroids. *Toxicol. appl. Pharmacol., 52,* 507-512

Codex Committee on Pesticide Residues (1990) *Guide to Codex Maximum Limits for Pesticide Residues,* Part 2, (CAC/PR 2—1990; CCPR Pesticide Classification No. 120), The Hague

DiNapoli, J.B., Austin, R.D., Englender, S.J., Gomez, M.P. & Barrett, J.F. (1988) Eradication of head lice with a single treatment. *Am. J. public Health, 78,* 978-980

Dyck, P.J., Shimono, M., Schoening, G.P., Lais, A.C., Oviatt, K.F. & Sparks, M.F. (1984) The evaluation of a new synthetic pyrethroid pesticide (permethrin) for neurotoxicity. *J. environ. Pathol. Toxicol. Oncol., 5,* 109-117

Elliot, M., Janes, N.F., Pulman, D.A., Gaughan, L.C., Unai, T. & Casida, J.E. (1976) Radiosynthesis and metabolism in rats of the 1R-isomers of the insecticide permethrin. *J. agric. Food Chem., 24,* 270-276

Fairfield American Corp. (1989) *Material Safety Data Sheet: Permethrin Technical,* Rutherford, NJ

FAO/WHO (1980) *Pesticide Residues in Food: 1979 Evaluations. The Monographs* (FAO Plant Production and Protection Paper 20 Sup.), Rome

FAO/WHO (1981) *Pesticide Residues in Food: 1980 Evaluations. The Monographs* (FAO Plant Production and Protection Paper 26 Sup.), Rome

FAO/WHO (1982) *Pesticide Residues in Food: 1981 Evaluations. The Monographs* (FAO Plant Production and Protection Paper 42), Rome

FAO/WHO (1983) *Pesticide Residues in Food: 1982 Evaluations. The Monographs* (FAO Plant Production and Protection Paper 49), Rome

FAO/WHO (1985a) *Pesticide Residues in Food: 1983 Evaluations. The Monographs* (FAO Plant Production and Protection Paper 61), Rome

FAO/WHO (1985b) *Pesticide Residues in Food: 1984 Evaluations. The Monographs* (FAO Plant Production and Protection Paper 67), Rome

FAO/WHO (1986) *Pesticide Residues in Food: 1985 Evaluations. The Monographs* (FAO Plant Production and Protection Paper 68), Rome

FAO/WHO (1987) *Pesticide Residues in Food: 1987 Evaluations. The Monographs. Report of the Joint Meeting of the FAO Panel of Experts on Pesticide Residues in Food and the Environment and a WHO Expert Group on Pesticide Residues* (FAO Plant Production and Protection Paper 84), Rome

FAO/WHO (1988) *Pesticide Residues in Food—1988 Evaluations. Part I—Residues* (FAO Plant Production and Protection Paper 93/1), Rome

FAO/WHO (1990) *Pesticide Residues in Food—1989 Evaluations. Part I—Residues* (FAO Plant Production and Protection Paper 100), Rome

Flannigan, S.A., Tucker, S.B., Key, M.M., Ross, C.E., Fairchild, E.J., II, Grimes, B.A. & Harrist, R.B. (1985) Synthetic pyrethroid insecticides: a dermatological evaluation. *Br. J. ind. Med., 42,* 363-372

Flodström, S., Wärngård, L., Ljungquist, S. & Ahlborg, U.G. (1988) Inhibition of metabolic cooperation *in vitro* and enhancement of enzyme altered foci incidence in rat liver by the pyrethroid insecticide fenvalerate. *Arch. Toxicol.*, *61*, 218-223

Gaughan, L.C., Unai, T. & Casida, J.E. (1977) Permethrin metabolism in rats. *J. agric. Food Chem.*, *25*, 9-17

Gaughan, L.C., Ackerman, M.E., Unai, T. & Casida, J.E. (1978) Distribution and metabolism of *trans*- and *cis*-permethrin in lactating Jersey cows. *J. agric. Food Chem.*, *26*, 613-618

Glickman, A.H., Weitman, S.D. & Lech, J.J. (1982) Different toxicity of *trans*-permethrin in rainbow trout and mice. I. Role of biotransformation. *Toxicol. appl. Pharmacol.*, *66*, 153-161

Government of Canada (1990) *Report on National Surveillance Data from 1984/85 to 1988/89*, Ottawa

Gupta, R.K., Mehr, Z.A., Korte, D.W., Jr & Rutledge, L.C. (1990) Mutagenic potential of permethrin in the *Drosophila melanogaster* (Diptera: Drosophilidae) sex-linked recessive lethal test. *J. Econ. Entomol.*, *83*, 721-724

Health and Welfare Canada (1990) *National Pesticide Residue Limits in Foods*, Ottawa, Bureau of Chemical Safety, Food Directorate, Health Protection Branch

Herrera, A. & Laborda, E. (1988) Mutagenic activity of synthetic pyrethroids in *Salmonella typhimurium*. *Mutagenesis*, *3*, 509-514

Hoellinger, H., Lecorsier, A., Sonnier, M., Leger, C., Do, C.-T. & Nguyen, H.-N. (1987) Cytotoxicity, cytogenotoxicity and allergenicity tests on certain pyrethroids. *Drug chem. Toxicol.*, *10*, 291-310

Hoffman, D.J. & Albers, P.H. (1984) Evaluation of potential embryotoxicity and teratogenicity of 42 herbicides, insecticides, and petroleum contaminants to mallard eggs. *Arch. environ. Contam. Toxicol.*, *13*, 15-27

Horiba, M., Kobayashi, A. & Murano, A. (1977) Gas-liquid chromatographic determination of a new pyrethroid, permethrin (S-3151) and its optical isomers. *Agric. biol. Chem.*, *41*, 581-586

Hunt, L.M. & Gilbert, B.N. (1977) Distribution and excretion rates of ^{14}C-labelled permethrin isomers administered orally to four lactating goats for 10 days. *J. agric. Food Chem.*, *25*, 673-676

IARC (1983) *IARC Monographs on the Evaluation of the Carcinogenic Risk of Chemicals to Humans*, Vol. 30, *Miscellaneous Pesticides*, Lyon, pp. 183-195

IARC (1987) *IARC Monographs on the Evaluation of Carcinogenic Risks to Humans*, Suppl. 7, *Overall Evaluations of Carcinogenicity: An Updating of* IARC Monographs *Volumes 1 to 42*, Lyon, p. 70

IARC (1989) *IARC Monographs on the Evaluation of Carcinogenic Risks to Humans*, Vol. 45, *Occupational Exposures in Petroleum Refining; Crude Oil and Major Petroleum Fuels*, Lyon, pp. 125-156

ICI Americas (1990) *Material Safety Data Sheet: Permethrin*, Wilmington, DE

Ishmael, J. & Litchfield, M.H. (1988) Chronic toxicity and carcinogenic evaluation of permethrin in rats and mice. *Fundam. appl. Toxicol.*, *11*, 308-322

Ivie, G.W. & Hunt, L.M. (1980) Metabolism of *cis*- and *trans*-permethrin in lactating goats. *J. agric. Food Chem.*, *28*, 1131-1138

Kalter, D.C., Sperber, J., Rosen, T. & Matarasso, S. (1987) Treatment of pediculosis pubis. Clinical comparison of efficacy and tolerance of 1% lindane shampoo vs 1% permethrin cream rinse. *Arch. Dermatol.*, *123*, 1315-1319

Kolmodin-Hedman, B., Swensson, Å. & Åkerbolm, N. (1982) Occupational exposure to some synthetic pyrethroids (permethrin and fenvalerate). *Arch. Toxicol.*, *50*, 27-33

Meister, R.T., ed. (1990) *Farm Chemicals Handbook '90*, Willoughby, OH, Meister Publishing Co., pp. C222-C223

Miyamoto, J. (1976) Degradation, metabolism and toxicity of synthetic pyrethroids. *Environ. Health Perspect.*, *14*, 15-28

Miyamoto, J., Beynon, K.I., Roberts, T.R., Hemingway, R.J. & Swaine, H. (1981) The chemistry, metabolism and residue analysis of synthetic pyrethroids. *Pure appl. Chem.*, *53*, 1967-2022

Moriya, M., Ohta, T., Watanabe, K., Miyazawa, T., Kato, K. & Shirasu, Y. (1983) Further mutagenicity studies on pesticides in bacterial reversion assay systems. *Mutat. Res.*, *116*, 185-216

Nassif, M., Brooke, J.P., Hutchinson, D.B.A., Kamel, O.M. & Savage, E.A. (1980) Studies with permethrin against bodylice in Egypt. *Pestic. Sci.*, *11*, 679-684

Nehmer, U. & Dimov, N. (1984) High-performance liquid chromatographic determination of kadethrin, permethrin and piperonyl butoxide in spray solutions. *J. Chromatogr.*, *288*, 227-229

Páldy, A. (1981) Examination of the mutagenic effect of synthetic pyrethroids on mouse bone-marrow cells. In: *Proceedings of the 21st Hungarian Annual Meeting on Biochemistry*, Budapest, National Institute of Public Health, pp. 227-228

Papadopoulou-Mourkidou, E. (1983) Analysis of established pyrethroid insecticides. *Residue Rev.*, *89*, 179-208

Pednekar, M.D., Gandhi, S.R. & Netrawali, M.S. (1987) Evaluation of mutagenic activities of endosulfan, phosalone, malathion and permethrin, before and after metabolic activation in the Ames *Salmonella* test. *Bull. environ. Contam. Toxicol.*, *38*, 925-933

Pluijmen, M., Drevon, C., Montesano, R., Malaveille, C., Hautefeuille, A. & Bartsch, H. (1984) Lack of mutagenicity of synthetic pyrethroids in *Salmonella typhimurium* strains and in V79 Chinese hamster cells. *Mutat. Res.*, *137*, 7-15

van der Rhee, H.J., Farquhar, J.A. & Vermeulen, N.P.E. (1989) Efficacy and transdermal absorption of permethrin in scabies patients. *Acta dermatol. venerol.*, *69*, 170-182

Roussel Bio Corp. (undated) *Technical Information Sheet: Pramex® (Permethrin) Synthetic Pyrethroid Insecticide*, Englewood Cliffs, NJ

Royal Society of Chemistry (1986) *European Directory of Agrochemical Products*, Vol. 3, *Insecticides, Acaricides, Nematicides*, Cambridge, pp. 453-465

Royal Society of Chemistry (1989) *The Agrochemicals Handbook* [Dialog Information Services (File 306)], Cambridge

Shah, P.V., Monroe, R.J. & Guthrie, F.E. (1981) Comparative rates of dermal penetration of insecticides in mice. *Toxicol. appl. Pharmacol.*, *59*, 414-423

Shah, P.V., Fisher, H.L., Sumler, M.R., Monroe, R.J., Chernoff, N. & Hall, L.L. (1987) Comparison of the penetration of 14 pesticides through the skin of young and adult rats. *J. Toxicol. environ. Health*, *21*, 353-366

Sidon, E.W., Moody, R.P. & Franklin, C.A. (1988) Percutaneous absorption of *cis*- and *trans*-permethrin in rhesus monkeys and rats: anatomic site and interspecies variation. *J. Toxicol. environ. Health*, *23*, 207-216

Sittig, M., ed. (1980) *Pesticide Manufacturing and Toxic Materials Control Encyclopedia*, Park Ridge, NJ, Noyes Data Corp., pp. 603-604

Spencer, F. & Berhane, Z. (1982) Uterine and fetal characteristics in rats following a post-implantational exposure to permethrin. *Bull. environ. Contam. Toxicol.*, *29*, 84-88

Swaine, H. & Tandy, M.J. (1984) Permethrin. In: Zweig, G. & Sherma, J., eds, *Analytical Methods for Pesticides and Plant Growth Regulators*, Vol. XIII, *Synthetic Pyrethroids and Other Pesticides*, New York, Academic Press, pp. 103-120

US Environmental Protection Agency (1989a) Method 508. Determination of chlorinated pesticides in water by gas chromatography with an electron capture detector. In: *Methods for the Determination of Organic Compounds in Drinking Water* (EPA Report No. EPA-600/4-88-039; US NTIS PB89-220461), Cincinnati, OH, Environmental Monitoring Systems Laboratory, pp. 171-198

US Environmental Protection Agency (1989b) Permethrin; tolerances for residues. *US Code fed. Regul., Title 40*, Part 180.378, pp. 356-357

US Environmental Protection Agency (undated) *Method 608.2: Analysis of Certain Organochlorine Pesticides in Wastewater by Gas Chromatography*, Cincinnati, OH, Environmental Monitoring and Support Laboratory

US Food and Drug Administration (1989) Permethrin. In: *Pesticide Analytical Manual*, Vol. II, *Methods Which Detect Multiple Residues*, Washington DC, US Department of Health and Human Services

WHO (1990) *Permethrin* (Environmental Health Criteria 94), Geneva

Woodruff, R.C., Phillips, J.P. & Irwin, D. (1983) Pesticide-induced complete and partial chromosome loss in screens with repair-defective females of *Drosophila melanogaster. Environ. Mutagenesis, 5*, 835-846

Worthing, C.R. & Walker, S.B., eds (1987) *The Pesticide Manual: A World Compendium*, 8th ed., Thornton Heath, British Crop Protection Council, pp. 647-648

FUNGICIDES

CAPTAFOL

1. Exposure Data

1.1 Chemical and physical data

1.1.1 *Synonyms, structural and molecular data*

Chem. Abstr. Serv. Reg. No.: 2425-06-1

Chem. Abstr. Name: 3α,4,7,7α-Tetrahydro-2-[(1,1,2,2-tetrachloroethyl)thiol]-1*H*-isoindole-1,3-(2*H*)dione

IUPAC Systematic Name: *N*-[(1,1,2,2-Tetrachloroethyl)thio]cyclohex-4-ene-1,2-dicarboximide

Synonyms: *N*-[(1,1,2,2-Tetrachloroethyl)thio]-4-cyclohexene-1,2-dicarboximide; tetrachloroethylthiotetrahydrophthalimide; *N*-(tetrachloroethylthio)tetrahydrophthalimide; *N*-(1,1,2,2-tetrachloroethylthio)-*delta*4-tetrahydrophthalimide; 3α,4,7,7α-tetrahydro-*N*-(1,1,2,2-tetrachloroethanesulfenyl)phthalimide

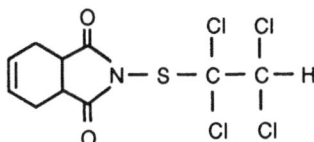

$C_{10}H_9Cl_4NO_2S$ Mol. wt: 349.06

1.1.2 *Chemical and physical properties*

 (*a*) *Description*: Colourless to pale-yellow crystals (Royal Society of Chemistry, 1989). The technical material is light-tan with a slight pungent odour (Pack, 1967).

 (*b*) *Melting-point*: 162°C (pure compound) (US Environmental Protection Agency, 1984a)

 (*c*) *Spectroscopy data*: Infrared spectroscopy data have been reported (US Environmental Protection Agency, 1975).

 (*d*) *Solubility*: Practically insoluble in water (1.4 mg/l at 20°C); slightly soluble in most organic solvents (g/kg): isopropanol, 13; benzene, 25; toluene, 17; xylene, 100; acetone, 43; methyl ethyl ketone, 44; dimethyl sulfoxide, 170 (Royal Society of Chemistry, 1989)

 (*e*) *Stability*: Slowly hydrolysed in aqueous emulsion or suspension; rapidly hydrolysed in acidic and alkaline media; decomposes slowly at the melting-point; corrosive to metals (Royal Society of Chemistry, 1989)

 (*f*) *Vapour pressure*: Negligible at room temperature (Royal Society of Chemistry, 1989)

 (*g*) *Conversion factor for airborne concentrations*[1]: mg/m³ = 14.28 × ppm

---

[1]Calculated from: mg/m³ = (molecular weight/24.45) × ppm, assuming standard temperature (25°C) and pressure (760 mm Hg [101.3 kPa])

1.1.3 *Trade names, technical products and impurities*

Some examples of common trade names are: Alfloc; Arborseal; CS 5623; Difolatan; Folcid; Foltaf; Haipen 50; Merpafol; Nalco 7046; Ortho 5865; Proxel EF; Santar SM; Terrazol (Worthing & Walker, 1987; Meister, 1990).

In the USA, the technical-grade product must contain at least 97% captafol as the sole active ingredient (US Environmental Protection Agency, 1984a). It has been formulated as dusts, emulsifiable concentrates, flowable suspensions, wettable powders and water-dispersible granules. The usual carriers are clay, talc (see IARC, 1987a), silica (see IARC, 1987b) and water (US Environmental Protection Agency, 1984b).

Formulated captafol products registered in European countries include coating agents, liquid formulations, pastes, suspension concentrates and wettable powders (Royal Society of Chemistry, 1986).

Captafol may be combined with most commonly used insecticides and fungicides, with the exception of strongly alkaline materials and oil sprays (Meister, 1990). It has been formulated in the USA in combination with triadimefon, carbendazim, folpet, ofurace, flutriafol, ethirimol, diclobutrazol, propiconazole, copper oxychloride, cymoxanil and halacrinate (Worthing & Walker, 1987). Formulations have also contained oxadiyl fenpropimorph, pyrazophos, captan (see IARC, 1983, 1987c), triadimenol and thiabendazole (Royal Society of Chemistry, 1986).

1.1.4 *Analysis*

Selected methods for the analysis of captafol in various matrices are given in Table 1.

Table 1. Methods for the analysis of captafol

Sample matrix	Sample preparation	Assay procedure[a]	Limit of detection	Reference
Specified fruits and vegetables	Extract with benzene; clean-up with thin-layer chromatography on silica gel or silicic acid column chromatography with or without preliminary hexane-aceto-nitrile partitioning	GC/ECD	0.1 ppm (mg/kg)	US Food and Drug Administration (1989a)
Maize, peanuts, tomatoes	Extract with ethyl acetate; clean-up by acetonitrile-hexane partitioning, aceto-nitrile-water-hexane partitioning and Florisil column chromatography	GC/ECD	0.1 ppm	US Food and Drug Administration (1989b)
Formulations	Extract with dichloromethane; centrifuge; filter	HPLC/UV	Not reported	Zweig & Sharma (1978)
Fruits, vegetables and oils	Extract with ethyl acetate; clean-up with either acetate-water, acetonitrile-hexane, or acetonitrile-water-hexane partitioning and Florisil column chromatography	GC/ECD or FID	Not reported	US Food and Drug Administration (1989c)

[a]Abbreviations: GC/ECD, gas chromatography/electron capture detection; GC/FID, gas chromatography/flame ionization detection; HPLC/UV, high-performance liquid chromatography/ultraviolet detection

1.2 Production and use

1.2.1 *Production*

Captafol is prepared by the reaction of tetrahydrophthalimide and 1,1,2,2-tetra-chloroethylsulfenyl chloride in the presence of aqueous sodium hydroxide (Pack, 1967). It was first produced commercially and registered for use in the USA in 1961 (County NatWest WoodMac, 1990). It is produced currently by two companies in India (Meister, 1990).

Production of captafol in the USA was estimated to be 3600-4500 tonnes (active ingredient) per year in 1979-81, of which half was exported (US Environmental Protection Agency, 1982). The sole US producer had a production of 6600 tonnes in 1985 (County NatWest WoodMac, 1990); that manufacturer ceased production in 1987 (Agriculture Canada, 1990).

1.2.2 *Use*

Captafol is a fungicide which has been used for the control of fungal diseases of fruits, vegetables, ornamental plants and turf grasses. It is also used to control certain seed- and soil-borne organisms (Pack, 1967). Captafol and/or its metabolites and degradrates are absorbed by roots and shoots of plants and translocated in plant tissue as a result of seed treatment, soil treatment and foliar application (US Environmental Protection Agency, 1984b).

Captafol is used to control scab of pome fruit, shot-hole of stone fruit, peach leaf curl, downy mildew and black rot of vines, early and late blights of potatoes, *Alternaria* and mildew of carrots, celery leaf spot, *Septoria* of wheat, *Rhynchosporium* of barley and various diseases of tomatoes, coffee, groundnuts, citrus fruit, pineapples, macadamia nuts, onions, cucurbits, maize, sorghum, etc. Captafol is also used as a seed treatment for control of *Pythium* and *Phoma* species and other emergence diseases of beetroot, cotton, groundnuts and rice. In addition, it is used as a protector for grafting and pruning wounds and cankers on trees and in the timber industry as a wood preservative (Royal Society of Chemistry, 1989).

Types and methods of application include dusting, spraying, misting and dipping under pressure for wood treatment (US Environmental Protection Agency, 1984b).

In the USA, annual use of captafol (active ingredient) as a pesticide in 1979-81 was about 500 tonnes for apples, 500 tonnes for cherries, 410 tonnes for citrus fruits, 240 tonnes for potatoes, 200 tonnes for tomatoes, 110 tonnes for sweet maize, 60 tonnes for plums, 10 tonnes for watermelon and 110 tonnes for other crops (US Environmental Protection Agency, 1982).

1.3 Occurrence

Some 1520 samples were analysed for captafol residues as part of the Canadian national surveillance programme between 1984 and 1989. Residues were found in nine samples: one of eight peaches, five of 200 pears and three of 97 tomatoes, at levels of 0.01-0.8 mg/kg (Government of Canada, 1990). Apples grown in Ontario (305 samples) were monitored for terminal residues of pest control chemicals on raw fruit offered for sale during the period 1978-86. On the 0.4% of crops treated with captafol, no residue was detected (detection limit, 0.02 mg/kg) (Frank *et al.*, 1989).

When fruit and vegetables were monitored in the United Kingdom at the point of sale, in 1981-82, residues of captafol at 0.02-0.7 mg/kg were found in six of 33 domestic potato samples and at 0.02-0.2 mg/kg in three of 16 imported potato samples (FAO/WHO, 1986a).

1.4 Regulations and guidelines

National and regional pesticide residue limits for captafol in foods are presented in Table 2.

Table 2. National and regional pesticide residue limits for captafol in food[a]

Country or region	Residue limit (mg/kg)	Commodities
Argentina	10	Sour cherries
	5	Cucumber, tomato, melon, peach, watermelon
	2	Plum, sweet cherry
	0.5	Grapefruit, mandarin, orange
	0.25	Apple, pear
Austria	0.1	Vegetables
Belgium	0[b] (0.05)	All foodstuffs of vegetable origin
Brazil	15	Peaches
	5	Apples, pears, eggplants, tomatoes
	2	Squash, honeydew melons, cucumbers, nectarines, watermelons
	1.0	Grapes, pineapples (treatment of seedlings)
	0.5	Carrots, citrus fruit, coffee, onions, peanuts (shelled), potatoes
	0.2	Wheat, rice
	0.1	Cottonseed, green beans, strawberries (treatment of seedlings)
	0.05	Peanuts
	0.04	Field beans
Chile	15	Peaches
	10	Plums
	5	Apples, pears, tomatoes
	2	Cherries
	0.5	Carrots, onions, potatoes
	0.2	Wheat
	0.1[c]	Carcasses[d] (sheep, hogs, goats and cattle), milk
Czechoslovakia[e]	15	Peaches
	10	Sour cherries
	5.0	Tomatoes
	2.0	Cherries, cucumbers, melons
Denmark	0.05[c]	All other foods, berries and small fruits, carrots, cereals, citrus fruits, leafy vegetables, other fruits, other root vegetables and onions, pome and stone fruits, potatoes
European Community	0.05	All products
Finland	2	Other (except cereal grains)
	0.5	Carrots, onions, potatoes
France	0.05	Cereal grains, fruits and vegetables
Germany	0.05	All foods of plant origin

Table 2 (contd)

Country or region	Residue limit (mg/kg)	Commodities
Hungary	15^e	Peaches
	10^e	Grapefruits, lemons, mandarins, oranges
	5	Apples, Brussels' sprouts, cabbage cauliflower, celery leaf, cherries, grapes, green beans, greenhouse tomatoes, green paprikas, kohlrabi, lettuce, pears, savoy, strawberries, tomatoes
	2.0	Cantaloupe, cucumbers, pumpkin, watermelons, wine grapes
	0.5	Beetroot, carrots, celery, horseradish, onion (green, red), parsley root, radish
Ireland	0.05	All products
Israel	5	Apples, eggplant, pears
	2	Pumpkin
	0.5	Carrots, onions, potatoes
	0.1	Almonds
Italy	8	Leafy garden vegetables, tobacco
	5	Hops, other fruit and garden vegetables
	2	Potatoes, root vegetables
	0.2	Cereals, sugar beets
	0.05	Fruit and garden vegetables
Japan	5	Apples, Japanese pear, fruit^f
	1.0	Cabbage, garden radish, garden radish leaves, potatoes^f, tea^f, vegetables^f, etc.
Kenya	15	Peaches
	10	Sour cherries
	5	Tomatoes
	2	Melons (whole), sweet cherries
	1.0	Cucumbers (whole)
	0.5	Apricots
	0.2	Plums
Netherlands	8	Leaf vegetables
	5	Fruit, other vegetables
	2	Root, tuber vegetables
	0.05^g	Cereals
	0 (0.05)^h	Other
Singapore	15	Apricots, nectarines, peaches
	5.0	Other fruits and vegetables
South Africa	10	Pineapples
	5	Avocados
	3	Coffee, tomatoes
	0.5	Potatoes
Spain	0.05^i	All plant products
Sweden	0.05^c	Cereals and hulled grains, flakes and flour made from cereals, fruits and vegetables, potatoes
Switzerland	0.1	Cereals, potatoes

Table 2 (contd)

Country or region	Residue limit (mg/kg)	Commodities
Taiwan	1.0	Berries, melons
	0.5	Citrus fruits, fruit vegetables, nut fruits, pome and stone fruits, tropical fruits
	0.1	Root vegetables
	0.01	Rice
United Kingdom	0.05[j]	Apples, bananas, barley, beans, black currants, Brussels' sprouts, cabbage, carrots, cauliflower, celery, cucumber, grapes, leeks, lettuce, maize, mushrooms, nectarines, oats, onions, oranges, other cereals, other citrus, paddy rice, pears, peaches, peas, plums, potatoes, raspberries, rye, strawberries, swedes, tomato, turnips, wheat
USA	50	Sour cherries
	35	Blueberries
	30	Apricots, peaches
	15	Tomatoes
	8	Cranberries
	5	Melons
	2	Cucumbers, nectarines, peanuts (hulls), plums (fresh prunes), sweet cherries
	0.5	Citrus fruits, potatoes
	0.25	Apples
	0.1	Fresh corn, macadamia nuts, onions, pineapples
	0.05	Peanuts (meats hulls removed)
	0.02	Taro (corn)
Yugoslavia	3.0	Fruit, vegetables
	0.1	Other food commodities

[a]From Health and Welfare Canada (1990)
[b]The figure in parentheses is the lower limit for determining residues in the corresponding product according to the standard method of analysis.
[c]Dose at detectable limit or close to same
[d]Muscle tissue including attached adipose tissue
[e]In imported produce
[f]Standards for witholding established registration
[g]A pesticide may be used on an eating or drinking ware or raw material without a demonstrable residue remaining behind. The value listed is considered the highest concentration at which this requirement is deemed to have been met.
[h]Residues shall be absent; value in parentheses indicates highest concentration at which requirement is met.
[i]Extraneous residue limit
[j]At the limit of detection except for peaches, nectarines and plums

International temporary maximum residue limits for captafol residues in raw agricultural commodities, ranging from 0.05 to 50 ppm (mg/kg), established by the Codex Committee on Pesticide Residues (US Environmental Protection Agency, 1984b) and the temporary acceptable daily intake values established by the Joint Meeting on Pesticide Residues in 1982 (FAO/WHO, 1983) were deleted in 1985 (FAO/WHO, 1986a).

The occupational exposure limit for captafol is 0.1 mg/m^3 (time-weighted average) in Denmark, Mexico, the Netherlands, Switzerland, the United Kingdom, the USA and Venezuela, with a skin notation in Mexico, the Netherlands, Switzerland, the United Kingdom and the USA (Cook, 1987; Arbejdstilsynet, 1988; American Conference of Governmental Industrial Hygienists, 1989; US Occupational Safety and Health Administration, 1989).

The FAO/WHO Joint Meeting on Pesticide Residues evaluated permethrin at its meetings in 1969, 1973, 1974, 1976, 1977, 1982 and 1985 (FAO/WHO, 1970, 1974, 1977, 1978, 1983, 1986a,b). The technical product captafol was classified by the WHO (1990) as 'extremely hazardous'. Several countries have banned the use of this pesticide, including Canada (1987) and Germany (1988) (Agriculture Canada, 1990; County NatWest WoodMac, 1990).

2. Studies of Cancer in Humans

No data were available to the Working Group.

3. Studies of Cancer in Experimental Animals

Oral administration

Mouse: Groups of 50-51 male and 50-51 female B6C3F$_1$ mice, six weeks old, were fed a diet containing captafol (94.9% pure; [impurities unspecified]) at 0, 0.075, 0.15 or 0.3% (maximum tolerated dose) for 96 weeks and the basal diet for a further eight weeks. Survivors were killed at 104 weeks. Dose-related retardation of body weight gain and increased mortality (particularly in the high-dose group) were observed. Mice surviving at week 104 were: males—33/50 control, 34/51 low-dose, 34/51 mid-dose and 0/51 high-dose; females—35/50 controls, 39/51 low-dose, 23/51 mid-dose and 0/51 high-dose. A dose-related increase in the incidence of heart haemangioendothelioma was observed in animals of each sex. Significant increases in the incidences of tumours were also seen at some other sites: forestomach papillomas in high-dose females and small intestinal adenoma, hepatocellular carcinoma and splenic angioma in males and females (Table 3). The increase in the incidence of small intestinal adenocarcinomas in males and females was possibly dose-related, although the incidence in the mid-dose group was higher than that in the high-dose group, probably due to earlier death in the latter, in which significant mortality was seen at approximately 80 weeks (Ito *et al.*, 1984).

Rat: Four groups of 49-50 male and 49-50 female Fischer 344 rats, four weeks of age, received a diet containing 0, 500, 2000 or 5000 mg/kg captafol (Merpafol; 97% pure) for 104 weeks, after which time they were killed. The high-dose group was sacrificed after 98 weeks of treatment, due to excess mortality (78% in males and 60% in females at week 96). A dose-related increase in the incidence of nonneoplastic renal lesions was found in males and females (tubular cystic dilatation, glomerulonephropathy, cystic tubules lined by cells with giant nuclei). Renal tumours were found only in treated males: one, three and 12 carcinomas in the low-, mid- and high-dose groups, respectively (positive trend, $p < 0.001$) (Nyska *et al.*, 1989).

Table 3. Occurrence of tumours in B6C3F$_1$ mice fed captafol in the diet^a

Site and type of tumour	Control	Concentration (%) of captafol		
		0.075	0.15	0.3
Males				
Effective number of mice	47	51	46	47
Heart haemangioendothelioma	0	1	4*	20***^{b}
Forestomach papilloma	0	2	3	2
Forestomach squamous cell carcinoma	0	0	1	2
Small intestinal adenoma	0	3	0	4*
Small intestinal adenocarcinoma	0	7**	32***	22***
Hepatocellular carcinoma	8	23**	15	1
Splenic haemangioma	0	0	5*	0
Females				
Effective number of mice	48	50	49	51
Heart haemangioendothelioma	0	2	2	11***^{b}
Forestomach papilloma	0	1	1	4*
Forestomach squamous cell carcinoma	0	0	0	1
Small intestinal adenoma	0	3	3	5*
Small intestinal adenocarcinoma	0	3	13***	7**
Hepatocellular carcinoma	2	13**	12**	0
Splenic haemangioma	0	2	4*	0

^{a}From Ito *et al.* (1984)
^{b}[Positive trend test ($p < 0.01$)]
*$p < 0.05$
**$p < 0.01$
***$p < 0.001$

Groups of 50 male and 50 female Fischer 344/DuCrj rats, six weeks of age, were fed diets containing 0, 750 or 1500 mg/kg captafol (97.5% pure) for 104 weeks and then the normal diet for a further eight weeks, after which time the experiment was terminated. Mean body weights in males and females of the high-dose group and in females of the low-dose group were reduced. There was no difference in survival times between control and treated rats; about 60% of rats survived to week 112. Statistically significant increased incidences of tumours of the kidney and liver were observed in treated rats, as shown in Table 4 (Tamano *et al.*, 1990).

4. Other Relevant Data

The toxicokinetics and toxicity of captafol have been reviewed (FAO/WHO, 1970, 1974, 1978, 1983, 1986a,b).

4.1 Absorption, distribution, metabolism and excretion

No published data were available to the Working Group.

Table 4. Occurrence of tumours in Fischer 344/DuCrj rats fed captafol in the diet[a]

Site and type of tumour	Control	Concentration (%) of captafol	
		750	1500
Males			
Effective number of rats	50	49	50
Renal-cell adenoma	0	26***	38***
Renal-cell carcinoma	0	1	8**
Hyperplastic (neoplastic) nodule (liver)	2	8*	21***
Hepatocellular carcinoma	2	0	1
Forestomach papilloma	0	0	3
Females			
Effective number of rats	50	50	50
Renal-cell adenoma	0	8**	6*
Renal-cell carcinoma	0	0	0
Hyperplastic (neoplastic) nodule (liver)	3	14**	34***
Hepatocellular carcinoma	0	0	4
Forestomach papilloma	0	1	0

[a]From Tamano *et al.* (1990)
*$p < 0.05$
**$p < 0.01$
***$p < 0.001$

4.2 Toxic effects

4.2.1 *Humans*

Contact dermatitis has been reported after exposure to captafol (Takamatsu *et al.*, 1968; Groundwater, 1977; Stoke, 1979; Matsushita *et al.*, 1980; Brown, 1984).

4.2.2 *Experimental systems*

The oral LD_{50} for captafol in rats is 2500-6200 mg/kg bw, and the dermal LD_{50} in rabbits is 15 400 mg/kg bw (Ben-Dyke *et al.*, 1970).

In rats, single intraperitoneal doses of captafol at 5 mg/kg bw decreased liver monoxygenase content and activity and increased plasma transaminase levels (Dalvi & Mutinga, 1990).

Captafol was given in the diet at 3000 mg/kg for six weeks, two weeks after a single intraperitoneal dose of N-nitrosodiethylamine (200 mg/kg bw) to male Fischer rats that were also subjected to a two-thirds hepatectomy three weeks after the start of the study. Significant increases were seen in the number and area of glutathione S-transferase-positive liver foci at eight weeks compared to rats treated with N-nitrosodiethylamine and partial hepatectomy alone (Ito *et al.*, 1988).

4.3 Reproductive and developmental effects

4.3.1 *Humans*

No data were available to the Working Group.

4.3.2 *Experimental systems*

Captafol has an *N*-substituted phthalimide-like structure similar to hydrolysis products of thalidomide. It was shown to have no teratogenic effect in two thalidomide-sensitive strains of rabbits (New Zealand white and Dutch belted) (Kennedy *et al.*, 1968) or in thalidomide-sensitive rhesus monkeys (Vondruska *et al.*, 1971). The rabbits received oral doses on days 6-16 of gestation of up to 75 mg/kg bw daily (Dutch belted) and on days 6-18 of up to 150 mg/kg bw daily (New Zealand). The monkeys received up to 25 mg/kg bw per day on days 22-32 of gestation. [The Working Group noted that the low doses used were reported to cause no systemic maternal toxicity in the monkeys, and no mention was made of the doses at which metabolites similar to those of thalidomide would occur in relevant concentrations.]

In Syrian hamsters, increased maternal and fetal lethality and teratogenic effects (fused ribs, short or curved tail, limb defects) were observed at oral doses of 200 mg/kg bw and above on days 7 or 8 of gestation (Robens, 1970).

4.4 Genetic and related effects (see also Table 5 and Appendices 1 and 2)

4.4.1 *Humans*

No data were available to the Working Group.

4.4.2 *Experimental systems*

Captafol caused DNA damage and gene mutation in bacteria; exogenous metabolic systems reduced or abolished the activity, as did rat blood or cysteine when captafol was tested in an *Escherichia coli* reverse mutation assay. [Only a few experiments have been performed with an exogenous metabolic system; their effect is supported by more extensive data on captan, a structural analogue.] In a single study with *Aspergillus nidulans*, captafol induced mitotic recombination and gene mutation, but not aneuploidy. Captafol induced sister chromatid exchange, micronucleus formation and chromosomal aberrations in cultured mammalian and human cell lines.

In dominant lethal tests in rats, captafol induced a small, but significant, trend towards increased numbers of early deaths per pregnancy (males treated intraperitoneally or orally). No such effect was observed in a single study in mice given one intraperitoneal injection of captafol. [The apparent species difference may be attributable to the doses and route of administration used.]

5. Summary of Data Reported and Evaluation

5.1 Exposure data

Captafol is a fungicide that has been widely used since 1961 for the control of fungal diseases in fruits, vegetables and some other plants.

Table 5. Genetic and related effects of captafol

Test system	Result[a] Without exogenous metabolic system	Result[a] With exogenous metabolic system	Dose[b] LED/HID	Reference
BSD, *Bacillus subtilis rec* strain (H17 *vs* M45), differential toxicity	+	0	0.1000	Shirasu *et al.* (1976)
SA0, *Salmonella typhimurium* TA100, reverse mutation	–	–	2500.0000	Moriya *et al.* (1983)
SAF, *Salmonella typhimurium* SV3, arabinose resistance	–	–	0.3000	Ruiz–Vásquez *et al.* (1978)
SA2, *Salmonella typhimurium* TA102, reverse mutation	+	+	0.0800	Barrueco & de la Peña (1988)
SA3, *Salmonella typhimurium* TA1530, reverse mutation (spot test)	+	0	0.0000	Seiler (1973)
SA4, *Salmonella typhimurium* TA102, reverse mutation	–	–	0.3000	Barrueco & de la Peña (1988)
SA5, *Salmonella typhimurium* TA1535, reverse mutation	–	0	0.0000	Kada *et al.* (1974)
SA5, *Salmonella typhimurium* TA1535, reverse mutatin	–	0	25.0000	Shirasu *et al.* (1976)
SA5, *Salmonella typhimurium* TA1535, reverse mutation (spot test)	–	0	200.0000	Carere *et al.* (1978)
SA5, *Salmonella typhimurium* TA1535, reverse mutation	–	–	2500.0000	Moriya *et al.* (1983)
SA7, *Salmonella typhimurium* TA1537, reverse mutation	–	0	0.0000	Kada *et al.* (1974)
SA7, *Salmonella typhimurium* TA1537, reverse mutation (spot test)	–	–	200.0000	Carere *et al.* (1978)
SA7, *Salmonella typhimurium* TA1537, reverse mutation	–	–	2500.0000	Moriya *et al.* (1983)
SA8, *Salmonella typhimurium* TA1538, reverse mutation	–	0	0.0000	Kada *et al.* (1974)
SA8, *Salmonella typhimurium* TA1538, reverse mutation (spot test)	–	–	200.0000	Carere *et al.* (1978)
SA8, *Salmonella typhimurium* TA1538, reverse mutation	–	–	2500.0000	Moriya *et al.* (1983)
SA9, *Salmonella typhimurium* TA98, reverse mutation	–	–	2500.0000	Moriya *et al.* (1983)
SAS, *Salmonella typhimurium his* G46, reverse mutation (spot test)	+	0	0.0000	Seiler (1973)
SAS, *Salmonella typhimurium* TA1531, reverse mutation (spot test)	–	0	0.0000	Seiler (1973)
SAS, *Salmonella typhimurium* TA1532, reverse mutation (spot test)	–	0	0.0000	Seiler (1973)
SAS, *Salmonella typhimurium* TA1534, reverse mutation (spot test)	–	0	0.0000	Seiler (1973)
SAS, *Salmonella typhimurium* TA1536, reverse mutation	–	0	0.0000	Kada *et al.* (1974)
SAS, *Salmonella typhimurium* TA1536, reverse mutation (spot test)	–	–	200.0000	Carere *et al.* (1978)
EC2, *Escherichia coli* B/r WP2, reverse mutation	+	0	50.0000	Kada *et al.* (1974)
EC2, *Escherichia coli* WP2, reverse mutation	+	0	25.0000	Shirasu *et al.* (1976)
EC2, *Escherichia coli* WP2 *hcr*, reverse mutation	+	0	25.0000	Shirasu *et al.* (1976)
EC2, *Escherichia coli* WP2 *hcr*, reverse mutation	+	0	26.0000	Moriya *et al.* (1978)
EC2, *Escherichia coli* WP2 *hcr* + cysteine, reverse mutation	–	0	26.0000	Moriya *et al.* (1978)

Table 5 (contd)

Test system	Result[a] Without exogenous metabolic system	Result[a] With exogenous metabolic system	Dose[b] LED/HID	Reference
EC2, *Escherichia coli* WP2 *hcr*, reverse mutation	+	+	2.5000	Moriya et al. (1983)
ANG, *Aspergillus nidulans*, genetic crossing–over	+	0	0.2000	Bignami et al. (1977)
Aspergillus nidulans, non–disjunction	–	0	2000.0000	Bignami et al. (1977)
ANF, *Aspergillus nidulans*, forward mutation	+	0	20.0000	Bignami et al. (1977)
SIC, Sister chromatid exchange, Chinese hamster V79 cells *in vitro*	+	0	0.7000	Tezuka et al. (1980)
SIC, Sister chromatid exchange, Chinese hamster Don cells *in vitro*	+	0	3.5000	Sasaki et al. (1980)
MIA, Micronucleus test, Chinese hamster Don cells *in vitro*	+	0	3.5000	Sasaki et al. (1980)
CIC, Chromosomal aberrations, Chinese hamster V79 cells *in vitro*	+	0	3.5000	Tezuka et al. (1980)
CIC, Chromosomal aberrations, Chinese hamster CHL cells *in vitro*	+	–	4.0000	Ishidate (1988)
SIH, Sister chromatid exchange, human HE 2144 cells *in vitro*	+	0	3.5000	Sasaki et al. (1980)
MIH, Micronucleus test, human HE 2144 cells *in vitro*	+	0	3.5000	Sasaki et al. (1980)
CIH, Chromosomal aberrations, human HE 2144 cells *in vitro*	+	0	3.5000	Sasaki et al. (1980)
HMM, Host-mediated assay, *Salmonella typhimurium* G46, CR mouse	–	0	250.0000 × 1 i.p.	Kennedy et al. (1975)
DLM, Dominant lethal test, CD mouse	–	0	3.0000 × i.p.	Kennedy et al. (1975)
DLR, Dominant lethal test, Osborne–Mendel rat	(+)	0	10.0000 × 5 i.p.	Collins (1972)
DLR, Dominant lethal test, Osborne–Mendel rat	(+)	0	200.0000 × 5 p.o.	Collins (1972)

*Not displayed on profile

[a] +, positive; (+), weakly positive; –, negative; 0, not tested; ?, inconclusive (variable response in several experiments within an adequate study)

[b] In-vitro tests, μg/ml; in-vivo tests, mg/kg bw

It has been formulated for use as dusts, emulsifiable concentrates, flowable suspensions and water-dispersible granules, and also in combination with other pesticides.

Exposure can occur during its production and application and, at much lower levels, from consumption of foods containing residues.

5.2 Carcinogenicity in humans

No data were available to the Working Group.

5.3 Carcinogenicity in experimental animals

Captafol was tested for carcinogenicity in one study in mice and in two studies in rats by oral administration. In mice, it produced a high incidence of adenocarcinomas of the small intestine and of vascular tumours of the heart and spleen; the increase in tumours of the heart was dose-related for animals of each sex. Increases in the incidence of hepatocellular carcinomas were also observed in animals of each sex. In two studies in rats, captafol produced a dose-related increase in the incidence of renal carcinomas in males; in one of these, it also induced dose-related increases in the incidence of benign renal tumours in females and of liver tumours in males and females.

5.4 Other relevant data

In one study, captafol increased the frequency of enzyme-positive foci in rat liver.

Captafol did not affect embryonic development in rabbits or monkeys but was embryolethal and teratogenic at high doses in hamsters.

No data were available on the genetic and related effects of captafol in humans.

Administration of captafol induced dominant lethal effects in rats. Captafol induced positive results in various short-term tests in human and mammalian cells *in vitro*, including gene mutation and chromosomal aberrations. It induced DNA damage and gene mutation in fungi and bacteria.

5.5 Evaluation[1]

No data were available from studies in humans.

There is *sufficient evidence* in experimental animals for the carcinogenicity of captafol.

In making the overall evaluation, the Working Group took into consideration the following supporting evidence: Captafol is active in a wide range of tests for genetic and related effects, including the generally insensitive in-vivo assay for dominant lethal mutation.

Overall evaluation

Captafol *is probably carcinogenic to humans (Group 2A).*

---

[1]For definition of the italicized terms, see Preamble, pp. 26-28.

6. References

Agriculture Canada (1990) *Cancellation of Captafol Fungicide*, Ottawa, Food Production and Inspection Branch, Pesticide Directorate

American Conference of Governmental Industrial Hygienists (1989) *Threshold Limit Values and Biological Exposure Indices for 1988-1989*, Cincinnati, OH, p. 13

Arbejdstilsynet (Labour Inspection) (1988) *Graensevaerdier for Stoffer og Materialer* (Limit Values for Compounds and Materials) (No. 3.1.0.2), Copenhagen, p. 13 (in Danish)

Barrueco, C. & de la Peña, E. (1988) Mutagenic evaluation of the pesticides captan, folpet, captafol, dichlofluanid and related compounds with the mutants TA102 and TA104 of *Salmonella typhimurium. Mutagenesis, 3*, 467-480

Ben-Dyke, R., Sanderson, D.M. & Noakes, D.N. (1970) Acute toxicity data for pesticides (1970). *World Rev. Pest Control, 9*, 119-127

Bignami, M., Anlicino, F., Velcich, A., Carere, A. & Morpurgo, G. (1977) Mutagenic and recombinogenic action of pesticides in *Aspergillus nidulans. Mutat. Res., 46*, 395-402

Brown, R. (1984) Contact sensitivity to difolatan (captafol). *Contact Derm., 10*, 181-182

Carere, A., Ortali, V.A., Cardamone, G., Torracca, A.M. & Raschetti, R. (1978) Microbiological mutagenicity studies of pesticides *in vitro. Mutat. Res., 57*, 277-286

Collins, T.F.X. (1972) Dominant lethal assay. II. Folpet and difolatan. *Food Cosmet. Toxicol., 10*, 363-371

Cook, W.A., ed. (1987) *Occupational Exposure Limits—Worldwide*, Washington DC, American Industrial Hygiene Association, pp. 20, 49, 85, 168-169

County NatWest WoodMac (1990) *Update of the Agrochemical Products Section*, Parts 1 and 2, London, County NatWest Securities Limited Incorporating Wood Mackenzie & Co., Agrochemical Service

Dalvi, R.R. & Mutinga, M.L. (1990) Comparative studies of the effects on liver and liver microsomal drug-metabolizing enzyme system by the fungicides captan, captafol and folpet in rats. *Pharmacol. Toxicol., 66*, 231-233

FAO/WHO (1970) *1969 Evaluations of Some Pesticide Residues in Food. The Monographs* (FAO/PL:1969/M/17/1; WHO/Food Add./70.38), Rome

FAO/WHO (1974) *1973 Evaluations of Some Pesticide Residues in Food. The Monographs* (FAO/AGP/1973/M/9/1; WHO Pesticide Residues Series No. 3), Rome

FAO/WHO (1977) *1976 Evaluations of Some Pesticide Residues in Food. The Monographs* (FAO/AGP/1976/M/14), Rome

FAO/WHO (1978) *Pesticide Residues in Food: 1977 Evaluations* (FAO Plant Production and Protection Paper 10 Sup.), Rome

FAO/WHO (1983) *Pesticide Residues in Food—1982. Report of the Joint Meeting of the FAO Panel of Experts on Pesticide Residues in Food and the Environment and the WHO Expert Group on Pesticide Residues* (FAO Plant Production and Protection Paper 46), Rome

FAO/WHO (1986a) *Pesticide Residues in Food—1985. Report of the Joint Meeting of the FAO Panel of Experts on Pesticide Residues in Food and the Environment and the WHO Expert Group on Pesticide Residues* (FAO Plant Production and Protection Paper 72/1), Rome

FAO/WHO (1986b) *Pesticide Residues in Food—1986. Report of the Joint Meeting of the FAO Panel of Experts on Pesticide Residues in Food and the Environment and a WHO Expert Group on Pesticide Residues* (FAO Plant Production and Protection Paper 77), Rome

Frank, R., Braun, H.E. & Ripley, B.D. (1989) Monitoring Ontario-grown apples for pest control chemicals used in their production, 1978-86. *Food Addit. Contam.*, *6*, 227-234

Government of Canada (1990) *Report on National Surveillance Data from 1984/85 to 1988/89*, Ottawa

Groundwater, J.R. (1977) Difolatan dermatitis in a welder; nonagricultural exposure. *Contact Derm.*, *3*, 104

Health and Welfare Canada (1990) *National Pesticide Residue Limits in Food*, Ottawa, Bureau of Chemical Safety, Food Directorate, Health Protection Branch

IARC (1983) *IARC Monographs on the Evaluation of the Carcinogenic Risk of Chemicals to Humans*, Vol. 30, *Miscellaneous Pesticides*, Lyon, pp. 295-318

IARC (1987a) *IARC Monographs on the Evaluation of Carcinogenic Risks to Humans*, Suppl. 7, *Overall Evaluations of Carcinogenicity: An Updating of* IARC Monographs *Volumes 1 to 42*, Lyon, pp. 349-350

IARC (1987b) *IARC Monographs on the Evaluation of Carcinogenic Risks to Humans*, Suppl. 7, *Overall Evaluations of Carcinogenicity: An Updating of* IARC Monographs *Volumes 1 to 42*, Lyon, pp. 341-343

IARC (1987c) *IARC Monographs on the Evaluation of Carcinogenic Risks to Humans*, Suppl. 7, *Overall Evaluations of Carcinogenicity: An Updating of* IARC Monographs *Volumes 1 to 42*, Lyon, p. 59

Ishidate, M., Jr (1988) *Data Book of Chromosomal Aberration Test In Vitro*, rev. ed., Amsterdam, Elsevier, p. 79

Ito, N., Ogiso, T., Fukushima, S., Shibata, M. & Hagiwara, A. (1984) Carcinogenicity of captafol in B6C3F$_1$ mice. *Gann*, *75*, 853-865

Ito, N., Tsuda, H., Tatematsu, M., Inoue, T., Tagawa, Y., Aoki, T., Uwagawa, S., Kagawa, M., Ogiso, T., Masui, T., Imaida, K., Fukushima, S. & Asamoto, M. (1988) Enhancing effect of various hepatocarcinogens on induction of preneoplastic glutathione S-transferase placental form positive foci in rats—an approach for a new medium-term bioassay system. *Carcinogenesis*, *9*, 387-394

Kada, T., Moriya, M. & Shirasu, Y. (1974) Screening of pesticides for DNA interactions by 'rec-assay' and mutagenesis testing, and frameshift mutagens detected. *Mutat. Res.*, *26*, 243-248

Kennedy, G., Fanchier, O.E. & Calandra, J.C. (1968) An investigation of the teratogenic potential of captan, folpet and difolatan. *Toxicol. appl. Pharmacol.*, *13*, 420-430

Kennedy, G.L., Jr, Arnold, D.W. & Keplinger, M.L. (1975) Mutagenicity studies with captan, captafol, folpet and thalidomide. *Food Cosmet. Toxicol.*, *13*, 55-61

Matsushita, T., Nomura, S. & Wakatsuki, T. (1980) Epidemiology of contact dermatitis from pesticides in Japan. *Contact Derm.*, *6*, 255-259

Meister, R.T., ed. (1990) *Farm Chemicals Handbook '90*, Willoughby, OH, Meister Publishing Company, p. C56

Moriya, M., Kato, K. & Shirasu, Y. (1978) Effects of cysteine and liver metabolic activation system on the activities of mutagenic pesticides. *Mutat. Res.*, *57*, 259-263

Moriya, M., Ohta, T., Watanabe, K., Miyazawa, T., Kato, K. & Shirasu, Y. (1983) Further mutagenicity studies on pesticides in bacterial reversion assay systems. *Mutat. Res.*, *116*, 185-216

Nyska, A., Waner, T., Pirak, M., Gordon, E., Bracha, P. & Klein, B. (1989) The renal carcinogenic effect of merpafor in the Fischer 344 rat. *Isr. J. med. Sci*, *25*, 428-432

Pack, D.E. (1967) Difolatan. In: Zweig, G., ed., *Analytical Methods for Pesticides, Plant Growth Regulators, and Food Additives*, Vol. 5, *Additional Principles and Methods of Analysis*, New York, Academic Press, pp. 293-304

Robens, J.F. (1970) Teratogenic activity of several phthalamide derivatives in the golden hamster. *Toxicol. appl. Pharmacol.*, *16*, 24-34

Royal Society of Chemistry (1986) *European Directory of Agrochemical Products*, Vol. 1, *Fungicides*, Cambridge, pp. 46-56

Royal Society of Chemistry (1989) *The Agrochemicals Handbook* [Dialog Information Services (File 306)], Cambridge

Ruiz-Vásquez, R., Pueyo, C. & Cerdá-Olmedo, E. (1978) A mutagen assay detecting forward mutations in an arabinose-sensitive strain of *Salmonella typhimurium*. *Mutat. Res.*, *54*, 121-129

Sasaki, M., Sugimura, K., Yoshida, M.A. & Abe, S. (1980) Cytogenetic effects of 60 chemicals on cultured human and Chinese hamster cells. *Kromosomo II*, *20*, 574-584

Seiler, J.P. (1973) A survey on the mutagenicity of various pesticides. *Experientia*, *29*, 622-623

Shirasu, Y., Moriya, M., Kato, K., Furuhashi, A. & Kada, T. (1976) Mutagenicity screening of pesticides in the microbial system. *Mutat. Res.*, *40*, 19-30

Stoke, J.C.J. (1979) Captafol dermatitis in the timber industry. *Contact Derm.*, *5*, 284-292

Takamatsu, M., Futatsuka, M., Arimatsu, Y., Maeda, H., Inuzuka, T. & Takamatsu, S. (1968) Epidemiological survey on dermatitis from a new fungicide used in tangerine orchards in Kumamoto Prefecture. *J. Kumamoto med. Soc.*, *42*, 854-859

Tamano, S., Kurata, Y., Yamada, M., Yamamoto, A., Hagiwara, A., Cabral, R. & Ito, N. (1990) Carcinogenicity of captafol in F344/DuCrj rats. *Jpn. J. Cancer Res.*, *81*, 1222-1231

Tezuka, H., Ando, N., Suzuki, R., Terahata, M., Moriya, M. & Shirasu, Y. (1980) Sister-chromatid exchanges and chromosomal aberrations in cultured Chinese hamster cells treated with pesticides positive in microbial reversion assays. *Mutat. Res.*, *78*, 177-191

US Environmental Protection Agency (1975) Infrared spectra of pesticides. In: *Manual of Chemical Methods for Pesticides and Devices*, Arlington, VA, Association of Official Analytical Chemists

US Environmental Protection Agency (1982) *Preliminary Quantitative Usage Analysis of Captafol*, Washington DC, Office of Pesticide Programs

US Environmental Protection Agency (1984a) *Guidance for the Registration of Pesticide Products Containing Captafol as the Active Ingredient* (EPA Case Number 116), Washington DC

US Environmental Protection Agency (1984b) *Pesticide Fact Sheet: Captafol*, Washington DC

US Food and Drug Administration (1989a) Captafol method II. In: *Pesticide Analytical Manual*, Vol. II, *Methods Which Detect Multiple Residues*, Washington DC, US Department of Health and Human Services, pp. 1-9

US Food and Drug Administration (1989b) Captafol method IIa. In: *Pesticide Analytical Manual*, Vol. II, *Methods Which Detect Multiple Residues*, Washington DC, US Department of Health and Human Services, pp. 10-14

US Food and Drug Administration (1989c) Captafol method A. In: *Pesticide Analytical Manual*, Vol. II, *Methods Which Detect Multiple Residues*, Washington DC, US Department of Health and Human Services, pp. 15-17

US Occupational Safety and Health Administration (1989) Air contaminants—permissible exposure limits. *US Code fed. Regul.*, *Title 29*, Part 1910.1000

Vondruska, J.F., Fanchier, O.E. & Calandra, J.C. (1971) An investigation into the teratogenic potential of captan, folpet and difolatan in nonhuman primates. *Toxicol. appl. Pharmacol.*, *18*, 619-624

WHO (1990) *The WHO Recommended Classification of Pesticides by Hazard and Guidelines to Classification 1990-91*, Geneva, p. 11

Worthing, C.R. & Walker, S.B., eds (1987) *The Pesticide Manual: A World Compendium*, 8th ed., Thornton Heath, British Crop Protection Council, pp. 121-122

Zweig, G. & Sherma, J., eds (1978) *Analytical Methods for Pesticides and Plant Growth Regulators*, Vol. X, *New and Updated Methods*, New York, Academic Press, pp. 171-173

PENTACHLOROPHENOL

This substance was considered by previous Working Groups, in 1978 (IARC, 1979), 1986 (IARC, 1986) and 1987 (IARC, 1987a). Since that time, new data have become available, and these have been incorporated into the monograph and taken into consideration in the present evaluation.

1. Exposure Data

1.1 Chemical and physical data

1.1.1 *Synonyms, structural and molecular data*

Chem. Abstr. Serv. Reg. No.: 87-86-5
Chem. Abstr. Name: Pentachlorophenol
IUPAC Systematic Name: Pentachlorophenol
Synonyms: Chlorophen; 1-hydroxypentachlorobenzene; PCP; penchlorol; penta; 2,3,4,5,6-pentachlorophenol

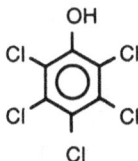

C_6HCl_5O Mol. wt: 266.34

1.1.2 *Chemical and physical properties*

(a) *Description*: Colourless to light-brown flakes or crystals with characteristic phenolic odour (Royal Society of Chemistry, 1989; WHO, 1989)
(b) *Boiling-point*: 309-310°C (decomposes) at 754 mm Hg [100.5 kPa] (Weast, 1989)
(c) *Melting-point*: 174°C (monohydrate); 191°C (anhydrous) (Weast, 1989)
(d) *Spectroscopy data:* Infrared (prism [279]; grating [96]), ultraviolet [112] and nuclear magnetic resonance (proton [39667]; C-13 [26001]) spectral data have been reported (Sadtler Research Laboratories, 1980, 1990).
(e) *Solubility*: Almost insoluble in water (8 mg/100 ml); soluble in acetone (215 g/l at 20°C), diethyl ether (150 g/l), benzene (150 g/l), ethanol (1200 g/l), methanol (1800 g/l), isopropanol (850 g/l), ethylene glycol (110 g/l); slightly soluble in cold petroleum ether, carbon tetrachloride and paraffins (WHO, 1987; Budavari, 1989; Royal Society of Chemistry, 1989)

(f) *Vapour pressure*: 1.5×10^{-5} mm Hg [0.2×10^{-5} kPa] at 20°C (WHO, 1989)

(g) *Stability*: Relatively stable and non-hygroscopic (Royal Society of Chemistry, 1989); decomposes on heating in the presence of water, forming corrosive fumes (hydrochloric acid); thermal degradation (at 600°C) products of technical pentachlorophenol include pentachlorobenzene, hexachlorobenzene, octachlorostyrene, octachloronaphthalene, decachlorobiphenyl, hexachlorodibenzofuran, octachlorodibenzofuran and octachlorodibenzodioxin (WHO, 1987). Sodium pentachlorophenate is degraded in water photolytically (Hiatt *et al.*, 1960). At pH 7.3, pentachlorophenol disappeared completely within 20 h (half-time, 3.5 h) but was more persistent at pH 3.3 (half-time, ~ 100 h) (Wong & Crosby, 1981).

(h) *Octanol/water partition coefficient* (P): log P = 3.32 at pH 7.2 (WHO, 1987)

(i) *Conversion factor for airborne concentrations*[1]: mg/m^3 = 10.89 × ppm

1.1.3 *Trade names, technical products and impurities*

Some examples of trade names are: Dowicide 7; Dowicide EC-7; Durotox; EP 30; Fungifen; Grundier Arbezol; Lauxtol; Liroprem; Permasan; Santophen 20; Witophen P; Weedone

Pentachlorophenol in aqueous solution can exist in ionized (phenate) or nonionized forms depending on pH. At pH 2.7, pentachlorophenol is only 1% ionized; at pH 6.7, it is 99% ionized. Technical-grade pentachlorophenol consists of brownish flakes, in some cases coated with a mixture of benzoin polyisopropyl and pine oil to suppress dust. Technical-grade sodium pentachlorophenate consists of cream-coloured beads (WHO, 1987). The formulated product is available as granules, wettable powder and oil-miscible liquid (Royal Society of Chemistry, 1989). Pentachlorophenol is also formulated as blocks, pellets, prills and concentrates (Meister, 1990). It is available as a liquid formulation in Finland and as granules in the Netherlands (Royal Society of Chemistry, 1986). In the USSR, it is manufactured as a 20% mineral oil concentrate (Izmerov, 1984).

Technical-grade pentachlorophenol has been shown to contain a large number of impurities, depending on the manufacturing method. Reported levels of impurities in commercial pentachlorophenol preparations are as follows: tetrachlorophenol (see IARC, 1987a), 4.4-10.2%; trichlorophenol (see IARC, 1987a), ≤ 1%; chlorinated phenoxyphenols, 5-6.2%; octachlorodibenzodioxin (see IARC, 1987b), 5.5-3600 mg/kg; heptachlorodibenzodioxin (see IARC, 1987b), 0.6-520 mg/kg; hexachlorodibenzodioxin (see IARC, 1987b), < 0.03-100 mg/kg; octachlorodibenzofuran, < 0.1-260 mg/kg; heptachlorodibenzofuran, < 0.1-400 mg/kg; hexachlorodibenzofuran, < 0.03-90 mg/kg; pentachlorodibenzofuran, < 0.03-40 mg/kg; and tetrachlorodibenzofuran < 0.02-0.45 mg/kg (Scow *et al.*, 1980; WHO, 1987). In addition, chlorinated cyclohexenones and cyclohexadienones, hexachlorobenzene (see IARC, 1987c) and polychlorinated biphenyls (see IARC, 1987d) are found (WHO, 1987).

The presence of the highly toxic 2,3,7,8-tetrachlorodibenzo-*para*-dioxin (see IARC, 1987e) has been confirmed only once in commercial pentachlorophenol samples. In the

---

[1]Calculated from: mg/m^3 = (molecular weight/24.45) × ppm, assuming standard temperature (25°C) and pressure (760 mm Hg [101.3 kPa])

course of a collaborative survey, one of five laboratories detected this dioxin in technical pentachlorophenol and sodium pentachlorophenate samples at concentrations of 0.25-0.26 and 0.89-1.10 μg/kg, respectively. Detectable amounts of tetrachlorodibenzo-*para*-dioxin (0.05-0.23 mg/kg) were reported in some samples of different technical pentachlorophenol products, but the identity of the compound could not be confirmed on re-analysis. In other cases, tetrachlorodibenzo-*para*-dioxin has not been identified, at detection limits of 0.001-0.2 mg/kg (WHO, 1987).

The higher polychlorinated dibenzodioxins and dibenzofurans are more characteristic of pentachlorophenol formulations. The 1,2,3,6,7,9-, 1,2,3,6,8,9-, 1,2,3,6,7,8- and 1,2,3,7,8,9-isomers of hexachlorodibenzo-*para*-dioxin have been detected in technical-grade pentachlorophenol. The 1,2,3,6,7,8- and 1,2,3,7,8,9-hexachlorodibenzo-*para*-dioxins predominated in commercial samples of technical-grade pentachlorophenol (Dowicide 7) and sodium pentachlorophenate. Octachlorodibenzo-*para*-dioxin is present in relatively high amounts in unpurified technical-grade products (WHO, 1987).

Suppliers of pentachlorophenol in the USA and Canada are now required to limit the hexachlorodibenzo-*para*-dioxin and 2,3,7,8-tetrachlorodibenzo-*para*-dioxin content to less than 4 ppm (mg/kg) and none detectable (< 0.001 ppm [mg/kg]), respectively (Agricultural Canadian Plant Research Centre, 1990).

The presence of 2-bromo-3,4,5,6-tetrachlorophenol as a major contaminant in three commercial pentachlorophenol samples (∼ 0.1%) has been reported. This manufacturing by-product has probably not been detected in other analyses because it is not resolved from the pentachlorophenol peak by traditional chromatographic methods (WHO, 1987).

For the treatment of wood in the USA, pentachlorophenol is usually administered as a 5% solution in a mineral spirit solvent, such as No. 2 fuel oil (see IARC, 1989) or kerosene (see IARC, 1989), or in dichloromethane (see IARC, 1987f), isopropyl alcohol (see IARC, 1987g) or methanol. Since pentachlorophenol is not very soluble in hydrocarbon solvents and tends to migrate to, and crystallize on, treated wood surfaces (a phenomenon known as 'blooming'), formulations may also contain co-solvents and anti-blooming agents. An aqueous solution of sodium pentachlorophenate is used commercially to control sapstain (WHO, 1987).

Chlorophenols may be combined with other active components, such as methylene bis-thiocyanate and copper naphthenate, in the formulation of pentachlorophenol pesticides. Conversely, pentachlorophenol is added to biocides, the primary active ingredient of which is another compound; for example, sodium fluoride formulations for wooden poles and posts may contain up to 10% technical pentachlorophenol (WHO, 1987).

1.1.4 *Analysis*

Most of the analytical methods used today involve acidification of the sample to convert pentachlorophenol to its nonionized form, extraction into an organic solvent, possible cleaning by back-extraction into a basic solution, and determination by gas chromatography with electron-capture detector or other chromatographic methods as ester or ether derivatives (e.g., acetyl-pentachlorophenol). Depending on sampling procedures and matrices, detection limits as low as 0.05 μg/m^3 in air and 0.01 μg/l in water can be achieved (WHO, 1987).

Selected methods for the analysis of pentachlorophenol in various matrices are given in Table 1.

Table 1. Methods for the analysis of pentachlorophenol

Sample matrix	Sample preparation	Assay procedure[a]	Limit of detection[b]	Reference
Air	Collect sample in bubble containing ethylene glycol; add methanol	HPLC/UV	8 µg per sample	Eller (1984a)
Drinking-water	Extract by passing sample through liquid-solid extractor; elute with dichloromethane; concentrate by evaporation	GC/MS	0.3 µg/l (I) 3.0 µg/l (M)	US Environmental Protection Agency (1988)
	Adjust to pH 12; wash with dichloromethane; acidify; extract with ethyl ether; derivatize with diazomethane	GC/ECD	0.076 µg/l	US Environmental Protection Agency (1989a)
Formulation	Dissolve sample in dioxane; inject aliquot	HPLC/UV	Not reported	Lawrence (1982)
Urine	Add concentrated hydrochloric acid and sodium bisulfite; boil; extract with benzene; concentrate; derivatize with diazomethane; add hexane and evaporate; clean up on alumina column	GC/ECD	1 µg/l	Eller (1984b)
Water	Adjust pH to > 11; extract sample with dichloromethane to remove base/neutral fraction; acidify to pH < 2; extract with dichloromethane to obtain acid fraction; dry; concentrate; analyse	GC/MS	3.6 µg/l	US Environmental Protection Agency (1989b)
Industrial municipal sludge	Acidify; extract with dichloromethane; dry extract; exchange solvent to 2-propanol during concentration of volume	GC/FID	0.59 µg/l	US Environmental Protection Agency (1989c)
Blood	Add 6 M sulfuric acid; add hexane and boil; extract with hexane; concentrate; derivatize with diazomethane; add hexane; evaporate; clean-up on alumina column	GC/ECD	1 µg/l	Eller (1984b)

[a]Abbreviations: GC/ECD, gas chromatography/electron capture detection; GC/FID, gas chromatography/flame ionization detection; GC/MS, gas chromatography/mass spectrometry; HPLC/UV, high-performance liquid chromatography/ultraviolet detection
[b]Abbreviations: (I), ion trap mass spectrometer; (M), magnetic sector mass spectrometer

1.2 Production and use

1.2.1 Production

Pentachlorophenol is prepared either by catalytic chlorination of phenol or by alkaline hydrolysis of hexachlorobenzene (see IARC, 1987g) (WHO, 1987).

World production of pentachlorophenol is estimated to be of the order of 30 000 tonnes per year (WHO, 1987). Four manufacturers in the USA produced a total of 18 000-23 000 tonnes of pentachlorophenol annually from 1945 to 1978. Less than 14 000 tonnes were produced in 1980 by two manufacturers. In 1987, about 12 000 tonnes were produced by the sole US producer; and in 1988, about 6000 tonnes were produced by the sole European producer. In 1985, about 3000 tonnes of sodium pentachlorophenate were produced by two European producers (Gjøs & Haegh, 1990).

1.2.2 *Use*

The main commercial use of pentachlorophenol is as a wood preservative; this use began in the late 1930s (WHO, 1987). It is used as a fungicide to protect wood from fungal decay and wood-boring insects. It is also used as a pre-harvest defoliant in cotton and as a general pre-emergence, non-selective contact herbicide (Worthing & Walker, 1987). It has been used as a bactericide in drilling fluids, as a fungicide in adhesives and textiles and for slime control in pulp and paper manufacture (WHO, 1987). Pentachlorophenol has also been used to control the snails that are the hosts of schistosomiasis (Meister, 1990).

Other reported applications of pentachlorophenol are in bactericidal soaps, laundry products, dental care products, leather tanning, mushroom culture, and as disinfectants for use in houses, farms and hospitals (WHO, 1987).

In the USA, it was estimated that 97% of the pentachlorophenol usage was as a wood preservative, 1% as a general herbicide and the remainder for miscellaneous smaller applications (Eckerman, 1986).

1.3 Occurrence

Pentachlorophenol is a ubiquitous environmental contaminant. Its widespread occurrence has been reviewed (WHO, 1987).

1.3.1 *Water*

Evaporation is commonly used for disposing of pentachlorophenol in wastewater at wood-preserving plants (WHO, 1987). Both temperature and pH influence the loss, since the phenate is non-volatile. At pH 5, the half-time is 328 h (30°C), whereas at pH 6 it increases to 3120 h (Klöpffer *et al.*, 1982). Wood-treatment factories contribute significantly to the pentachlorophenol load in surface water, which ranges from non-detectable to 10 500 µg/l. The majority of water samples analysed contained less than 10 µg/l, and most contained less than 1 µg/l. Extreme levels of up to 10 500 µg/l were reported in a polluted stream near an industrial area in the vicinity of Philadelphia (USA) (Fountaine *et al.*, 1976) .

Levels of pentachlorophenol in a man-made lake in Mississipi, USA, increased from a background of 0.3 µg/l to 16-81 µg/l immediately after an accidental overflow from a pole-treatment plant and to 29-147 a month after the accident. After four months, levels had returned to 5-16 µg/l (Pierce & Victor, 1978). Pignatello *et al.* (1983) showed that aquatic microflora can adapt to pentachlorophenol and become the most important factor for clearing pentachlorophenol from contaminated surface water.

Municipal sewage contains only low concentrations of pentachlorophenol, as opposed to industrial wastewater from wood-treatment factories (see Table 2). Levels of pentachlorophenol in industrial and municipal discharges in different countries ranged from 0.1 to 75 000 μg/l (WHO, 1987).

The pentachlorophenol input into the German Bight near the River Weser was calculated to be about 1000 kg per year, assuming an average level of pentachlorophenol of 0.1 μg/l per year and a water flow of 300 m^3/sec. The total load in all surface water in western Germany was estimated to be 60 tonnes per year, with 30-40 tonnes transported by the Rhine (as reported by WHO, 1987).

In general, sediments contain much higher levels of pentachlorophenol than the overlying waters. At several freshwater and marine sites in British Columbia, Canada, receiving effluents from the wood-treatment industry, average pentachlorophenol levels in the sediments ranged from not detectable to 590 μg/kg, while the corresponding range for the overlying waters was from not detectable to 7.3 μg/l (as reported by WHO, 1987).

Pentachlorophenol levels in surface water in various countries are given in Table 2.

Table 2. Concentrations of pentachlorophenol (PCP) in surface waters of different countries[a]

Country	Surface water and location	PCP (μg/l) Range	Mean
Germany	Weser River and estuary	0.05-0.5	
	German Bight	< 0.002-0.026	
	Ruhr River	< 0.1-0.2	0.1
	River Rhine, Cologne	0.1	
Japan	Tama River, Tokyo	0.1-0.9	
		0.01-0.09	
	Sumida River, Tokyo	1-9	
	River water, Tokyo area	0.18 ± 0.14	
Netherlands	River Rhine 1976	Max 2.4	0.7
	River Rhine 1977	Max 11.0	1.1
	River Meuse 1976	Max 1.4	0.3
	River Meuse 1977	Max 10.0	0.8
South Africa	124 sampling points	ND-0.85	
Sweden	River water downstream from a pulp mill	9	
	Lake receiving discharges	3	
USA	Willamette River	0.1-0.7	
	Estuary in Galveston Bay, Texas	ND-0.01	
	Pond in Mississippi contaminated by waste from pole-treatment plant	< 1-82	

[a]From WHO (1987)
ND, not detectable

1.3.2 Soil

Soil samples from four sites near a Swiss pentachlorophenol-producing facility contained 25-140 μg/kg (dry weight) at depths of 0-10 cm and 33-184 μg/kg at 20-30 cm.

These levels were greater than those at a reference site ($<$ 35 μg/kg for both depths) (as reported by WHO, 1987).

Soil surrounding Finnish sawmills was heavily contaminated, with up to 45.6 mg/kg at 0-5 cm depth near the treatment basin and up to 0.14 mg/kg in the area for storing treated wood. The background level was 0.012 mg/kg (Valo et al., 1984). Average pentachlorophenol levels in soil samples at 2.5, 30.5 and 152.5 cm from poles treated with pentachlorophenol were 658, 3.4 and 0.26 mg/kg, respectively (Arsenault, 1976). The background level (0.26 mg/kg) was considered to be high and could have resulted from contamination of the soil or of analytical samples (WHO, 1987).

Both pentachlorophenol and sodium pentachlorophenate are readily leached from soils. Substantial quantities of pentachlorophenol were found in waters leaching from contaminated soil, and residues ranging from 3.0 to 23 μg/l were detected in groundwater within saw-mill areas. A level as high as 3.35 mg/l was found in groundwater near a wood-preserving plant (WHO, 1987), and levels of pentachlorophenol of $<$ 1 μg/l were detected in water seeping from a landfill site (Kotzias et al., 1975).

1.3.3 Food

In Canada, a total of 881 pork liver tissue samples revealed a gradual decline of pentachlorophenol levels in 1988-89 from those in previous years. Some 6.6% of the samples contained levels in excess of 0.1 mg/kg, the highest level being 0.72 mg/kg. Of 51 beef liver samples, 2.0 % had levels in excess of 0.1 mg/kg, the maximal level being 0.35 mg/kg. Examination of 214 chicken and 68 turkey liver samples showed only one with a level above 0.1 mg/kg; this incident was traced to the use of wood shavings as bedding (Agriculture Canada, 1989).

The amount of pentachlorophenol that enters the food chain and the long-term average daily intake of pentachlorophenol by the general population in the USA was estimated using six-compartment environmental partitioning models. Pentachlorophenol partitions mainly into soil (96.5%), and food chains, especially fruits, vegetables and grains, account for 99.9% of human exposure to pentachlorophenol. The long-term, average daily intake of pentachlorophenol is estimated to be 16 μg/day (Hattemer-Frey & Travis, 1989).

1.3.4 Humans

The mean levels of pentachlorophenol in samples collected from the general population in Barcelona, Spain, in 1982-83 were 25 ng/ml (50 samples) in urine and 21.9 ng/ml (100 samples) in serum (Gómez-Catalán et al., 1987).

A family living in a wooden house in Germany was subjected to continual minor illnesses following the application of wood protection agents. These included nearly 12 kg pentachlorophenol and 3 kg lindane. While the air concentrations were low, the textiles in the house, comprising mostly clothing and bed linen, were highly contaminated, and extensive contact with these materials resulted in high dermal absorption (Gebefügi, 1989).

1.3.5 Occupational exposure

Aerial spraying of farm crops gave rise to levels of pentachlorophenol of 0.9 mg/m^3 in the cockpit of the spray plane, 38 mg/m^3 in the vicinity of the signal man and 1-4 mg/m^3 outside the treated field (Demidenko, 1969).

In general, studies of pentachlorophenol in human tissues and body fluids are discussed in section 4.1.1 of this monograph. Table 6 shows the concentrations of pentachlorophenol found in workers involved in the production of pentachlorophenol and treatment of wood with pentachlorophenol. In pressure treatment of wood, workers are exposed to pentachlorophenol when opening the door of pressure vessels. In non-pressure treatment, there is continuous evaporation of pentachlorophenol into the air, and consequently the residues in the urine of these workers are higher. People using the treated timber, such as carpenters and boat builders, have lower exposures.

1.4 Regulations and guidelines

In the USSR, the maximum allowable single concentration of pentachlorophenol in the air of communities is 0.005 mg/m^3, and the median daily concentration is 0.001 mg/m^3 (Izmerov, 1984).

The maximum allowable concentration of pentachlorophenol in drinking-water is 0.06 mg/l in Canada (Ritter & Wood, 1989) and 0.3 mg/l in the USSR (Izmerov, 1984). WHO (1984) recommended a drinking-water quality guideline value of 10 µg/l for pentachlorophenol based on 10% of the acceptable daily intake of 3 µg/kg bw.

In the USA, the acceptable daily intake of pentachlorophenol from food is 3 µg/kg bw per day (WHO, 1987).

National pesticide residue limits for pentachlorophenol in foods are presented in Table 3.

Table 3. National pesticide residue limits for pentachlorophenol in foods[a]

Country	Residue limit (mg/kg)	Commodities
Australia	0.01[b]	Citrus, grapes, mushrooms, pineapples, potatoes
Austria	0.05	Foods of vegetable origin
Belgium	0.05[c]	Mushrooms
	0 (0.01)[d]	Other foodstuffs of vegetable origin
Germany	0.01	All foods of plant origin
Israel	0.05	Mushrooms, other foods
Netherlands	0.05	Mushrooms
	0 (0.01)[d]	Other crops and foods
Switzerland	0.05[e]	Milk
USSR	Not permitted	
Yugoslavia	0.01	Crops and food

[a]From Health and Welfare Canada (1990)
[b]Including the sodium salt
[c]Including salts
[d]Residues shall be absent while value in parentheses indicates highest concentration at which requirement has been met.
[e]Includes 'TCP' as an impurity; upper limit value beyond which food is unfit for human consumption

Occupational exposure limits for pentachlorophenol in some countries and regions are given in Table 4. Each limit has a notation indicating a hazard for absorption through skin.

Table 4. Occupational exposure limits to pentachlorophenol[a]

Country	Year	Concentration	Interpretation[b]
Austria	1987	0.5	TWA
Belgium	1987	0.5	TWA
Denmark	1987	0.5	TWA
Finland	1987	0.5	TWA
	1987	1.5	STEL (15 min)
Germany	1989	0.05	TWA
Hungary	1987	0.2	TWA
	1987	0.4	STEL
Indonesia	1987	0.5	TWA
Italy	1987	0.5	TWA
Mexico	1987	0.5	TWA
Netherlands	1987	0.5	TWA
Poland	1987	0.5	TWA
Romania	1987	0.5	TWA
	1987	1	STEL
Sweden	1987	0.5	TWA
	1987	1.5	STEL
Switzerland	1987	0.5	TWA
Taiwan	1987	0.5	TWA
United Kingdom	1987	0.5	TWA
	1987	1.5	STEL (10 min)
USA			
ACGIH	1989	0.5	TWA
OSHA	1989	0.5	TWA
USSR	1987	0.1	TWA
Venezuela	1987	0.5	TWA
	1987	1.5	Ceiling
Yugoslavia	1987	0.5	TWA

[a]From Cook (1987); American Conference of Governmental Industrial Hygienists (ACGIH) (1989); Deutsche Forschungsgemeinschaft (1989); US Occupational Safety and Heath Administration (OSHA) (1989)
[b]TWA, time weighted average; STEL, short–term exposure limit

Some countries have restricted the use of pentachlorophenol. Sweden banned all use of pentachlorophenol in 1977, and Germany banned all uses in 1987. The USA cancelled its registration for herbicidal and anti-microbial use and for the preservation of wood in contact with food, feed, domestic animals and livestock; the sale and use of pentachlorophenol is restricted to certified applicators. The agricultural use of pentachlorophenol has also been suspended or restricted in other countries, including Canada and Japan. Canada and the Netherlands have suspended its use for indoor wood treatment (WHO, 1987).

2. Studies of Cancer in Humans

Exposure to pentachlorophenol usually occurs concomitantly with exposure to other chlorophenols. The effects of exposure to chlorophenols as a group were evaluated in Volume 41 of the *Monographs* (IARC, 1986). In this monograph, only those studies in which exposure to pentachlorophenol was reported specifically are reviewed.

2.1 Case reports

Bishop and Jones (1981) reported two cases of non-Hodgkin's lymphoma of the scalp in a cohort of 158 workers handling pentachlorophenol.

Greene *et al.* (1978) reported the occurrence of Hodgkin's disease in three siblings and a first cousin. Two of the brothers had been employed by a fence installation company for 12 and 15 years, respectively, and had worked primarily with wood products immersed in pentachlorophenol. They had prepared the preservative by hand without protective clothing, and the one sibling still employed at the time of the study had high levels of pentachlorophenol in his serum and urine. There were no similar exposures in the remaining two familial cases.

2.2 Case-control studies

Risk from exposure to chlorophenols in farming was estimated in three population-based case-control studies based on data from the New Zealand Cancer Registry (Smith *et al.*, 1984; Pearce *et al.*, 1986a, 1987). The authors reported that sodium pentachlorophenate is used for treating sawn timber and, to a lesser extent, fencing materials against sap stain. Vacuum-pressure impregnation with copper chrome arsenate is the principal method for preserving fencing timber in New Zealand, but, in the past, pentachlorophenol was also used (on less than 1% of posts) (Pearce *et al.*, 1986b). Thus, sawmill workers who reported handling treated timber were considered potentially to have been exposed to sodium pentachlorophenate, whereas fencing workers were considered to be exposed predominantly to copper chrome arsenate rather than chlorophenols.

In the case-control study on soft-tissue sarcomas, 82 male patients registered during 1976-80 (or their next of kin) were interviewed regarding their occupational history, and the findings were compared with those for 92 age-matched male controls with other types of cancer selected from the National Cancer Registry. The response rate was 84% for cases and 83% for controls. Work in a sawmill or timber company was reported for 12 cases and 11 controls (odds ratio, 1.3; 90% confidence interval [CI], 0.6-2.9). Of these, three cases and five controls were considered potentially to have been exposed to chlorophenols [presumably sodium pentachlorophenate (see above)] (odds ratio, 0.7; 90% CI, 0.1-2.7). Work as a fencing contractor was reported for five cases and three controls (1.9; 0.5-8.6), whereas 20 cases and 26 controls were farmers who had carried out fencing work (0.8; 0.4-1.5). These results were not affected by stratification on year of birth, year of registration or whether the patient or next-of-kin was interviewed (Smith *et al.*, 1984).

The second study included 183 cases of non-Hodgkin's lymphoma registered in 1977-81 and 338 cancer registry controls (other than soft-tissue sarcoma, Hodgkin's disease and multiple myeloma) (Pearce *et al.*, 1985), with response rates of 85 and 81%, respectively. All analyses were adjusted for age and whether the patient or next-of-kin had been interviewed. The odds ratio for work in a sawmill or timber company was 0.9 (24 exposed cases, 45 exposed cancer controls; 90% CI, 0.6-1.5), and that for potential exposure to chlorophenols [presumably sodium pentachlorophenate (see above)] in these occupations was 1.0 (11 exposed cases, 18 exposed controls; 90% CI, 0.5-2.0). The odds ratio for fencing work was 1.4 (68 exposed cases, 93 exposed controls; 90% CI, 1.0-2.0) (Pearce *et al.*, 1987).

The third study involved interviews with 76 patients with multiple myeloma registered in 1977-81 (or their next-of-kin) and 315 controls with cancers other than soft-tissue sarcoma, Hodgkin's disease and non-Hodgkin's lymphoma, who were also included in the control group for the study on non-Hodgkin's lymphoma of Pearce *et al.* (1987). Response rates were 82 and 81%, respectively, for cases and controls. All analyses were adjusted for age and whether the patient or next-of-kin had been interviewed. Work in a sawmill or timber company was reported for 11 cases and 42 controls (odds ratio, 1.1; 95% CI, 0.5-2.3), and potential exposure to chlorophenols [presumably sodium pentachlorophenate (see above)] was reported for five of the cases and 16 of the controls (odds ratio, 1.4; 95% CI, 0.5-3.9). Fencing work was reported for 29 cases and 87 controls (1.6; 0.9-2.7) (Pearce *et al.*, 1986a).

A population-based case-control study in central Sweden comprised 237 cases of soft-tissue sarcoma and 237 controls matched for age, gender and county of residence. The design is described in detail in the monograph on occupational exposure in spraying and application of insecticides (p. 70). Exposure to pentachlorophenol more than five years before the date of diagnosis for one week or more continuously or at least one month in total was reported from interviews with patients or next-of-kin for 11 cases and three controls (odds ratio, 3.9; 95% CI, 1.2-12.9). This analysis excluded cases and controls for whom exposure to phenoxyacetic herbicides was reported (Eriksson *et al.*, 1990).

2.3 Cohort studies

A cohort study of workers in the sawmill industry in the province of Kymi in Finland (Jäppinen *et al.*, 1989) comprised 721 men and 502 women who had been employed for at least one year during 1945-61. Cancer incidence during the period 1953-80 was identified through the cancer registries of Finland, Sweden and Norway, but the incidence figures for Kymi were used as reference. There were 90 cases of cancer in men (standardized incidence ratio (SIR), 1.1; 95% CI, 0.87-1.3) and 55 cases in women (SIR, 1.2; 95% CI, 0.93-1.6). Several cancer types occurred in excess in both men and women, including skin cancer (ICD, 173) (8 cases [SIR, 2.7; 95% CI, 1.2-5.3]), cancer of the lip, mouth and pharynx (7 cases [1.6; 0.7-3.4]) and leukaemia (7 cases [2.3; 0.9-4.8]). One case of soft-tissue sarcoma was observed (0.6 expected). The chlorophenols used for wood treatment in this industry, however, contained predominantly 2,3,4,6-tetrachlorophenol and only 5-9% pentachlorophenol by weight.

3. Studies of Cancer in Experimental Animals

The Working Group was aware of a study in mice by the US National Technical Information Service (1968) and Innes *et al.* (1969) and a study in rats by Schwetz *et al.* (1978), which were considered in the previous monograph (IARC, 1979). Because of deficiencies in design, performance and/or reporting, the present Working Group did not consider these studies informative for an evaluation.

Oral administration

Mouse: Groups of 50 male and 50 female B6C3F$_1$ mice, nine weeks old, were fed technical-grade pentachlorophenol (90.4% pure; tetrachlorophenol, 3.8%; nonachloro-hydroxydiphenyl ether, 3.56%; octachlorohydroxydiphenyl ether, 1.91%; heptachloro-hydroxydibenzofuran, 0.47%; trichlorophenol, 0.01%) at 100 or 200 mg/kg of diet or Dowicide EC-7 (a technical-grade formulation: 91% pure; tetrachlorophenol, 9.4%) at 100, 200 or 600 mg/kg of diet for two years. Two groups of 35 male and 35 female mice were fed control diets. Animals were killed at the age of 112 weeks. Survival was similar in treated and control groups, except that the survival of low-dose females was significantly reduced after 628 days with the EC-7 formulation. A significant, dose-related increase in the incidence of hepatocellular adenomas and carcinomas was observed in male mice treated with either formulation of pentachlorophenol; and a significant, dose-related increase in the incidence of hepatocellular adenomas was seen in females treated with EC-7 (Table 5). There was also a dose-related increase in the incidence of adrenal phaeochromocytomas in male mice exposed to either formulation and in females exposed to the high dose of EC-7. Female mice exposed to high doses of either formulation had a significantly higher incidence of haemangiosarcomas of the spleen and/or liver (US National Toxicology Program, 1989).

Table 5. Study of the carcinogenicity of two grades of pentachlorophenol fed in the diet for 103 weeks in B6C3F$_1$ mice[a]

Material	Sex	Experimental parameter/ observation	Group				Statistical conclusion (trend test)[b]
			0	1	2	3	
Technical-grade	M	Dose (mg/kg of diet)	0	100	200		
		Liver adenomas	5/32	20/47	33/48***		$p < 0.001$
		Liver carcinomas	2/32	10/47	12/48		
		Phaeochromocytomas	0/31	10/45*	23/45***		$p < 0.001$
	F	Dose (mg/kg of diet)	0	100	200		
		Liver adenomas	3/33	8/49	8/50		NS
		Liver carcinomas	0/33	1/49	1/50		NS
		Haemangiosarcomas	0/35	3/50	6/50*		$p < 0.05$
EC-7	M	Dose (mg/kg of diet)	0	100	200	600	
		Liver adenomas	5/35	13/48	17/48**	32/49***	$p < 0.001$
		Liver carcinomas	1/35	7/48*	7/48*	9/49*	
		Phaeochromocytomas	0/34	4/48	21/48***	44/49***	$p < 0.001$

Table 5 (contd)

Material	Sex	Experimental parameter/ observation	Group				Statistical conclusion (trend test)[b]
			0	1	2	3	
EC-7	F	Dose (mg/kg of diet)	0	100	200	600	
(contd)		Liver adenomas	1/34	3/50	6/49	30/48***	$p < 0.001$
		Liver carcinomas	0/34	1/50	0/49	2/48	ND
		Haemangiosarcomas	0/35	1/50	3/50	8/49*	$p < 0.01$

[a]From US National Toxicology Program (1989)
[b]Incidental tumour test (adjusted for survival)

*$p < 0.05$
**$p < 0.01$
***$p < 0.001$
NS, not signifiicant

4. Other Relevant Data

4.1 Absorption, distribution, metabolism and excretion

The pharmacokinetics of pentachlorophenol has been reviewed (Ahlborg & Thunberg, 1980; Exon, 1984; WHO, 1987) and shows great variation between studies and across species. Data are available for humans, monkeys, rats and, to a lesser extent, mice.

4.1.1 *Humans*

Dermal and pulmonary absorption of pentachlorophenol may occur during occupational exposure (Truhaut et al., 1952; Menon, 1958; Robson et al., 1969; Kauppinen & Lindroos, 1985).

The half-time for absorption of orally administered sodium pentachlorophenate (0.1 mg/kg bw) to healthy volunteers was found to be 1.3 ± 0.4 h. The decrease in the plasma concentration (maximum plasma concentration occurring 4 h after ingestion) fitted a first-order, one-compartment model with a half-time of 30.2 ± 4.0 h. Maximal urinary excretion occurred 40 h after ingestion, with a half-time of excretion of 33.1 ± 5.4 h (Braun et al., 1979). These results were challenged in another study in which the blood half-time of orally administered pentachlorophenol (0.98 mg ^{13}C-labelled compound) to a presumably healthy volunteer was found to be 16 ± 2.5 days. In the same subject, the urine half-time was 18 ± 2.4 days, whereas in another subject given 18.8 mg/kg bw pentachlorophenol orally it was 20 ± 3.4 days (Uhl et al., 1986). These authors calculated similar figures for comparable data obtained from the literature: a urinary half-time of 16 days could be calculated from the urinary concentrations measured after accidental skin exposure (Bevenue et al., 1967), and half-times for both plasma and urine of 12 days were calculated from measurements before and after holidays in workers occupationally exposed to pentachlorophenol (Begley et al., 1977). Finally, in a case of intentional ingestion (Haley, 1977), an elimination half-time of about 10 days could be calculated (WHO, 1987). Uhl et al. (1986) concluded that elimination behaviour does not depend on the extent of the exposure. The long elimination half-time of pentachlorophenol cannot be explained by enterohepatic circulation (biliary levels of pentachlorophenol were in the same range as those in plasma and urine in patients with biliary drainage) but rather by the extensive plasma protein binding of the compound (> 96%) and by its very effective tubular reabsorption, as shown *in vivo* by changing urinary pH. From these results, it can be calculated that urinary levels in humans will reach a steady state within approximately three months.

Data on tissue distribution in humans have been derived from examination of autopsy samples from unexposed and poisoned subjects (WHO, 1987). Decreasing tissue concentrations of pentachlorophenol have been found in liver, kidney and brain of people with no known exposure. Data from cases of poisoning resulting in death show large variations among different organs.

Pentachlorophenol is metabolized *in vitro* by human liver microsomes to tetrachlorohydroquinone (Juhl *et al.*, 1985), which has been found in the urine of workers exposed to pentachlorophenol (Ahlborg *et al.*, 1974). Pentachlorophenol glucuronide is also formed *in vitro* by human liver microsomes (Lilienblum, 1985), but its concentration in urine as compared with that of the parent compound may vary and is probably underestimated owing to the instability of the conjugate at urinary pH.

Many data are available on blood and urinary levels of pentachlorophenol in occupationally exposed workers, nonoccupationally exposed subjects, including residents of log homes treated with pentachlorophenol, and subjects with no known exposure; these were summarized (WHO, 1987). Studies in which levels of pentachlorophenol were measured both in air and in the serum, plasma or urine of exposed people are summarized in Tables 6 and 7. Studies in which levels were measured in the serum or plasma of people with no known exposure are summarized in Table 8.

4.1.2 *Experimental systems*

The absorption rate constants of ^{14}C-labelled pentachlorophenol after oral administration to male and female rats (10 mg/kg bw) were found to be 1.95 and 1.52/h, respectively. Maximal plasma concentrations were reached 4-6 h after administration (Braun *et al.*, 1977). The average half-times of absorption in male and female rhesus monkeys were 3.6 and 1.8 h, respectively, with a plasma peak concentration within 12-24 h after administration (Braun & Sauerhoff, 1976). Rapid absorption of pentachlorophenol also occurred in rats after inhalation (Hoben *et al.*, 1976).

Conflicting results have been reported on elimination kinetics (*via* urine or urine and faeces) in mammals after administration of single oral doses of pentachlorophenol (WHO, 1987). Besides interspecies variation, there also appeared to be sex differences. Monophasic elimination was reported in male rats after inhalation of 5.7 mg/kg bw (Hoben *et al.*, 1976) and in female rats after an oral dose of 100 mg/kg bw (Braun *et al.*, 1977). Biphasic elimination was reported in female rats after oral doses of 37-41 mg/kg bw and 10 mg/kg bw (Larsen *et al.*, 1972; Braun *et al.*, 1977) and in male rats after oral doses of 10 or 100 mg/kg bw pentachlorophenol (Braun *et al.*, 1977). The half-times for the single and the rapid phase were between 10 and 27 h, whereas for the slow phase they were between 33 h and 102 days.

Table 6. Levels of pentachlorophenol in the air and in the serum or plasma and urine of individuals exposed occupationally[a]

Exposure	No. of subjects	Length of exposure (years)	Air ($\mu g/m^3$) Mean	Air Range	Serum (mg/l) Mean	Serum Range	Urine (mg/l) Mean	Urine Range
Lumber, dipping	NS	NS	19	3-63	NA		2.83	0.12-9.68
Lumber dipping, spraying or brushing	18	NS	NA		5.14	0.43-14	1.31	0.09-3.3
6th day of vacation	18	NS	NA		4.92	0.50-13	1.36	0.18-3.5
20th day of vacation	18	NS	NA		2.19	0.32-5.3	0.59	0.05-1.4
51st day of renewed work	13	NS	NA		2.61	0.19-8.1	0.95	0.03-3.6
Lumber, general	3	5 (2-11)	1[b]	< 1-15	1.11[b]	0.35-3	0.15[b]	0.044-0.47
Lumber, office	1	10	2[b]	< 1-3	0.65[b]	0.42-0.75	0.06[b]	0.04-0.11
Lumber, pressure treatment	1	5	6[b]	< 1-15	2.29[b]	1.51-3.55	0.30[b]	0.09-0.76
Airborne and dermal	NS	NS	14[c]	4-1000	NA		1.24	0.17-5.57
Airborne	10	5-10	55.6	± 89	0.71	± 0.38	0.11	± 0.02
Airborne	8	5-10	66.7	± 100	0.24	± 0.23	0.05	± 0.02
Lumber, spraying	NS	NS	6[c]	3-69	NA		0.98	0.13-2.58
Pentachlorophenol application	23	3[d] (0.5-12)	2.4	0.3-8	1[d,e]	0.2-2.4	NS	
Pentachlorophenol processing[f]	18	10[d] (0.2-31)	17.5	2-50	0.25[d,e]	0.02-1.5	NS	
Pentachlorophenol processing factory[f]	18	12 (0.3-31)	NS	2.2-55.5	0.25[d]	0.02-1.5	0.112[d]	0.013-1.224
Pentachlorophenol production	8	NS	< 100- > 500[g]		4.73 ± 3.41		2.38 ± 1.91	
	18	NS	270-4000		NA		0.72 ± 0.55	
Sodium pentachlorophenol production	14	NS	< 100- > 500[h]		2.23 ± 1.51		0.84 ± 0.65	
	50	NS	0-50		NA		0.35 ± 0.30	

[a]Selected from WHO (1987)
[b]Calculated from sampling data collected over 5 months
[c]Air at 'maximum exposure' sites, next to sources, contained 26 $\mu g/m^3$ (lumber spraying site) and 297 $\mu g/m^3$ (pressure treatment site).
[d]Median
[e]Plasma
[f]Overlapping studies
[g]Of 67 samples, 18 were < 100 and 10 > 500 $\mu g/m^3$
[h]Of 55 samples, 7 were < 100 and 8 > 500 $\mu g/m^3$
NA, not analysed
NS, not specified

Table 7. Levels of pentachlorophenol in the air and in the serum or plasma and urine of individuals exposed non-occupationally[a]

Exposure	No. of subjects	Length of exposure (years)	Air (µg/m³) Mean	Air (µg/m³) Range	Serum (mg/l) Mean	Serum (mg/l) Range	Urine (mg/l) Mean	Urine (mg/l) Range
Indoor application of pentachlorophenol solutions	16	NS	NS	1–10	NA		NS	0.030–0.150
Residence in log homes treated with pentachlorophenol solutions	5	NS	0.29[b]	0.20–0.38	1.126	0.580–1.750	0.084	0.047–0.216
Indoor application of an average of 40 litres pentachlorophenol solution	989	NS (< 9 years)	6.1[c] 4.9[d]	ND–25 2.5–0.5	NA		0.044 0.029[d]	0.013–0.071
Men < 18 years	16	NS	≤ 5		NA		0.047[d]	0.017–0.107
Men ≥ 18 years	39	NS	≤ 5		NA		0.023[d]	0.011–0.052
Women < 18 years	22	NS	≤ 5		NA		0.033[d]	0.016–0.066
Women ≥ 18 years	39	NS	≤ 5		NA		0.026[d]	0.015–0.059
Men < 18 years	23	NS	> 5		NA		0.079[d]	0.014–0.125
Men ≥ 18 years	31	NS	> 5		NA		0.043[d]	0.011–0.146
Women < 18 years	25	NS	> 5		NA		0.059[d]	0.011–0.103
Women ≥ 18 years	43	NS	> 5		NA		0.039[d]	0.021–0.125
Indoor application of about 70 litres pentachlorophenol solution								
Before ventilation	6	6	0.60	0.14–1.20	NA		0.032	0.0007–0.0078
After ventilation	6	–	0.08	ND–0.24	0.080[e]	0.025–0.190	0.0033	0.0018–0.0080
Indoor application of about 75 litres pentachlorophenol solution	2	0.5	0.15	ND–0.40	0.033[e]	0.031–0.034	NA	
Indoor application of about 100 litres pentachlorophenol solution	2	1	0.67	0.44–0.95	0.565[e]	0.47–0.66	NA	

[a]Selected from WHO (1987)

[b]Samples taken on 1st and 2nd floors of a two-storey log house; a sample of interior surface wood contained 1132 mg/kg pentachlorophenol (0.11%)

[c]104 indoor air samples taken

[d]Median (2/3 range)

[e]Plasma

NA, not analysed; ND, not detectable; NS, not specified

Table 8. Levels of pentachlorophenol (PCP) in the serum or urine of individuals with no known exposure[a]

Exposure	No. of subjects	Serum (mg/l)		Urine (mg/l)	
		Mean	Range	Mean	Range
US National Human Monitoring Program for Pesticides	418	NA		0.0063	ND-0.193
Control group for non-occupational exposure (indoor application of PCP solutions)	12	NA		0.0135	0.006-0.023
Control group for non-occupational exposure (residents of log homes treated with PCP solutions)					
January 1980 'conventional' homes	42	NS	0.004-0.068	NS	0.0007-0.011
March 1980 untreated log homes	2	0.051	0.034-0.075	0.0014	0.001-0.002
March 1980 'conventional' homes	11	0.048	0.015-0.055	0.025	0.001-0.007
Control group for non-occupational indoor air levels below detection limit of 0.1 μg/m^3 (indoor application of 40 litres PCP solution)	207	NA		0.0127 0.0102[c]	0.0038-0.0214
Control group for non-occupational exposure (indoor application of PCP solution, 70-100 litres)	99	0.129 0.088[b]	<0.05-1.10	NA	
Non-specifically exposed persons	12 30	0.025	0.019-0.036	0.014	0.007-0.034[c]

[a]Selected from WHO (1987)
[b]Median (2/3 range)
[c]Assuming a daily urine volume of 1.4 litres
NA, not analysed; ND, not detectable; NS, not specified

The half-time value for clearance of pentachlorophenol from plasma was 83.5 h for female and 72 h for male rhesus monkeys given 10 mg/kg bw of a ^{14}C-labelled compound orally. The half-times for urinary excretion were 92.4 h for females and 40.8 h for males. Slow, steady elimination of the compound in the faeces of monkeys suggests a role of enterohepatic circulation (Braun & Sauerhoff, 1976).

Pentachlorophenol was shown to be 99% bound to plasma protein in rats (Braun *et al.*, 1977).

Concentrations of pentachlorophenol in tissues account for only a small fraction of the administered dose, because it is usually rapidly excreted in urine. Total-body recovery of radiolabel from rats nine days after a single oral dose of 10 mg/kg bw of ^{14}C-labelled compound was less than 0.5%, most of which was concentrated in the liver (Braun *et al.*, 1977). Similar results were obtained in mice after subcutaneous and intraperitoneal injection of ^{14}C-labelled compound (15-37 mg/kg bw) (Jakobson & Yllner, 1971) and in lactating dairy cows after oral administration (Kinzell *et al.*, 1985). The total tissue concentration of radiolabel recovered from monkeys 360 h after administration was about 11% of a dose of 10 mg/kg bw ^{14}C-pentachlorophenol (Braun & Sauerhoff, 1976).

Very little pentachlorophenol crosses the placenta in rats. When ^{14}C-pentachlorophenol was administered orally on day 15 of pregnancy (60 mg/kg bw), the maximal amount of specific radiolabel in maternal blood was 1.1% of the dose, while it never exceeded 0.3% in the placenta and 0.1% in the fetuses (Larsen et al., 1975).

Biotransformation of pentachlorophenol in rats involves its urinary excretion as the glucuronic acid conjugate and its hydrolytic dechlorination to tetrachlorohydroquinone, which is excreted free or conjugated with glucuronic acid in the urine (Ahlborg et al., 1978). Trichlorohydroquinone is also formed in rats by reductive dechlorination of tetrachloro-hydroquinone and excreted as the glucuronate in urine (Ahlborg & Thunberg, 1978, 1980). Free and conjugated pentachlorophenol and free tetrachlorohydroquinone have been identified in the urine of mice administered pentachlorophenol (Jakobson & Yllner, 1971). In contrast to rodents, rhesus monkeys eliminate pentachlorophenol in urine unchanged (Braun & Sauerhoff, 1976). A number of drugs that affect liver microsomal enzymes have also been shown to influence the biotransformation of pentachlorophenol selectively (Ahlborg & Thunberg, 1978; Ahlborg et al., 1978; Van Ommen et al., 1986).

4.2 Toxic effects

The toxicology of pentachlorophenol has been reviewed (Ahlborg & Thunberg, 1980; Williams, 1982; Exon, 1984; WHO, 1987).

4.2.1 Humans

Several cases of acute accidental, suicidal and occupational poisoning have been reported and reviewed (WHO, 1987). Symptoms of acute poisoning include central nervous system disorders, dyspnoea and hyperpyrexia; the cause of death is cardiac arrest, and poison victims usually show marked rigor mortis. Examination post mortem shows nonspecific organ damage. One case of fatal poisoning was associated with higher pentachlorophenol concentrations in bile and kidney (Wood et al., 1983). The minimal lethal dose of pentachlorophenol in man has been estimated to be 29 mg/kg bw. Occupational exposures to technical-grade pentachlorophenol resulted in various disorders of the skin and mucous membranes (WHO, 1987). The incidence of chloracne was highest in people who had had confirmed direct skin contact (O'Malley et al., 1990). Several health and biomonitoring surveys of workers with plasma pentachlorophenol concentrations ranging from nanograms to milligrams per litre showed some minor and often transitory changes in various biochemical, haematological and electrophysiological parameters, but no clinical effect was seen (Klemmer et al., 1980; Triebig et al., 1981; Zober et al., 1981). Anecdotal exposure to pentachlorophenol has been associated with aplastic anaemia and/or red-cell aplasia (Roberts, 1983).

4.2.2 Experimental systems

Data on the acute toxicity in experimental animals of pentachlorophenol given by various routes have been summarized (WHO, 1987).

The oral LD_{50} was 36-177 mg/kg bw in mice (Ahlborg & Larsson, 1978; Borzelleca et al., 1985), 27-175 mg/kg bw in rats (Deichmann et al., 1942; Gaines, 1969) and 168 mg/kg bw in hamsters (Cabral et al., 1979, abstract). Cutaneous minimal lethal doses ranged from

39-170 mg/kg bw in rabbits (Kehoe *et al.*, 1939; Deichmann *et al.*, 1942) to 300 mg/kg bw in rats (Gaines, 1969). The acute toxicities of some known and possible metabolites of pentachlorophenol have also been reported (Borzelleca *et al.*, 1985; Renner *et al.*, 1986).

Symptoms of acute toxicity are similar to those in humans, including hyperpyrexia and neurological and respiratory dysfunction (WHO, 1987). Furthermore, palmitoylpentachlorophenol, which has been isolated from human fat (Ansari *et al.*, 1985), causes selective pancreatic toxicity in rats after single oral doses of 100 mg/kg bw (Ansari *et al.*, 1987).

A number of toxic effects described in acute and short-term toxicity studies have been attributed to impurities present in technical-grade pentachlorophenol preparations. The toxicity of impurities became clear when comparative studies with pure and technical-grade pentachlorophenol products were reported (Johnson *et al.*, 1973; Goldstein *et al.*, 1977; Kimbrough & Linder, 1978). Rats receiving 500 ppm [mg/kg] technical-grade pentachlorophenol in the diet for eight months had slow growth rates, liver enlargement, porphyria and increased activities of some liver microsomal enzymes (Goldstein *et al.*, 1977); rats fed purified pentachlorophenol at the same dose and for the same period of time showed only a reduction of growth rate and increased liver glucuronyl transferase activity. Analogous results were reported in a similar study (Kimbrough & Linder, 1978). Technical-grade pentachlorophenol, but not the pure compound, caused a porphyria similar to that due to hexachlorobenzene when given orally to rats for several months at increasing doses (Wainstok de Calmanovici & San Martin de Viale, 1980).

Several toxic effects of pentachlorophenol have been explained by the uncoupling effect of pentachlorophenol on oxidative phosphorylation (Ahlborg & Thunberg, 1980). Studies of structure–activity relationships among a series of chlorinated phenols showed that the effect increases with increasing chlorination of the phenol ring (Farquharson *et al.*, 1958). Pentachlorophenol and other chlorophenols inhibited some liver microsomal enzymes (Arrhenius *et al.*, 1977a,b), and pentachlorophenol strongly inhibited sulfotransferase activity in rat and mouse liver cytosol (Boberg *et al.*, 1983).

Reduced humoral immunity was observed in mice exposed to technical-grade pentachlorophenol, as well as impairment of T-cell cytolytic activity *in vitro* (Kerkvliet *et al.*, 1982a,b). In rats exposed to technical-grade pentachlorophenol, decreased cell-mediated and humoral immunity was demonstrated, while phagocytosis by macrophages and numbers of induced peritoneal macrophages were increased (Exon & Koller, 1983). Dioxin and furan contaminants are thought to be the chemical species responsible for the immunotoxicity of technical-grade pentachlorophenol (Kerkvliet *et al.*, 1985).

4.3 Reproductive and developmental effects

4.3.1 *Humans*

No data were available to the Working Group.

4.3.2 *Experimental systems*

Purified and commercial grades of pentachlorophenol were administered orally to rats at doses ranging from 5 to 50 mg/kg bw per day at various intervals during days 6-15 of pregnancy. A dose-related increase in the incidence of resorptions, subcutaneous oedema, dilated ureters and anomalies of the skull, ribs, vertebrae and sternebrae was observed. Early organogenesis was the most sensitive period. The no-effect dose level of the commercial grade was 5 mg/kg bw per day; purified pentachlorophenol given at the same dose level caused a statistically significant increase in the incidence of delayed ossification of the skull bones but had no other effect on embryonal or fetal development (Schwetz et al., 1974). Ingestion of 3 mg/kg bw per day of a commercially available purified grade of pentachlorophenol had no effect on reproduction, neonatal growth, survival or development (Schwetz et al., 1978).

In Charles River CD rats given a single oral dose of 60 mg/kg bw pentachlorophenol (purity, > 99%) at various times on one of days 8-13 of gestation, the incidence of resorptions was not significantly greater than that in controls. Malformations were observed (5.8% of 51 fetuses examined after exposure on day 9 versus 0% in controls), including, for example, exencephaly and lack of tail, but the number was considered minimal, and the authors suggested that the effect could have been due to indirect toxic effects of the compound on the dams. No maternal mortality was reported (Larsen et al., 1975).

Two later studies (Exon & Koller, 1982; Welsh et al., 1987) in Sprague-Dawley rats administered pentachlorophenol in the feed throughout mating and pregnancy confirmed findings of embryo- and fetotoxicity and lethality, as judged by decreased litter size, and, at 13 mg/kg bw per day for 181 days (Welsh et al., 1987), decreased body weight and crown–rump length and an increase in skeletal variations.

Pentachlorophenol was reported not to be embryolethal or teratogenic in CD rats given 75 mg/kg bw per day on days 7-18 of gestation (Courtney et al., 1976).

As reported in an abstract, fetal deaths and/or resorptions were observed in three of six test groups of Syrian golden hamsters after oral administration of doses varying from 1.25 to 20.0 mg/kg bw per day on days 5-10 of gestation (Hinkle, 1973). Sea urchin eggs exposed to pentachlorophenol (0.2 mg/l medium or above) had delayed development and were malformed (Ozretić & Krajnović-Ozretić, 1985).

4.4 Genetic and related effects (see also Table 9 and Appendices 1 and 2)

The genotoxicity of pentachlorophenol has been reviewed (Seiler, 1991).

4.4.1 Humans

Sister chromatid exchange and chromosomal aberrations were analysed in peripheral lymphocytes from 22 exposed male workers with 1-30 years of exposure at a pentachlorophenol plant. Exposure to pentachlorophenol and sodium pentachlorophenate was estimated by measurements of concentrations in blood and urine. A matched control group of 22 unexposed workers was used, although matching was not quite complete since all exposed workers but only nine of the 22 controls were smokers. [The Working Group noted that pentachlorophenol was not measured in controls.] A total of 300 first-division metaphases were evaluated from each exposed and 500 from each unexposed person. Significant increases in the frequencies of dicentric chromosomes and of acentric fragments were observed in exposed versus control men, and the increases were not influenced by smoking habits. When smoking was controlled for, there was no effect of exposure to pentachlorophenol or its sodium salt upon the frequency of sister chromatid exchange (Bauchinger et al., 1982).

In a study of 20 workers, with exposures to pentachlorophenol ranging from three to 34 years, divided into two groups according to their main occupation, exposure was estimated by measurement of the serum concentration of pentachlorophenol. No difference in the frequency of chromosomal aberration or of sister chromatid exchange was detected in peripheral lymphocytes from the two groups (Ziemsen et al., 1987). [The Working Group noted that no unexposed control was used and that the time of culturing for metaphase analysis was not given]. Biological monitoring data showed exposure to be much lower than in the study of Bauchinger et al. (1982).

4.4.2 Experimental systems

In bacteria, pentachlorophenol gave equivocal results in tests for DNA damage and mostly negative results for induction of gene mutation. It was inactive in a host-mediated assay in mice with bacteria as the indicator organism. In yeast, pentachlorophenol induced gene mutation and mitotic gene conversion, but not mitotic recombination. It did not induce aneuploidy or, in the form of the sodium salt, recessive lethal mutation in Drosophila melanogaster. Pentachlorophenol did not induce gene mutation at the hprt locus in Chinese hamster V79 cells. It marginally increased the frequency of sister chromatid exchange in Chinese hamster CHO cells in vitro but not in human peripheral lymphocytes in vitro. Pentachlorophenol induced chromosomal aberrations in cultured Chinese hamster CHO cells but not in cultured human peripheral lymphocytes.

Pentachlorophenol exhibited a weak, but apparently dose-dependent effect in the mouse coat colour spot test for somatic gene mutation. It was reported in one study that high doses of pentachlorophenol did not induce sperm abnormality in mice. [The Working Group noted that no positive control was used.]

5. Summary of Data Reported and Evaluation

5.1 Exposure data

Since its introduction in the 1930s, pentachlorophenol has been used in large quantities, mainly as a wood preservative. It has also found minor use as a herbicide, defoliant, bactericide and molluscicide. In recent years, its use in agriculture has been restricted in many countries.

Pentachlorophenol is usually formulated and applied to wood with a hydrocarbon diluant. Technical-grade pentachlorophenol has been shown to contain a large number of impurities, including tetrachlorophenols and, to a much lesser extent, polychloro-dibenzodioxins, polychlorodibenzofurans, polychlorodiphenyl ethers, polychlorophenoxy phenols and chlorinated hydrocarbons.

Pentachlorophenol has been detected in fruits, vegetables, meats, water and soils. It has been detected in the urine of the general population in several countries and at higher levels in the urine of workers in wood treatment plants.

Exposure to pentachlorophenol can occur during its production and use; from contact with pentachlorophenol-treated wood; at lower levels, from consumption of foods and water containing residues; and as a result of its ubiquitous presence as an environmental contaminant.

Table 9. Genetic and related effects of pentachlorophenol

Test system	Result[a] Without exogenous metabolic system	Result[a] With exogenous metabolic system	Dose[b]	Reference
PRB, prophage induction	(+)	(+)	12.0000	DeMarini et al. (1990)
PRB, PM2 phage, DNA strand breaks	–	0	26600.0000	Witte et al. (1985)
BSD, Bacillus subtilis rec strain, differential toxicity (spot test)	+	0	5.0000	Shirasu et al. (1976)
BSD, Bacillus subtilis rec strain, differential toxicity	–	–	2.2000	Matsui et al. (1989)
SA0, Salmonella typhimurium TA100, reverse mutation	–	–	5.0000	Nishimura et al. (1982)
SA0, Salmonella typhimurium TA100, reverse mutation	–	–	5.0000	Nishimura & Oshima (1983)
SA0, Salmonella typhimurium TA100, reverse mutation	–	–	15.0000	US National Toxicology Program (1989)
SA5, Salmonella typhimurium TA1535, reverse mutation	–	–	15.0000	US National Toxicology Program (1989)
SA7, Salmonella typhimurium TA1537, reverse mutation	–	–	15.0000	US National Toxicology Program (1989)
SA9, Salmonella typhimurium TA98, reverse mutation	–	+	5.0000	Nishimura et al. (1982)
SA9, Salmonella typhimurium TA98, reverse mutation	–	+	5.0000	Nishimura & Oshima (1983)
SA9, Salmonella typhimurium TA98, reverse mutation	–	–	15.0000	US National Toxicology Program (1989)
SCG, Saccharomyces cerevisiae, mitotic gene conversion	+	0	50.0000	Fahrig (1974)
SCG, Saccharomyces cerevisiae MP1, mitotic gene conversion	+	0	400.0000	Fahrig et al. (1978)
SCH, Saccharomyces cerevisiae MP1, mitotic crossing–over	+	0	400.0000	Fahrig et al. (1978)
SCF, Saccharomyces cerevisiae MP1, gene mutation	+	0	400.0000	Fahrig et al. (1978)
DMX, Drosophila melanogaster, sex-linked recessive lethal mutation	–	0	1860.0000	Vogel & Chandler (1974)
DMN, Drosophila melanogaster, chromosomal loss	–	0	400.0000	Ramel & Magnusson (1979)
DIA, DNA damage, Chinese hamster ovary cells in vitro	–	0	10.0000	Ehrlich (1990)
G9H, Gene mutation, Chinese hamster lung V79 cells in vitro, hprt locus	–	0	15.0000	Hattula & Knuutinen (1985)
G9H, Gene mutation, Chinese hamster lung V79 cells in vitro, hprt locus	–	0	50.0000	Jansson & Jansson (1986)
SIC, Sister chromatid exchange, Chinese hamster CHO cells in vitro	(+)	–	3.0000	Galloway et al. (1987)
CIC, Chromosomal aberrations, Chinese hamster CHO cells in vitro	–	(+)	100.0000	Galloway et al. (1987)
CIC, Chromosomal aberrations, Chinese hamster CHO cells in vitro	+	+	240.0000	Ishidate (1988)
SHL, Sister chromatid exchange, human lymphocytes in vitro	–	0	90.0000	Ziemsen et al. (1987)

Table 9 (contd)

Test system	Result[a] Without exogenous metabolic system	With exogenous metabolic system	Dose[b]	Reference
CHL, Chromosomal aberrations, human lymphocytes *in vitro*	–	0	90.0000	Ziemsen *et al.* (1987)
HMM, Host-mediated assay, *Salmonella typhimurium* G46, NMRI mouse	–	0	75.0000	Buselmaier *et al.* (1972)
HMM, Host-mediated assay, *Serratia marcescens* 21a, NMRI mouse	–	0	75.0000	Buselmaier *et al.* (1972)
MST, Spot test, C57Bl/6JHan×T mouse	(+)	0	50.0000	Fahrig *et al.* (1978)
SPM, Sperm morphology, (C57Bl/6×C3H)F₁ mouse	–	0	50.0000 × 5 i.p.	Osterloh *et al.* (1983)
SLH, Sister chromatid exchange, human lymphocytes *in vivo*	+	0	4.7300	Bauchinger *et al.* (1982)
CLH, Chromosomal aberrations, human lymphocytes *in vivo*	+	0	4.7300	Bauchinger *et al.* (1982)

[a] +, positive; (+), weakly positive; –, negative; 0, not tested; ?, inconclusive (variable response in several experiments within an adequate study)
[b] In-vitro tests, μg/ml; *in-vivo* tests, mg/kg bw

5.2 Carcinogenicity in humans

Two population-based case-control studies of soft-tissue sarcoma and non-Hodgkin's lymphoma in New Zealand found no increased risk associated with potential exposure to sodium pentachlorophenate through work in a sawmill or timber company. A similar study of multiple myeloma showed a slightly increased risk. A Swedish population-based case-control study found an increased risk for soft-tissue sarcoma associated with self-reported exposure to pentachlorophenol.

Excess incidences of cancers of the skin and of the lip, mouth and pharynx and of leukaemia were found in a cohort study of sawmill workers in Finland. Pentachlorophenol constituted only a minor proportion of the chlorophenols to which the workers were exposed.

5.3 Carcinogenicity in experimental animals

Two different pentachlorophenol formulations were tested for carcinogenicity by oral administration in two separate experiments in mice. A dose-related increase in the incidence of hepatocellular adenomas and carcinomas was observed in males exposed to either formulation and of hepatocellular adenomas in females exposed to one of the formulations. A dose-related increase in the incidence of adrenal phaeochromocytomas was observed in male mice exposed to either formulation, and an increase was also seen in females exposed to one of the formulations at the highest dose. A dose-related increase in the incidence of malignant vascular tumours of the liver and spleen was seen in female mice exposed to either formulation.

5.4 Other relevant data

Pentachlorophenol was embryotoxic and embryolethal and caused a slight increase in the number of malformations in rats.

Significant increases in the incidence of dicentric chromosomes and acentric fragments were detected in the peripheral lymphocytes of workers exposed occupationally to pentachlorophenol in one study, but no increase in the frequency of sister chromatid exchange was observed.

Pentachlorophenol gave negative results in most tests for genetic and related effects. It gave weakly positive results for somatic gene mutation in a mouse spot test. It induced chromosomal aberrations in cultured rodent cells but not in human cells and caused gene conversion in yeast.

5.5 Evaluation[1]

There is *inadequate evidence* in humans for the carcinogenicity of pentachlorophenol.

There is *sufficient evidence* in experimental animals for the carcinogenicity of pentachlorophenol.

Overall evaluation

Pentachlorophenol *is possibly carcinogenic to humans (Group 2B)*.

---

[1]For definition of the italicized terms, see Preamble, pp. 26-28.

6. References

Agriculture Canada (1989a) *Annual Report on Residue and Formula Compliance Monitoring for Fiscal Year 1988/89*, Ottawa, Agri-Food Safety Division, Food Inspection Directorate

Agricultural Canadian Plant Research Centre (1990) *Upgraded Product Quality for Pentachlorophenol*, Ottawa

Ahlborg, U.G. & Larsson, K. (1978) Metabolism of tetrachlorophenols in the rat. *Arch. Toxicol.*, *40*, 63-74

Ahlborg, U.G. & Thunberg, T. (1978) Effects of 2,3,7,8-tetrachlorodibenzo-*p*-dioxin on the in vivo and in vitro dechlorination of pentachlorophenol. *Arch. Toxicol.*, *40*, 55-61

Ahlborg, U.G. & Thunberg, T. (1980) Chlorinated phenols: occurrence, toxicity, metabolism and environmental impact. *Crit. Rev. Toxicol.*, *7*, 1-35

Ahlborg, U.G., Lindgren, J.-E. & Mercier, M. (1974) Metabolism of pentachlorophenol. *Arch. Toxicol.*, *32*, 271-281

Ahlborg, U.G., Larsson, K. & Thunberg, T. (1978) Metabolism of pentachlorophenol *in vivo* and *in vitro*. *Arch. Toxicol.*, *40*, 45-53

American Conference of Governmental Industrial Hygienists (1989) *Threshold Limit Values and Biological Exposure Indices for 1988-1989*, Cincinnati, OH, p. 29

Ansari, G.A.S., Britt, S.G. & Reynolds, E.S. (1985) Isolation and characterization of palmitoylpentachlorophenol from human fat. *Bull. environ. Contam. Toxicol.*, *34*, 661-667

Ansari, G.A.S., Kaphalia, B.S. & Boor, P.J. (1987) Selective pancreatic toxicity of palmitoylpentachlorophenol. *Toxicology*, *46*, 57-63

Arrhenius, E., Renberg, L. & Johansson, L. (1977a) Subcellular distribution, a factor in risk evaluation of pentachlorophenol. *Chem.-biol. Interactions*, *18*, 23-34

Arrhenius, E., Renberg, L., Johansson, L. & Zetterqvist, M.-A. (1977b) Disturbance of microsomal detoxication mechanisms in liver by chlorophenol pesticides. *Chem.-biol. Interactions*, *18*, 35-46

Arsenault, R.D. (1976) Pentachlorophenol and contained chlorinated dibenzodioxins in the environment. A study of environmental fate, stability and significance when used in wood preservation. *Am. Wood Preserv. Assoc.*, *20*, 122-148

Bauchinger, M., Dresp, J., Schmid, E. & Hauf, R. (1982) Chromosome changes in lymphocytes after occupational exposure to pentachlorophenol (PCP). *Mutat. Res.*, *102*, 83-88

Begley, J., Reichert, E.L., Rashad, M.N. & Klemmer, H.W. (1977) Association between renal function tests and pentachlorophenol exposure. *Clin. Toxicol.*, *11*, 97-106

Bevenue, A., Haley, T.J. & Klemmer, H.W. (1967) A note on the effects of a temporary exposure of an individual to pentachlorophenol. *Bull. environ. Contam. Toxicol.*, *2*, 293-296

Bishop, C.M. & Jones, A.H. (1981) Non-Hodgkin's lymphoma of the scalp in workers exposed to dioxins (Letter to the Editor). *Lancet*, *ii*, 369

Boberg, E.W., Miller, E.C., Miller, J.A., Poland, A. & Liem, A. (1983) Strong evidence from studies with brachymorphic mice and pentachlorophenol that 1'-sulfooxysafrole is the major ultimate electrophilic and carcinogenic metabolite of 1'-hydroxysafrole in mouse liver. *Cancer Res.*, *43*, 5163-5173

Borzelleca, J.F., Hayes, J.R., Condie, L.W. & Egle, J.L., Jr (1985) Acute toxicity of monochlorophenols, dichlorophenols and pentachlorophenol in the mouse. *Toxicol. Lett.*, *29*, 39-42

Braun, W.H. & Sauerhoff, M.W. (1976) The pharmacokinetic profile of pentachlorophenol in monkeys. *Toxicol. appl. Pharmacol.*, *38*, 525-533

Braun, W.H., Young, J.D., Blau, G.E. & Gehring, P.J. (1977) The pharmacokinetics and metabolism of pentachlorophenol in rats. *Toxicol. appl. Pharmacol.*, *41*, 395-406

Braun, W.H., Blau, G.E. & Chenoweth, M.B. (1979) The metabolism/pharmacokinetics of pentachlorophenol in man, and a comparison with the rat and monkey. In: Deichman, W.B., ed., *Toxicology and Occupational Medicine*, New York, Elsevier, pp. 289-296

Budavari, S., ed. (1989) *The Merck Index*, 11th ed., Rahway, NJ, Merck & Co., p. 1126

Buselmaier, W., Röhrborn, G. & Propping, P. (1972) Mutagenicity investigations with pesticides in the host-mediated assay and with the dominant lethal test in the mouse (Ger.). *Biol. Zbl.*, *91*, 311-325

Cabral, J.R.P., Raitano, F., Mollner, T., Bronczyk, S. & Shubik, P. (1979) Acute toxicity of pesticides in hamsters (Abstract No. 384). *Toxicol. appl. Pharmacol.*, *48*, A-192

Cook, W.A., ed. (1987) *Occupational Exposure Limits—Worldwide*, Washington DC, American Industrial Hygiene Association, pp. 32, 63, 148, 149, 206

Courtney, K.D., Copeland, M.F. & Robbins, A. (1976) The effects of pentachloronitrobenzene, hexachlorobenzene, and related compounds on fetal development. *Toxicol. appl. Pharmacol.*, *35*, 239-256

Deichmann, W., Machle, W., Kitzmiller, K.V. & Thomas, G. (1942) Acute and chronic effects of pentachlorophenol and sodium pentachlorophenate upon experimental animals. *J. Pharmacol. exp. Ther.*, *76*, 104-117

DeMarini, D.M., Brooks, H.G. & Parkes, D.G., Jr (1990) Induction of prophage lambda by chlorophenols. *Environ. mol. Mutagenesis*, *15*, 1-9

Demidenko, N.M. (1969) Materials for establishing the maximum permissible concentrations in air (Russ.). *Gig. Tr. Prof. Zabol.*, *7*, 58-60

Deutsche Forschungsgemeinschaft (1989) *Maximum Concentrations at the Workplace and Biological Tolerance Values for Working Materials. 1989* (Report No. XXV), Commission for the Investigation of Health Hazards of Chemical Compounds in the Work Area, Weinheim, VCH-Verlagsgesellschaft, p. 52

Eckerman, D.E. (1986) *Preliminary Quantitative Usage Analysis of Pentachlorophenol*, Washington DC, Office of Pesticide Programs, US Environmental Protection Agency

Ehrlich, W. (1990) The effect of pentachlorophenol and its metabolite tetrachlorohydroquinone on cell growth and the induction of DNA damage in Chinese hamster ovary cells. *Mutat. Res.*, *244*, 299-302

Eller, P.M., ed. (1984a) *NIOSH Manual of Analytical Methods*, 3rd ed., Vol. 2 (DHHS (NIOSH) Publ. No. 84-100), Washington DC, US Government Printing Office, pp. 5512-1—5512-3

Eller, P.M., ed. (1984b) *NIOSH Manual of Analytical Methods*, 3rd ed., Vol. 1 (DHHS (NIOSH) Publ. 84-100), Washington DC, US Government Printing Office, pp. 8001-1—8001-4, 8303-1—8303-4

Eriksson, M., Hardell, L. & Adami, H.-O. (1990) Exposure to dioxins as a risk factor for soft tissue sarcoma: a population-based case-control study. *J. natl Cancer Inst.*, *82*, 486-490

Exon, J.H. (1984) A review of chlorinated phenols. *Vet. hum. Toxicol.*, *26*, 508-519

Exon, J.H. & Koller, L.D. (1982) Effects of transplacental exposure to chlorinated phenols. *Environ. Health Perspect.*, *46*, 137-140

Exon, J.H. & Koller, L.D. (1983) Effects of chlorinated phenols on immunity in rats. *Int. J. Immunopharmacol.*, *5*, 131-136

Fahrig, R. (1974) Comparative mutagenicity studies with pesticides. In: Rosenfeld, C. & Davis, W., eds, *Environmental Pollution and Carcinogenic Risks* (IARC Scientific Publications No. 10), Lyon, IARC, pp. 161-181

Fahrig, R., Nilsson, C.-A. & Rappe, C. (1978) Genetic activity of chlorophenols and chlorophenol impurities. *Environ. Sci. Res.*, *12*, 325-338

Farquharson, M.E., Gage, J.C. & Northover, J. (1958) The biological action of chlorophenols. *Br. J. Pharmacol.*, *13*, 20-24

Fountaine, J.E., Joshipura, P.B. & Keliher, P.N. (1976) Some observations regarding pentachlorophenol levels in Haverford township, Pennsylvania. *Water Res.*, *10*, 185-188

Gaines, T.B. (1969) Acute toxicity of pesticides. *Toxicol. appl. Pharmacol.*, *14*, 515-534

Galloway, S.M., Armstrong, M.J., Reuben, C., Colman, S., Brown, B., Cannon, C., Bloom, A.D., Nakamura, F., Ahmed, M., Duk, S., Rimpo, J., Margolin, B.H., Resnick, M.A., Anderson, B. & Zeiger, Z. (1987) Chromosome aberrations and sister chromatid exchanges in Chinese hamster ovary cells: evaluations of 108 chemicals. *Environ. mol. Mutagenesis*, *10* (Suppl. 10), 1-175

Gebefügi, I. (1989) Chemical exposure in enclosed environments. *Toxicol. environ. Chem.*, *20-21*, 121-127

Gjøs, N. & Haegh, G.S. (1990) *OECD Co-operation on Existing Chemicals Clearing House Activity on Chlorinated Phenols*, Paris, Organisation for Economic Co-operation and Development

Goldstein, J.A., Friesen, M., Linder, R.E., Hickman, P., Hass, J.R. & Bergman, H. (1977) Effects of pentachlorophenol on hepatic drug-metabolizing enzymes and porphyria related to contamination with chlorinated dibenzo-*p*-dioxins and dibenzofurans. *Biochem. Pharmacol.*, *26*, 1549-1557

Gómez-Catalán, J., To-Figueras, J., Planas, J., Rodamilans, J. & Corbella, J. (1987) Pentachlorophenol and hexachlorobenzene in serum and urine of the population of Barcelona. *Hum. Toxicol.*, *6*, 397-400

Greene, M.H., Brinton, L.A., Fraumeni, J.F. & D'Amico, R. (1978) Familial and sporadic Hodgkin's disease associated with occupational wood exposure. *Lancet*, *ii*, 626-627

Haley, T.J. (1977) Human poisoning with pentachlorophenol and its treatment. *Ecotoxicol. environ. Saf.*, *1*, 343-347

Hattemer-Frey, H.A. & Travis, C.C. (1989) Pentachlorophenol: environmental partitioning and human exposure. *Arch. environ. Contam. Toxicol.*, *18*, 482-489

Hattula, M.-L. & Knuutinen, J. (1985) Mutagenesis of mammalian cells in culture by chlorophenols, chlorocatechols and chloroguaiacols. *Chemosphere*, *14*, 1617-1625

Health and Welfare Canada (1990) *National Pesticide Residue Limits in Food*, Ottawa, Bureau of Chemical Safety, Food Directorate, Health Protection Branch

Hiatt, C.W., Haskins, W.T. & Olivier, L. (1960) The action of sunlight on sodium pentachlorophenate. *Am. J. trop. Med. Hyg.*, *9*, 527-531

Hinkle, D.K. (1973) Fetotoxic effects of pentachlorophenol in the golden Syrian hamster (Abstract No. 42). *Toxicol. appl. Pharmacol.*, *25*, 455

Hoben, H.J., Ching, S.A. & Casarett, L.J. (1976) A study of inhalation of pentachlorophenol by rats. IV. Distribution and excretion of inhaled pentachlorophenol. *Bull. environ. Contam. Toxicol.*, *15*, 466-474

IARC (1977) *IARC Monographs on the Evaluation of the Carcinogenic Risk of Chemicals to Man*, Vol. 15, *Some Fumigants, the Herbicides 2,4-D and 2,4,5-T, Chlorinated Dibenzodioxins and Miscellaneous Industrial Chemicals*, Lyon, pp. 41-102

IARC (1979) *IARC Monographs on the Evaluation of the Carcinogenic Risk of Chemicals to Humans*, Vol. 20, *Some Halogenated Hydrocarbons*, Lyon, pp. 303-326

IARC (1986) *IARC Monographs on the Evaluation of the Carcinogenic Risk of Chemicals to Humans*, Vol. 41, *Some Halogenated Hydrocarbons and Pesticide Exposures*, Lyon, pp. 319-356

IARC (1987a) *IARC Monographs on the Evaluation of Carcinogenic Risks to Humans*, Suppl. 7, *Overall Evaluations of Carcinogenicity: An Updating of* IARC Monographs *Volumes 1 to 42*, Lyon, pp. 154-156

IARC (1987b) *IARC Monographs on the Evaluation of Carcinogenic Risks to Humans*, Suppl. 7, *Overall Evaluations of Carcinogenicity: An Updating of* IARC Monographs *Volumes 1 to 42*, Lyon, p. 59

IARC (1987c) *IARC Monographs on the Evaluation of Carcinogenic Risks to Humans*, Suppl. 7, *Overall Evaluations of Carcinogenicity: An Updating of* IARC Monographs *Volumes 1 to 42*, Lyon, pp. 219-220

IARC (1987d) *IARC Monographs on the Evaluation of Carcinogenic Risks to Humans*, Suppl. 7, *Overall Evaluations of Carcinogenicity: An Updating of* IARC Monographs *Volumes 1 to 42*, Lyon, pp. 322-326

IARC (1987e) *IARC Monographs on the Evaluation of Carcinogenic Risks to Humans*, Suppl. 7, *Overall Evaluations of Carcinogenicity: An Updating of* IARC Monographs *Volumes 1 to 42*, Lyon, pp. 350-354

IARC (1987f) *IARC Monographs on the Evaluation of Carcinogenic Risks to Humans*, Suppl. 7, *Overall Evaluations of Carcinogenicity: An Updating of* IARC Monographs *Volumes 1 to 42*, Lyon, pp. 194-195

IARC (1987g) *IARC Monographs on the Evaluation of Carcinogenic Risks to Humans*, Suppl. 7, *Overall Evaluations of Carcinogenicity: An Updating of* IARC Monographs *Volumes 1 to 42*, Lyon, p. 229

IARC (1989) *IARC Monographs on the Evaluation of Carcinogenic Risks to Humans*, Vol. 45, *Occupational Exposures in Petroleum Refining; Crude Oil and Major Petroleum Fuels*, Lyon, pp. 239-270

Innes, J.R.M., Ulland, B.M., Valerio, M.G., Petrucelli, L., Fishbein, L., Hart, E.R., Pallotta, A.J., Bates, R.R., Falk, H.L., Gart, J.J., Klein, M., Mitchell, I. & Peters, J. (1969) Bioassay of pesticides and industrial chemicals for tumorigenicity in mice: a preliminary note. *J. natl Cancer Inst.*, *42*, 1101-1114

Ishidate, M., Jr (1988) *Data Book of Chromosomal Aberration Test In Vitro*, Amsterdam, Elsevier, pp. 312-313

Izmerov, N.F., ed. (1984) *International Register of Potentially Toxic Chemicals. Scientific Reviews of Soviet Literature on Toxicity and Hazards of Chemicals: Pentachlorophenol* (Issue 75), Moscow, Centre of International Projects, United Nations Environment Programme

Jakobson, I. & Yllner, S. (1971) Metabolism of ^{14}C-pentachlorophenol in the mouse. *Acta pharmacol. toxicol.*, *29*, 513-524

Jansson, K. & Jansson, V. (1986) Inability of chlorophenols to induce 6-thioguanine-resistant mutants in V79 Chinese hamster cells. *Mutat. Res.*, *171*, 165-168

Jäppinen, P., Pukkala, E. & Tola, S. (1989) Cancer incidence of workers in a Finnish sawmill. *Scand. J. Work Environ. Health*, *15*, 18-23

Johnson, R.L., Gehring, P.J., Kociba, R.J. & Schwetz, B.A. (1973) Chlorinated dibenzodioxins and pentachlorophenol. *Environ. Health Perspect.*, *5*, 171-175

Juhl, U., Witte, I. & Butte, W. (1985) Metabolism of pentachlorophenol to tetrachlorohydroquinone by human liver homogenate. *Bull. environ. Contam. Toxicol.*, *35*, 596-601

Kauppinen, T. & Lindroos, L. (1985) Chlorophenol exposure in sawmills. *Am. ind. Hyg. Assoc. J.*, *46*, 34-38

Kehoe, R.A., Deichmann-Gruebler, W. & Kitzmiller, K.V. (1939) Toxic effects upon rabbits of pentachlorophenol and sodium pentachlorophenate. *J. ind. Hyg. Toxicol.*, *21*, 160-172

Kerkvliet, N.I., Baecher-Steppan, L., Claycomb, A.T., Craig, A.M. & Sheggeby, G.G. (1982a) Immunotoxicity of technical pentachlorophenol (PCP-T): depressed humoral immune responses to T-dependent and T-independent antigen stimulation in PCP-T exposed mice. *Fundam. appl. Toxicol.*, 2, 90-99

Kerkvliet, N.I., Baecher-Steppan, L. & Schmitz, J.A. (1982b) Immunotoxicity of pentachlorophenol (PCP): increased susceptibility to tumor growth in adult mice fed technical PCP-contaminated diets. *Toxicol. appl. Pharmacol.*, 62, 55-64

Kerkvliet, N.I., Brauner, J.A. & Matlock, J.P. (1985) Humoral immunotoxicity of polychlorinated diphenyl ethers, phenoxyphenols, dioxins and furans present as contaminants of technical grade pentachlorophenol. *Toxicology*, 36, 307-324

Kimbrough, R.D. & Linder, R.E. (1978) The effect of technical and purified pentachlorophenol on the rat liver. *Toxicol. appl. Pharmacol.*, 46, 151-162

Kinzell, J.J., McKenzie, R.M., Olson, B.A., Kirsch, D.G. & Shull, L.R. (1985) Metabolic fate of [U-^{14}C]pentachlorophenol in a lactating dairy cow. *J. agric. Food Chem.*, 33, 827-833

Klemmer, H.W., Wong, L., Sato, M.M., Reichert, E.L., Korsak, R.J. & Rashad, M.N. (1980) Clinical findings in workers exposed to pentachlorophenol. *Arch. environ. Contam. Toxicol.*, 9, 715-725

Klöpffer, W., Kaufmann, G., Rippon, G. & Poremski, H.-J. (1982) A laboratory model for testing the volatility from aqueous solution: first results and comparison with theory. *Ecotoxicol. environ. Saf.*, 6, 545-559

Kotzias, D., Klein, W. & Korte, F. (1975) Occurrence of xenobiotica in infiltrating waters of landfalls (Ger.). *Chemosphere*, 5, 301-306

Larsen, R.V., Kirsch, L.E., Shaw, S.M., Christian, J.E. & Born, G.S. (1972) Excretion and tissue distribution of uniformly labeled ^{14}C-pentachlorophenol in rats. *J. pharm. Sci.*, 61, 2004-2006

Larsen, R.V., Born, G.S., Kessler, W.V., Shaw, S.M. & Van Sickle, D.C. (1975) Placental transfer and teratology of pentachlorophenol in rats. *Environ. Lett.*, 10, 121-128

Lawrence, J.F. (1982) *High Pressure Liquid Chromatography of Pesticides*, New York, Academic Press, pp. 111-113

Lilienblum, W. (1985) Formation of pentachlorophenol glucuronide in rat and human liver microsomes. *Biochem. Pharmacol.*, 34, 893-894

Matsui, S., Yamamoto, R. & Yamada, H. (1989) The *Bacillus subtilis*/microsome rec-assay for the detection of DNA damaging substances which may occur in chlorinated and ozonated waters. *Water Sci. Technol.*, 21, 875-887

Meister, R.T., ed. (1990) *Farm Chemicals Handbook '90*, Willoughby, OH, Meister Publishing Company, p. C221

Menon, J.A. (1958) Tropical hazards associated with the use of pentachlorophenol. *Br. med. J.*, i, 1156-1158

Nishimura, N. & Oshima, H. (1983) Mutagenicity of pentachlorophenol, dinitro-*o*-cresol and their related compounds (Jpn.). *Jpn. J. ind. Health*, 25, 510-511

Nishimura, N., Nishimura, H. & Oshima, H. (1982) Survey on mutagenicity of pesticides by the *Salmonella* microsome test. *J. Aichi med. Univ. Assoc.*, 10, 305-312

O'Malley, M.A., Carpenter, A.V., Sweeney, M.H., Fingerhut, M.A., Marlow, D.A., Halperin, W.E. & Mathias, C.G. (1990) Chloracne associated with employment in the production of pentachlorophenol. *Am. J. ind. Med.*, 17, 411-421

Osterloh, J., Letz, G., Pond, S. & Becker, C. (1983) An assessment of the potential testicular toxicity of 10 pesticides using the mouse-sperm morphology assay. *Mutat. Res.*, 116, 407-415

Ozretić, B. & Krajnović-Ozretić, M. (1985) Morphological and biochemical evidence of the toxic effect of pentachlorophenol on the developing embryos of the sea urchin. *Aquat. Toxicol.*, 7, 255-263

Pearce, N.E., Smith, A.H. & Fisher, D.O. (1985) Malignant lymphoma and multiple myeloma linked with agricultural occupations in a New Zealand cancer registry-based study. *Am. J. Epidemiol.*, 121, 225-237

Pearce, N.E., Smith, A.H., Howard, J.K., Sheppard, R.A., Giles, H.J. & Teague, C.A. (1986a) Case-control study of multiple myeloma and farming. *Br. J. Cancer*, 54, 493-500

Pearce, N.E., Smith, A.H., Howard, J.K., Sheppard, R.A., Giles, H.J. & Teague, C.A. (1986b) Non-Hodgkin's lymphoma and exposure to phenoxyherbicides, chlorophenols, fencing work, and meat works employment: a case-control study. *Br. J. ind. Med.*, 43, 75-83

Pearce, N.E., Sheppard, R.A., Smith, A.H. & Teague, C.A. (1987) Non-Hodgkin's lymphoma and farming: an expanded case-control study. *Int. J. Cancer*, 39, 155-161

Pierce, R.H., Jr & Victor, D.M. (1978) The fate of pentachlorophenol in an aquatic ecosystem. In: Rao, K.R., ed., *Pentachlorophenol Chemistry, Pharmacology and Environmental Toxicology*, New York, Plenum Press, pp. 41-52

Pignatello, J.J., Martinso, M.M., Steiert, J.C., Carlson, R.E. & Crawford, R.L. (1983) Biodegradation and photolysis of pentachlorophenol in artificial freshwater streams. *Appl. environ. Microbiol.*, 46, 1024-1031

Ramel, C. & Magnusson, J. (1979) Chemical induction of nondisjunction in *Drosophila*. *Environ. Health Perspect.*, 31, 59-66

Renner, G., Hopfer, C. & Gokel, J.M. (1986) Acute toxicities of pentachlorophenol, pentachloro-anisole, tetrachlorohydroquinone, tetrachlorocatechol, tetrachlororesorcinol, tetrachloro-dimethoxybenzenes and tetrachlorobenzenediol diacetates administered to mice. *Toxicol. environ. Chem.*, 11, 37-50

Ritter, L. & Wood, G. (1989) Evaluation and regulation of pesticides in drinking water: a Canadian approach. *Food. Addit. Contam.*, 6 (Suppl. 1), S87-S94

Roberts, H.J. (1983) Aplastic anemia and red cell aplasia due to pentachlorophenol. *South med. J.*, 76, 45-48

Robson, A.M., Kissane, J.M., Elvick, N.H. & Pundavela, L. (1969) Pentachlorophenol poisoning in a nursery for newborn infants. 1. Clinical features and treatment. *J. Pediatr.*, 75, 309-316

Royal Society of Chemistry (1986) *European Directory of Agrochemical Products*, Vol. 1, *Fungicides*, Cambridge, p. 375

Royal Society of Chemistry (1989) *The Agrochemicals Handbook* [Dialog Information Services (File 306)], Cambridge

Sadtler Research Laboratories (1980) *The Sadtler Standard Spectra. 1980 Cumulative Index*, Philadelphia, PA

Sadtler Research Laboratories (1990) *The Sadtler Standard Spectra. 1981-1990 Supplementary Index*, Philadelphia, PA

Schwetz, B.A., Keeler, P.A. & Gehring, P.J. (1974) The effect of purified and commercial grade pentachlorophenol on rat embryonal and fetal development. *Toxicol. appl. Pharmacol.*, 28, 151-161

Schwetz, B.A., Quast, J.F., Keeler, P.A., Humiston, C.G. & Kociba, R.J. (1978) Results of two-year toxicity and reproduction studies on pentachlorophenol in rats. In: Ranga Rao, K., ed., *Pentachlorophenol*, New York, Plenum Press, pp. 301-309

Scow, K., Goyer, M., Payne, E., Perwak, J., Thomas, R., Wallace, D., Walker, P. & Wood, M. (1980) *An Exposure and Risk Assessment for Pentachlorophenol* (EPA Report No. EPA-440/4-81-021; US NTIS PB85-211944/XAB), Washington DC, Office of Water Regulations and Standards, pp. 165-182

Seiler, J.P. (1991) Pentachlorophenol. *Mutat. Res.*, *257*, 27-47

Shirasu, Y., Moriya, M., Kato, K., Furuhashi, A. & Kada, T. (1976) Mutagenicity screening of pesticides in the microbial system. *Mutat. Res.*, *40*, 19-30

Smith, A.H., Pearce, N.E., Fisher, D.O., Giles, H.J., Teague, C.A. & Howard, J.K. (1984) Soft tissue sarcoma and exposure to phenoxyherbicides and chlorophenols in New Zealand. *J. natl Cancer Inst.*, *73*, 1111-1117

Triebig, G., Krekeler, H., Gossler, K. & Valentin, H. (1981) Investigations on neurotoxicity of chemical substances at the work-place. II. Determination of motor and sensory nerve conduction velocity in persons exposed to pentachlorophenol (Ger.). *Int. Arch. occup. environ. Health*, *48*, 357-367

Truhaut, R., L'Epée, P. & Boussemart, E. (1952) Studies on the toxicology of pentachlorophenol. II. Occupational intoxication in the wood industry. Observation of two fatal cases (Fr.). *Arch. Mal. prof.*, *13*, 567-569

Uhl, S., Schmid, P. & Schlatter, C. (1986) Pharmacokinetics of pentachlorophenol in man. *Arch. Toxicol.*, *58*, 182-186

US Environmental Protection Agency (1988) Method 525. Determination of organic compounds in drinking water by liquid-solid extraction and capillary column gas chromatography/mass spectrometry. In: *Methods for the Determination of Organic Compounds in Drinking Water* (EPA Report No. EPA-600/4-88/039; US NTIS PB89-220461), Cincinnati, OH, Environmental Monitoring Systems Laboratory, pp. 325-356

US Environmental Protection Agency (1989a) Method 515-1. Determination of chlorinated acids in water by gas chromatography with an electron capture detector. In: *Methods for the Determination of Organic Compounds in Drinking Water* (EPA Report No. EPA-600/4-88/039; US NTIS PB89-220461), Cincinnati, OH, Environmental Monitoring Systems Laboratory, pp. 221-253

US Environmental Protection Agency (1989b) Appendix A. Methods for organic chemical analysis of municipal and industrial wastewater. Method 625—Base neutrals and acids. *US Code fed. Regul.*, *Title 40*, Part 136

US Environmental Protection Agency (1989c) Appendix A. Methods for organic chemical analysis of municipal and industrial wastewater. Method 604—phenols. *US Code fed. Regul.*, *Title 40*, Part 136

US National Technical Information Service (1968) *Evaluation of Carcinogenic, Teratogenic and Mutagenic Activities of Selected Pesticides and Industrial Chemicals*, Vol. 1, *Carcinogenic Study*, Washington DC, US Department of Commerce

US National Toxicology Program (1989) *Toxicology and Carcinogenesis Studies of Two Pentachlorophenol Technical-grade Mixtures (CAS No. 87-86-5) in B6C3F₁ Mice (Feed Studies)* (Technical Report Series No. 349; NIH Publ. No. 89-2804), Research Triangle Park, NC

US Occupational Safety and Health Administration (1989) Air contaminants—permissible exposure limits. *US Code fed. Regul.*, *Title 29*, Part 1910.1000

Valo, R., Kitunen, V., Salkinoja-Salonen, N. & Raisanen, S. (1984) Chlorinated phenols as contaminants of soil and water in the vicinity of 2 Finnish sawmills. *Chemosphere*, *13*, 835-844

Van Ommen, B., Adang, A., Müller, F. & Van Bladeren, P.J. (1986) The microsomal metabolism of pentachlorophenol and its covalent binding to protein and DNA. *Chem.-biol. Interactions, 60,* 1-11

Vogel, E. & Chandler, J.L.R. (1974) Mutagenicity testing of cyclamate and some pesticides in *Drosophila melanogaster. Experientia, 30,* 621-623

Wainstok de Calmanovici, R. & San Martin de Viale, L.C. (1980) Effect of chlorophenols on porphyrin metabolism in rats and chick embryo. *Int. J. Biochem., 12,* 1039-1044

Weast, R.C., ed. (1989) *CRC Handbook of Chemistry and Physics,* 70th ed., Boca Raton, FL, CRC Press, p. C-414

Welsh, J.J., Collins, T.F.X., Black, T.N., Graham, S.L. & O'Donnell, M.W., Jr (1987) Teratogenic potential of purified pentachlorophenol and pentachloroanisole in subchronically exposed Sprague-Dawley rats. *Food chem. Toxicol., 25,* 163-172

WHO (1984) *Guidelines for Drinking-water Quality,* Vol. 1, *Recommendations,* Geneva, pp. 75-76

WHO (1987) *Pentachlorophenol* (Environmental Health Criteria 71), Geneva

WHO (1989) *Pentachlorophenol Health and Safety Guide* (Health and Safety Guide No. 19), Geneva

Williams, P.L. (1982) Pentachlorophenol, an assessment of the occupational hazard. *Am. ind. Hyg. Assoc. J., 43,* 799-810

Witte, I., Juhl, U. & Butte, W. (1985) DNA-damaging properties and cytotoxicity in human fibroblasts of tetrachlorohydroquinone, a pentachlorophenol metabolites. *Mutat. Res., 145,* 71-75

Wong, A.S. & Crosby, D.G. (1981) Photodecomposition of pentachlorophenol in water. *J. agric. Food Chem., 29,* 125-130

Wood, S., Rom, W.N., White, G.L., Jr & Logan, D.C. (1983) Pentachlorophenol poisoning. *J. occup. Med., 25,* 527-530

Worthing, C.R. & Walker, S.B., eds (1987) *The Pesticide Manual: A World Compendium,* 8th ed., Thornton Heath, British Crop Protection Council, pp. 641-64

Ziemsen, B., Angerer, J. & Lehnert, G. (1987) Sister chromatid exchange and chromosomal breakage in pentachlorophenol (PCP) exposed workers. *Int. Arch. occup. environ. Health, 59,* 413-419

Zober, A., Schaller, K.H., Gossler, K. & Krekeler, H.J. (1981) Pentachlorophenol and liver function: a pilot study on occupationally exposed groups (Ger.). *Int. Arch. occup. environ. Health, 48,* 347-356

THIRAM

This substance was considered by a previous Working Group, in 1976 (IARC, 1976a). Since that time, new data have become available, and these have been incorporated into the monograph and taken into consideration in the present evaluation.

1. Exposure Data

1.1 Chemical and physical data

1.1.1 *Synonyms, structural and molecular data*

Chem. Abstr. Serv. Reg. No.: 137-26-8

Replaced CAS Reg. Nos: 12680-07-8; 12680-62-5; 39456-80-9; 66173-72-6; 93196-73-7

Chem. Abstr. Name: Tetramethylthioperoxydicarbonic diamide

IUPAC Systematic Name: Tetramethylthiuram disulphide

Synonyms: Bis(dimethylthiocarbamoyl)disulfide; bis(dimethylthiocarbamyl)disulfide; tetramethylthioperoxydicarbonic diamide; tetramethylthiuram bisulfide; *N,N,N',N'*-tetramethylthiuram disulfide; thiuram disulfide, tetramethyl-; thiuram TMTD; thiuramyl; TMT; TMTD; TMTDS

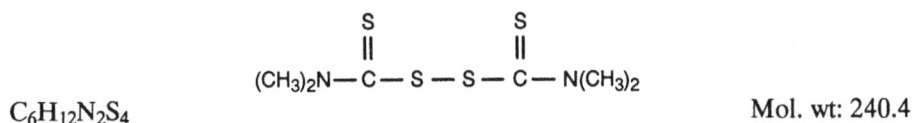

$$(CH_3)_2N - \overset{\overset{\displaystyle S}{\|}}{C} - S - S - \overset{\overset{\displaystyle S}{\|}}{C} - N(CH_3)_2$$

$C_6H_{12}N_2S_4$ Mol. wt: 240.4

1.1.2 *Chemical and physical properties*

  (a) *Description*: White or yellow monoclinic crystals (Weast, 1989)
  (b) *Boiling-point*: 129°C at 20 mm Hg [2.7 kPa] (Weast, 1989)
  (c) *Melting-point*: 155.6°C (Weast, 1989)
  (d) *Spectroscopy data*: Infrared (prism [10588]; grating [21299]), nuclear magnetic resonance (proton [6403]), ultraviolet and mass spectral data have been reported (Benson & Damico, 1968; Brinkhoff & Grotens, 1971; Gore *et al.*, 1971; US Environmental Protection Agency, 1975; Sadtler Research Laboratories, 1980).
  (e) *Solubility*: Insoluble in water; soluble in chloroform (230 g/l), ethanol and diethyl ether (< 2%), acetone (80 g/l), benzene (2.5%); slightly soluble in carbon disulfide (Meister, 1990; Budavari, 1989; Royal Society of Chemistry, 1989)
  (f) *Vapour pressure*: Negligible at room temperature (Royal Society of Chemistry, 1989)
  (g) *Stability*: Decomposes in acidic media (Royal Society of Chemistry, 1989); some deterioration on prolonged exposure to heat, air or moisture (Worthing & Walker, 1987)

(h) *Conversion factor for airborne concentrations*[1]: mg/m^3 = 9.83 × ppm

1.1.3 *Trade names, technical products and impurities*

Some common trade names are: Aapirol; Aatiram; Accel TMT; Accelerant T; Accelerator Thiuram; Accelerator T; Aceto TETD; Aules; Apirol; Arasan; Atiram; Basultra; Betoxin; Delsan; Ekagom TB; Falitiram; Ferna-Col; Fernasan; Fernide; Formalsol; Hermal; Hermat TMT; Heryl; Hexathir; Kregasan; Mercuram; Methyl Thiram; Methyl Tuads; Metiurac; Nobecutan; Nocceler TT; Normersan; Panoram 75; Pol-Thiuram; Polyram ultra; Pomarsol; Pomasol; Puralin; Radothiram; Radotiram; Rezifilm; Rhenogran TMTD; Rhodiauram; Robac TMT; Royal TMTD; Sadoplon; Sadoplon 75; Soxinol TT; Spotrete; SQ 1489; Tersan; Tetrasipton; Thillate; Thiosan; Thioscabin; Thiotox; Thirasan; Thiride; Thiulin; Thiurad; Thiuram; Thylate; Tigam; Tiradin; Tiuramyl; Trametan; Tridipam; Tripomol; Tuads; TUEX; Tulisan; Tutan; Tyradin; VUAgT-I-4; Vucafor; Vulcacit thiuram; Vulkacit Th; Zaprawa Nasienna T; Zupa S 80

In the USA, thiram is formulated as dusts, wettable powder and flowable suspensions. The usual carriers are marl, talc (see IARC, 1987a), clays, petroleum oils, graphite, vermiculite, mineral oil (see IARC, 1987b), charcoal and water (US Environmental Protection Agency, 1984). Formulated thiram products registered in European countries include dustable powders, dry seed treatments, flowable concentrates for seed treatment, liquids, liquid seed treatments, pastes, powders, suspension concentrates, water-dispersible granules, wettable powders and slurries for seed treatment (Royal Society of Chemistry, 1986).

Thiram can be combined in formulations with most fungicides and insecticides. In the USA, such products include thiram with phenylmercury-dimethyldithiocarbamate, malachite green, thiophanate, zineb (see IARC, 1976b, 1987c), molybdenum, vinclozolin and carboxin (Anon., 1989; Meister, 1990). Formulated thiram products registered in European countries include in addition, combinations with trichloronat, ziram (see monograph, p. 423), cycloheximide, benomyl, permethrin, fonofos, carbendazim, rotenone, thiophanate methyl, bendiocarb, thiabendazole, lindane (see IARC, 1987d), 4-indol-3-yl butyric acid, methyl 2-(1-naphthyl)acetate, 2-(1-naphthyl)acetamide and dicloran (Royal Society of Chemistry, 1986; Worthing & Walker, 1987).

In the USSR, technical-grade thiram contains 95-98% thiram. Thiram is formulated as a dust and as an aqueous suspension (Izmerov, 1982).

1.1.4 *Analysis*

Selected methods for the analysis of thiram in various matrices are given in Table 1.

---

[1]Calculated from: mg/m^3 = (molecular weight/24.45) × ppm, assuming standard temperature (25°C) and pressure (760 mm Hg [101.3 kPa])

Table 1. Methods for the analysis of thiram

Sample matrix	Sample preparation	Assay procedure[a]	Limit of detection	Reference
Air	Collect on filter; extract with acetonitrile	HPLC/UV	0.005 mg per sample	Eller (1984)
	Collect on filter; extract with chloroform; measure absorbance at 440 nm	Spectrophotometric	0.5 mg/m^3	Taylor (1977)
Fruits and vegetables	Extract with chloroform; treat with copper iodide; measure absorbance at 440 nm	Spectrophotometric	Not reported	Williams (1984a)
Specified crop samples and water	Extract with chloroform; evaporate, dissolve in methanol; add to a mixture of methanolic 0.2% haematoxylin, aqueous 0.4% chloramine-T and phosphate buffer solution at pH 7.0; heat; dilute with water; read absorbance at 555 nm	Spectrophotometric	Not reported	Sastry et al. (1988)
Formulations (technical, dusts, dispersible powders)	Decompose by boiling with acetic acid and zinc acetate; pass through cadmium sulfate scrubber into absorption system containing methanol/potassium hydroxide; titrate with aqueous iodine	Colorimetric	Not reported	Williams (1984b)

[a]Abbreviation: HPLC/UV, high-performance liquid chromatography/ultraviolet detection

1.2 Production and use

1.2.1 *Production*

Thiram was first produced commercially in the USA in 1925 (US Tariff Commission, 1926). It is produced by passing chlorine gas through a solution of sodium dimethyldithiocarbamate (Wenyon, 1972), by the oxidation of sodium dimethyldithiocarbamate with hydrogen peroxide (see IARC, 1985, 1987e) or iodine (Spencer, 1973), from iron oxide (see IARC, 1987f), hydrogen peroxide, sodium hydroxide, dimethylamine and carbon disulfide (Japanese Ministry of Agriculture and Forestry, 1975) or by continuous mixing of cyanochloride and aqueous solution of sodium dimethyldithiocarbamate at pH 7.9 (Izmerov, 1982).

US production was 2000 tonnes in 1960 (US Tariff Commission, 1961) and 7900 tonnes in 1973 (US International Trade Commission, 1975a). In 1974, four US companies reported total production of 5800 tonnes (US International Trade Commission, 1975b). In 1981, an estimated 1360 tonnes of thiram were produced in the USA (Vlier, 1982). Thiram is produced currently in Belgium, the Netherlands, Spain and the USA (Meister, 1990). One company in India produced 300 tonnes of thiram for pesticide use in 1989 (Indian Ministry of Petroleum and Chemicals, 1990). In Japan, commercial production of thiram began in 1953; in 1970, four companies reported production of 140 tonnes and in 1974, 240 tonnes (Japanese Ministry of Agriculture and Forestry, 1975).

1.2.2 *Use*

The major use of thiram is in rubber processing as an accelerator and vulcanizing agent (see IARC, 1982). It is also used as a seed treatment to protect against fungal diseases and by foliar application for control of diseases on fruit and vegetable crops and on lawns and turf (Izmerov, 1982; Vlier, 1982). In the USA, it was estimated that the following amounts of thiram (active ingredient) were used in 1981 for seed treatment: small grains (wheat, oats, barley and rye), 220 tonnes; soya beans, 60 tonnes; maize, 23 tonnes; cotton, 23 tonnes; sweet maize, 7 tonnes; beans, 5 tonnes; sorghum, 5 tonnes; and peanuts, 2 tonnes. About 55 tonnes were estimated to have been used for foliar treatment of apples, 170 tonnes for treatment of golf courses and 55 tonnes for treatment of sod (Vlier, 1982). Thiram has also been used for mould control in textiles and polyurethane (US Environmental Protection Agency, 1984), for slime control in the manufacture of paper and as a bacteriostat in soap (IARC, 1976).

1.3 Occurrence

Thiram can be found in the environment as a degradation product of ferbam (Lowen, 1961) and ziram (see monograph, p. 423).

The dermal and respiratory exposure of personnel operating commercial seed treating equipment was examined in eight industrial plants in the USA, where a liquid formulation of thiram and carboxin was applied to small grain cereals. It was estimated that there was no dermal exposure *via* the chest or arms, but hands were exposed to levels ranging from not detectable (< 0.5 mg/h) at four plants to a maximum of 3.7 mg/h at the remaining plants. One case of respiratory exposure at 0.75 mg/h was reported (Grey *et al.*, 1983).

Thiram has been found as a dust in the work room air of formulating plants in Italy. Levels of thiram in the air were 0.06 mg/m^3 in the packing room and 0.04 mg/m^3 in the mixing room (Maini & Boni, 1986).

1.4 Regulations and guidelines

The FAO/WHO Joint Meeting on Pesticide Residues evaluated thiram at its meetings in 1965, 1967, 1970, 1974, 1977, 1980, 1983, 1984, 1985, 1987, 1988 and 1989 (FAO/WHO, 1965, 1968, 1971, 1975, 1978, 1981, 1984, 1985, 1986, 1988a,b, 1989). A temporary acceptable daily intake for man of 0.005 mg/kg bw was valid until 1985, when it was withdrawn (FAO/WHO, 1986).

In the USSR, the maximum allowable concentration in drinking-water is 1 mg/ml. Thiram is permitted for use only for seed disinfection (Izmerov, 1982).

National and regional pesticide residue limits for thiram in foods are presented in Table 2.

Occupational exposure limits for thiram in air are given in Table 3. The limit in the USA is proposed to be revised to 1 mg/m^3 (American Conference of Governmental Industrial Hygienists, 1989; US Occupational Safety and Health Administration, 1989).

2. Studies of Cancer in Humans

In a group of 223 workers (42 men and 181 women) in the USSR, mostly aged between 20-50 years, who had been engaged in the manufacture of thiram for more than three years, one case of a malignant lesion of the thyroid was reported among 105 workers examined (Cherpak *et al.*, 1971; Kaskevich & Bezugly, 1973).

Table 2. National and regional pesticide residue limits for thiram in foods[a]

Country or region	Residue limit (mg/kg)	Commodities
Argentina	5[b]	Grapes
	3[b]	Broccoli, Brussels' sprouts, cabbage, cauliflower, celery, Damson plums, eggplants, escarole, lettuce, peaches, peppers, spinach, sweet maize, tomatoes
	2[b]	Apples, pears
	1.0[b]	Cherries, cucumbers, marrows, melons, plums, watermelons
	0.5[b]	Beans (with pods), chick peas, lentils, onions, peas, sugar beets (root), table beets (root)
	0.1[b]	Carrots, potatoes, sweet potatoes, turnips
Australia	7	Fruits, vegetables
Austria	25[b,c]	Hops
	2[c]	Fruit, vegetables
	0.05[b,c]	Other
Belgium	2[c]	Fruit, other vegetables
	0.5[c]	Bulb vegetables, grains
	0.2[c]	Potatoes
	0 (0.02)[c,d]	Other foodstuffs of vegetable origin
Brazil	7	Peas, string beans
	1.0	Bananas (peeled)
	0.5	Garlic, onions, tobacco
Canada	7	Apples, celery, peaches, strawberries, tomatoes
	1.0	Bananas (edible pulp)
	Negligible	Barley, maize, flax, oats, plums, safflower (oil), wheat
Chile	5[b,c]	Grapes
	3[b,c]	Apples, peaches, pears, tomatoes
	1.0[b,c]	Cherries, lettuce, plums
	0.5[b,c]	Carrots
	0.2[b,c]	Wheat
	0.1[b,c]	Potatoes
European Community	3.8[e]	Lettuce, strawberries
	3.0[e]	Other products
Finland	1.0[b]	Other (except cereal grains)
	0.5[b]	Carrots
	0.1[b]	Bananas, potatoes

Table 2 (contd)

Country or region	Residue limit (mg/kg)	Commodities
Germany	25[b]	Hops
	2[b]	Fruit, oilseed, raw coffee, spices, tea, tea–like products, vegetables (except cucumbers and tomatoes)
	1.0[b]	Cucumbers, tomatoes
	0.2[b]	Other vegetable foodstuffs
Greece	3.4	Grapes, strawberries
	3.0	Other fruit and vegetables
Ireland	4	Grapes, strawberries
	3	Other food products
Israel	5[b,c]	Celery, currants (black, red), grapes
	3[b,c]	Apples, peaches, pears, strawberries, tomatoes
	1.0[b,c]	Bananas (whole), cherries, plums
	0.5[b,c]	Endive, lettuce, melons
	0.2[b,c]	Beans (in pods), carrots, cucumber
	0.1[b,c]	Wheat, banana pulp, potatoes
Italy	3.8	Grapes, strawberries
	3.0	Other fruits, vegetables
	2.0	Potatoes, tobacco
Japan	1.0	Apples
	0.5	Peaches, pears, persimmons
Kenya	7	Apples, celery, peaches, strawberries, tomatoes
	1.0	Bananas (edible pulp)
	0.5	Onions (dry bulb)
Mexico	7	Apples, celery, peaches, strawberries, tomatoes
	0.5	Onions
Netherlands	4[c]	Lettuce
	3[c]	Berries, small fruit
	2[c]	Other fruit, other vegetables
	1.0[c]	Cucumber, melon
	0.5[c]	Bulb vegetables, cereals
	0.2[c]	Potatoes, pulses
	0 (0.2)[f]	Other
New Zealand	7[c]	Fruit, vegetables
Singapore	3	Fruit, grain, vegetables
South Africa	3[b]	Apples, apricots, peaches, pears, plums
Spain	4[g]	Grapes, hops, strawberries
	3[g]	Other fruits and vegetables (except potatoes)
	0.2[g]	Potatoes and other plant products

Table 2 (contd)

Country or region	Residue limit (mg/kg)	Commodities
Sweden	1.0[h]	Fruit and vegetables
	0.5[h]	Carrots
	0.1[h,i]	Potatoes
Switzerland	50[b,c]	Tobacco
	2[b,c]	Fruit, lettuce, vegetables (except potatoes)
	0.5[b,c]	Bananas (pulp)
	0.1[b,c]	Cereals
	0.05[b,c]	Potatoes
USA	7[j]	Apples, bananas (not more than 1 ppm in pulp after peel is removed), celery, peaches, strawberries, tomatoes
	0.5[j]	Onions (dry bulb)
USSR	Not permitted	
Yugoslavia	2[c]	Fruit, tobacco, vegetables
	0.05[c]	Other food commodities

[a]From Health and Welfare Canada (1990)
[b]Calculated as carbon disulfide
[c]As dithiocarbamates
[d]The figure in parentheses is the lower limit for determining residues in the corresponding product according to the standard method of analysis.
[e]These values should be reviewed (Commission of the European Communities, 1990)
[f]Residues shall be absent; the value in parentheses is the highest concentration at which this requirement is still deemed to have been met.
[g]Sum of dithiocarbamates expressed as carbon disulfide
[h]Sum of dimethyl-, ethylenebis-, and propylenebis-dithiocarbamates expressed as carbon disulfide
[i]At the limit of detection
[j]From US Environmental Protection Agency (1989)

Table 3. Occupational exposure limits for thiram[a]

Country	Year	Concentration (mg/m^3)	Interpretation[b]
Austria	1987	5	TWA
Belgium	1987	5	TWA
Denmark	1987	2	TWA
Finland	1987	5, skin notation	TWA
		10, skin notatin	STEL
Germany	1989	5[c]	TWA
Indonesia	1987	5	TWA
Italy	1987	5	TWA
Mexico	1987	5	TWA
Netherlands	1987	5	TWA
Poland	1987	0.5	TWA

Table 3 (contd)

Country	Year	Concentration (mg/m^3)	Interpretation[b]
Romania	1987	2	TWA
		5	MAC
Switzerland	1987	5	TWA
United Kingdom	1987	5	TWA
		10	STEL (10 min)
USSR	1982	0.5	MAC
Venezuela	1987	5	TWA
		10	Ceiling
Yugoslavia	1987	5	TWA

[a]From Izmerov (1982); Cook (1987); Deutsche Forschungsgemeinschaft (1989)
[b]TWA, time-weighted average; STEL, short-term exposure limit; MAC, maximum allowable concentration
[c]Calculated as total dust

3. Studies of Cancer in Experimental Animals

Several studies on the carcinogenicity of thiram were summarized in a previous monograph (IARC, 1976), but, because of deficiencies in various aspects of study design, performance and/or reporting, the present Working Group did not consider them further. The studies in question are those of the US National Technical Information Service (1968), Innes *et al.* (1969) and Chernov *et al.* (1972).

3.1 Oral administration

Rat: Groups of 50 male and 50 female SPF Fischer 344 rats, eight weeks old, were fed thiram (purity, 99.8%) at 0, 0.05 or 0.1% (the maximum tolerated dose was estimated to be > 0.06%) in the diet for 104 weeks and basal diet for an additional eight weeks, at which time all survivors were killed. There was no significant difference in survival between treated and control animals. The incidences of leukaemia were decreased: males—10/50 control, 4/49 low-dose and 2/50 high-dose ($p < 0.05$); females—14/49 control, 6/50 low-dose ($p < 0.05$) and 2/50 high-dose ($p < 0.01$). The incidence of pituitary chromophobe adenomas in females was significantly lower in both treated groups: control, 22/49; low-dose, 11/50 ($p < 0.05$) and high-dose, 10/50 ($p < 0.01$); and that of C-cell adenomas of the thyroid was significantly lower ($p < 0.01$) in high-dose females (0/50 *versus* 7/49 controls). There was no statistically significant difference in the incidence of tumours at other sites (Takahashi *et al.*, 1983; Hasegawa *et al.*, 1988).

Groups of 24 male and 24 female Fischer 344 rats, 7-8 weeks old, were fed 0 or 500 mg/kg (750 mg/kg for the first three weeks) of diet thiram [purity unspecified] for 104 weeks. The experiment was terminated at week 130. Average time to death was 122-127 weeks in the treated animals and 107-122 weeks in the controls. There was a significant decrease in the incidence of monocytic leukaemia in treated rats (treated females, 1/24;

control females, 11/24 [$p < 0.001$]; treated males, 4/24; control males, 12/24 [$p < 0.02$]). The concentration used was considered by the author to be a maximum tolerated dose, since, in a prelimary experiment, 1000 mg/kg of diet were not acceptable to the animals and 750 mg/kg of diet were poorly consumed in this experiment (Lijinsky, 1984). [The Working Group noted the small number of animals used.]

3.2 Combination with nitrite

Rat: Groups of 24 male and 24 female Fischer 344 rats, 7-8 weeks of age, were fed 0 or 500 mg/kg (750 mg/kg for the first three weeks) of diet thiram alone or in combination with 2000 mg/kg of diet sodium nitrite for 104 weeks in order to assess the possibility of formation of carcinogenic *N*-nitroso compounds (*N*-nitrosodimethylamine) *in vivo*. Of the rats receiving the combined treatment, 18/24 males and 15/24 females developed tumours of the nasal cavity (adenocarcinoma, adenoma, olfactory carcinoma, squamous-cell carcinoma). No nasal cavity tumour was found in untreated rats or in rats receiving thiram or sodium nitrite alone. Five male and five female rats receiving combined treatment developed squamous-cell papillomas of the forestomach; 2/24 males and 1/24 females receiving sodium nitrite alone, but none of the untreated or thiram-treated rats, developed forestomach papillomas (Lijinsky, 1984). [The Working Group noted that this study was not directly relevant to an evaluation of the carcinogenicity of thiram.]

4. Other Relevant Data

The toxicology of dithiocarbamates has been reviewed (WHO, 1988).

4.1 Absorption, distribution, metabolism and excretion

4.1.1 *Humans*

No data were available to the Working Group.

4.1.2 *Experimental systems*

Administration of thiram with nitrite to guinea-pigs by gavage resulted in the formation of *N*-nitrosodimethylamine (Sen *et al.*, 1974). Similarly, thiram reacted with nitrite *in vitro* at acid pH to form *N*-nitrosodimethylamine (Elespuru & Lijinsky, 1973; Sen *et al.*, 1974).

In rats administered thiram intraperitoneally, carbon disulfide was found in expired air in a dose-dependent fashion (Dalvi & Deoras, 1986).

4.2 Toxic effects

4.2.1 *Humans*

In a group of 223 workers (42 men and 181 women) in the USSR, mostly aged between 20 and 50 years, engaged in the manufacture of thiram generally for more than three years, various clinical and pathological manifestations, including ocular irritation, coughing, thoracic pain, tachycardia, epistaxis, dermal lesions, myocardiodystrophia, clinical and subclinical liver dysfunction and asthaenia, were reported, often in excess of those seen in a group of 193 persons not in contact with thiram. Thyroid gland disorders were more common in the exposed group (7.6% *versus* 1.04%); one case of a malignant lesion of the thyroid and seven of enlarged thyroid gland were reported among 105 workers examined (Cherpak *et al.*, 1971; Kaskevich & Bezugly, 1973).

Contact dermatitis has been reported after exposure to thiram (Penneys *et al.*, 1976; Rudzki & Napiórkowska, 1980; Kruis-de Vries *et al.*, 1987).

4.2.2 *Experimental systems*

Oral LD_{50} values for thiram in mice of 1500-2000 mg/kg bw (Kirchheim, 1951), 2300 mg/kg bw (Matthiaschk, 1973) and 3300-4500 mg/kg bw (Lee *et al.*, 1978), in rats of 865 mg/kg bw (Lehman, 1951), 375-1000 mg/kg bw (Ben-Dyke *et al.*, 1970) and 1400-5400 mg/kg bw (Lee *et al.*, 1978) and in rabbits of 210 mg/kg bw (Worthing & Walker, 1987) have been reported. The dermal LD_{50} in rats is more than 2000 mg/kg bw (Ben-Dyke *et al.*, 1970).

Intraperitoneal administration of 120 mg/kg bw thiram to rats caused an increase in plasma transaminase activity 24 h after treatment, which was associated with a reduction in hepatic microsomal benzphetamine *N*-demethylase and cytochrome P450 activities (Dalvi *et al.*, 1984). Different results were reported in another study, which showed impairment of microsomal aniline hydroxylase and carboxylesterase activities 24 h after oral administration of thiram (1 g/kg) to rats, whereas cytochrome P450 and ethylmorphine *N*-demethylase activities were unchanged (Zemaitis & Greene, 1979). Epoxide hydrolase activity was enhanced in rat liver after exposure to thiram (1 mmol/kg bw [240 mg/kg bw]) by gavage; glutathione *S*-transferase activity was slightly enhanced by doses of up to 4 mmol/kg [960 mg/kg bw] (Schreiner & Freundt, 1985).

Like most dithiocarbamates, thiram induced the accumulation of acetaldehyde in the blood of rats administered ethanol (see WHO, 1988).

Chronic feeding of rats with thiram (about 60 mg/kg bw per day) caused neurotoxicity, with onset of ataxia in some animals, 5-19 months from the beginning of exposure. Morphological examination showed chromatolysis of motor neurones. Some behavioural changes, not related to morphological changes, were also observed (Lee & Peters, 1976).

Thiram was given in the diet at 1000 mg/kg for six weeks, two weeks after a single intraperitoneal dose of *N*-nitrosodiethylamine (200 mg/kg bw) to male Fischer rats that were also subjected to a two-thirds hepatectomy three weeks after the start of the study. A marginal increase in the number and area of glutathione *S*-transferase-positive liver foci was seen at eight weeks compared to rats treated with the nitrosamine and partial hepatectomy alone (Ito *et al.*, 1988).

4.3 Reproductive and developmental effects

4.3.1 *Humans*

No data were available to the Working Group.

4.3.2 *Experimental systems*

Pregnant NMRI mice given daily oral doses of thiram at 10-30 mg/animal on days 5-15 or 6-17 of gestation had increased resorptions during the intermediate and late stages of organogenesis. Fetal malformations were characterized by cleft palate, micrognathia, wavy ribs and distorted bones (Roll, 1971; Matthiaschk, 1973).

Daily administration of 132 mg/kg bw thiram in the feed for 13 weeks decreased fertility in male Charles River CD rats; daily administration of 96 mg/kg bw to female rats for 14 days prolonged the dioestrous phase of the oestrus cycle. These effects were accompanied by loss of body weight. Daily administration of 136-200 mg/kg bw thiram to rats by gavage during the organogenetic period (gestation days 6-15) increased the mortality rate of conceptuses; the weight of surviving embryos was decreased at doses as low as 40 mg/kg bw per day. In Swiss-Webster mice, no significant developmental effect was observed with doses of up to 300 mg/kg bw per day given by gavage on days 6-14 of gestation. A number of female rats died during the experiment. Administration to dams of 0.1% in feed during pre- and postnatal periods reduced the growth and survival of pups (Short et al., 1976).

In Syrian hamsters, administration of thiram at doses of 250 mg/kg bw and higher on day 7 or 8 of gestation resulted in an increased rate of resorptions, decreased fetal weight and an increased number of terata (Robens, 1969).

Administration of 250 ppm [mg/kg] and above of thiram in the diet to laying hens for one week decreased the weight of ovaries (Serio et al., 1984). As reported in an abstract, administration of 8.8 mg/kg bw per day to quail reduced egg laying by 50% (Wedig et al., 1968). The ED_{50} value for embryolethality was 1.9 μg/egg when thiram was injected into the air chamber of hens' eggs prior to incubation (Gebhardt & van Logten, 1968). Injection of 20 μg/egg and above on day 3 of incubation increased early embryonic death and caused malformations (small eye cup, lid and corneal defects and open coelom) in chick embryos (Korhonen et al., 1982).

4.4 Genetic and related effects (see also Table 4 and Appendices 1 and 2)

4.4.1 Humans

No data were available to the Working Group.

4.4.2 Experimental systems

Thiram induced point mutation in bacteria, but data on the induction of DNA damage were conflicting. In Aspergillus nidulans, thiram induced gene mutation and aneuploidy; both mutation and chromosomal aberrations were induced in plants. Recessive lethal mutation was induced in Drosophila melanogaster, but the response was not dose-related.

Testing for mutation at the hprt locus of Chinese hamster V79 cells gave a negative result in one study and a positive result in another, in which a six-fold higher concentration was used and survival was less than 3%. In other studies with cultured mammalian cells, a negative response was obtained in an assay for sister chromatid exchange and there was a weak response in a test for chromosomal aberration. In single studies with human lymphocytes, thiram induced unscheduled DNA synthesis and sister chromatid exchange, but only in the presence of an exogenous metabolic activation system.

Thiram induced micronucleus formation in mouse bone marrow, chromosomal aberrations in mouse spermatocytes and morphologically abnormal sperm in mice in vivo. A negative response was obtained in one of three studies of micronucleus formation. [This difference may be attributable to the use of Chinese hamsters rather than mice.]

Table 4. Genetic and related effects of thiram

Test system	Result[a] Without exogenous metabolic system	Result[a] With exogenous metabolic system	Dose[b] LED/HID	Reference
PRB, Prophage induction	-	-	10.0000	Zdzienicka et al. (1981)
SAD, Salmonella typhimurium, repair (TA1538 vs TA1978)	+	-	50.0000	Zdzienicka et al. (1981)
BSD, Bacillus subtilis rec strain, differential toxicity	(+)	0	2.0000	Shirasu et al. (1976)
BSD, Bacillus subtilis rec strain, differential toxicity	-	-	800.0000	Ueno & Ishizaki (1984)
SA0, Salmonella typhimurium TA100, reverse mutation	+	+	5.0000	Byeon et al. (1976)
SA0, Salmonella typhimurium TA100, reverse mutation	+	+	2.5000	Hedenstedt et al. (1979)
SA0, Salmonella typhimurium TA100, reverse mutation	+	0	25.0000	Zdzienicka et al. (1979)
SA0, Salmonella typhimurium TA100, reverse mutation	+	0	50.0000	Zdzienicka et al. (1981)
SA0, Salmonella typhimurium TA100, reverse mutation	+	-	25.0000	Moriya et al. (1983)
SA0, Salmonella typhimurium TA100, reverse mutation	+	+	25.0000	Rannug & Rannug (1984)
SA0, Salmonella typhimurium TA100, reverse mutation	-	+	20.0000	Crebelli et al. (1985)
SA5, Salmonella typhimurium TA1535, reverse mutation	(+)	(+)	25.0000	Byeon et al. (1976)
SA5, Salmonella typhimurium TA1535, reverse mutation	+	0	2.5000	Hedenstedt et al. (1979)
SA5, Salmonella typhimurium TA1535, reverse mutation	+	0	25.0000	Zdzienicka et al. (1979)
SA5, Salmonella typhimurium TA1535, reverse, mutation	+	0	50.0000	Zdzienicka et al. (1981)
SA5, Salmonella typhimurium TA1535, reverse mutation	(+)	-	2500.0000	Moriya et al. (1983)
SA7, Salmonella typhimurium TA1537, reverse mutation	+	0	5.0000	Hedenstedt et al. (1979)
SA7, Salmonella typhimurium TA1537, reverse mutation	-	-	2500.0000	Moriya et al. (1983)
SA8, Salmonella typhimurium TA1538, reverse mutation	-	-	25.0000	Byeon et al. (1976)
SA8, Salmonella typhimurium TA1538, reverse mutation	+	0	5.0000	Hedenstedt et al. (1979)
SA8, Salmonella typhimurium TA1538, reverse mutation	-	+	25.0000	Zdzienicka et al. (1979)
SA8, Salmonella typhimurium TA1538, reverse mutation	-	(+)	50.0000	Zdzienicka et al. (1981)
SA8, Salmonella typhimurium TA1538, reverse mutation	-	-	2500.0000	Moriya et al. (1983)
SA9, Salmonella typhimurium TA98, reverse mutation	-	-	25.0000	Byeon et al. (1976)
SA9, Salmonella typhimurium TA98, reverse mutation	+	0	2.5000	Hedenstedt et al. (1979)
SA9, Salmonella typhimurium TA98, reverse mutation	-	+	25.0000	Zdzienicka et al. (1979)
SA9, Salmonella typhimurium TA98, reverse mutation	-	-	50.0000	Zdzienicka et al. (1981)
SA9, Salmonella typhimurium TA98, reverse mutation	-	-	2500.0000	Moriya et al. (1983)

Table 4 (contd)

Test system	Result[a]		Dose[b] LED/HID	Reference
	Without exogenous metabolic system	With exogenous metabolic system		
SA9, *Salmonella typhimurium* TA98, reverse mutation	−	+	20.0000	Crebelli et al. (1985)
EC2, *Escherichia coli* WP2 hcr, reverse mutation	−	−	2500.0000	Moriya et al. (1983)
ANF, *Aspergillus nidulans*, forward mutation	+	−	0.5000	Zdzienicka et al. (1981)
ANN, *Aspergillus nidulans*, chromosomal nondisjunction (aneuploidy)	+	0	20.0000	Upshall & Johnson (1981)
PLM, *Triticum* (spring wheat), chlorophyll mutations	+	0	0.0000	Mamalyga et al. (1974)
HSC, *Hordeum vulgare*, chromosomal aberrations	+	0	250.0000	George et al. (1970)
DMX, *Drosophila melanogaster*, sex-linked recessive lethal mutation	+	0	1000.0000	Donner et al. (1983)
G9H, Gene mutation, Chinese hamster lung V79 cells *in vitro*, *hprt* locus	−	−	1.6000	Donner et al. (1983)
G9H, Gene mutation, Chinese hamster lung V79 cells *in vitro*, *hprt* locus	+	0	5.0000	Paschin & Bakhitova (1985)
SIC, Sister chromatid exchange, Chinese hamster CHO cells *in vitro*	−	−	2.4000	Donner et al. (1983)
CIC, Chromosomal aberrations, Chinese hamster CHL cells *in vitro*	(+)	+	0.4000	Ishidate (1988)
UHL, Unscheduled DNA synthesis, human lymphocytes *in vitro*	−	+	5.0000	Perocco et al. (1989)
SHL, Sister chromatid exchange, human lymphocytes *in vitro*	−	+	15.0000	Perocco et al. (1989)
MVM, Micronucleus test, BALB/c mouse *in vivo*	+	0	500.0000 × 2 i.p.	Dulout et al. (1982)
MVM, Micronucleus test, (CBA×C57Bl/6J)F$_1$ mouse *in vivo*	+	0	100.0000 × 1 i.p.	Paschin & Bakhitova (1985)
MVC, Micronucleus test, Chinese hamsters *in vivo*	−	0	0.5000 × 1 i.p.	Donner et al. (1983)
CGC, Chromosomal aberrations, primary spermatocytes, Swiss mouse	+	0	80.0000 × 3 p.o.	Prasad et al. (1987)
SPM, Sperm morphology, (CFW×C57Bl)F$_1$ mouse	+	0	50.0000 × 1 i.p.	Zdzienicka et al. (1981)
SPM, Sperm morphology, (CFW×C57Bl)F$_1$ mouse	+	0	50.0000 × 1 i.p.	Zdzienicka et al. (1982)
SPM, Sperm morphology, (CFW×C57Bl)F$_1$ mouse	+	0	30.0000 × 5 i.p.	Zdzienicka et al. (1982)
SPM, Sperm morphology, Swiss mouse	+	0	80.0000 × 3 p.o.	Prasad et al. (1987)

[a] +, positive; (+), weakly positive; −, negative; 0, not tested; ?, inconclusive (variable response in several experiments within an adequate study)

[b] In-vitro tests, μg/ml; in-vivo tests, mg/kg bw

5. Summary of Data Reported and Evaluation

5.1 Exposure data

The major use of thiram is as an accelerator and vulcanization agent in the rubber industry. It is also used as a fungicide on seeds and as a foliar fungicide on turf, fruit and vegetables. It has been in commercial use since 1925.

Thiram has been formulated for use as dusts, wettable powders and flowable suspensions and also in combination with other pesticides.

Exposure may occur during its production, its use in the rubber industry and its application as a fungicide, and, at much lower levels, from consumption of foods containing residues. Thiram is also an environmental degradation product of the two fungicides, ferbam and ziram.

5.2 Carcinogenicity in humans

No adequate data were available to the Working Group.

5.3 Carcinogenicity in experimental animals

Thiram was tested adequately for carcinogenicity by oral administration in one study in rats. No increase in incidence was seen for tumours at any site.

When thiram was administered orally to rats in combination with nitrite, a high incidence of tumours of the nasal cavity was observed in males and females.

5.4 Other relevant data

Thyroid abnormalities were observed in a group of subjects exposed occupationally to thiram.

Thiram marginally increased the frequency of enzyme-positive foci in rat liver. It decreased fertility in rats and caused embryolethality and embryotoxicity in rats and hamsters and malformations in mice and hamsters.

No data were available on the genetic and related effects of thiram in humans.

Thiram induced various kinds of chromosomal damage and altered sperm morphology in rodents *in vivo*. It induced unscheduled DNA synthesis and sister chromatid exchange in cultured human cells. It was genotoxic to insects, plants, fungi and bacteria.

5.5 Evaluation[1]

There is *inadequate evidence* in humans for the carcinogenicity of thiram.

There is *inadequate evidence* in experimental animals for the carcinogenicity of thiram.

Overall evaluation

Thiram *is not classifiable as to its carcinogenicity to humans (Group 3)*.

---

[1]For definition of the italicized terms, see Preamble, pp. 26-28.

6. References

American Conference of Governmental Industrial Hygienists (1989) *Threshold Limit Values and Biological Exposure Indices for 1988-1989*, Cincinnati, OH, p. 35

Anon. (1989) *Crop Protection Chemicals Reference*, 5th ed., New York, Chemical and Pharmaceutical Press, p. 2201

Ben-Dyke, R., Sanderson, D.M. & Noakes, D.N. (1970) Acute toxicity data for pesticides. *World Rev. Pest Control, 9*, 119-127

Benson, W.R. & Damico, J.N. (1968) Mass spectra of some carbamates and related ureas. II. *J. Assoc. off. anal. Chem., 51*, 347-365

Brinkhoff, H.C. & Grotens, A.M. (1971) IR and NMR studies of symmetrically and unsymmetrically bonded N,N-dialkyldithiocarbamates. *Recl. Trav. Chim. Pays-Bas, 90*, 252-257

Budavari, S., ed. (1989) *The Merck Index*, 11th ed., Rahway, NJ, Merck & Co., p. 1476

Byeon, W.-H., Hyun, H.H. & Lee, S.Y. (1976) Mutagenicity of pesticides in the *Salmonella*/microsome system (Korean). *Korean J. Microbiol., 14*, 128-134

Chernov, O.V., Khitsenko, I.I. & Balin, P.N. (1972) Blastomogenic properties of some derivatives of dithiocarbamic acid and their metabolites (Russ.). *Onkologiya, 3*, 123-126

Cherpak, V.V., Bezugly, V.P. & Kaskevich, L.M. (1971) Sanitary-hygienic characteristics of working conditions and health of persons working with tetramethylthiuram disulfide (TMTD) (Russ.). *Vrach. Delo, 10*, 136-139

Commission of the European Communities (1990) *Agriculture. Report of the Scientific Committee for Pesticides*, 3rd Series (EUR 13081 EN), Luxembourg, pp. 43-52

Cook, W.A., ed. (1987) *Occupational Exposure Limits—Worldwide*, Washington DC, American Industrial Hygiene Association, pp. 35, 67, 154-155, 218-219

Crebelli, R., Paoletti, A., Falcone, E., Aquilina, G., Fabri, G. & Carere, A. (1985) Mutagenicity studies in a tyre plant: in vitro activity of workers' urinary concentrates and raw material. *Br. J. ind. Med., 42*, 481-487

Dalvi, R.R. & Deoras, D.P. (1986) Metabolism of a dithiocarbamate fungicide thiram to carbon disulfide in the rat and its hepatoxic implications. *Acta pharmacol. toxicol., 58*, 38-42

Dalvi, R.R., Robbins, T.J., Williams, M.K., Deoras, D.P., Donastorg, F. & Banks, C. (1984) Thiram-induced toxic liver injury in male Sprague-Dawley rats. *J. environ. Sci. Health, B19*, 703-712

Deutsche Forschungsgemeinschaft (German Research Society) (1989) *Maximale Arbeitsplatzkonzentrationen und Biologische Arbeitsstofftoleranzwerte 1989* [Maximal Concentrations in the Workplace and Biological Tolerance Values for Working Materials 1989] (Report No. XXV), Weinheim, VCH Verlagsgesellschaft, p. 59 (in German)

Donner, M., Husgafvel-Pursiainen, K., Jenssen, D. & Rannug, A. (1983) Mutagenicity of rubber additives and curing fumes. *Scand. J. Work Environ. Health, 9* (Suppl. 2), 27-37

Dulout, F.N., Olivero, O.A. & Pastori, M.C. (1982) The mutagenic effect of thiram analysed by the micronucleus test and the anaphase-telophase test. *Mutat. Res., 105*, 409-412

Elespuru, R.K. & Lijinsky, W. (1973) The formation of carcinogenic nitroso compounds from nitrite and some types of agriculture chemicals. *Food Cosmet. Toxicol., 11*, 807-817

Eller, P.M., ed. (1984) *NIOSH Manual of Analytical Methods*, 3rd ed., Vol. 2 (DHHS (NIOSH) Publ. 84-100), Washington DC, US Government Printing Office, pp. 5005-1—505-3

FAO/WHO (1965) *Evaluation of the Toxicity of Pesticide Residues in Food* (FAO Meeting Report No. PL/1965/10/1; WHO/Food Add./27.65), Rome

FAO/WHO (1968) *1967 Evaluations of Some Pesticide Residues in Food* (FAO/PL:1967/M/11/1; WHO/Food Add./68.30), Rome

FAO/WHO (1971) *1970 Evaluations of Some Pesticide Residues in Food* (AGP:1970/M/12/1; WHO/Food Add./71.42), Rome

FAO/WHO (1975) *1974 Evaluations of Some Pesticide Residues in Food* (WHO Pesticide Residues Series No. 4), Geneva

FAO/WHO (1978) *Pesticide Residues in Food: 1977 Evaluations* (FAO Plant Production and Protection Paper 10 Sup.), Rome

FAO/WHO (1981) *Pesticide Residues in Food: 1980 Evaluations. The Monographs* (FAO Plant Production and Protection Paper 26 Sup.), Rome

FAO/WHO (1984) *Pesticide Residues in Food: 1983 Evaluations* (FAO Plant Production and Protection Paper 56), Rome

FAO/WHO (1985) *Pesticide Residues in Food: 1984 Evaluations* (FAO Plant Production and Protection Paper 62), Rome

FAO/WHO (1986) *Pesticide Residues in Food: 1985 Evaluations* (FAO Plant Production and Protection Paper 68), Rome

FAO/WHO (1988a) *Pesticide Residues in Food: 1987 Evaluations* (FAO Plant Production and Protection Paper 86/1), Rome

FAO/WHO (1988b) *Pesticide Residues in Food: 1988 Evaluations* (FAO Plant Production and Protection Paper 93/1), Rome

FAO/WHO (1989) *Pesticide Residues in Food: 1989 Evaluations* (FAO Plant Production and Protection Paper 99), Rome

Gebhardt, D.O.E. & van Logten, M.J. (1968) The chick embryo test as used in the study of the toxicity of certain dithiocarbamates. *Toxicol. appl. Pharmacol.*, 13, 316-324

George, M.K., Anlakh, K.S. & Dhesi, J.S. (1970) Morphological and cytological changes induced in barley (*Hordeum vulgare*) seedlings following seed treatment with fungicides. *Can. J. genet. Cytol.*, 12, 415-419

Gore, R.C., Hannah, R.W., Pattacini, S.C. & Porro, T.J. (1971) Infrared and ultraviolet spectra of seventy-six pesticides. *J. Assoc. off. anal. Chem.*, 54, 1040-1082

Grey, W.E., Marthre, D.E. & Rogers, S.J. (1983) Potential exposure of commercial seed-treating applicators to the pesticides carboxin-thiram and lindane. *Bull. environ. Contam. Toxicol.*, 31, 244-250

Hasegawa, R., Takahashi, M., Furukawa, F., Toyoda, K., Sato, H., Jang, J.J. & Hayashi, Y. (1988) Carcinogenicity study of tetramethylthiuram disulfide (Thiram) in F344 rats. *Toxicology, 51*, 155-165

Hedenstedt, A., Rannug, U., Ramel, C. & Wachtmeister, C.A. (1979) Mutagenicity and metabolism studies on 12 thiuram and dithiocarbamate compounds used as accelerators in the Swedish rubber industry. *Mutat. Res.*, 68, 313-325

Health and Welfare Canada (1990) *National Pesticide Residue Limits in Food*, Ottawa, Bureau of Chemical Safety, Food Directorate, Health Protection Branch

IARC (1976a) *IARC Monographs on the Evaluation of Carcinogenic Risk of Chemicals to Man*, Vol. 12, *Some Carbamates, Thiocarbamates and Carbazides*, Lyon, pp. 225-236

IARC (1976b) *IARC Monographs on the Evaluation of Carcinogenic Risk of Chemicals to Man*, Vol. 12, *Some Carbamates, Thiocarbamates and Carbazides*, Lyon, pp. 245-257

IARC (1982) *IARC Monographs on the Evaluation of the Carcinogenic Risk of Chemicals to Humans*, Vol. 28, *The Rubber Industry*, Lyon

IARC (1985) *IARC Monographs on the Evaluation of the Carcinogenic Risk of Chemicals to Humans*, Vol. 36, *Allyl Compounds, Aldehydes, Epoxides and Peroxides*, Lyon, pp. 285-314

IARC (1987a) *IARC Monographs on the Evaluation of Carcinogenic Risks to Humans*, Suppl. 7, *Overall Evaluations of Carcinogenicity: An Updating of* IARC Monographs, *Volumes 1 to 42*, Lyon, pp. 349-459

IARC (1987b) *IARC Monographs on the Evaluation of Carcinogenic Risks to Humans*, Suppl. 7, *Overall Evaluations of Carcinogenicity: An Updating of* IARC Monographs, *Volumes 1 to 42*, Lyon, pp. 252-254

IARC (1987c) *IARC Monographs on the Evaluation of Carcinogenic Risks to Humans*, Suppl. 7, *Overall Evaluations of Carcinogenicity: An Updating of* IARC Monographs, *Volumes 1 to 42*, Lyon, p. 74

IARC (1987d) *IARC Monographs on the Evaluation of Carcinogenic Risks to Humans*, Suppl. 7, *Overall Evaluations of Carcinogenicity: An Updating of* IARC Monographs, *Volumes 1 to 42*, Lyon, pp. 220-222

IARC (1987e) *IARC Monographs on the Evaluation of Carcinogenic Risks to Humans*, Suppl. 7, *Overall Evaluations of Carcinogenicity: An Updating of* IARC Monographs, *Volumes 1 to 42*, Lyon, p. 64

IARC (1987f) *IARC Monographs on the Evaluation of Carcinogenic Risks to Humans*, Suppl. 7, *Overall Evaluations of Carcinogenicity: An Updating of* IARC Monographs, *Volumes 1 to 42*, Lyon, pp. 216-219

Indian Ministry of Petroleum and Chemicals (1990) *Production Capacity of Technical Grade Pesticides in the Organized Sector as on 1-7-1989*, New Delhi, Department of Chemicals and Petrochemicals

Innes, J.R.M., Ulland, B.M., Valerio, M.G., Petrucelli, L., Fishbein, L., Hart, E.R., Pallotta, A.J., Bates, R.R., Falk, H.L., Gart, J.J., Klein, M., Mitchell, I. & Peters, J. (1969) Bioassay of pesticides and industrial chemicals for tumorigenicity in mice: a preliminary note. *J. natl Cancer Inst.*, 42, 1101-1114

Ishidate, M., Jr (1988) *Data Book of Chromosomal Aberration Test In Vitro*, rev. ed., Amsterdam, Elsevier, p. 47

Ito, N., Tsuda, H., Tatematsu, M., Inoue, T., Tagawa, Y., Aoki, T., Uwagawa, S., Kagawa, M., Ogiso, T., Masui, T., Imaida, K., Fukushima, S. & Asamoto, M. (1988) Enhancing effect of various hepatocarcinogens on induction of preneoplastic glutathione S-transferase placental form positive foci in rats—an approach for a new medium-term bioassay system. *Carcinogenesis*, 9, 387-394

Izmerov, N.F., ed. (1982) *International Register of Potentially Toxic Chemicals, Scientific Reviews of Soviet Literature on Toxicity and Hazards of Chemicals: Thiram* (No. 12), Moscow, Centre of International Projects, United Nations Environment Programme

Japanese Ministry of Agriculture and Forestry (1975) *Noyaku Yoran (Agricultural Chemicals Annual), 1975*, Takeo Endo, Division of Plant Disease Prevention, pp. 17-20, 22, 26, 86, 89, 101, 254, 267-269, 271, 275, 301

Kaskevich, L.M. & Bezugly, V.P. (1973) Clinical aspects of intoxications induced by TMTD (Russ.). *Vrach. Delo*, 6, 128-130

Kirchheim, D. (1951) Toxicity and action of some thiuram disulfide compounds on the metabolism of alcohol (Ger.). *Arch. exp. Pathol. Pharmakol.*, 214, 59-66

Korhonen, A., Hemminki, K. & Vainio, H. (1982) Application of the chicken embryo in testing for embryotoxicity. Thiurams. *Scand. J. Work Environ. Health*, 8, 63-69

Kruis-de Vries, M.H., Coenraads, P.J. & Nater, J.P. (1987) Allergic contact dermatitis due to rubber chemicals in haemodialysis equipment. *Contact Derm.*, *17*, 303-305

Lee, C.-C. & Peters, P.J. (1976) Neurotoxicity and behavioral effects of thiram in rats. *Environ. Health Perspect.*, *17*, 35-43

Lee, C.-C., Russell, J.Q. & Minor, J.L. (1978) Oral toxicity of ferric dimethyldithiocarbamate (ferbam) and tetramethylthiuram disulphide (thiram) in rodents. *J. Toxicol. environ. Health*, *4*, 93-106

Lehman, A.J. (1951) Chemicals in foods: a report to the Association of Food and Drug Officials on current developments. II. Pesticides. *Q. Bull. Assoc. Food Drug Off. USA*, *15*, 122-133

Lijinsky, W. (1984) Induction of tumors of the nasal cavity in rats by concurrent feeding of thiram and sodium nitrite. *J. Toxicol. environ. Health*, *13*, 609-614

Lowen, W.K. (1961) Determination of thiram in ferbam. *J. Assoc. off. agric. Chem.*, *44*, 584-585

Maini, P. & Boni, R. (1986) Gas chromatographic determination of dithiocarbamate fungicides in workroom air. *Bull. environ. Contam. Toxicol.*, *37*, 931-937

Mamalyga, V.S., Kulik, M.I. & Logvinenko, V.F. (1974) Induced chlorophyll mutations in hard spring wheat (Russ.). *Dokl. Akad. Nauk SSSR*, *215*, 211-213

Matthiaschk, G. (1973) Influence of L-cysteine on the teratogenicity of thiram in NMRI mice (Ger.). *Arch. Toxikol.*, *30*, 251-262

Meister, R.T., ed. (1990) *Farm Chemicals Handbook '90*, Willoughby, OH, Meister Publishing Company, p. C 286

Moriya, M., Ohta, T., Watanabe, K., Miyazawa, T., Kato, K. & Shirasu, Y. (1983) Further mutagenicity studies on pesticides in bacterial reversion assay systems. *Mutat. Res.*, *116*, 185-216

Paschin, Y.V. & Bakhitova, L.M. (1985) Mutagenic effects of thiram in mammalian somatic cells. *Food chem. Toxicol.*, *23*, 373-375

Penneys, N.S., Edwards, L.S. & Katsikas, J.L. (1976) Allergic contact sensitivity to thiuram compounds in a hemodialysis unit. *Arch. Dermatol.*, *112*, 811-813

Perocco, P., Santucci, M.A., Campani, A.G. & Forti, G.C. (1989) Toxic and DNA-damaging activities of the fungicides mancozeb and thiram (TMTD) on human lymphocytes *in vitro*. *Teratog. Carcinog. Mutagenesis*, *9*, 75-81

Prasad, M.H., Pushpavathi, K., Rita, P. & Reddy, P.P. (1987) The effect of thiram on the germ cells of male mice. *Food chem. Toxicol.*, *25*, 709-711

Rannug, A. & Rannug, U. (1984) Enzyme inhibition as a possible mechanism of the mutagenicity of dithiocarbamic acid derivatives in *Salmonella typhimurium*. *Chem.-biol. Interactions*, *49*, 329-340

Robens, J.F. (1969) Teratologic studies of carbaryl, diazinon, norea, disulfiran and thiram in small laboratory animals. *Toxicol. appl. Pharmacol.*, *15*, 152-163

Roll, R. (1971) Teratological studies with thiram (TMTD) in two strains of mice (Ger.). *Arch. Toxikol.*, *27*, 173-186

Royal Society of Chemistry (1986) *European Directory of Agrochemical Products*, Vol. 1, *Fungicides*, Cambridge, pp. 441-451

Royal Society of Chemistry (1989) *The Agrochemicals Handbook* [Dialog Information Services (File 306)], Cambridge

Rudzki, E. & Napiórkowska, T. (1980) Dermatitis caused by the Polish fungicide Sadoplon 75. *Contact Derm.*, *6*, 300-301

Sadtler Research Laboratories (1980) *The Sadtler Standard Spectra. 1980 Cumulative Index*, Philadelphia, PA

Sastry, C.S.P., Satyanarayana, P., Rao, A.R. & Sinch, N.R. (1988) Spectrophotometric determination of thiram, ziram and zineb in formulations, water, grains and vegetables using oxidized haematoxylin. *J. Food Sci. Technol.*, 25, 377-378

Schreiner, E. & Freundt, K.J. (1985) Activities of hepatic epoxide hydrolase and glutathione S-transferase in rats under the influence of tetramethyl thiuramdisulfide, tetramethyl thiurammonosulfide or dimethyl dithiocarbamate. *Toxicol. Lett.*, 25, 147-152

Sen, N.P., Donaldson, B.A. & Charbonneau, C. (1974) Formation of nitrosodimethylamine from the interaction of certain pesticides and nitrite. In: Bogovski, P. & Walker, E.A., eds, *N-Nitroso Compounds in the Environment* (IARC Scientific Publications No. 9), Lyon, IARC, pp. 75-79

Serio, R., Long, R.A., Taylor, J.E., Tolman, R.L., Weppelman, R.M. & Olson, G. (1984) The antifertility and antiadrenergic actions of thiocarbamate fungicides in laying hens. *Toxicol. appl. Pharmacol.*, 72, 333-342

Shirasu, Y., Moriya, M., Kato, K., Furuhashi, A. & Kada, T. (1976) Mutagenicity screening of pesticides in the microbial system. *Mutat. Res.*, 40, 19-30

Short, R.D., Jr, Russel, J.Q., Minor, J.L. & Lee, C.-C. (1976) Developmental toxicity of ferric dimethyldithiocarbamate and bis(dimethylthiocarbamoyl)disulfide in rats and mice. *Toxicol. appl. Pharmacol.*, 35, 83-94

Spencer, E.Y. (1973) *Guide to the Chemicals Used in Crop Protection*, 6th ed. (Publication 1093), London, Ontario, University of Western Ontario, Research Branch, Agriculture Canada

Takahashi, M., Kokubo, T., Furukawa, F., Nagano, K., Maekwawa, A., Kurowa, Y. & Hayashi, Y. (1983) Inhibition of spontaenous leukemia in F344 rats by tetramethylthiuram disulfide (Thiram). *Gann*, 74, 810-813

Taylor, D.G. (1977) *NIOSH Manual of Analytical Methods*, 2nd ed., Vol. 1 (DHEW (NIOSH) Publ. No. 77/157-A; US NTIS PB-274845), Washington DC, US Government Printing Office, pp. 228-1—228-6

Ueno, S. & Ishizaki, M. (1984) Mutagenicity of organic rubber additives (Jpn). *Jpn. J. ind. Health*, 26, 147-154

Upshall, A. & Johnson, P.E. (1981) Thiram-induced abnormal chromosome segregation in *Aspergillus nidulans*. *Mutat. Res.*, 89, 297-301

US Environmental Protection Agency (1975) Infrared spectra of pesticides. In: *Manual of Chemical Methods for Pesticides and Devices*, Arlington, VA, Association of Official Analytical Chemists

US Environmental Protection Agency (1984) *Pesticide Fact Sheet No. 29; Thiram*, Washington DC, Office of Pesticide Programs

US Environmental Protection Agency (1989) Thiram: tolerances for residues. Tolerances and exemptions from tolerances for pesticide chemicals in or on raw agricultural commodities. *US Code fed. Regul.*, Title 40, Part 180.132

US International Trade Commission (1975a) *Synthetic Organic Chemicals, US Production and Sales, 1973* (ITC Publication 728), Washington DC, US Government Printing Office, pp. 137, 141

US International Trade Commission (1975b) *Synthetic Organic Chemicals, US Production and Sales of Rubber-Processing Chemicals, 1974 Preliminary*, Washington DC, US Government Printing Office, pp. 4, 8

US National Technical Information Service (1968) *Evaluation of Carcinogenic, Teratogenic and Mutagenic Activities of Selected Pesticides and Industrial Chemicals*, Vol. 1, *Carcinogenic Study*, Washington DC, US Department of Commerce

US Occupational Safety and Health Administration (1989) Air contaminants—permissible exposure limits. *US Code fed. Regul.*, Title 29, Part 1910.1000

US Tariff Commission (1926) *Census of Dyes and Other Synthetic Organic Chemicals, 1925* (Tariff Information Series No. 34), Washington DC, US Government Printing Office, p. 148

US Tariff Commission (1961) *Synthetic Organic Chemicals, US Production and Sales, 1960* (TC Publication 34), Washington DC, US Government Printing Office, p. 43

Vlier, L.K. (1982) *Preliminary Quantitative Usage Analysis of Thiram*, Washington DC, Office of Pesticide Programs, US Environmental Protection Agency

Weast, R.C., ed. (1989) *CRC Handbook of Chemistry and Physics*, 70th ed., Boca Raton, FL, CRC Press, p. C-247

Wedig, J., Cowan, A. & Hartung, R. (1968) Some of the effects of tetramethylthiuram disulfide (TMTD) on reproduction of the bobwhite quail (*Colinus virginianus*) (Abstract No. 21). *Toxicol. appl. Pharmacol.*, *12*, 293

Wenyon, C.E. (1972) Organic sulfur compounds. In: *Chemical Technology: An Encyclopedic Treatment*, Vol. 4, *Petroleum and Organic Chemicals*, New York, Barnes & Noble, pp. 621-623

WHO (1988) *Dithiocarbamate Pesticides, Ethylenethiourea and Propylenethiourea—A General Introduction* (Environmental Health Criteria 78), Geneva

Williams, S., ed. (1984a) *Official Methods of Analysis of the Association of Official Analytical Chemists*, 14th ed., Washington DC, Association of Official Analytical Chemists, p. 562

Williams, S., ed. (1984b) *Official Methods of Analysis of the Association of Official Analytical Chemists*, 14th ed., Washington DC, Association of Official Analytical Chemists, p. 144

Worthing, C.R. & Walker, S.B., eds (1987) *The Pesticide Manual: A World Compendium*, 8th ed., Thornton Heath, British Crop Protection Council, pp. 807-808

Zdzienicka, M., Zieleńska, M., Tudek, B. & Szymczyk, T. (1979) Mutagenic activity of thiram in Ames tester strains of *Salmonella typhimurium*. *Mutat. Res.*, *68*, 9-13

Zdzienicka, M., Zieleńska, M., Hryniewicz, M., Trojanowska, M., Zalejska, M. & Szymczyk, T. (1981) The mutagenicity of the fungicide thiram. *Progr. Mutat. Res.*, *2*, 79-86

Zdzienicka, M., Hryniewicz, M. & Pienkowska, M. (1982) Thiram-induced sperm-head abnormalities in mice. *Mutat. Res.*, *102*, 261-264

Zemaitis, M.A. & Greene, F.E. (1979) In vivo and in vitro effects of thiuram disulfides and dithiocarbamates on hepatic microsomal drug metabolism in the rat. *Toxicol. appl. Pharmacol.*, *48*, 343-350

ZIRAM

This substance was considered by a previous Working Group, in 1976 (IARC, 1976). Since that time, new data have become available, and these have been incorporated into the monograph and taken into consideration in the present evaluation.

1. Exposure Data

1.1 Chemical and physical data

1.1.1 Synonyms, structural and molecular data

Chem. Abstr. Serv. Reg. No.: 137-30-4
Replaced CAS Reg. Nos: 111922-61-3; 12768-61-5; 98391-07-2; 12773-04-5; 55870-88-7; 31300-71-7; 8059-74-3; 8070-07-3; 14459-91-7; 17125-91-6; 19488-81-4
Chem. Abstr. Name: (T-4)-Bis(dimethylcarbamodithioato-S,S')-zinc
IUPAC Systematic Name: Zinc bis(dimethyldithiocarbamate)
Synonyms: Bis(dimethyldithiocarbamato)zinc; dimethylcarbamodithioic acid, zinc complex; dimethylcarbamodithioic acid, zinc salt; zinc, bis(dimethyldithiocarbamate); zinc dimethyldithiocarbamate

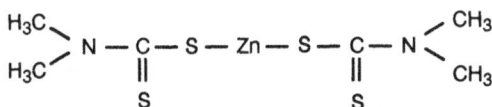

$$H_3C \diagdown \atop H_3C \diagup N - C - S - Zn - S - C - N \diagup CH_3 \atop \diagdown CH_3 ; \quad \underset{S}{\overset{\|}{}} \quad \underset{S}{\overset{\|}{}}$$

C$_6$H$_{12}$N$_2$S$_4$Zn   Mol. wt: 305.83

1.1.2 Chemical and physical properties

(a) *Description*: Crystalline white solid (Meister, 1990)
(b) *Melting-point*: 250°C (Budavari, 1989)
(c) *Density*: 1.66 at 25°C (Royal Society of Chemistry, 1989)
(d) *Spectroscopy data*: Infrared (prism [1296, 11231]; grating [15318] and nuclear magnetic resonance (proton [35587]) spectral data have been reported (US Environmental Protection Agency, 1975; Sadtler Research Laboratories, 1980, 1990).
(e) *Solubility*: Practically insoluble in water (65 mg/l); soluble at 25°C in ethanol (< 2 g/100 ml), acetone (< 0.5 g/100 ml), benzene (< 0.5 g/100 ml), carbon tetrachloride (< 0.2 g/100 ml) and dilute caustic solutions (Zweig, 1972; Budavari, 1989; Royal Society of Chemistry, 1989)

(f) *Vapour pressure*: Negligible at room temperature (Royal Society of Chemistry, 1989)
(g) *Stability*: Decomposed by acids and by ultraviolet irradiation; corrosive to iron and copper (Royal Society of Chemistry, 1989); hydrolysed slowly in water and stable in acidic media (Izmerov, 1982)
(h) *Conversion factor for airborne concentrations*[1]: mg/m^3 = 12.51 × ppm

1.1.3 *Trade names, technical products and impurities*

Some common trade names are: Aaprotect; Aavolex; Aazira; Accelerator L; Aceto ZDED; Aceto ZDMD; Alcobam ZM; Carbazinc; Corozate; Crittam; Cuman; Cymate; Eptac 1; Fuclasin; Fuklasin; Hermat ZDM; Hexazir; Karbam White; Methasan; Methazate; Methyl zimate; Methyl zineb; Methyl Ziram; Mezene; Milbam; Molurame; Mycronil; Nocceler PZ; Orchard brand Ziram; Pomarzol Z-forte; Rhodiacid; Rodisan; Soxinal PZ; Soxinol PZ; Trikagol; Vancide; Vulcacure ZM; Vulkacite L; Z 75; Zarlate; Z-C Spray; Zerlate; Zirberk; Ziride; Zirthane.

Ziram is formulated in the USA as a wettable powder, a paste and as water-dispersible granules (Anon., 1989). In Europe, it is also formulated as a dustable powder, in liquid formulations and as suspension concentrates (Royal Society of Chemistry, 1986).

Ziram is combined in formulations with many fungicides and insecticides (Royal Society of Chemistry, 1989). A wettable powder is available in Europe that is a combination of ziram and copper(II) oxychloride. In the past, a product was available that contained ziram, methyl-arsinediyl bis(dimethyldithiocarbamate) and thiram (see monograph, p. 403) (Worthing & Walker, 1987).

1.1.4 *Analysis*

Selected methods for the analysis of ziram in various matrices are presented in Table 1.

1.2 Production and use

1.2.1 *Production*

Ziram was introduced around 1931 as a fungicide (WHO, 1988). It is prepared from zinc oxide, dimethylamine and carbon disulfide (Budavari, 1989).

Ziram is produced currently in Belgium, India, Italy, Spain and the USA (Meister, 1990). One company in the USA produced approximately 320 tonnes in 1989, 230 tonnes in 1985, 450 tonnes in 1980 and approximately 135 tonnes in 1975. In 1981, an estimated 350-400 tonnes of ziram were produced in the USA (Luttner, 1981). Ziram is produced in Spain for use in the rubber industry.

1.2.2 *Use*

Ziram has principal uses as an accelerator in the process of rubber vulcanization (Wolfe, 1971; see IARC, 1982) and as a protective foliar fungicide on fruit, nuts, vines, vegetables and ornamental plants. It is used extensively on almond and peaches to control shot hole, brown rot and peach leaf curl (Luttner, 1981). It is also used on pecans, apples and pears to control

---

[1]Calculated from: mg/m³ = (molecular weight/24.45) × ppm, assuming standard temperature (25°C) and pressure (760 mm Hg [101.3 kPa])

Table 1. Methods for the analysis of ziram

Sample matrix	Sample preparation	Assay procedure	Limit of detection	Reference
Industrial and municipal wastewaters	Digest with acid to hydrolyse; trap evolved carbon disulfide in colour reagent; measure absorbance at 380 and 435 nm	Colorimetric	1.9 µg/l	Pressley & Longbottom (1982)
Specified crop samples	Decompose with the evolution of carbon disulfide, which is swept through a trap containing a solution of copper acetate and an amine to remove hydrogen sulfide; read absorbance of the coloured dithiocarbamate complex formed	Colorimetric	Not reported	US Food and Drug Administration (1989)
Specified crop samples and water	Extract with chloroform; evaporate; dissolve in methanol; add to mixture of methanolic 0.2% haematoxylin, aqueous 0.4% chloramine-T, and phosphate buffer solution at pH 7.0; heat; dilute with water; read absorbance at 555 nm	Spectro-photometric	Not reported	Sastry et al. (1988)
Formulations	Digest with acid; evolved carbon disulfide is trapped in methanolic potassium hydroxide; add phenolphthalein and starch indicator; titrate	Titrimetric	Not reported	Williams (1984)

scab and bull's-eye rot (Meister, 1990). The following amounts of ziram (active ingredient) were used in the USA in 1980 (tonnes): almonds, 320; peaches, 25-50; pears, 4-15; apricots, 5-10; and apples, 4-5. In the USA, ziram is registered for use as a fungicide in the following industrial applications: cooling-water slime control, paper-mill slime control, provision of mould resistance to paper and paperboard, and preservation of adhesives, textiles, paper coatings and industrial yarn and fabrics (Luttner, 1981). It is used as a wildlife repellant, when smeared as a paste onto tree trunks or sprayed onto ornamental plants, dormant fruit trees and other crops (Royal Society of Chemistry, 1989). In the USSR, ziram is used on potatoes for combatting phytophthora infection; other agricultural uses are prohibited. It is also used as a curing agent in the rubber industry (Izmerov, 1982).

1.3 Occurrence

1.3.1 *Water*

When precipitated to the bottom of bodies of water, thiram persisted for months. During cooking, ziram decomposed to thiram, tetramethylthiourea and dimethylamine dimethyl-dithiocarbamate (Izmerov, 1982).

1.3.2 *Food*

In the USSR, within two to five weeks after spraying with a 0.8-2.0% suspension of ziram, residual amounts in grapes and tomatoes were 0.1-0.8 mg/kg. Peelings of unwashed apples contained 1.0 mg/kg, and pulp of washed apples contained 0.04 mg/kg of ziram. The degradation products of ziram (thiram, dimethylamine dimethyldithiocarbamate and sulfur) were detected in fruit in the USSR two to three months after treatment (Izmerov, 1982).

1.4 Regulations and guidelines

The USSR has established a MAC in industrial air of 0.05 mg/m^3 and a recommended maximum concentration of 0.01 mg/l in water reservoirs used as sources for drinking-water (Izmerov, 1982).

National pesticide residue limits for ziram in foods are presented in Table 2 and Codex maximum residue limits in Table 3.

Table 2. National pesticide residue limits for ziram in foods[a]

Country	Residue limit (mg/kg)	Commodities
Australia	7	Fruit, vegetables
Austria	25[b]	Hops
	2[b]	Fruit, vegetables
	0.05[b]	Other
Belgium	2[c]	Fruit, other vegetables
	0.5[c]	Bulb vegetables, grains
	0.2[c,d]	Potatoes
	0[c,e] (0.02)	Other
Brazil	7[f]	Citrus fruit, broccoli, kale, cabbage, squash, watermelons, peanuts
	5[f]	Grapes
	3[f]	Apples, peaches, pears, strawberries, tomatoes, figs, guava, papaya, coffee
	1.0[f]	Honeydew melon
	0.5[f]	Cucumbers
	0.2[f]	Wheat, rice, cashew nuts, kaki
	0.1[f]	Potatoes
Canada	7[g]	Apples, apricots, beans, beetroot, blackberries, black-eyed peas, blueberries (huckleberries), broccoli, Brussels' sprouts, cabbage, carrots, cauliflower, celery, cherries, collards, cranberries, cucumbers, eggplants, gooseberries, grapes, kale, kohlrabi, lettuce, loganberries, melons, onions, peaches, peanuts, pears, peas, peppers, pumpkins, quinces, radishes, raspberries, rutabagas, spinach, squash, strawberries, summer squash, tomatoes, turnips
Chile	5[b]	Grapes
	3[b]	Apples, peaches, pears, tomatoes
	1.0[b]	Lettuce, cherries, plums
	0.5[b]	Carrots
	0.2[b]	Wheat
	0.1[b]	Potatoes
Finland	1.0[b]	Others (except cereal grains)
	0.5[b]	Carrots
	0.1[b]	Bananas, potatoes

Table 2 (contd)

Country	Residue limit (mg/kg)	Commodities
Germany	25^b	Hops
	2^b	Vegetables (except cucumbers, tomatoes), fruit, spices, raw coffee, tea, tea-like products, oilseed
	1.0^b	Cucumbers, tomatoes
	0.2^b	Other vegetable foodstuffs
Israel	5^b	Celery, currants (black, red), grapes
	3^b	Apples, peaches, pears, strawberries, tomatoes
	1.0^b	Bananas (whole), cherries, plums
	0.5^b	Endives, lettuce, melons
	0.2^b	Beans (in pods), carrots, cucumber
	0.1^b	Wheat, banana pulp, potatoes
Italy	2^h	Fruit, garden vegetables, cereals
	0.2^h	Other products intended for food use
Japan	1.0	Persimmon, pear, peach, apple
Kenya	7	Apples, apricots, beans, beetroot, blackberries, blueberries, boysenberries, broccoli, Brussels' sprouts, cabbage, carrots, cauliflower, celery, cherries, collards, cranberries, cucumbers, dewberries, eggplants, gooseberries, grapes, kale, kohlrabi, lettuce, loganberries, melons, nectarines, onions, peaches, peanuts, pears, peas, peppers, pumpkins, quinces, radishes, raspberries, rutabagas, spinach, squash, strawberries, summer squash, tomatoes, turnips, youngberries
	0.1	Almonds
Netherlands	4^c	Lettuce
	3^c	Berries, small fruit
	2^c	Other fruit, other vegetables
	1.0^c	Cucumbers, melons
	0.5^c	Bulb vegetables, cereals
	$0.2^{c,i}$	Pulses, potatoes
	$0^{c,e}$ (0.2)	Other
Singapore	5	Fruit, grains, vegetables
Spain	4^b	Grapes, hops, strawberries
	3^b	Other fruit and vegetables (except potatoes)
	0.2^b	Potatoes and other plant products
Sweden	1.0^b	Fruit and vegetables
	0.5^b	Carrots
	$0.1^{b,d}$	Potatoes, cereals and hulled grain, flakes and flour made from cereal
Switzerland	50^b	Tobacco
	2^b	Fruit, vegetables (except potatoes), lettuce
	0.5^b	Bananas (pulp)
	0.1^b	Cereals
	0.05^b	Potatoes

Table 2 (contd)

Country	Residue limit (mg/kg)	Commodities
USA	7[g]	Apples, apricots, beans, beetroot (with or without tops) or beetroot greens alone, blackberries, blueberries (huckleberries), boysenberries, broccoli, Brussels sprouts, cabbage, carrots, cauliflower, celery, cherries, collards, cranberries, cucumbers, dewberries, eggplants, gooseberries, grapes, kale, kohlrabi, lettuce, loganberries, melons, nectarines, onions, peaches, peanuts, pears, peas, peppers, pumpkins, quinces, radishes (with or without tops) or radish tops, raspberries, rutabagas (with or without tops) or rutabaga tops, spinach, squash, strawberries, summer squash, tomatoes, turnips (with or without tops) or turnip greens, youngberries
	0.1[g]	Almonds, pecans
USSR[j]	0.03	Foodstuffs
Yugoslavia	2[c]	Fruit, vegetables, tobacco
	0.05[c]	Other food commodities

[a]From Health and Welfare Canada (1990)
[b]Dithiocarbamates determined and expressed as carbon disulfide
[c]As dithiocarbamates
[d]The figure in parentheses is the lower limit for determining residues in the corresponding product according to the standard method of analysis.
[e]Residues shall be absent; the value in parentheses is the highest concentration at which this requirement is still deemed to have been met.
[f]Provisional tolerance
[g]Calculated as zineb
[h]Residues expressed as carbon sulfide; alone or combined with dithiocarbamates
[i]A pesticide may be used on an eating or drinking ware or raw material without a demonstrable residue remaining behind. The value listed is considered the highest concentration at which this requirement is deemed to have been met.
[j]From Izmerov (1982)

Table 3. Codex maximum residue limits for ziram[a]

Commodity	Maximum residue limit[b] (mg/kg)
Apples	3
Bananas	1
Carrots	0.5
Celery	5
Cherries	1
Common beans	0.5
Cucumbers	0.5
Currants (black, red, white)	5
Endives	1
Grapes	5
Lettuce, head	5

Table 3 (contd)

Commodity	Maximum residue limit[b] (mg/kg)
Melons, except watermelon	1
Peaches	3
Pears	3
Plums (including prunes)	1
Potatoes	0.1
Strawberries	3
Tomatoes	3
Wheat	0.2

[a]From Codex Committee on Pesticide Residues (1990); as dimethyl dithiocarbamates resulting from use of ferbam or ziram
[b]Determined and expressed as mg/kg carbon disulfide. The Joint Meeting on Pesticide Residues of 1980 (FAO/WHO, 1981) required further information on use patterns and data from residue trials before its estimates could be confirmed; as these requirements have not been met, the proposed limits, except that for lettuce (head), should be regarded as temporary. The proposal for lettuce (head) was made in 1985 without a requirement for further work or information.

Ziram was evaluated at the joint meetings of the FAO/WHO Expert Committee on Pesticide Residues in 1965, 1967, 1974, 1977 and 1980 (FAO/WHO, 1965, 1968, 1975, 1978, 1981). In 1977, the Committee established an acceptable daily intake for humans of 0.02 mg/kg bw (FAO/WHO, 1978), which was confirmed in 1980 for ziram and for the sum of ferbam and ziram (FAO/WHO, 1981; Codex Committee on Pesticide Residues, 1990).

2. Studies of Cancer in Humans

No data were available to the Working Group.

3. Studies of Cancer in Experimental Animals

Several studies on the carcinogenicity of ziram were summarized in a previous monograph (IARC, 1976), but, because of deficiencies in various aspects of study design, performance and/or reporting, the present Working Group did not consider them further. The studies in question are those of Hodge *et al.* (1956), the US National Technical Information Service (1968), Chernov and Khitsenko (1969) and Andrianova and Alekseev (1970).

Oral administration

Mouse: Groups of 49-50 male and 50 female B6C3F$_1$ mice, six weeks of age, were fed diets containing 600 or 1200 mg/kg ziram (89% pure, with 6.5% thiram, 2% other zinc salts and 2% unidentified impurity) for 103 weeks; survivors were killed one to three weeks later.

A group of 50 males and 50 females served as untreated controls. Survival was comparable in the treated and control groups. The incidence of lesions described by the authors as alveolar/bronchiolar adenomas was significantly ($p < 0.05$, trend) increased in female mice: control, 2/50; low-dose, 5/49; and high-dose, 10/50 ($p < 0.05$). The incidence of alveolar/bronchiolar carcinomas in female mice was: control, 2/50; low-dose, 1/49; and high-dose, 1/50. No increase in the incidence of tumours at any site was observed in males (US National Toxicology Program, 1983).

Rat: Groups of 50 male and 50 female Fischer 344/N rats, five weeks old, were fed diets containing 300 or 600 mg/kg commercial-grade ziram (89% pure, with 6.5% thiram, 2% other zinc salts and 2% unidentified impurity) for 103 weeks; survivors were killed one to four weeks later. A group of 50 males and 50 females served as untreated controls. Survival at the end of the experiment was: males—control, 33/50; low-dose, 34/50; and high-dose, 40/50; females—control, 37/50; low-dose, 44/50; and high-dose, 46/50. The incidence of C-cell carcinomas of the thyroid was significantly higher in high-dose males ($p < 0.05$) than in controls, with a significant positive trend (controls, 0/50; low-dose, 2/49; and high-dose, 7/49; $p < 0.01$). The combined incidence of C-cell adenomas and carcinomas in male rats also showed a significant positive trend (control, 4/50; low-dose, 9/49; and high-dose, 12/49; $p < 0.05$). No increase was observed in the incidence of tumours at any other site in males or in females (US National Toxicology Program, 1983).

4. Other Relevant Data

The toxicology of dithiocarbamates has been reviewed (WHO, 1988).

4.1 Absorption, distribution, metabolism and excretion

4.1.1 *Humans*

No data were available to the Working Group.

4.1.2 *Experimental systems*

Water-soluble metabolites were found in the blood, kidneys, liver, ovaries, spleen and thyroid of female rats 24 h after oral administration of radiolabelled ziram; unchanged ziram was excreted in the faeces (Izmirova, 1972; Izmirova & Marinov, 1972).

Administration of ziram with nitrite in aqueous solution by stomach tube to rats led to the formation of detectable amounts of N-nitrosodimethylamine in the stomach contents after 15 min (Eisenbrand *et al.*, 1974).

4.2 Toxic effects

4.2.1 *Humans*

Ingestion of 0.5 litre of a solution of ziram of unknown concentration was fatal within a few hours; nonspecific pathology was observed (Buklan, 1974). A case of contact dermatitis has also been reported (Manuzzi *et al.*, 1988).

4.2.2 *Experimental systems*

The oral LD_{50} of ziram in rats was 1400 mg/kg bw, and lethal oral doses in guinea-pigs and rabbits were in the range 100-150 and 100-1020 mg/kg bw, respectively. The intraperitoneal LD_{50} in rats was 23-33 mg/kg bw, and lethal intraperitoneal doses in guinea-pigs and rabbits were in the range 20-30 and 5-50 mg/kg bw, respectively. A dog tolerated doses of 25 mg/kg bw per day for one month (Hodge *et al.*, 1952); convulsions occurred in animals given this dose daily for one year (Hodge *et al.*, 1956).

A glycogenolytic response was elicited in rats after an intraperitoneal injection of 10 mg/kg bw ziram (Dailey *et al.*, 1969). Like most dithiocarbamates, ziram induces the accumulation of acetaldehyde in the blood of rats administered ethanol concurrently (van Logten, 1972).

In a 24-month chronic feeding study in rats, epiphyseal abnormalities in the long bones of the hind legs were observed in males and females at the highest dose tested (2000 ppm [mg/kg] in the diet; Enomoto *et al.*, 1989).

Ziram was reported to inhibit epoxide hydrolase and glutathione *S*-transferase in rat liver both *in vivo* and *in vitro* (Schreiner & Freundt, 1986).

4.3 Reproductive and developmental effects

4.3.1 *Humans*

No data were available to the Working Group.

4.3.2 *Experimental systems*

Administration of ziram at 50 or 100 mg/kg bw per day by gastric intubation to CD rats during the first five days of pregnancy reduced fetal weight by day 21 of gestation. Treatment at 25 mg/kg bw per day and above on days 6-15 resulted in embryotoxicity in the presence of maternal toxicity; at 100 mg/kg bw, a slight increase in the incidence of visceral malformations was observed (Giavini *et al.*, 1983).

Injection of ziram into the air chamber of eggs prior to incubation was embryolethal to chicks (LD_{50}; 2.1 μg/egg) (Gebhardt & van Logten, 1968).

4.4 Genetic and related effects (see also Table 4 and Appendices 1 and 2)

4.4.1 *Humans*

Peripheral blood lymphocytes from four male and five female workers who handled and packaged ziram were analysed for chromosomal aberrations. Average concentrations of ziram dust in the air of the work place were estimated to be 1.95 mg/m^3 in the store and 3.7 mg/m^3 in the packing area, but some were up to 71.3 mg/m^3. Despite protective measures (respirators and rubber gloves), ziram was detected on the skin of the workers' hands at concentrations of approximately 0.02 mg/m^2. Four controls (three women and one man) were matched with respect to age and residence. A marked increase in chromatid- and chromosome-type aberrations was observed in the exposed people as compared to the controls. The increase was about six-fold, and the exposed person in each pair had a significantly increased aberration frequency over the mean control level (Pilinskaya, 1970). [The Working Group noted the small number of individuals investigated in this study.]

4.4.2 *Experimental systems*

Ziram caused DNA damage and point mutation in bacteria, and these effects were increased by the presence of exogenous metabolic systems. It induced neither gene

Table 4. Genetic and related effects of ziram

Test system	Result[a]		Dose[b] LED/HID	Reference
	Without exogenous metabolic system	With exogenous metabolic system		
BSD, Bacillus subtilis rec strain, differential toxicity	+	0	0.6000	Shirasu et al. (1976)
SA0, Salmonella typhimurium TA100, reverse mutation	+	+	2.5000	Hedenstedt et al. (1979)
SA0, Salmonella typhimurium TA100, reverse mutation	-	+[c]	30.0000	Wideman & Nazar (1982)
SA0, Salmonella typhimurium TA100, reverse mutation	+	+	17.0000	Haworth et al. (1983)
SA0, Salmonella typhimurium TA100, reverse mutation	+		15.0000	Moriya et al. (1983)
SA0, Salmonella typhimurium TA100, reverse mutation	(+)	(+)	20.0000	Brooks et al. (1983)
SA5, Salmonella typhimurium TA1535, reverse mutation	+	+	5.0000	Hedenstedt et al. (1979)
SA5, Salmonella typhimurium TA1535, reverse mutation	+		10.0000	Brooks et al. (1983)
SA5, Salmonella typhimurium TA1535, reverse mutation	-	(+)	50.0000	Haworth et al. (1983)
SA5, Salmonella typhimurium TA1535, reverse mutation	-	-	2500.0000	Moriya et al. (1983)
SA7, Salmonella typhimurium TA1537, reverse mutation	-	0	50.0000	Hedenstedt et al. (1979)
SA7, Salmonella typhimurium TA1537, reverse mutation	+	+	46.0000	Brooks et al. (1983)
SA7, Salmonella typhimurium TA1537, reverse mutation	(+)	(+)	50.0000	Haworth et al. (1983)
SA7, Salmonella typhimurium TA1537, reverse mutation	-	-	2500.0000	Moriya et al. (1983)
SA8, Salmonella typhimurium TA1538, reverse mutation	-	0	50.0000	Hedenstedt et al. (1979)
SA8, Salmonella typhimurium TA1538, reverse mutation	-	-	80.0000	Brooks et al. (1983)
SA8, Salmonella typhimurium TA1538, reverse mutation	-	-	2500.0000	Moriya et al. (1983)
SA9, Salmonella typhimurium TA98, reverse mutation	+	+	50.0000	Hedenstedt et al. (1979)
SA9, Salmonella typhimurium TA98, reverse mutation	(+)	(+)	30.0000	Wideman & Nazar (1982)
SA9, Salmonella typhimurium TA98, reverse mutation	+	-	10.0000	Brooks et al. (1983)
SA9, Salmonella typhimurium TA98, reverse mutation	-	(+)	50.0000	Haworth et al. (1983)
SA9, Salmonella typhimurium TA98, reverse mutation	-	-	2500.0000	Moriya et al. (1983)
EC2, Escherichia coli WP2 hcr, reverse mutation	-	-	2500.0000	Moriya et al. (1983)
SCG, Saccharomyces cerevisiae, mitotic gene conversion	-	0	1000.0000	Siebert et al. (1970)
HSC, Hordeum vulgare (barley), chromosomal aberrations	-	0	500.0000	George et al. (1970)
DMM, Drosophila melanogaster, somatic mutation	+	0	130.0000 larval feeding	Tripathy et al. (1989)
DMX, Drosophila melanogaster, sex-linked recessive lethal mutation	-	0	50.0000 adult injection	Benes & Sram (1969)

Table 4 (contd)

Test system	Result[a] Without exogenous metabolic system	With exogenous metabolic system	Dose[b] LED/HID	Reference
DMX, *Drosophila melanogaster*, sex-linked recessive lethal mutation	+	0	500.0000 adult feeding	Donner et al. (1983)
DMX, *Drosophila melanogaster*, sex-linked recessive lethal mutation	+	0	54.0000 larval feeding[d]	Hemavathy & Krishnamurthy (1989)
DMX, *Drosophila melanogaster*, sex-linked recessive lethal mutation	+	0	130.0000 larval feeding	Tripathy et al. (1989)
DMH, *Drosophila melanogaster*, translocation	–	0	162.0000 larval feeding[d]	Hemavathy & Krishnamurthy (1989)
* *Drosophila melanogaster*, germ-cell mutation	+	0	130.0000 larval feeding	Tripathy et al. (1989)
G9H, Gene mutation, Chinese hamster lung V79 cells *in vitro*, *hprt* locus	–	–	0.0800	Donner et al. (1983)
G5T, Gene mutation, mouse lymphoma L5178Y cells *in vitro*, *tk* locus	+	0	0.1000	McGregor et al. (1988)
SIC, Sister chromatid exchange, Chinese hamster CHO cells *in vitro*	–	–	1.7500	Gulati et al. (1989)
CIC, Chromosomal aberrations, Chinese hamster CHO cells *in vitro*	+	+	0.0250	Gulati et al. (1989)
TCL, Cell transformation, BHK hamster cells	0	–	0.0500	Brooks et al. (1983)
CHL, Chromosomal aberrations, human lymphocytes *in vitro*	+	0	0.0030	Plinskaya (1971)
MVM, Micronucleus test, Swiss mouse bone marrow *in vivo*	+	0	95.0000 × 2 po[d]	Hemavathy & Krishnamurthy (1988)
CGC, Chromosomal aberrations, germ cells, Swiss mouse	+	0	95.0000 × 5 po[d]	Hemavathy & Krishnamurthy (1988)
DLM, Dominant lethal test, C3H mouse	(+)	0	2.0000 × 21 po	Cilievici et al. (1983)
DLM, Dominant lethal test, AK mouse	(+)	0	2.0000 × 21 po	Cilievici et al. (1983)
CVH, Chromosomal aberrations, human lymphocytes *in vivo*	+	0	0.0000	Plinskaya (1970)

*Not displayed on profile

[a]+, positive; (+), weakly positive; –, negative; 0, not tested; ?, inconclusive (variable response in several experiments within an adequate study)

[b]In-vitro tests, μg/ml; in-vivo tests, mg/kg bw

[c]Positive with plant activation system also

[d]Cuman L (27% ziram) was tested; dose represents ziram concentration

conversion in yeast nor chromosomal aberrations in *Hordeum vulgare*. In *Drosophila melanogaster*, ziram induced gene mutation in feeding studies but not when given by injection; it did not induce chromosomal translocation. Gene mutation was induced in mouse lymphoma L5178Y cells at the *tk* locus but not in Chinese hamster V79 cells at the *hprt* locus. [The Working Group noted that this discrepancy may be due to the different concentrations used and the difference in sensitivity of these two tests.] Chromosomal aberrations were induced in cultured rodent and human cells, whereas there was no induction of either sister chromatid exchange or anchorage-independent growth in rodent cells (Brooks *et al.*, 1983).

In vivo, ziram induced micronuclei in mouse bone marrow and chromosomal aberrations in mouse spermatogonia. Weak activity was reported in tests for dominant lethal mutation in male mice. [The Working Group noted the very low doses given in the latter tests.]

5. Summary of Data Reported and Evaluation

5.1 Exposure data

Ziram is used primarily as a rubber vulcanization accelerator but is also used as a foliar fungicide, mainly on fruit and nuts. It has been in commercial use since the 1930s.

Ziram has been formulated for use as a wettable powder, a paste and water-dispersible granules and also in combination with other pesticides.

Exposure can occur during its production, its use in the rubber industry and its application as a fungicide, and, at much lower levels, from consumption of foods containing residues.

5.2 Carcinogenicity in humans

No data were available in the Working Group.

5.3 Carcinogenicity in experimental animals

Ziram was tested adequately for carcinogenicity by oral administration in one study in mice and one study in rats. In mice, the incidence of benign lung tumours was increased in females. In rats, a dose-related increase in the incidence of C-cell thyroid carcinomas was observed in males.

5.4 Other relevant data

In single studies, ziram caused embryotoxicity and minor malformations in rats and embryolethality in chicks hatched from injected ova.

An increased frequency of chromatid and chromosomal aberrations was seen in peripheral blood lymphocytes of workers who handled and packaged ziram.

Ziram was clastogenic in mammalian cells *in vivo* and *in vitro* and induced mutations in cultured rodent cells and in insects and bacteria.

5.5 Evaluation[1]

No data were available from studies in humans.

There is *limited evidence* in experimental animals for the carcinogenicity of ziram.

Overall evaluation

Ziram *is not classifiable as to its carcinogenicity to humans (Group 3).*

6. References

Andrianova, M.M. & Alekseev, I.V. (1970) On the carcinogenic properties of the pesticides sevine, maneb, ziram and zineb (Russ.). *Vop. Pitan.*, *29*, 71-74

Anon. (1989) *Crop Protection Chemicals Reference*, 5th ed., New York, Chemical and Pharmaceutical Press, pp. 1244-1245, 1816-1819

Benes, V. & Sram, R. (1969) Mutagenic activity of some pesticides in *Drosophila melanogaster*. *Ind. Med.*, *38*, 442-444

Brooks, T.M., Meyer, A.L. & Dean, B.J. (1983) Genotoxicity studies with a blend of zinc dialkyl-dithiophosphate lubricant additives. *Mutat. Res.*, *124*, 129-143

Budavari, S., ed. (1989) *The Merck Index*, 11th ed., Rahway, NJ, Merck & Co., p. 1602

Buklan, A.I. (1974) Acute ziram poisoning (Russ.). *Sud.-med. Ekspert.*, *17*, 51

Chernov, O.V. & Khitsenko, I.I. (1969) Blastomogenic properties of some derivatives of dithio-carbamic acid (herbicides—zineb and ziram) (Russ.). *Vopr. Onkol.*, *15*, 71-74

Cilievici, O., Crăcium, C. & Ghidus, E. (1983) Decreased fertility, increased dominant lethals, skeletal malformations induced in the mouse by ziram fungicide. *Rev. Roum. Morphol. Embryol. Physiol.*, *29*, 159-165

Codex Committee on Pesticide Residues (1990) *Guide to Codex Maximum Limits for Pesticide Residues*, Part 2 (CAC/PR 2—1990; CCPR Pesticide Classification No. 119), The Hague

Dailey, R.E., Leavens, C.L. & Walton, M.S. (1969) Effect of certain dimethyldithiocarbamate salts on some intermediates of the glycolytic pathway *in vivo*. *J. agric. Food Chem.*, *17*, 827-828

Donner, M., Husgafvel-Pursiainen, K., Jenssen, D. & Rannug, A. (1983) Mutagenicity of rubber additives and curing fumes. Results from five short-term bioassays. *Scand. J. Work Environ. Health*, *9* (Suppl. 2), 27-37

Eisenbrand, G., Ungerer, O. & Preussmann, R. (1974) Rapid formation of carcinogenic *N*-nitro-samines by interaction of nitrite with fungicides derived from dithiocarbamic acid *in vitro* under simulated gastric conditions and *in vivo* in the rat stomach. *Food Cosmet. Toxicol.*, *12*, 229-232

Enomoto, A., Harada, T., Maita, K. & Shirasu, Y. (1989) Epiphyseal lesions of the femur and tibia in rats following oral chronic administration of zinc dimethyldithiocarbamate (ziram). *Toxicology*, *54*, 45-58

FAO/WHO (1965) *1965 Evaluations of Some Pesticide Residues in Food* (WHO/Food Add./27.65), Geneva

FAO/WHO (1968) *1967 Evaluations of Some Pesticide Residues in Food* (FAO/PL/1967/M/11/1; WHO/Food Add./68.30), Geneva

---

[1]For definition of the italicized terms, see Preamble, pp. 26-28.

FAO/WHO (1975) *1974 Evaluations of Some Pesticide Residues in Food* (FAO/AGP/1974/M/11; WHO Pesticide Residues Series No. 4), Geneva

FAO/WHO (1978) *Pesticide Residues in Food: 1977 Evaluations. The Monographs* (FAO Plant Production and Protection Paper 10 Sup.), Rome

FAO/WHO (1981) *Pesticide Residues in Food: 1980 Evaluations* (FAO Plant Production and Protection Paper 26 Sup.), Rome

Gebhardt, D.O.E. & van Logten, M.J. (1968) The chick embryo test as used in the study of the toxicity of certain dithiocarbamates. *Toxicol. appl. Pharmacol.*, *13*, 316-324

George, M.K., Aulakh, K.S. & Dhesi, J.S. (1970) Morphological and cytological changes induced in barley (*Hordeum vulgare*) seedlings following seed treatment with fungicides. *Can. J. Genet. Cytol.*, *12*, 415-419

Giavini, E., Vismara, C. & Broccia, M.L. (1983) Pre- and postimplantation embryotoxic effects of zinc dimethyldithiocarbamate (ziram) in the rat. *Ecotoxicol. environ. Saf.*, *7*, 531-537

Gulati, D.K., Witt, K., Anderson, B., Zeiger, E. & Shelby, M.D. (1989) Chromosome aberrations and sister chromatid exchange tests in Chinese hamster ovary cells *in vitro*. III: Results with 27 chemicals. *Environ. mol. Mutagenesis*, *13*, 133-193

Haworth, S., Lawlor, T., Mortelmans, K., Speck, W. & Zeiger, E. (1983) *Salmonella* mutagenicity test results for 250 chemicals. *Environ. Mutagenesis, Suppl. 1*, 3-142

Health and Welfare Canada (1990) *National Pesticide Residue Limits in Food*, Ottawa, Bureau of Chemical Safety, Food Directorate, Health Protection Branch

Hedenstedt, A., Rannug, U., Ramel, C. & Wachtmeister, C.A. (1979) Mutagenicity and metabolism studies on 12 thiuram and dithiocarbamate compounds used as accelerators in the Swedish rubber industry. *Mutat. Res.*, *68*, 313-325

Hemavathy, K.C. & Krishnamurthy, N.B. (1988) Cytogenetic effects of Cuman L, a dithiocarbamate fungicide. *Mutat. Res.*, *208*, 57-60

Hemavathy, K.C. & Krishnamurthy, N.B. (1989) Genotoxicity studies with Cuman L in *Drosophila melanogaster*. *Environ. mol. Mutagenesis*, *14*, 252-253

Hodge, H.C., Maynard, E.A., Downs, W., Blancher, H.J., Jr & Jones, C.K. (1952) Acute and short-term oral toxicity tests of ferric dimethyldithiocarbamate (ferbam) and zinc dimethyldithiocarbamate (ziram). *J. Am. pharm. Assoc.*, *41*, 662-665

Hodge, H.C., Maynard, E.A., Downs, W., Coye, R.D., Jr & Steadman, L.T. (1956) Chronic oral toxicity of ferric dimethyldithiocarbamate (ferbam) and zinc dimethyldithiocarbamate (ziram). *J. Pharmacol. exp. Ther.*, *118*, 174-181

IARC (1976) *IARC Monographs on the Evaluation of Carcinogenic Risk of Chemicals to Man*, Vol. 12, *Some Carbamates, Thiocarbamates and Carbazides*, Lyon, pp. 259-270

IARC (1982) *IARC Monographs on the Evaluation of the Carcinogenic Risks of Chemicals to Humans*, Vol. 28, *The Rubber Industry*, Lyon

Izmerov, N.F., ed. (1982) *International Register of Potentially Toxic Chemicals. Scientific Reviews of Soviet Literature on Toxicity and Hazards of Chemicals: Ziram* (Issue 15), Moscow, Centre of International Projects, United Nations Environment Programme

Izmirova, N. (1972) A study on the water-soluble and chloroform metabolites of ^{35}S-ziram by means of paper and thin-layer chromatography (Russ.). *Eksp. Med. Morfol.*, *11*, 240-243

Izmirova, N. & Marinov, V. (1972) Distribution and excretion of ^{35}S-ziram and metabolic products after 24 hours following oral administration of the preparation in female rats (Russ.). *Eksp. Med. Morfol.*, *11*, 152-156 van Logten, M.J. (1972) *The Dithiocarbamate–Alcohol Reaction in the Rat*, Amsterdam, Bedrifj FA Lammers, p. 40 (in Dutch)

Luttner, M.A. (1981) *Preliminary Quantitative Usage of Analysis of Ziram*, Washington DC, US Environmental Protection Agency

Manuzzi, P., Borrello, P., Misciali, C. & Guerra, L. (1988) Contact dermatitis due to ziram and maneb (Short communication). *Contact Derm.*, *19*, 148

McGregor, D.B., Brown, A., Cattanach, P., Edwards, I., McBride, D., Riach, C. & Caspary, W.J. (1988) Responses of the L5178Y tk⁺/tk⁻ mouse lymphoma cell forward mutation assay: III. 72 coded chemicals. *Environ. mol. Mutagenesis*, *12*, 85-154

Meister, R.T., ed. (1990) *Farm Chemicals Handbook '90*, Willoughby, OH, Meister Publishing Company, pp. C311-C312

Moriya, M., Ohta, T., Watanabe, K., Miyazawa, T., Kato, K. & Shirasu, Y. (1983) Further mutagenicity studies on pesticides in bacterial reversion assay systems. *Mutat. Res.*, *116*, 185-216

Pilinskaya, M. (1970) Chromosomal aberrations in persons handling ziram under industrial conditions (Russ.). *Genetika*, *6*, 157-163

Pilinskaya, M. (1971) Cytogenetic action of the fungicide ziram in a culture of human lymphocytes *in vitro* (Russ.). *Genetika*, *7*, 138-143

Pressley, T.A. & Longbottom, J.E. (1982) *The Detection of Dithiocarbamate Pesticides in Industrial and Municipal Wastewaters: Method 630* (EPA-600/4-82-011; US NTIS PB82-156050), Cincinnati, OH, Environmental Monitoring Systems Laboratory, US Environmental Protection Agency

Royal Society of Chemistry (1986) *European Directory of Agrochemical Products*, Vol. 1, *Fungicides*, Cambridge, pp. 486-489

Royal Society of Chemistry (1989) *The Agrochemicals Handbook* [Dialog Information Services (File 306)], Cambridge

Sadtler Research Laboratories (1980) *The Standard Spectra, 1980 Cumulative Index*, Philadelphia, PA

Sadtler Research Laboratories (1990) *The Standard Spectra, 1990 Cumulative Index*, Philadelphia, PA

Sastry, C.S.P., Satyanarayana, P., Rao, A.R. & Sinch, N.R. (1988) Spectrophotometric determination of thiram, ziram and zineb in formulations, water, grains and vegetables using oxidized haematoxylin. *J. Food Sci. Technol.*, *25*, 377-378

Schreiner, E. & Freundt, K.J. (1986) Inhibition of hepatic epoxide hydrolase and glutathione S-transferase in rats by bis(dimethyldithiocarbamato)zinc (ziram). *Bull. environ. Contam. Toxicol.*, *37*, 53-54

Shirasu, Y., Moriya, M., Kato, K., Furuhashi, A. & Kada, T. (1976) Mutagenicity screening of pesticides in the microbial system. *Mutat. Res.*, *40*, 19-30

Siebert, D., Zimmermann, F.K. & Lemperle, E. (1970) Genetic effects of fungicides. *Mutat. Res.*, *10*, 533-543

Tripathy, N.K., Majhi, B., Dey, L. & Das, C.C. (1989) Genotoxicity of ziram established through wing, eye and female germ-line mosaic assays and the sex-linked recessive lethal test in *Drosophila melanogaster*. *Mutat. Res.*, *224*, 161-169

US Environmental Protection Agency (1975) Infrared spectra of pesticides. In: *Manual of Chemical Methods for Pesticides and Devices*, Arlington, VA, Association of Official Analytical Chemists

US Food and Drug Administration (1989) Dithiocarbamates. In: *Pesticide Analytical Manual*, Vol. II, *Methods Which Detect Multiple Residues*, Washington DC, US Department of Health and Human Services, p. 1

US National Technical Information Service (1968) *Evaluation of Carcinogenic, Teratogenic and Mutagenic Activities of Selected Pesticides and Industrial Chemicals*, Vol. 1, *Carcinogenic Study*, Washington DC, US Department of Commerce

US National Toxicology Program (1983) *Carcinogenesis Bioassay of Ziram (CAS No. 137-30-4) in F344/N Rats and B6C3F1 Mice (Feed Study)* (NTP Technical Report Series No. 238), Research Triangle Park, NC

WHO (1988) *Dithiocarbamate Pesticides, Ethylenethiourea and Propylenethiourea. A General Introduction* (Environmental Health Criteria 78), Geneva

Wildeman, A.G. & Nazar, R.N. (1982) Significance of plant metabolism in the mutagenicity and toxicity of pesticides. *Can. J. Genet. Cytol.*, 24, 437-449

Williams, S., ed. (1984) *Official Methods of Analysis of the Association of the Official Analytical Chemists*, 14th ed., Washington DC, Association of Official Analytical Chemists, pp. 139-140

Wolfe, J.R., Jr (1971) Vulcanization. In: Bikalis, N.M., ed., *Encyclopedia of Polymer Science and Technology*, Vol. 14, New York, Interscience, pp. 740-71, 747-748

Worthing, C.R. & Walker, S.B., eds (1987) *The Pesticide Manual: A World Compendium*, 8th ed., Thornton Heath, British Crop Protection Council, pp. 850-851

Zweig, G., ed. (1972) *Analytical Methods for Pesticides and Plant Growth Regulators*, Vol. VI, *Gas Chromatographic Analysis*, New York, Academic Press, p. 561

HERBICIDES

ATRAZINE

1. Exposure Data

1.1 Chemical and physical data

1.1.1 Synonyms, structural and molecular data

Chem. Abstr. Serv. Reg. No.: 1912-24-9
Replaced CAS Reg. Nos: 11121-31-6, 12040-45-8, 12797-72-7, 39400-72-1, 69771-31-9, 93616-39-8
Chem. Abstr. Name: 6-Chloro-*N*-ethyl-*N'*-(1-methylethyl)-1,3,5-triazine-2,4-diamine
IUPAC Systematic Name: 6-Chloro-N^2-ethyl-N^4-isopropyl-1,3,5-triazine-2,4-diamine
Synonyms: 2-Chloro-4-ethylamino-6-isopropylamino-1,3,5-triazine; 2-chloro-4-(ethyl-amino)-6-(isopropylamino)triazine; 2-chloro-4-(ethylamino)-6-(isopropylamino)-*s*-triazine

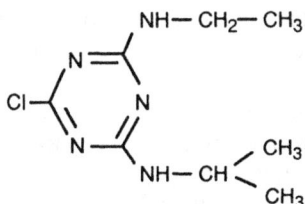

$C_8H_{14}ClN_5$ Mol. wt: 215.69

1.1.2 Chemical and physical properties

(a) *Description*: Colourless crystals (Royal Society of Chemistry, 1989)
(b) *Melting-point*: 175-177°C (Worthing & Walker, 1987)
(c) *Spectroscopy data*: Infrared (prism [35712]; grating [13706]) and ultraviolet [16141] spectral data have been reported (Sadtler Research Laboratories, 1980).
(d) *Solubility*: Very slightly soluble in water (30 mg/l at 20°C) and hydrocarbon solvents; moderately soluble in ether (1.2%), chloroform (5.2%), methanol (1.8%), ethyl acetate (2.8%), dimethyl sulfoxide (18.3%) and octanol (1%) (Worthing & Walker, 1987; Royal Society of Chemistry, 1989)
(e) *Vapour pressure*: 3×10^{-7} mm Hg [0.4×10^{-7} kPa] at 20°C (Royal Society of Chemistry, 1989)
(f) *Stability*: Forms salts with acids; stable in slightly acidic or basic media; slowly hydrolysed to inactive hydroxy derivative at 70°C under neutral conditions, more rapidly in alkali or mineral acids (Worthing & Walker, 1987; Royal Society of Chemistry, 1989)

(g)   Conversion factor for airborne concentrations[1]: $mg/m^3 = 8.82 \times ppm$

1.1.3   Trade names, technical products and impurities

Some common trade names include: A 361; Aatrex; Akticon; Aktikon; Aktinit A; Argezin; Atrataf; Atrazin; ATZ; CET; Chromozin; Cyazin; G 30027; Gesaprim; Herbatoxol; Hungazin; Oleogesaprim; Primatol A; Radazin; Triazine A 1294; Wonuk; Zeapos; Zeazin; Zeazine; Zeopos

In the USA, technical-grade products contain at least 94% atrazine as the sole active ingredient; the percentage of related compounds must also be stated (US Environmental Protection Agency, 1983).

Atrazine is available in the USA as a wettable powder, as water-dispersible granules and in liquid formulations (Anon., 1989a). Formulated atrazine products registered in European countries include, in addition, emulsifiable concentrates, emulsions, suspension concentrates and other granular formulations (Royal Society of Chemistry, 1986).

In the USA, atrazine is also formulated in combination with pendimethalin, metolachlor, cyanazine, *S*-ethyl diisobutylthiocarbamate, *N,N*-diallyl-2,2-dichloroace-tamide, alachlor, propachlor, bromoxynil octanoate, sodium chlorate, sodium metaborate and the potassium salt of dicamba. Several products contain some ethylene glycol and formaldehyde (see IARC, 1987a) (Anon., 1989a,b).

Combination atrazine products registered in European countries include atrazine with bentazone, bromofenoxim, bromoxynil, butylate, cyanazine, 2,4-D (see IARC, 1987b), dalapon sodium, dicamba, dichlobenil, dichlormid, dichlormidcyanazine, dichlorprop, diuron, *S*-ethyl dipropylthiocarbamate, ethalfluralin, fenteracol, fenuron, linuron, MCPA (see IARC, 1987b), methabenzthiazuron, metolachlor, paraquat dichloride, pendimethalin, petroleum oils, picloram (see monograph, p. 481), prometryne, propachlor, pyridate, simazine (see monograph, p. 495), sodium chlorate, tallow amine ethoxylate, sodium trichloroacetate, terbumeton, terbuthylazine, terbutryn and thiazafluron (Royal Society of Chemistry, 1986).

In the USSR, atrazine is available as a wettable powder, as a paste and in combination with prometryne (Izmerov, 1982).

1.1.4   Analysis

Selected methods for the analysis of atrazine in various matrices are given in Table 1.

1.2   Production and use

1.2.1   Production

Atrazine was introduced in 1957 (Funari *et al.*, 1988). It is produced through consecutive substitution of ethylamine and isopropylamine on cyanuric chloride in the presence of alkali (Izmerov, 1982).

---

[1]Calculated from: $mg/m^3 = $ (molecular weight/24.45) $\times$ ppm, assuming standard temperature (25°C) and pressure (760 mm Hg [101.3 kPa])

Table 1. Methods for the analysis of atrazine

Sample matrix	Sample preparation	Assay procedure[a]	Limit of detection[b]	Reference
Formulation (80% wettable powder)	Dissolve in chloroform; centrifuge	GC/FID	Not reported	Williams (1984)
Drinking-water	Extract in liquid-solid extractor; elute with dichloromethane; concentrate by evaporation	GC/MS	0.1 µg/l (I) 0.3 µg/l (M)	US Environmental Protection Agency (1988)
	Extract with dichloromethane; isolate extract; dry; concentrate with methyl *tert*-butyl ether	GC/NPD	0.13 µg/l (estimated detection limit)	US Environmental Protection Agency (1989a)
	Extract with hexane; inject extract	GC/ECD	2.4 µg/l	US Environmental Protection Agency (1989b)
Forage (all crops)	Extract with chloroform (green forage) or acetonitrile:water (9:1) (dry forage); partition with dichloromethane (dry forage); evaporate to dryness; partition with hexane and acetonitrile; clean-up on alumina column (for all forages)	GC/MCD	0.05-0.1 ppm	US Food and Drug Administration (1989)

[a]Abbreviations: GC/ECD, gas chromatography/electron capture detection; GC/FID, gas chromatography/flame ionization detection; GC/MCD, gas chromatography/microcoulometric detection; GC/MS, gas chromatography/mass spectrometry; GC/NPD, gas chromatography/nitrogen-phosphorous detection
[b]Abbreviations: (I), ion trap mass spectrometer; (M), magnetic sector mass spectrometer

It is produced currently in Argentina, Israel, Mexico, Switzerland and the USA (Meister, 1990). Production in the USA in 1980 was estimated to be 50 000 tonnes, 10 000 tonnes of which were exported (US Environmental Protection Agency, 1980). The major US producer reported production of 40 000-50 000 tonnes per annum between 1981 and 1989.

1.2.2 *Use*

Worldwide, atrazine has been one of the most heavily used herbicides over the past 30 years. It is a selective pre- and early post-emergent herbicide (Worthing & Walker, 1987), which acts mainly through root absorption to control many annual broadleaf and grass weeds. The most important use is as a selective herbicide on maize; other crops include sorghum, sugar-cane and pineapple. It is used in heavier doses for non-selective residual control of most annual and many perennial broadleaf and grass weeds in non-crop areas (Royal Society of Chemistry, 1986, 1989). Atrazine is also used on turf for fairways, lawns, sod production and similar areas and on established conifers prior to or after transplanting (Anon., 1989b).

In the USA in 1980, use of atrazine (active ingredient) was as follows (tonnes): maize, 32 000–36 000; sorghum, 4100–5500; sugar-cane, 340–570; sweet maize, 270–360; soya beans, 180–270; wheat, 180–270; cotton, 50–70; and other crops, 90–180 (US Environmental

Protection Agency, 1980). Approximately 34–45 thousand tonnes of atrazine (active ingredient) were used in the USA in 1987 (US Environmental Protection Agency, 1990).

1.3 Occurrence

1.3.1 *Water*

Atrazine has been found in surface water and in groundwater due to its mobility in soil. It is relatively stable in aquatic environments (half-time measured in months) but is degraded by photolysis (US Environmental Protection Agency, 1988).

A monitoring study of Mississippi River water (USA) indicated the presence of atrazine residues at a maximum level of 17 μg/l. Residues were detected throughout the year, with the highest concentrations in June and July (US Environmental Protection Agency, 1988).

Triazine herbicide residues were monitored in central European streams by methods with a limit of detection usually of 0.4 mg/m^3. Residues were found in 80% of samples at below 0.4 mg/m^3, in 14% at 0.4-1 mg/m^3, in 6% at 1-10 mg/m^3 and in 0.3% at levels higher than 10 mg/m^3. Detectable residues consisted mainly of atrazine from downstream sampling sites and mainly peaked during June (Hörmann *et al.*, 1979).

Atrazine was found in 4123 of 10 942 surface water samples in the USA and in 343 of 3208 groundwater samples. The 85th percentile of the residues in the positive samples was 2.3 μg/l in surface water and 1.9 μg/l in groundwater, with maximum concentrations of 2.3 mg/l and 0.7 mg/l, respectively. Atrazine was found in the surface water of 31 states and in groundwater in 13 states in the USA (US Environmental Protection Agency, 1988).

Some 600 000 kg of atrazine are used annually on maize, which is grown extensively in the Lombardy area of Italy. Groundwater from almost 3000 wells was analysed for atrazine residues in 1986: of 2005 public wells, 29 had levels greater than 1.0 μg/l, 281 wells had levels > 0.1-1.0 μg/l, the remaining wells having < 0.1 μg/l. Of the private wells, 61 had levels > 1.0 μg/l, 536 in the range 0.1–1.0 μg/l and the remainder, < 0.1 μg/l. The soil type is thought to play an important role in the contamination of groundwater by atrazine (Funari *et al.*, 1988).

Atrazine residues have also been reported in groundwater in Pennsylvania, Iowa, Nebraska, Wisconsin and Maryland (USA); typical levels ranged from 0.3 to 3 μg/l (Cohen *et al.*, 1986).

1.3.2 *Soil*

Atrazine is degraded in soil by photolysis and microbial processes; the products are dealkylated metabolites, hydroxyatrazine and nonextractable residues. Atrazine and its dealkylated metabolites are relatively mobile, whereas hydroxyatrazine is not.

A study of aerobic soil metabolism in Lakeland sandy loam, Hagerstown silty clay loam and Wehadkee silt loam soils showed conversion of atrazine to hydroxyatrazine after eight weeks to be 38%, 40% and 47%, respectively (Harris, 1967).

The half-time of atrazine in soil ranged from 20 to 101 days. In California, Minnesota and Tennessee (USA) soils, no leaching of atrazine or of metabolites was observed below 15-30.5 cm of soil. The water-holding capacity of a soil is one factor that affects the rate of degradation of atrazine (US Environmental Protection Agency, 1988). For a sandy soil with

4%, 35% and 70% water-holding capacity, the half-times were 151, 37 and 36 days, respectively (Hurle & Kibler, 1976).

In a Mississippi (USA) field study, atrazine in silt loam soil had a half-time of less than 30 days. In loam-to-silt loam soil in Minnesota, phytotoxic atrazine residues persisted for more than one year and were detected in maximum-depth samples (76-107 cm). Phytotoxic residues persisted in Nebraska silty clay and loam soils for 16 months and were found at depths of 30.5-61 cm (US Environmental Protection Agency, 1988).

Atrazine was also found to persist for up to three years on the sides and bottom of irrigation ditches at the maximal depths sampled (67.5-90 cm; Smith et al., 1975).

1.3.3 Food

No residue of atrazine was detected in a Canadian national surveillance study in 1984-89 of 1075 samples, which included fruit, vegetables, grain, dairy products and wine (Government of Canada, 1990).

No atrazine residue (< 0.05 ppm [mg/kg]) was reported in a survey of various foods and feeds over the period 1981-86 in 19 851 samples in the USA (Luke et al., 1988).

1.3.4 Occupational exposure

A study was carried out in the USA to determine the exposure of four men when applying 4 litres of atrazine at 4.5 kg active ingredient/ha by boom sprayer towed by an all-terrain vehicle. Dermal exposure was higher during mixing-loading operations than boom operations, with levels of 272 and 3 µg/kg active ingredient, respectively. Respiratory exposure was similar in both operations at 12 µg/kg active ingredient. The specific area of greatest exposure was the forearm during mixing-loading, which had significantly greater concentrations (686 µg/kg active ingredient) than all other sampling areas (Reed et al., 1990).

Exposure to atrazine during its industrial production was assessed by air monitoring and by measuring free atrazine in the urine of four workers. Ambient air concentrations of atrazine during production and bagging varied from 0.07 to 0.53 mg/m^3 (8-h time-weighted average), and skin deposition (whole body) from 4.11 to 10.66 mg/h. Urinary excretion in exposed workers showed a pattern consistent with exposure, with maximal excretion rates of 0.1-0.3 µg/h during the work shift, which decreased to 0.01-0.04 µg/h 12 h after the workshift (Catenacci et al., 1990).

1.4 Regulations and guidelines

WHO (1987) recommended a drinking-water guideline of 2 µg/l for atrazine. The maximum allowable concentration of atrazine in Canadian drinking-water is 2 µg/l (Health and Welfare Canada, 1990).

An acceptable daily intake of 0.7 µg/kg bw was established by the WHO (1987). National and regional limits for residues of atrazine in foods are given in Table 2.

Occupational exposure limits for atrazine are given in Table 3.

Table 2. National and regional pesticide residue limits for atrazine in foods[a]

Country or region	Residue limit (mg/kg)	Commodities
Argentina	0.25	Maize, sorghum, sweet maize
Australia	0.1[b]	Citrus, grapes, maize, pineapples, sorghum, sugar-cane, sweet maize
	0.02[b]	Lupins
	0.01[b]	Meat, milk, milk products, potatoes
Austria	1.0	Asparagus
	0.5	Maize
	0.1	Other foods of vegetable origin
Belgium	0.1	Fruit, vegetables, maize
	0[c] (0.05)	Other
Brazil	1.0	Conifers, rubber plants, sisal
	0.2	Maize, sorghum, pineapple, sugar-cane, avocados, bananas, mangos, peaches, apples, citrus fruit, nuts, tea, cocoa, coffee
	0.1	Black pepper
Canada	Negligible	Blueberries, maize
European Community	0.1	All products
Finland	0.2	General
France	0.1	Fruit, vegetables
	0.05	Maize
Germany	10	Wild mushrooms
	1.0	Sweet maize
	0.5	Maize
	0.1	Other foods of plant origin
Greece	1.0	Fruit and vegetables
Hungary	0.1	All crops
Ireland	0.1	All products
Israel	15	Maize fodder, sorghum fodder
	10	Wheat fodder and straw
	0.25	Fresh maize, maize grain, sorghum grain
	0.02	Eggs, milk, meat, fat and meat by-products
Italy	0.5	Maize, sorghum
	0.1	Fruit, garden vegetables
Japan	0.02	Oats, etc. and minor cereals; fruit, vegetables, sugar-cane
Kenya	0.25	Maize grain, sorghum grain, sugar-cane, wheat grain
	0.02	Eggs, milk, meat, fat and meat products of cattle, goats, hogs, horses, poultry and sheep

Table 2 (contd)

Country or region	Residue limit (mg/kg)	Commodities
Mexico	15	Maize (forage), sorghum (forage)
	10	Pineapple (forage)
	5	Wheat (straw)
	0.25	Maize (fresh and grain), pineapple, sorghum (grain), sugar-cane, wheat (grain)
Netherlands	0.1	Maize, fruit, vegetables
	0[d] (0.05)	Other
Spain	1.0	Maize and sorghum forage
	0.25	Maize and sorghum grain
	0.1	Other plant products
Switzerland	0.5	Asparagus, grapes
	0.1	All crops except asparagus and grapes
Taiwan	0.5	Field crops, tropical fruits
USA[e]	15	Maize forage or fodder (including field maize, sweet maize, popcorn), sorghum fodder and forage, perennial rye grass
	10	Pineapple fodder and forage
	5	Wheat fodder and straw, millet forage, fodder and straw
	0.25	Fresh maize including sweet maize (kernels plus cobs with husks removed), maize grain, macadamia nuts, pineapples, sorghum grain, sugar-cane, sugar-cane fodder and forage, wheat grain
	0.05	Guava
	0.02	Eggs, milk, meat, fat and meat by-products of cattle, goats, hogs, horses, poultry and sheep (negligible residues)
	15[f]	Orchard grass (hay)
	5.0[c]	Proso millet (fodder, forage, straw)
	4.0[c]	Grass (range)
	0.25[f]	Proso millet, grain
Yugoslavia	0.5	Maize
	0.1	Fruit, vegetables
	0.03	Milk and other dairy products (fat basis)
	0.02	Meat and meat products (fat basis), eggs (shell-free basis)

[a]From Health and Welfare Canada (1990)
[b]Maximum residue limit set at or about the limit of analytical determination
[c]The figure in parentheses is the lower limit for determining residues in the corresponding product according to the standard method of analysis.
[d]Residues shall be absent; the value in parentheses is the highest concentration at which this requirement is still deemed to have been met.
[e]From US Environmental Protection Agency (1989c)
[f]Atrazine and its metabolites

Table 3. Occupational exposure limits for atrazine[a]

Country	Year	Concentration (mg/m³)	Interpretation[b]
Belgium	1987	10	TWA
Denmark	1987	5	TWA
Finland	1987	10	TWA
		20	STEL
Germany	1989	2	TWA
Mexico	1987	10	TWA
Netherlands	1987	10	TWA
Switzerland	1987	2	TWA
United Kingdom	1987	10	TWA
USA	1989		
OSHA		5	TWA
ACGIH		5	Guideline
USSR	1987	2	MAC

[a]From Cook (1987); American Conference of Governmental Industrial Hygienists (ACGIH) (1989); US Occupational Safety and Health Administration (OSHA) (1989)
[b]TWA, time-weighted average; STEL, short-term exposure limit; MAC, maximum allowable concentration

2. Studies of Cancer in Humans

2.1 Case-control studies of cancer of the ovary

According to local agricultural experts, triazines are used as herbicides in all maize cultivation in Alessandria province in northern Italy. About 10 times more atrazine than simazine was sold in the province in 1970, according to the National Institute of Statistics (Donna *et al.*, 1989). In a study of herbicide exposure, all 66 incident cases of histologically confirmed primary ovarian tumours diagnosed between 1 January 1974 and 30 June 1980 in the city hospital of Alessandria were considered. Fifty patients still alive in 1981 were interviewed, and information was obtained from next-of-kin for 10 dead cases; the remaining six cases were untraced. Controls were incident cases of cancer at sites other than the ovary from the same hospital, matched by year of diagnosis, age and district of residence: 135 controls were obtained, of whom 127 were interviewed in 1982. Definite herbicide exposure (i.e., self-reported personal herbicide use) was found for eight cases and no control, and probable exposure (i.e., employment as farmer after 1960 and residence in areas of herbicide use) for 10 cases and 14 controls. The relative risk (RR) for ovarian tumours associated with any herbicide exposure was 4.4 (95% confidence interval [CI], 1.9-16.1). The risk was mostly confined to younger subjects; the RR was 9.1 (95% CI, 3.0-28.3) for women under 55 years of age (Donna *et al.*, 1984).

A second study of a different time period in the same area covered women who were at risk of ovarian cancer, aged 20-69 years, and residents in 143 municipalities in the province.

Cases were histologically confirmed primary malignant epithelial tumours of the ovary diagnosed from 1 July 1980 to 30 June 1985. Two controls per case of the same age were selected randomly from the electoral rolls of the study area. Of the 69 eligible cases, 42 were alive and interviewed; relatives were interviewed for 23 of the 27 dead cases. Of the 150 controls selected, 13 could not be interviewed and 11 were excluded because they had undergone a bilateral oophorectomy. In the calculation of odds ratios, adjustment was made for age, number of live births and use of oral contraceptives. Seven cases and seven controls were defined as having been definitely exposed to triazine (preparation or use of triazine herbicides or worked in maize cultivation with reported use of herbicides), giving an odds ratio of 2.7 (90% CI, 1.0-6.9); the numbers of women who had possibly been exposed (acknowledged personal exposure to herbicides or who had worked in some job possibly involving herbicide exposure or who denied personal use of herbicides but worked in maize cultivation after 1964) were 14 cases and 20 controls, giving an odds ratio of 1.8 (0.9-3.5). These odds ratios were slightly higher for women definitely exposed for > 10 years (2.9; 0.9-8.7) than for women exposed for < 10 years (2.3; 0.4-12.3). The same pattern was seen for women who had possibly been exposed. Among subjects definitely exposed to triazine, 4/7 had used triazines and 3/7 had worked in herbicide-treated fields; the equivalent numbers for the controls were 6/7 and 1/7; 5/7 cases and 5/7 controls were also exposed to other herbicides (Donna *et al.*, 1989). [Although risk estimates were not given for exposure to individual triazines, the Working Group noted that the predominant triazine exposure was probably to atrazine; there may also have been exposure to simazine.]

The interpretation of this study was discussed through correspondence (Crosignani *et al.*, 1990; Minder, 1990). In particular, Minder questioned the exposure classification, because 'definitely exposed' included both use of and exposure in the fields to triazines. The authors said that, since triazines are stable chemicals, they had no reason to suppose that preparation and distribution of these herbicides would have led to cumulative exposure greater than that occurring during work carried out in the fields where herbicides were used.

2.2 Case-control studies of lymphatic and haematopoietic malignancies

Parallel population-based case-control interview studies of leukaemia and non-Hodgkin's lymphoma were conducted in Iowa and Minnesota, USA, during 1981-84. In the study of leukaemia (for detailed description, see the monograph on occupational exposures in spraying and application of insecticides, p. 68), 38 cases and 108 controls reported use of atrazine (odds ratio, 1.0; 95% CI, 0.6-1.5) (Brown *et al.*, 1990). In the study of non-Hodgkin's lymphoma, reported in an abstract, small-cell lymphocytic lymphoma was associated with reported use of atrazine (odds ratio, 1.6), as was farming in general (odds ratio, 1.4) [numbers of exposed persons and confidence intervals not given] (Cantor *et al.*, 1985).

In the case-control study undertaken in Kansas, USA, of soft-tissue sarcoma, Hodgkin's disease and non-Hodgkin's lymphoma, described in detail in the monograph on occupational exposures in spraying and application of insecticides (p. 66), 14 cases of non-Hodgkin's lymphoma and 43 controls reported use of triazines (atrazine was one of six triazines mentioned) (odds ratio, 2.5; 95% CI, 1.2-5.4). The odds ratio for non-Hodgkin's lymphoma associated with exposure to triazines was slightly lower in the absence of exposure to phenoxyacetic acid herbicides and uracils (2.2; 95% CI, 0.4-9.1, based on three cases and

11 controls) (Hoar *et al.*, 1986). [The Working Group noted that no information was given about the proportion of triazines represented by atrazine.]

A population-based case-control study was conducted in eastern Nebraska, USA, to evaluate agricultural risk factors for non-Hodgkin's lymphoma (Hoar Zahm *et al.*, 1990). A detailed description of the study design is given in the monograph on occupational exposures in spraying and application of insecticides (p. 66). In an abstract of this study (Hoar Zahm *et al.*, 1988), self-reported use of atrazine was associated with a slightly increased risk (odds ratio, 1.4; 95% CI, 0.8-2.2). Odds ratios by years of atrazine use were 0.9 for 1-5 years, 0.8 for 6-15 years, 2.0 for 16-20 years and 2.0 for 21 or more years. [Although the description is incomplete, the Working Group assumed that these odds ratio were not adjusted for exposures to other chemicals.]

2.3 Case-control study of cancer of the colon

A case-control study from Kansas, USA (reported as a letter to the Editor of *The Lancet*) covered 57 pathologically confirmed cases of colon cancer diagnosed in 1976-82 and 948 population controls selected by random digit dialling, who were interviewed about farming history. Employment on a farm was associated with a slight increase in the incidence of colon cancer (odds ratio, 1.6; 95% CI, 0.8-3.5). The same was true for reported use of triazine (odds ratio, 1.4; 95% CI, 0.2-7.9, based on two exposed cases and 43 exposed controls) (Hoar *et al.*, 1985). [The Working Group noted that apparently the same controls were used as in the study of Hoar *et al.* (1986) and that no information was given about the proportion of triazines represented by atrazine.]

3. Studies of Cancer in Experimental Animals

3.1 Oral administration

Rat: Groups of 53-56 male and 50-55 female Fischer 344/LATI rats, weighing 150-180 g, were fed pelleted diets containing 0 (control), 500 (low dose) or 1000 mg/kg (high dose) atrazine (purity, 98.9%) during the first eight weeks of the study. Because of toxicity, the high dose was reduced to 750 mg/kg of diet and the low dose to 375 mg/kg of diet for life. The experiment was terminated at week 126, when the four surviving males were killed. Six surviving females were killed at week 123. There was no difference in the survival rates in females of all groups; males in the treated groups lived longer than controls. In males of the high-dose group, there was a significantly increased incidence of mammary gland tumours, all but one of which were benign: males—control, 1/48; low-dose, 1/51; and high-dose, 9/53 ($p < 0.05$) (test for trend; $p < 0.01$). In females, a significantly increased incidence of uterine adenocarcinomas was noted: control, 6/45; low-dose, 8/52; and high-dose, 13/45 ($p < 0.05$ trend test). In addition, a few malignant mesenchymal tumours of the uterus were found only in the treated groups: 2/52 low-dose and 1/45 high-dose group. An increased incidence of tumours of the lymphatic and haematopoietic system was noted in females; the numbers of leukaemias and lymphomas combined were 12/44 control, 16/52 low-dose and 22/51 high-dose ($p < 0.05$, trend test) (Pintér *et al.*, 1990).

3.2 Intraperitoneal administration

Mouse: A group of 30 male Swiss mice, four weeks old, received intraperitoneal injections of 'pure' atrazine every third day for 13 injections (total dose, 0.26 mg/kg bw). Two control groups of 50 mice each were treated with saline or were untreated. The experiment was terminated after 375 days, when all surviving animals were killed. The incidence of lymphomas was 6/30 ($p < 0.001$) in the atrazine-treated group and 1/50 in the untreated controls; no tumour was observed in the saline control group (Donna *et al.*, 1986). [The Working Group noted the incomplete reporting of information on survival.]

A group of 25 female Swiss albino mice, seven weeks old, received up to 13 injections of Fogard S (a formulation containing 25% atrazine and 37.5% simazine) at three-day intervals for a total dose of 0.0065 mg of active principle per mouse. One group of 50 saline controls was available. The animals were kept under observation for seven months from the beginning of the treatment. Serial killings took place from one month after the end of treatment to the end of experiment at 15-day intervals. Lymphomas occurred in 2/20 [$p = 0.02$] treated animals; none occurred in the controls (Donna *et al.*, 1981). [The Working Group noted the short duration of treatment and observation, the incomplete reporting of the study and the report of animal losses due to intercurrent disease.]

3.3 Subcutaneous administration

Mouse: A group of 25 female Swiss albino mice, seven weeks old, received 13 subcutaneous injections of Fogard S (a formulation containing 25% atrazine and 37.5% simazine) at three-day intervals for a total dose of 0.0065 mg active principle per mouse. One group of 50 saline controls was also available. All animals were kept under observation for a period of seven months from the beginning of treatment. One animal from each group was sacrificed every 15 days from one month after the end of treatment to the end of the experiment. Lymphomas occurred in 3/24 treated animals compared with none in the controls [$p < 0.01$]. Another mouse had a mesothelioma of the peritoneum (Donna *et al.*, 1981). [The Working Group noted the short duration of treatment and observation, the incomplete reporting of the study and the report of animal losses due to intercurrent disease.]

4. Other Relevant Data

4.1 Absorption, distribution, metabolism and excretion

4.1.1 *Humans*

Workers occupationally exposed to atrazine excreted some unchanged atrazine in their urine (Catenacci *et al.*, 1990). The majority of an absorbed dose was recoverable in urine as the fully dealkylated metabolite, 2-chloro-4,6-diamino-*s*-triazine, and the monodealkylated metabolite, 2-chloro-4-amino 6-(ethylamino)-*s*-triazine; practically none of the other monodealkylated metabolite, 2-chloro-4-amino-6-(isopropylamino)-*s*-triazine, was found (Ikonen *et al.*, 1988). Neither study identified any of the mercapturate metabolites found in the urine of rats exposed to atrazine.

4.1.2 *Experimental systems*

Atrazine was well absorbed after oral dosing in rats; 72-h urinary recoveries were similar (66%) after administration of either 30 mg/kg bw uniformly labelled ^{14}C-atrazine in corn oil

(Timchalk *et al.*, 1990) or approximately 1.5 mg/kg bw ^{14}C-[ring]-atrazine in ethanol (Bakke *et al.*, 1972). Moderate, inverse dose-dependent absorption (3-8% adults; 3-10% juveniles) through the skin was demonstrated in Fischer F344 rats (Shah *et al.*, 1987).

In rats, less than 0.1% of an oral radioactive dose was detected in expired air. At 72 h after dosing, the retention of radioactivity in the carcass ranged from 4% (Timchalk *et al.*, 1990) to 16% (Bakke *et al.*, 1972). Relative tissue retentions were: liver, kidney, lung > heart, brain > > muscle, fat (Bakke *et al.*, 1972).

A one-compartment model adequately describes the kinetics of atrazine in the plasma of rats. The plasma concentration peaked 8-10 h after dosing, with an apparent absorption half-time of 2.6 h, and there was mono-exponential elimination with a half-time of 10.8 h. Neither the kinetic characteristics nor dose recoveries were affected by concurrent administration of 60 mg/kg bw tridiphane, a herbicidal synergist in plants which blocks glutathione transferase-mediated conjugation (Timchalk *et al.*, 1990).

N-Dealkylation and conjugation with glutathione are the main metabolic pathways in various species *in vivo* and *in vitro* (Böhme & Bär, 1967; Adams *et al.*, 1990; Timchalk *et al.*, 1990). 2-Chloro-4,6-diamino-1,3,5-triazine is the major urinary metabolite (64-67%) in rats, and mercapturates of the mono- and di-dealkylated products are the other major urinary metabolites (13-14% and 9%, respectively) (Timchalk *et al.*, 1990). Minor metabolic pathways in rats may include alkyl side-chain oxidation (Böhme & Bär, 1967). Oxidative dechlorination to 2-hydroxyatrazine, a metabolite formed in plants, did not occur in rat liver homogenates (Dauterman & Muecke, 1974), despite the fact that Bakke *et al.* (1972) claimed to have found some 2-hydroxyatrazine in rat urine and showed that it was metabolized along similar pathways to atrazine.

N-Nitrosoatrazine is formed from atrazine in acidic aqueous nitrite solutions and by the action of nitrogen oxides at an air:solid interface (Wolfe *et al.*, 1976; Janzowski *et al.*, 1980). *N*-Nitrosoatrazine was hydrolytically stable in aqueous solutions at pH > 4, although it was relatively susceptible to photolysis (Wolfe *et al.*, 1976). While there was virtually no formation of *N*-nitrosoatrazine in acid nitrated soils treated with 2 ppm (mg/kg) atrazine, exogenously added *N*-nitrosoatrazine was found to be relatively immobile in such soil systems and to degrade over a period of several weeks (Kearney *et al.*, 1977).

4.2 Toxic effects

4.2.1 *Humans*

No data were available to the Working Group.

4.2.2 *Experimental systems*

The oral LD$_{50}$ of atrazine was reported to be 2000 mg/kg bw in rats (Ben-Dyke *et al.*, 1970) and 672, 737 and 2310 mg/kg bw in adult female, male and weanling male rats, respectively. The dermal LD$_{50}$ was > 2500 mg/kg bw in rats of each sex (Gaines & Linder, 1986).

Administration of atrazine by oral gavage at 100-600 mg/kg bw per day to Wistar rats for seven or 14 days induced both nephrotoxicity and hepatotoxicity (Santa Maria *et al.*, 1986, 1987). Hepatotoxic effects included a dose-related reduction in blood sugar levels and increases in the activity of serum alanine aminotransferase and alkaline phosphatase and in the level of total serum lipids. Electron micrographs showed degeneration of the smooth endoplasmic reticulum, lipid droplet accumulation and swollen mitochondria (Santa Maria *et al.*, 1987). There was no liver toxicity at the lowest dose tested. Renal toxicity, in the form of a dose-related proteinurea, reduced creatinine clearance and increased urinary electrolyte output, was evident at all dose levels (Santa Maria *et al.*, 1986).

Hormonal imbalances induced by atrazine may be of significance to the interpretation of possible carcinogenic effects in hormonally sensitive tissues. Most work has been directed towards the effects of atrazine on the pituitary–gonadal axis. Steroid hormone metabolism was found to be impaired by atrazine, which inhibits 5-α-steroid reductase in the anterior pituitary of rats (Kniewald *et al.*, 1979). Subsequently, it was shown in male rats that atrazine (at 120 mg/kg bw per day orally for seven days) increased [~ 60-70%] the wet weight of the anterior pituitary and caused hyperaemia and hypertrophy of the chromophobic cells and reductions of 37%, 39% and 46%, respectively, in 5α-steroid reductase, 3α- and 17β-hydroxysteroid dehydrogenase activities *in vivo*. The de-ethylated metabolite was approximately equipotent in reducing 5α-steroid reductase activity after administration *in vivo*. Only 5α-steroid reductase and 17β-hydroxysteroid dehydrogenase were inhibited by either compound in the hypothalamus *in vivo*; deethylatrazine was the more potent inhibitor of these enzymes in the hypothalamus *in vitro* (Babić-Gojmerac *et al.*, 1989). Treatment prenatally with atrazine or de-ethylatrazine (16.6 mg/kg bw subcutaneously) did not alter pituitary metabolism in male rat pups, but atrazine increased 5α-steroid reductase activity in female pups. Treatment pre- and postnatally with atrazine and its metabolite decreased 3α-hydroxysteroid dehydrogenase activity, and atrazine decreased 5α-steroid reductase activity in male pups; both compounds decreased the number of androgen-specific binding sites in the prostate. Neither atrazine nor its metabolite had any effect on female pituitary androgen metabolism (Kniewald *et al.*, 1987). Other studies conducted *in vitro* have demonstrated inhibition of androgen metabolism by atrazine when incubated with rat pituitary homogenates (Kniewald *et al.*, 1979; Babić-Gojmerac *et al.*, 1989).

4.3 Reproductive and developmental effects

4.3.1 *Humans*

No data were available to the Working Group.

4.3.2 *Experimental systems*

In a teratology study, 10, 70 or 700 mg/kg bw technical atrazine were administered by gavage to Charles River rats once a day on gestation days 6-15, and 1, 5 or 75 mg/kg bw was administered by gavage to New Zealand white rabbits on gestation days 7-19. Incomplete ossification of the skeleton increased with the intermediate dose (70 mg/kg bw) and above; other effects on the rat fetus were observed only at maternally toxic doses, in the form of decreased fetal weight (700 mg/kg bw). In rabbits, increased resorption rate, decreased litter size, lowered fetal weight and a higher rate of non-ossification were observed at the high dose (75 mg/kg bw), which was maternally toxic. It was concluded that on a milligram per kilogram basis, pregnant rabbits are more sensitive than pregnant rats and that atrazine is not teratogenic (Infurna *et al.*, 1988).

Embryotoxicity was reported in rats after subcutaneous injection of 1000 or 2000 mg/kg bw atrazine per day on days 3, 6 and 9 of gestation, but not after administration at concentrations of up to 1000 ppm (mg/kg) in the feed from day 1 throughout gestation. Maternal toxicity was not reported (Peters & Cook, 1973).

Application of atrazine to fertile mallard eggs, by immersing them for 30 sec in an aqueous solution, resulted in embryonic death at exposure levels calculated to be more than 67 times that expected after usual application in the field, i.e., more than 400 lb/acre (448 kg/ha) (Hoffman & Albers, 1984).

Perinatal effects on sex steroid metabolism are discussed in section 4.2.2.

4.4 Genetic and related effects (see also Table 4 and Appendices 1 and 2)

4.4.1 *Humans*

No data were available to the Working Group.

4.4.2 *Experimental systems*

Atrazine did not induce mutation in bacteriophage, bacteria, *Saccharomyces cerevisiae* or *Nicotiana tabacum*, whereas mutations were induced in *Schizosaccharomyces pombe*, *Aspergillus nidulans* and *Zea mays*; conflicting results were obtained in *Hordeum vulgare*. In *Drosophila melanogaster*, sex-linked recessive lethal mutations were induced in one study but not in another. 6-Thioguanine-resistant mutants were induced in cultured Chinese hamster lung V79 cells, only in the presence of microsomes from potato, and not in the presence of an exogenous metabolic activation system from rat liver.

Gene conversion was not induced in *S. cerevisiae* or *A. nidulans*. Mitotic recombination was not increased by atrazine in *S. cerevisiae*, while conflicting results were obtained in *A. nidulans*. Aneuploidy was induced in *Neurospora crassa*, *A. nidulans* and *D. melanogaster*.

Dominant lethal effects were induced in *D. melanogaster*. Chromosomal aberrations were induced in the majority of plants studied. In cultured rodent or human cells, atrazine did not induce chromosomal aberrations, sister chromatid exchange or unscheduled DNA synthesis.

Atrazine induced ampicillin-resistant mutations in *Escherichia coli* in a mouse host-mediated assay. In mammals *in vivo*, atrazine induced DNA strand breakage in rat stomach, liver and kidney cells, but not in lung cells, following oral dosing. It induced dominant lethal effects in mouse spermatids but did not induce morphological abnormalities in mouse sperm heads.

5. Summary of Data Reported and Evaluation

5.1 Exposure data

Atrazine was introduced in 1957. It is now one of the most extensively used herbicides worldwide, with US production of at least 50 000 tonnes per annum since 1980. It is widely used on maize and to a lesser extent on a variety of other crops.

Atrazine has been formulated as wettable powders, granules and liquid formulations.

Table 4. Genetic and related effects of atrazine

Test system	Result[a]		Dose[b] LED/HID	Reference
	Without exogenous metabolic system	With exogenous metabolic system		
BPF, Bacteriophage T4, forward mutation	–	0	20.0000	Andersen et al. (1972)
BPR, Bacteriophage, reverse mutation	–	0	1000.0000	Andersen et al. (1972)
SAF, Salmonella typhimurium, forward mutation	–	–	250.0000	Adler (1980)
SA0, Salmonella typhimurium TA100, reverse mutation	0	–	2500.0000	Simmon et al. (1977)
SA0, Salmonella typhimurium TA100, reverse mutation	–	–	50.0000	Lusby et al. (1979)
SA0, Salmonella typhimurium TA100, reverse mutation	0	–	500.0000	Bartsch et al. (1980)
SA0, Salmonella typhimurium TA100, reverse mutation	–	–	0.0000	Ishidate et al. (1981)
SA0, Salmonella typhimurium TA100, reverse mutation	0	–[c]	15000.0000	Sumner et al. (1984)
SA0, Salmonella typhimurium TA100, reverse mutation	–	–	500.0000	Kappas (1988)
SA0, Salmonella typhimurium TA100, reverse mutation	0	+[c]	0.0000	Means et al. (1988)
SA0, Salmonella typhimurium TA100, reverse mutation	–	–	500.0000	Mersch–Sundermann et al. (1988)
SA0, Salmonella typhimurium TA100, reverse mutation	–	–	500.0000	Zeiger et al. (1988)
SA0, Salmonella typhimurium TA100, reverse mutation	–	0	1000.0000	Butler & Hoagland (1989)
SA2, Salmonella typhimurium TA102, reverse mutation	–	–	500.0000	Mersch–Sundermann et al. (1988)
SA3, Salmonella typhimurium TA1530, reverse mutation (spot test)	–	0	0.0000	Seiler (1973)
SA5, Salmonella typhimurium TA1535, reverse mutation	–	–	2500.0000	Simmon et al. (1977)
SA5, Salmonella typhimurium TA1535, reverse mutation	–	–	50.0000	Lusby et al. (1979)
SA5, Salmonella typhimurium TA1535, reverse mutation	–	–	500.0000	Kappas (1988)
SA5, Salmonella typhimurium TA1535, reverse mutation	–	–	500.0000	Zeiger et al. (1988)
SA7, Salmonella typhimurium TA1537, reverse mutation	0	–	2500.0000	Simmon et al. (1977)
SA7, Salmonella typhimurium TA1537, reverse mutation	–	–	0.0000	Ishidate et al. (1981)
SA7, Salmonella typhimurium TA1537, reverse mutation	–	–	500.0000	Kappas (1988)
SA7, Salmonella typhimurium TA1537, reverse mutation	–	–	500.0000	Zeiger et al. (1988)
SA8, Salmonella typhimurium TA1538, reverse mutation	0	–	2500.0000	Simmon et al. (1977)
SA8, Salmonella typhimurium TA1538, reverse mutation	–	–	500.0000	Kappas (1988)

Table 4 (contd)

Test system	Result[a]		Dose[b] LED/HID	Reference
	Without exogenous metabolic system	With exogenous metabolic system		
SA8, *Salmonella typhimurium* TA1538, reverse mutation	–	–	500.0000	Zeiger et al. (1988)
SA9, *Salmonella typhimurium* TA98, reverse mutation	0	–	2500.0000	Simmon et al. (1977)
SA9, *Salmonella typhimurium* TA98, reverse mutation	–	–	50.0000	Lusby et al. (1979)
SA9, *Salmonella typhimurium* TA98, reverse mutation	0	–	500.0000	Bartsch et al. (1980)
SA9, *Salmonella typhimurium* TA98, reverse mutation	–	–	0.0000	Ishidate et al. (1981)
SA9, *Salmonella typhimurium* TA98, reverse mutation	–	–	500.0000	Kappas (1988)
SA9, *Salmonella typhimurium* TA98, reverse mutation	–	–	500.0000	Mersch–Sundermann et al. (1988)
SA9, *Salmonella typhimurium* TA98, reverse mutation	–	0	1000.0000	Butler & Hoagland (1989)
SAS, *Salmonella typhimurium*, reverse mutation	–	0	0.0000	Andersen et al. (1972)
SAS, *Salmonella typhimurium his* G46, reverse mutation (spot test)	–	0	0.0000	Seiler (1973)
SAS, *Salmonella typhimurium* TA1531, reverse mutation (spot test)	–	0	0.0000	Seiler (1973)
SAS, *Salmonella typhimurium* TA1532, reverse mutation (spot test)	–	0	0.0000	Seiler (1973)
SAS, *Salmonella typhimurium* TA1534, reverse mutation (spot test)	–	0	0.0000	Seiler (1973)
SAS, *Salmonella typhimurium*, reverse mutation	–	–	0.0000	Adler (1980)
SAS, *Salmonella typhimurium* TA97, reverse mutation	–	0	1000.0000	Butler & Hoagland (1989)
SAS, *Salmonella typhimurium* TM677, reverse mutation	0	–[c]	1000.0000	Sumner et al. (1984)
SAS, *Salmonella typhimurium* TA97, reverse mutation	–	–	500.0000	Kappas (1988)
SAS, *Salmonella typhimurium* TA97, reverse mutation	–	–	500.0000	Mersch–Sundermann et al. (1988)
SAS, *Salmonella typhimurium* TA97, reverse mutation	–	–	500.0000	Zeiger et al. (1988)
SCG, *Saccharomyces cerevisiae*, gene conversion	–	+[c]	10.0000	Plewa & Gentile (1976)
SCG, *Saccharomyces cerevisiae*, gene conversion	–	–	2000.0000	Adler (1980)
SCG, *Saccharomyces cerevisiae*, gene conversion	–	–	4000.0000	de Bertoldi et al. (1980)
SCG, *Saccharomyces cerevisiae*, mitotic recombination	–	0	50.0000	Emnova et al. (1987)

Table 4 (contd)

Test system	Result[a] Without exogenous metabolic system	Result[a] With exogenous metabolic system	Dose[b] LED/HID	Reference
ANG, *Aspergillus nidulans*, gene conversion	−	0	8000.0000	de Bertoldi et al. (1980)
ANG, *Aspergillus nidulans*, mitotic recombination	−	+	0.0000	Adler (1980)
ANG, *Aspergillus nidulans*, mitotic recombination	−	−	1000.0000	Kappas (1988)
SCF, *Saccharomyces cerevisiae*, forward mutation	−	0	50.0000	Emnova et al. (1987)
SZR, *Schizosaccharomyces pombe*, reverse mutation	+	0	17.5000	Mathias (1987)
SZR, *Schizosaccharomyces pombe*, reverse mutation	+	+[c]	70.0000	Mathias et al. (1989)
ANF, *Aspergillus nidulans*, forward mutation	−	+	2500.0000	Benigni et al. (1979)
ANN, *Aspergillus nidulans*, aneuploidy	−	+	2000.0000	Benigni et al. (1979)
NCN, *Neurospora crassa*, aneuploidy	+	0	0.0000	Griffiths (1979)
HSM, *Hordeum vulgare*, mutation	+	0	1000.0000	Wuu & Grant (1966)
HSM, *Hordeum vulgare*, mutation	−	0	200.0000	Stroyev (1968)
PLM, *Zea mays*, mutation	+	0	200.0000	Morgun et al. (1982)
PLM, *Zea mays*, mutation	+	0	0.0000	Plewa et al. (1984)
PLM, *Nicotiana tabacum*, mutation	−	0	0.0000[d]	Bříza (1989)
TSI, *Tradescantia paludosa*, micronuclei	−	0	200.0000	Ma et al. (1984)
HSC, *Hordeum vulgare*, chromosomal aberrations	+	0	500.0000 spray	Wuu & Grant (1967a)
HSC, *Hordeum vulgare*, chromosomal aberrations	−	0	2000.0000	Müller et al. (1972)
* *Hordeum vulgare*, decrease in chiasma frequency	+	0	1000.0000	Sharma et al. (1982)
VFC, *Vicia faba*, chromosomal aberrations	+	0	400.0000	Wuu & Grant (1967b)
VFC, *Vicia faba*, chromosomal aberrations	−	0	200.0000	Müller et al. (1972)
PLC, *Sorghum* sp, chromosomal aberrations	+	0	0.0000[d]	Liang & Liang (1972)
PLC, *Sorghum* sp, chromosomal aberrations	−	0	0.0000	Müller et al. (1972)
PLC, *Sorghum* sp, chromosomal aberrations	+	0	0.0000	Lee et al. (1974)
PLC, *Nigella damascena*, chromosomal aberrations	−	0	320.0000	Mathias (1987)
PLC, *Nigella damascena*, chromosomal aberrations	+	0	40.0000[d]	Mathias (1987)
PLC, *Zea mays*, chromosomal aberrations	−	0	200.0000	Morgun et al. (1982)
DMX, *Drosophila melanogaster*, sex-linked recessive lethal mutation	+	0	100.0000	Murnik & Nash (1977)

Table 4 (contd)

Test system	Result[a] Without exogenous metabolic system	With exogenous metabolic system	Dose[b] LED/HID	Reference
DMX, *Drosophila melanogaster*, sex–linked recessive lethal mutation	−	0	2000.0000	Adler (1980)
DML, *Drosophila melanogaster*, dominant lethal mutation	+	0	100.0000	Murnik & Nash (1977)
DMN, *Drosophila melanogaster*, aneuploidy	+	0	100.0000	Murnik & Nash (1977)
G9H, Gene mutation, Chinese hamster lung V79 cells *in vitro*, *hprt* locus	−	−[e]	2000.0000	Adler (1980)
SIC, Sister chromatid exchange, Chinese hamster CHO cells *in vitro*	−	−	2000.0000	Adler (1980)
CIC, Chromosomal aberrations, Chinese hamster CHO cells *in vitro*	−	−	2000.0000	Adler (1980)
CIC, Chromosomal aberrations, Chinese hamster cells *in vitro*	−	0	250.0000	Ishidate (1988)
UHF, Unscheduled DNA synthesis, human EUE cells *in vitro*	−	−[e]	650.0000	Adler (1980)
SHL, Sister chromatid exchanges, human lymphocytes *in vitro*	−	0	0.0000	Ghiazza *et al.* (1984)
HMM, Host–mediated assay, *Escherichia coli* ampr in mouse	+	0	100.0000 × 1 p.o.	Adler (1980)
DVA, DNA strand breaks, rat stomach, liver and kidney *in vivo*	+	0	875.0000 × 1 p.o.	Pino *et al.* (1988)
DVA, DNA strand breaks, rat stomach, liver and kidney *in vivo*	+	0	350.0000 × 15 p.o.	Pino *et al.* (1988)
DVA, DNA strand breaks, rat lung *in vivo*	−	0	875.0000 × 1 p.o.	Pino *et al.* (1988)
DVA, DNA strand breaks, rat lung *in vivo*	−	0	350.0000 × 15 p.o.	Pino *et al.* (1988)
DLM, Dominant lethal mutation, mouse spermatids	(+)	0	1500.0000 × 1 p.o.	Adler (1980)
SPM, Sperm morphology, mouse	−	0	600.0000	Osterloh *et al.* (1983)

*Not displayed on profile

[a] +, positive; (+), weakly positive; −, negative; 0, not tested; ?, inconclusive (variable response in several experiments within an adequate study)

[b] In–vitro tests, μg/ml; in–vivo tests, mg/kg bw

[c] Tested with extracts of atrazine–treated *Zea mays*

[d] Commercial pesticide

[e] Positive with potato microsomes at doses up to 3 mM

Exposure can occur during production and application of atrazine and *via* contaminated ground- and surface water. Exposure could also occur from consumption of foods containing residues. Atrazine residues were not detected in large-scale surveys of foods products in Canada and the USA.

5.2 Carcinogenicity in humans

One population-based case-control study in northern Italy found an elevated risk for ovarian cancer in women considered to have been exposed to triazine herbicides. A hospital-based case-control study in the same area found an elevated risk for ovarian tumours among women exposed to herbicides, including triazine herbicides.

A case-control study from Kansas, USA, indicated an association between self-reported use of triazine herbicides and risk for non-Hodgkin's lymphoma. A nonsignificant doubling of the risk was found in the absence of exposure to phenoxyacetic acid herbicides and uracils. In another study in Kansas, USA, in which apparently the same controls were used, self-reported use of triazine herbicides was associated with a slight excess risk of colon cancer, as was employment on a farm in general.

In two case-control studies from Iowa and Minnesota, USA, there was no association between self-reported use of atrazine and leukaemia, whereas a slightly increased risk was suggested for a subgroup of lymphomas.

In a case-control study in Nebraska, USA, a nonsignificant elevation in risk for non-Hodgkin's lymphoma was associated with self-reported use of atrazine. Risks were greater among men with 16 or more years of use than among those with a shorter duration.

These seven studies were considered to provide some evidence for the carcinogenicity of exposure to triazine herbicides. Complex exposures and insufficient reporting made it difficult to evaluate the carcinogenicity of individual triazine herbicides, including atrazine.

5.3 Carcinogenicity in experimental animals

Atrazine was tested for carcinogenicity in one experiment by oral administration to rats, producing increased incidences of mammary tumours (mainly benign) in males and of uterine adenocarcinomas and tumours of the haematopoietic system in females. It was also tested by intraperitoneal administration to mice; it was stated in a preliminary report to have produced an increase in the incidence of lymphomas.

5.4 Other relevant data

Atrazine was embryotoxic and embryolethal but not teratogenic in rats and rabbits when administered at maternally toxic doses.

Atrazine and its de-ethylated metabolite have been shown to alter the activity of some testosterone-metabolizing enzymes in the rat pituitary and hypothalamus, and to decrease hormone-receptor binding in the prostate.

No data were available on the genetic and related effects of atrazine in humans.

Atrazine induced DNA strand breaks in stomach, liver and kidney cells but not lung cells of rats treated orally. Chromosomal aberrations were induced in plants and insects, but not in cultured rodent cells. Aneuploidy was induced in *Drosophila melanogaster* and fungi. Atrazine induced gene mutation in plants, but not in bacteria or cultured rodent cells.

5.5 Evaluation[1]

There is *inadequate evidence* in humans for the carcinogenicity of atrazine.

There is *limited evidence* in experimental animals for the carcinogenicity of atrazine.

In making the overall evaluation, the Working Group took into consideration the following supporting evidence. The increased risks for tumours that are known to be associated with hormonal factors, which were observed in studies of both animals and human beings, are consistent with the known effects of atrazine on the hypothalamic–pituitary–gonadal axis.

Overall evaluation

Atrazine *is possibly carcinogenic to humans (Group 2B).*

6. References

Adams, N.H., Levi, P.E. & Hodgson, E. (1990) In vitro studies of the metabolism of atrazine, simazine and terbutryn in several vertebrate species. *J. agric. Food Chem.*, *38*, 1411-1417

Adler, I.D. (1980) A review of the coordinated research effort on the comparison of test systems for the detection of mutagenic effects sponsored by the EEC. *Mutat. Res.*, *74*, 77-93

American Conference of Governmental Industrial Hygienists (1989) *Threshold Limit Values and Biological Exposure Indices for 1988-1989*, Cincinnati, OH, p. 12

Andersen, K.J., Leighty, E.G. & Takahashi, M.K. (1972) Evaluation of herbicides for possible mutagenic properties. *J. agric. Food Chem.*, *20*, 649-656

Anon. (1989a) *MSDS Reference for Crop Protection 1988/1989*, New York, Chemical and Pharmaceutical Press, pp. 71-72, 118-126, 133-138, 142-147, 309-313, 346-351, 358-363, 705-709, 861-865, 912-915, 1115-1118, 1381-1385

Anon. (1989b) *Crop Protection Chemicals Reference*, 5th ed., New York, Chemical and Pharmaceutical Press, pp. 402-405, 513-536, 541-550, 741-746, 811-824, 827-860, 1419-1424, 1655-1660, 1706-1709, 1868-1870, 2129-2132

Babić-Gojmerac, T., Kniewald, Z. & Kniewald, J. (1989) Testoterone metabolism in neuroendocrine organs in male rats under atrazine and deethylatrazine influence. *J. steroid Biochem.*, *33*, 141-146

Bakke, J.E., Larson, J.D. & Price, C.E. (1972) Metabolism of atrazine and 2-hydroxyatrazine by the rat. *J. agric. Food Chem.*, *20*, 602-607

Bartsch, H., Malaveille, C., Camus, A.-M., Martel-Planche, G., Brun, G., Hautefeuille, A., Sabadie, N., Barbin, A., Kuroki, T., Drevon, C., Piccoli, C. & Montesano, R. (1980) Validation and comparative studies on 180 chemicals with *S. typhimurium* strains and V79 Chinese hamster cells in the presence of various metabolizing systems. *Mutat. Res.*, *76*, 1-50

Ben-Dyke, R., Sanderson, D.M. & Noakes, D.N. (1970) Acute toxicity data for pesticides (1970). *World Rev. Pest Control*, *9*, 119-127

Benigni, R., Bignami, M., Camoni, I., Carere, A., Conti, G., Iachetta, R., Morpurgo, G. & Ortali, V.A. (1979) A new in vitro method for testing plant metabolism in mutagenicity studies. *J. Toxicol. environ. Health*, *5*, 809-819

---

[1]For definition of the italicized terms, see Preamble, pp. 26-28.

de Bertoldi, M., Griselli, M., Giovannetti, M. & Barale, R. (1980) Mutagenicity of pesticides evaluated by means of gene-conversion in *Saccharomyces cerevisiae* and in *Aspergillus nidulans*. *Environ. Mutagenesis*, *2*, 359-370

Böhme, C. & Bär, F. (1967) The transformation of triazine herbicides in the animal organism (Ger.). *Food Cosmet. Toxicol.*, *5*, 23-28

Bříza, J. (1989) Estimation of mutagenicity and metabolic activation after recurrent exposures of *Nicotiana tabacum* L. var. *xanthi* to 14 pesticides. *Biol. Plant. (Prague)*, *31*, 145-151

Brown, L.M., Blair, A., Gibson, R., Everett, G.D., Cantor, K.P., Schuman, L.M., Burmeister, L.F., Van Lier, S.F. & Dick, F. (1990) Pesticide exposures and other agricultural risk factors for leukemia among men in Iowa and Minnesota. *Cancer Res.*, *50*, 6585-6591

Butler, M.A. & Hoagland, R.E. (1989) Genotoxicity assessment of atrazine and some major metabolites in the Ames test. *Bull. environ. Contam. Toxicol.*, *43*, 797-804

Cantor, K., Everett, G., Blair, A., Gibson, R., Schuman, L. & Isacson, P. (1985) Farming and non-Hodgkin's lymphoma (Abstract). *Am. J. Epidemiol.*, *122*, 535

Catenacci, G., Maroni, M., Cottica, D. & Pozzoli, L. (1990) Assessment of human exposure to atrazine through the determination of free atrazine in urine. *Bull. environ. Contam. Toxicol.*, *44*, 1-7

Cohen, S.Z., Eiden, C. & Lorber, M.N. (1986) Monitoring ground water for pesticides. In: *Evaluation of Pesticides in Ground Water* (ACS Symposium Series No. 315), Washington DC, American Chemical Society

Cook, W.A., ed. (1987) *Occupational Exposure Limits—Worldwide*, Washington DC, American Industrial Hygiene Association, pp. 18, 128, 162-163

Crosignani, P., Donna, A. & Berrino, F. (1990) Triazine herbicides and ovarian epithelial neoplasms. The authors' reply (Letter to the Editor). *Scand. J. Work Environ. Health*, *16*, 446-447

Dauterman, W.C. & Muecke, W. (1974) In vitro metabolism of atrazine by rat liver. *Pestic. Biochem. Physiol.*, *4*, 212-219

Donna, A., Betta, P.G., Gagliardi, F., Ghiazza, G.F., Gallareto, M. & Gabutto, V. (1981) Preliminary experimental contribution to the study of possible carcinogenic activity of two herbicides containing atrazine-simazine and trifluralin as active principles. *Pathologica*, *73*, 707-721

Donna, A., Betta, P.-G., Robutti, F., Crosignani, P., Berrino, F. & Bellingeri, D. (1984) Ovarian mesothelial tumors and herbicides: a case-control study. *Carcinogenesis*, *5*, 941-942

Donna, A., Betta, P.G., Robutti, F. & Bellingeri, D. (1986) Carcinogenicity testing of atrazine: preliminary report on a 13-month study on male Swiss albino mice treated by intraperitoneal administration. *Med. Lav.*, *8*, 119-121

Donna, A., Crosignani, P., Robutti, F., Betta, P.G., Bocca, R., Mariani, N., Ferrario, F., Fissi, R. & Berrino, F. (1989) Triazine herbicides and ovarian epithelial neoplasms. *Scand. J. Work Environ. Health*, *15*, 47-53

Emnova, E.E., Mereniouk, G.V. & Tsourkan, L.G. (1987) Genetic study of simazine-triazine herbicides on *Saccharomyces cerevisiae* (Russ.). *Tsitol. Genet.*, *21*, 127-130

Funari, E., Brambillia, A.L., Camani, I., Canuti, A., Cavallaro, A., Chierici, S., Cialella, G., Donati, G., Iaforte, A., Prandi, L., Salamana, V., Silano, V. & Zapponi, G.A. (1988) Extensive atrazine pollution of drinking water in the Lombardia region and related public health aspects. *Biomed. environ. Sci.*, *1*, 350-355

Gaines, T.B. & Linder, R.E. (1986) Acute toxicity of pesticides in adult and weanling rats. *Fundam. appl. Toxicol.*, *7*, 299-308

Ghiazza, G., Zavarise, G., Lanero, M. & Ferraro, G. (1984) SCE (sister chromatid exchanges) induced in chromosomes of human lymphocytes by trifluralin, atrazine and simazine (Ital.). *Boll. Soc. It. Biol. sper.*, *60*, 2149-2153

Government of Canada (1990) *Report on National Surveillance Data from 1984/85 to 1988/89*, Ottawa

Griffiths, A.J.F. (1979) Neurospora prototroph selection system for studying aneuploid production. *Environ. Health Perspect.*, *31*, 75-80

Harris, C.I. (1967) Fate of 2-chloro-*s*-triazine herbicides in soil. *J. agric. Food Chem.*, *15*, 157-162

Health and Welfare Canada (1990) *National Pesticide Residue Limits in Food*, Ottawa, Bureau of Chemical Safety, Food Directorate, Health Protection Branch

Hoar, S.K., Blair, A., Holmes, F.F., Boysen, C. & Robel, R.J. (1985) Herbicides and colon cancer (Letter to the Editor). *Lancet*, *i*, 1277-1278

Hoar, S.K., Blair, A., Holmes, F.F., Boysen, C., Robel, R.J., Hoover, R. & Fraumeni, J.F. (1986) Agricultural herbicide use and risk of lymphoma and soft-tissue sarcoma. *J. Am. med. Assoc.*, *256*, 1141-1147

Hoar Zahm, S., Weisenburger, D.D., Babbitt, P.A., Saal, R.C., Cantor, K.P. & Blair, A. (1988) A case-control study of non-Hodgkin's lymphoma and agricultural factors in eastern Nebraska (Abstract). *Am. J. Epidemiol.*, *128*, 901

Hoar Zahm, S., Weisenburger, D.D., Babbitt, P.A., Saal, R.C., Vaught, J.B., Cantor, K.P. & Blair, A. (1990) A case-control study of non-Hodgkin's lymphoma and the herbicide 2,4-dichlorophenoxyacetic acid (2,4-D) in eastern Nebraska. *Epidemiology*, *1*, 349-356

Hoffman, D.J. & Albers, P.H. (1984) Evaluation of potential embryotoxicity and teratogenicity of 42 herbicides, insecticides, and petroleum contaminants to mallard eggs. *Arch. environ. Contam. Toxicol.*, *13*, 15-27

Hörmann, W.D., Tournayre, J.C. & Egli, H. (1979) Triazine herbicide residues in central European streams. *Pestic. Monit. J.*, *13*, 128-131

Hurle, K. & Kibler, E. (1976) The effect of changing moisture conditions on the degradation of atrazine in soil. In: *Proceedings of the British Crop Protection Conference on Weeds*, Vol. 2, Thornton Heath, British Crop Protection Council, pp. 627-633

IARC (1987a) *IARC Monographs on the Evaluation of Carcinogenic Risks to Humans*, Suppl. 7, *Overall Evaluations of Carcinogenicity: An Updating of* IARC Monographs *Volumes 1 to 42*, Lyon, pp. 211-216

IARC (1987b) *IARC Monographs on the Evaluation of Carcinogenic Risks to Humans*, Suppl. 7, *Overall Evaluations of Carcinogenicity: An Updating of* IARC Monographs *Volumes 1 to 42*, Lyon, pp. 156-160

Ikonen, R., Kangas, J. & Savolainen, H. (1988) Urinary atrazine metabolites as indicators for rat and human exposure to atrazine. *Toxicol. Lett.*, *44*, 109-112

Infurna, R., Levy, B., Meng, C., Yau, E., Traina, V., Rolofson, G., Stevens, J. & Barnett, J. (1988) Teratological evaluations of atrazine technical, a triazine herbicide, in rats and rabbits. *J. Toxicol. environ. Health*, *24*, 307-319

Ishidate, M., Jr (1988) *Data Book of Chromosomal Aberration Test In Vitro*, rev. ed., Amsterdam, Elsevier, p. 34

Ishidate, M., Jr, Sofuni, T. & Yoshikawa, K. (1981) Chromosomal aberration tests *in vitro* as a primary screening tool for environmental mutagens and/or carcingens. *Gann*, *27*, 95-108

Izmerov, N.F., ed. (1982) *International Register of Potentially Toxic Chemicals, Scientific Reviews of Soviet Literature on Toxicity and Hazards of Chemicals: Atrazine* (Issue 18), Moscow, Centre of International Projects, United Nations Environment Programme

Janzowski, C., Klein, R. & Preussmann, R. (1980) Formation of N-nitroso compounds of the pesticides atrazine, simazine and carbaryl with nitrogen oxides. In: Walker, E.A., Griciute, L., Castegnaro, M. & Börzsönyi, M., eds, N-*Nitroso Compounds: Analysis, Formation and Occurrence* (IARC Scientific Publications No. 31), Lyon, IARC, pp. 329-339

Kappas, A. (1988) On the mutagenic and recombinogenic activity of certain herbicides in *Salmonella typhimurium* and in *Aspergillus nidulans. Mutat. Res.*, *214*, 615-621

Kearney, P.C., Oliver, J.E., Helling, C.S., Isensee, A.R. & Konston, A. (1977) Distribution, movement, persistence and metabolism of *N*-nitrososatrazine in soils and a model aquatic system. *J. agric. Food Chem.*, *25*, 1177-1181

Kniewald, J., Mildner, P. & Kniewald, Z. (1979) Effects of *s*-triazine herbicides on hormone-receptor complex formation, 5α-reductase and 3α-hydroxysteroid dehydrogenase activity at the anterior pituitary level. *J. Steroid Biochem.*, *11*, 833-838

Kniewald, J., Peruzovic, M., Gojmerac, T., Milković, K. & Kniewald, Z. (1987) Indirect influence of *s*-triazines on rat gonadotropic mechanism at early postnatal period. *J. Steroid Biochem.*, *27*, 1095-1100

Lee, K.C., Rao, G.M., Barnett, F.L. & Liang, G.H. (1974) Further evidence of meiotic instability induced by atrazine in grain sorghum. *Cytologia*, *34*, 697-702

Liang, G.H. & Liang, Y.T.S. (1972) Effects of atrazine on chromosomal behavior in sorghum. *Can. J. Genet. Cytol.*, *14*, 423-427

Luke, M.A., Masumoto, M.T., Cairns, T. & Hundley, H.K. (1988) Levels and incidences of pesticide residues in various foods and animals feeds analyzed by the Luke multiresidue methodology for fiscal years 1982-1986. *J. Assoc. off. anal. Chem.*, *71*, 415-420

Lusby, A.F., Simmons, Z. & McGuire, P.M. (1979) Variation in mutagenicity of *s*-triazine compounds tested on four *Salmonella* strains. *Environ. Mutagenesis*, *1*, 287-290

Ma, T.H., Harris, M.M., Anderson, V.A., Ahmed, I., Mohammad, K., Bare, J.L. & Lin, G. (1984) Tradescantia-micronucleus (Trad-MCN) tests on 140 health-related agents. *Mutat. Res.*, *138*, 157-167

Mathias, M. (1987) Comparison of the genotoxicity of two atrazine preparations in the yeast *Schizosaccharomyces pombe* Lindner and in the plant *Nigella damascena* L. (Fr.). *Bull. Soc. R. Sci. Liège*, *56*, 425-432

Mathias, M., Gilot-Delhalle, J. & Moutschen, J. (1989) Mutagenicity of atrazine in *Schizosaccharomyces pombe* Lindner with and without metabolic activation by maize. *Environ. exp. Bot.*, *29*, 237-240

Means, J.C., Plewa, M.J. & Gentile, J.M. (1988) Assessment of the mutagenicity of fractions from *s*-triazine-treated *Zea mays. Mutat. Res.*, *197*, 325-326

Meister, R.T., ed. (1990) *Farm Chemicals Handbook '90*, Willoughby, OH, Meister Publishing Company, pp. C4-C5, C27-C28

Mersch-Sundermann, V., Dickgiesser, N., Hablizel, U. & Gruber, B. (1988) Examination of the mutagenicity of organic microcontaminations in the environment. I. Mutagenicity of selected herbicides and insecticides with the *Salmonella*-microsome test (Ames test) with consideration of the pathogenic potency of contaminated ground- and drinking water (Ger.). *Zbl. Bakt. Hyg. B.*, *186*, 247-260

Minder, C.E. (1990) Triazine herbicides and ovarian epithelial neoplasms (Letter to the Editor). *Scand. J. Work Environ. Health*, *16*, 445-446

Morgun, V.V., Logvinenko, V.F., Merezhinskii, Y.G., Lapina, T.V. & Grigorenko, N.V. (1982) Cytogenetic and genetic activity of the herbicides atrazine, simazine, prometrin and linuron (Russ.). *Tsitol. Genet.*, *16*, 38-41

Müller, A., Ebert, E. & Gast, A. (1972) Cytogenetic studies with atrazine (2-chloro-4-ethyl-amino-6-isopropylamino-s-triazine) on plants. *Experientia*, *28*, 704-705

Murnik, M.R. & Nash, C.L. (1977) Mutagenicity of the triazine herbicides atrazine, cyanazine and simazine in *Drosophila melanogaster*. *J. Toxicol. environ. Health*, *3*, 691-697

Osterloh, J., Letz, G., Pond, S. & Becker, C. (1983) An assessment of the potential testicular toxicity of 10 pesticides using the mouse-sperm morphology assay. *Mutat. Res.*, *116*, 407-415

Peters, J.W. & Cook, R.M. (1973) Effects of atrazine on reproduction in rats. *Bull. environ. Contam. Toxicol.*, *9*, 301-304

Pino, A., Maura, A. & Grillo, P. (1988) DNA damage in stomach, kidney, liver and lung of rats treated with atrazine. *Mutat. Res.*, *209*, 145-147

Pintér, A., Török, G., Börzsönyi, M., Surján, A., Csik, M., Kelecsényi, Z. & Kocsis, Z. (1990) Long-term carcinogenicity bioassay of the herbicide atrazine in F344 rats. *Neoplasma*, *37*, 533-544

Plewa, M.J. & Gentile, J.M. (1976) Mutagenicity of atrazine: a maize-microbe bioassay. *Mutat. Res.*, *18*, 287-292

Plewa, M.J., Wagner, E.D., Gentile, G.J. & Gentile, J.M. (1984) An evaluation of the genotoxic properties of herbicides following plant and animal activation. *Mutat. Res.*, *136*, 233-245

Reed, J.R., Hall, F.R. & Krueger, H.R. (1990) Measurement of ATV applicator exposure to atrazine using an Eliza method. *Bull. environ. Contam. Toxicol.*, *44*, 8-12

Royal Society of Chemistry (1986) *European Directory of Agrochemical Products*, Vol. 2, *Herbicides*, Cambridge, pp. 51-79

Royal Society of Chemistry (1989) *The Agrochemicals Handbook* [Dialog Information Services (File 306)], Cambridge

Sadtler Research Laboratories (1980) *The Standard Spectra, 1980, Cumulative Index*, Philadelphia, PA

Santa Maria, C., Vilas, M.G., Muriana, F.G. & Relimpio, A. (1986) Subacute atrazine effects on rat renal function. *Bull. environ. Contam. Toxicol.*, *36*, 325-331

Santa Maria, C., Moreno, J. & Lopez-Campos, J.L. (1987) Hepatotoxicity induced by the herbicide atrazine in the rat. *J. appl. Toxicol.*, *7*, 373-378

Seiler, J.P. (1973) A survey on the mutagenicity of various pesticides. *Experientia*, *29*, 622-623

Shah, P.V., Fisher, H.L., Sumler, M.R., Monroe, R.J., Chernoff, N. & Hall, L.L. (1987) Comparison of the penetration of 14 pesticides through the skin of young and adult rats. *J. Toxicol. environ. Health*, *21*, 353-366

Sharma, C.B.S.R., Rao, A.A., Murty, K.V. & Raju, D.S.S. (1982) Induced variation in chiasma frequency in barley in response to atrazine and simazine treatments. *Indian J. exp. Biol.*, *20*, 97-98

Simmon, V.F., Kauhanen, K. & Tardiff, R.G. (1977) Mutagenic activity of chemicals identified in drinking water. In: Scott, D., Bridges, B.A. & Sobels, F.H., eds, *Progress in Genetic Toxicology*, Amsterdam, North-Holland Biomedical Press, pp. 249-258

Smith, A.E., Grover, R., Emmond, G.S. & Korven, H.C. (1975) Persistence and movement of atrazine, bromocil, monuron, and simazine in intermittently filled irrigation ditches. *Can. J. Plant Sci.*, *55*, 809-816

Stroyev, V.S. (1968) The mutagenic effect by the action of herbicides on the barley (Russ.). *Genetika*, *4*, 164-167

Sumner, D.D., Cassidy, J.E., Szolics, I.M., Marco, G.J., Bakshi, K.S. & Brusick, D.J. (1984) Evaluation of the mutagenic potential of corn (*Zea mays* L.) grown in untreated and atrazine (AATREX) treated soil in the field. *Drug chem. Toxicol.*, *7*, 243-257

Timchalk, C., Dryzga, M.D., Langvardt, P.W., Kastl, P.E. & Osborne, D.W. (1990) Determination of the effect of tridiphane on the pharmacokinetics of [^{14}C]-atrazine following oral administration to male Fischer 344 rats. *Toxicology*, *61*, 27-40

US Environmental Protection Agency (1980) *Preliminary Quantitative Usage Analysis of Atrazine*, Washington DC, Office of Pesticide Programs

US Environmental Protection Agency (1983) *Guidance for the Reregistration of Pesticide Products Containing Atrazine as the Active Ingredient*, Washington DC

US Environmental Protection Agency (1988) Method 525. Determination of organic compounds in drinking water by liquid-solid extraction and capillary column gas chromatography/mass spectrometry. In: *Methods for the Determination of Organic Compounds in Drinking Water* (EPA Report No. EPA-600/4-88/039; US NTIS PB89-220461), Cincinnati, OH, Environmental Monitoring Systems Laboratory, pp. 325-356

US Environmental Protection Agency (1989a) Method 507. Determination of nitrogen- and phosphorus-containing pesticides in water by gas chromatography with a nitrogen-phosphorus detector. In: *Methods for the Determination of Organic Compounds in Drinking Water* (EPA Report No. EPA-600/4-88/039; US NTIS PB89-220461), Cincinnati, OH, Environmental Monitoring Systems Laboratory, pp. 143-170

US Environmental Protection Agency (1989b) Method 505. Analysis of organohalide pesticides and commercial polychlorinated biphenyl (PCB) products in water by microextraction and gas chromatography. In: *Methods for the Determination of Organic Compounds in Drinking Water* (EPA Report No. EPA-600/4-88/039; US NTIS PB89-220461), Cincinnati, OH, Environmental Monitoring Systems Laboratory, pp. 109-141

US Environmental Protection Agency (1989c) Atrazine: tolerances for residues. Tolerances and exemptions from tolerances for pesticide chemicals in or on raw agricultural commodities. *US Code fed. Regul.*, *Title 40*, Part 180-220

US Environmental Protection Agency (1990) *Pesticides Industry Sales and Usage: 1988 Market Estimates*, Washington DC, Office of Pesticide Programs

US Food and Drug Administration (1989) Atrazine. In: *Pesticide Analytical Manual*, Vol. II, *Methods Which Detect Multiple Residues*, Washington DC, US Department of Health and Human Services, pp. 1-7

US Occupational Safety and Health Administration (1989) Air contaminants—permissible exposure limits. *US Code fed. Regul., Title 29*, Part 1910.1000

WHO (1987) *Drinking-water Quality: Guidelines for Selected Herbicides* (Environmental Health Criteria 27), Copenhagen, p. 4

Williams, S., ed. (1984) *Official Methods of Analysis of the Association of Official Analytical Chemists*, 14th ed., Washington DC, Association of Official Analytical Chemists, pp. 145-146

Wolfe, N.L., Zepp, R.G., Gordon, J.A. & Fincher, R.C. (1976) N-Nitrosamine formation from atrazine. *Bull. environ. Contam. Toxicol.*, *15*, 342-347

Worthing, C.R. & Walker, S.B., eds (1987) *The Pesticide Manual: A World Compendium*, 8th ed., Thornton Heath, British Crop Protection Council, pp. 36-37

Wuu, K.D. & Grant, W.F. (1966) Morphological and somatic chromosomal aberrations induced by pesticides in barley (*Hordeum vulgare*). *Can. J. Genet. Cytol.*, *8*, 481-501

Wuu, K.D. & Grant, W.F. (1967a) Chromosomal aberrations induced by pesticides in meiotic cells of barley. *Cytologia, 32,* 31-41

Wuu, K.D. & Grant, W.F. (1967b) Chromosomal aberrations induced in somatic cells of *Vicia faba* by pesticides. *Nucleus, 10,* 37-46

Zeiger, E., Anderson, B., Haworth, S., Lawlor, T. & Mortelmans, K. (1988) *Salmonella* mutagenicity tests: IV. Results from the testing of 300 chemicals. *Environ. mol. Mutagenesis, 11* (Suppl. 12), 1-158

MONURON

This substance was considered by a previous Working Group, in 1976 (IARC, 1976). Since that time, new data have become available, and these have been incorporated into the monograph and taken into consideration in the present evaluation.

1. Exposure Data

1.1 Chemical and physical data

1.1.1 Synonyms, structural and molecular data

Chem. Abstr. Serv. Reg. No.: 150-68-5

Chem. Abstr. Name: N'-(4-Chlorophenyl)-N,N-dimethylurea

IUPAC Systematic Name: 3-(4-Chlorophenyl)-1,1-dimethylurea; 3-(4-chlorophenyl)-1,1-dimethyluronium trichloroacetate

Synonyms: Chlorfenidim; N-(*para*-chlorophenyl)-N',N'-dimethylurea; N-(4-chlorophenyl)-N',N'-dimethylurea; 1-(4-chlorophenyl)-3,3-dimethylurea; 1-(*para*-chlorophenyl)-3,3-dimethylurea; 3-(*para*-chlorophenyl)-1,1-dimethylurea; CMU; 1,1-dimethyl-3-(*para*-chlorophenyl)urea; 1,1-dimethyl-3-(4-chlorophenyl)urea; N,N-dimethyl-N'-(4-chlorophenyl)urea

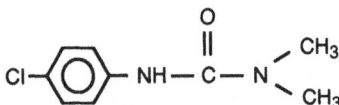

C$_9$H$_{11}$ClN$_2$O   Mol. wt: 198.65

1.1.2 Chemical and physical properties

(a) *Description*: Colourless crystals with a slight odour (Budavari, 1989; Royal Society of Chemistry, 1989)

(b) *Melting-point*: 174-175°C (Royal Society of Chemistry, 1989)

(c) *Spectroscopy data*: Infrared (prism [10667]; grating [28355]), ultraviolet [20884] and nuclear magnetic resonance (proton [16056]) spectral data have been reported (Sadtler Research Laboratories, 1980).

(d) *Solubility*: Slightly soluble in water (230 mg/l at 25°C) and benzene (3 g/kg at 27°C); moderately soluble in methanol (177 g/kg at 25°C), ethanol, acetone (52 g/kg at 27°C); practically insoluble in hydrocarbon solvents (Budavari, 1989; Royal Society of Chemistry, 1989)

(e) *Vapour pressure*: 5×10^{-7} mm Hg [0.7×10^{-7} kPa] at 25°C (Budavari, 1989)

(f)   *Stability*: Stable toward oxygen and moisture under ordinary conditions at neutral pH; elevated temperatures and more acid or alkaline conditions increase the rate of hydrolysis (Budavari, 1989; Royal Society of Chemistry, 1989)

(g)   *Conversion factor for airborne concentration*[1]: $mg/m^3 = 8.12 \times ppm$

1.1.3   *Trade names, technical products and impurities*

Some examples of trade names are: Karmex Monuron Herbicide; Karmex W. Monuron Herbicide; Telvar; Telvar Monuron Weedkiller; Televar W. Monuron Weedkiller

Monuron is available as a technical product at 97% active ingredient (US Environmental Protection Agency, 1983). A technical-grade sample of monuron analysed by liquid chromatography contained small amounts of 1,3-bis(4-chlorophenyl)urea (0.78%) and diuron (0.34%) as impurities (Sidwell & Ruzicka, 1976).

Monuron has been formulated as a wettable powder and as granules of monuron or monuron trichloroacetate or as an oil/water miscible liquid concentrate containing monuron trichloroacetate plus 2,4-D (see IARC, 1987). In the USSR, the commercial product usually contains 99% of the active ingredient (Izmerov, 1984; Royal Society of Chemistry, 1986; Worthing & Walker, 1987). Isomeric compounds may be present as impurities when monuron is produced by direct halogenation of aryldialkylureas (Izmerov, 1984).

1.1.4   *Analysis*

Selected methods for the analysis of monuron in various matrices are given in Table 1.

Table 1. Methods for the analysis of monuron

Sample matrix	Sample preparation	Assay procedure[a]	Reference
Specified fruit and vegetables	Alkaline hydrolysis to release *para*-chloroaniline; diazotize; couple with *N*-(1-naphthyl)ethylene-diamine; clean-up and separate resulting dyes on cellulose column	TLC	US Food and Drug Administration (1989)
Residues	Hydrolyse to *para*-chloroaniline using sodium hydroxide; distil; acidify distillate; wash with hexane or dichloromethane; neutralize; extract with hexane	GC/FID	Zweig (1964)

[a]Abbreviations: GC/FID, gas chromatography/flame ionization detector; TLC, thin-layer chromatography

1.2   Production and use

1.2.1   *Production*

Monuron was introduced in 1952 (US National Toxicology Program, 1988) and is prepared by reaction of *para*-chlorophenylisocyanate with dimethylamine (Izmerov, 1984).

---

[1]Calculated from: $mg/m^3 = $ (molecular weight/24.45) $\times$ ppm, assuming standard temperature (25°C) and pressure (760 mm Hg [101.3 kPa])

In 1973, production in the USA was 230-400 tonnes, but larger quantities were produced earlier when its use was permitted on food crops (IARC, 1976). Production of monuron and its trichloroacetate salt was discontinued in Israel in 1984 and in the USA in 1988 (Meister, 1990).

1.2.2 *Use*

Monuron is a non-selective systemic herbicide which inhibits photosynthesis and is applied either pre- or post-emergence. It has been used for the control of many grasses and weeds in non-cropland areas, such as rights-of-way, industrial sites and drainage ditch banks (US Environmental Protection Agency, 1975; US National Technical Information Service, Environmental Protection Agency, 1983; Worthing & Walker, 1987; Royal Society of Chemistry, 1989).

Izmerov (1984) reported that, in some countries, monuron was used on potatoes, soya beans, peas and beans. In the USSR, monuron has been used on non-crop areas at doses ranging from 20-30 kg/ha, and at lower application rates on certain crops. Crops to which it has been applied include cotton, sugar-cane, pip gardens, vineyards, tea plantations, apple and pear trees and citrus plants at least three years old. Monuron has also been used in combination with other herbicides, such as chlorpropham and simazine (see monograph, p. 495), to control resistant weeds.

1.3 Occurrence

1.3.1 *Air*

In the air of the working zone of a sower, the highest concentrations of monuron ranged from 8.6 to 11 mg/m^3; monuron vapours were not detectable in the breathing zone of a tractor driver (Izmerov, 1984).

1.3.2 *Water*

In one investigation of the persistence of monuron in river water, acetone solutions of monuron were injected into water samples, which were exposed to natural and artificial light at room temperature. By the end of one week, 40% of the monuron remained; at two weeks, 30%; at four weeks, 20%; and at eight weeks none was detected (US Environmental Protection Agency, 1975).

1.3.3 *Soil*

Phytotoxic concentrations of monuron disappeared from the soil within one year. When applied at non-selective rates for total vegetation control, e.g., on rights-of-way, it retained its phytotoxic activity for several seasons. Heavier applications (20-200 lb/acre [23-230 kg/ha]) required up to three years to dissipate (US Environmental Protection Agency, 1975).

Monuron moves fast in light (sandy loam) soils. At large doses and on soils with a high moisture content (up to 75%), it may penetrate as deeply as 40 cm. Monuron applied at rates of 20-60 kg/ha persists in soil for 1.7 years or longer. At an application rate of 1.8 kg/ha, all of an applied dose of monuron is broken down within 1 year; at 3.6 kg/ha, only 85-90% of the chemical decomposes within the same time. In the hottest months, 36% of an applied dose was degraded, compared to 14% in cool months (Izmerov, 1984).

1.3.4 *Plants*

When citrus plants were treated with monuron at a rate of 10-16 kg/ha, it was found to have accumulated to 0.21-0.41 mg/kg in leaves two months later, in May; in September, accumulation ranged from 0.12 to 0.2 mg/kg. At application rates as high as 16 kg/ha, the peel of unripe fruits exhibited levels of monuron ranging from 0.01 to 0.02 mg/kg; no residue was detected in ripe fruit (Izmerov, 1984).

1.4 Regulations and guidelines

In the USSR, the maximum allowable concentration of monuron in workplace air is 2 mg/m^3. In the air of communities, the maximum allowable single concentration is 0.02 mg/m^3. The maximum allowable concentration for drinking-water is 5 mg/l (Izmerov, 1984).

National pesticide residue limits for monuron in foods are presented in Table 2.

Table 2. National pesticide residue limits for monuron in foods[a]

Country	Residue limit (mg/kg)	Commodities
Austria	1.0	Asparagus
	0.2	Fruit, potatoes, other vegetables
	0.1	Cereals
	0.05	Other
Belgium[b]	0.5	Pome fruit, cabbages and related plants
	0.2	Other vegetables
	0.1	Grains
	0.05[c]	Other fruit
	0[d] (0.05)	Other foodstuffs of vegetable origin
Germany[e]	1.0	Asparagus
	0.2	Vegetables (except asparagus), potatoes, fruit
	0.1	Cereals
	0.05	Other foods of plant origin
Italy[f]	0.1	Fruit, vegetables
Kenya	7	Asparagus
	1.0	Avocados, citrus fruits, grapes, grapefruit, cottonseed, kumquats, lemons, limes, oranges, pineapple, spinach, sugar-cane, tangerines
Netherlands[b]	0.5	Cabbage, pome fruits
	0.2	Other vegetables
	0.1	Cereals, potatoes
	0.05[c]	Other fruit
	0[d] (0.05)	Other
Spain[g]	0.5	Asparagus
	0.2	Other vegetables
	0.05	Potatoes
	0.02	Other plant products

Table 2 (contd)

Country	Residue limit (mg/kg)	Commodities
USSR[h]	0.005	Vegetables, pears, apples, grapes, citruses, tea, cotton-seed oil
	0	Potatoes

[a]From Health and Welfare Canada (1990)
[b]Calculated as 4-chloroaniline
[c]This figure is also the lower limit for determining residues in the corresponding product according to the standard method of analysis; traces of residues below the lower limit indicated for determining residues may be found in the product.
[d]Residues should not be present; the number in parentheses is the lower limit for residue determination according to the standard method of analysis, this limit having been used to reach the no-residue conclusion.
[e]Including decomposition and reaction products that still contain the 4-chloroaniline group, calculated in total as 4-chloroaniline
[f]From Royal Society of Chemistry (1989)
[g]Sum of monolinuron, buturon and monuron, expressed as 4-chloroaniline; not registered for agricultural use
[h]From Izmerov (1984)

2. Studies of Cancer in Humans

No data were available to the Working Group.

3. Studies of Cancer in Experimental Animals

The Working Group was aware of two studies in rats (Hodge *et al.*, 1958; Rubenchik *et al.*, 1970) and one study in mice (Rubenchik *et al.*, 1970) that were reported in the previous monograph (IARC, 1976). They did not consider these studies informative for the evaluation.

Oral administration

Mouse: In a screening study on a large number of compounds, groups of 18 male and 18 female (C57Bl/6 × C3H/Anf)F_1 and (C57Bl/6 × AKR)F_1 mice, seven days of age, received 215 mg/kg bw commercial monuron (95% pure) in 0.5% gelatine by stomach tube daily [not adjusted for increasing body weight] up to four weeks of age; subsequently, they were fed 517 mg/kg of diet. The dose was the maximum tolerated dose for infant and young mice but not necessarily for adults. The experiment was terminated when the mice were about 78 weeks of age, at which time there was no difference in survival. A significant increase in the incidence of lung adenomas was observed in males of the second strain (6/16) compared with combined controls (9/90) [$p < 0.01$]; in gelatin controls the incidence was 2/18 (US National Technical Information Service, 1968; Innes *et al.*, 1969).

Groups of 50 male and 50 female B6C3F_1 mice, seven to nine weeks old, were fed 0, 5000 or 10 000 mg/kg of diet monuron (purity, > 99%) for 103 weeks. Mean body weights of treated female mice were significantly lower than those of controls. Survival of both control and low-dose male and female mice was significantly shorter than that of the high-dose group. In male mice, a dose-related decrease in the incidences of hepatocellular adenomas or carcinomas (control, 12/50; low-dose, 8/49; and high-dose 6/50) ($p < 0.05$, trend test) was noted. In female mice, there was also a decrease in the incidence of hepatocellular tumours; however, this was not dose-related. The incidence of malignant lymphomas was significantly reduced in treated females (control, 16/50; low-dose, 8/50; and high dose, 7/50) ($p < 0.01$ life-table test for trend) (US National Toxicology Program, 1988).

Rat: Groups of 50 male and 50 female Fischer 344/N rats, seven weeks old, were fed 0, 750 or 1500 mg/kg of diet monuron (purity, $> 99\%$) for 103 weeks. The mean body weights of treated male and female rats were lower than those of controls throughout the study. Survival rates were higher in treated than in control animals, since 11 control male rats died at week 93 due to a malfunction in the room thermostat. In male rats, administration of monuron was associated with an increase in the incidence of renal tubular-cell adenomas (control, 0/50; low-dose, 2/50; high-dose, 7/50) and of renal tubular-cell adenocarcinomas (control, 0/50; low-dose, 1/50; high-dose, 8/50). The combined incidence of renal tumours in males was: control, 0/50; low-dose, 3/50; and high-dose, 15/50 ($p < 0.001$, incidental tumour test for trend). No such tumour was observed in females. The most frequent other change observed in the kidney of both male and female treated rats was cytomegaly of renal tubular epithelial cells (nuclear enlargement, multiple nucleoli and nuclei with many anaplastic characteristics). In the liver, the combined incidence of neoplastic nodules or carcinoma in males was: 1/50 control, 6/49 low-dose and 9/50 high-dose (incidental tumour test, $p = 0.04$). Significant negative trends were noted in the incidences of mononuclear cell leukaemia in male and female rats, of adrenal gland phaeochromocytomas ($p < 0.01$) and thyroid C-cell carcinomas ($p < 0.04$) in male rats and of mammary gland fibroadenomas ($p < 0.02$) in female rats (US National Toxicology Program, 1988).

4. Other Relevant Data

4.1 Absorption, distribution, metabolism and excretion

4.1.1 *Humans*

No data were available to the Working Group.

4.1.2 *Experimental systems*

Monuron is metabolized mainly by oxidative N-demethylation and aromatic hydroxylation, but some chlorinated aniline derivatives are also produced (Ernst & Bohme, 1965; Ernst, 1969). The principal urinary metabolites in rats are N-(4-chlorophenyl)urea (14.5% of dose), N-(2-hydroxy-4-chlorophenyl)urea (6.5%), N-(2-hydroxy-4-chloro-phenyl)-N'-methylurea (1.5%), N-(3-hydroxy-4-chlorophenyl)urea (2.2%), N-(4-chloro-phenyl)-N'-methylurea, N-(2-hydroxy-4-chlorophenyl)-N,N'-dimethylurea and 2-aceta-mido-5-chlorophenol. The metabolite yields indicate that hydroxylation favours the 2-position rather than the 3-position. Phenolic metabolites were excreted in the urine as conjugates. 4-Chloro-2-hydroxyaniline was excreted as the N-acetyl conjugate.

The detection of 4-chloroaniline-haemoglobin adducts by gas chromatography-mass spectrometry (estimated to be equivalent to 0.56% of the dose in rats given 1 mmol/kg monuron orally) confirms the availability of an aromatic amine metabolite *in vivo* (Sabbioni & Neumann, 1990).

There is indirect evidence that the *N*-demethylation reaction occurs *via* a relatively stable *N*-hydroxymethyl intermediate, which has been identified from mouse hepatic microsomal incubates *in vitro* and as conjugates from mouse urine *in vivo* (Ross *et al.*, 1981).

4.2 Toxic effects

4.2.1 *Humans*

No data were available to the Working Group.

4.2.2 *Experimental systems*

The oral LD_{50} for monuron in rats was 1480-3700 mg/kg bw, and the dermal LD_{50} in rabbits was > 2500 mg/kg bw (Ben-Dyke *et al.*, 1970).

Rats fed monuron for two years at 25-2500 mg/kg per day in the diet (0.0025-0.25%) developed only mild toxicity at the higher dose; slight growth retardation, mild anaemia and, in females only, slight splenic and hepatic enlargement were observed (Hodge *et al.*, 1958). In subsequent feeding studies (US National Toxicology Program, 1988), at dietary intakes of monuron (> 99% pure) of up to 12 000 ppm (mg/kg) in Fischer 344 rats and 50 000 ppm (mg/kg) in B6C3F$_1$ mice for 13 weeks and 750 and 500 ppm (mg/kg) (rats) and 5000 and 10 000 ppm (mg/kg) (mice) for two years, the kidney, liver and lympho/haematopoietic systems were targets for toxicity. The lymphocytic and haematopoietic tissue atrophy seen in both rats and mice at high doses in the 13-week studies was not seen in the two-year feeding studies. In the two-year studies, renal tubular epithelial hypertrophy was noted at high incidence in rats (48/50 low-dose males and 50/50 high-dose males; 12/50 low-dose females and 49/50 high-dose females). The nuclei of these cells were greatly enlarged, had anaplastic features and were sometimes multiple. In mice, there was no remarkable kidney lesion. Dose-dependent hepatocytic changes and degeneration observed in males (but not females) of both species and splenic haemosiderosis in female rats were the only other toxic effects clearly related to treatment in the two-year studies.

Short-term (2-18 weeks) feeding of monuron at 450 mg/kg to rats caused hepatocyte mitochondrial changes associated with altered activity of glycolytic enzymes (Rubenchik *et al.*, 1969).

In dogs, feeding of monuron at 2.5-25 mg/kg bw per day in the diet for one year produced no toxicity attributable to treatment (Hodge *et al.*, 1958).

The number and volume fraction of enzyme-specific altered foci in rat liver were increased when monuron was used as a promoter (750 or 1500 ppm [mg/kg] in the diet) subsequent to a single injection of *N*-nitrosodiethylamine (10 mg/kg bw intraperitoneally) 24 h after partial hepatectomy. The incidence of foci was not increased when monuron was used as an initiator (125 or 250 mg/kg bw intraperitoneally in a single dose after partial hepatectomy) followed by promotion with dietary phenobarbital (Maronpot *et al.*, 1989).

4.3 Reproductive and developmental effects

No data were available to the Working Group.

4.4 Genetic and related effects (see also Table 3 and Appendices 1 and 2)

4.4.1 *Humans*

No data were available to the Working Group.

4.4.2 *Experimental systems*

Monuron did not induce gene mutation in bacteria or yeast but did in plants. In mouse lymphoma L5178Y cells, conflicting results were obtained for mutation at the *tk* locus. Chromosomal aberrations were induced in plants, insects and cultured mammalian cells. Monuron induced sister chromatid exchange and morphological transformation but not unscheduled DNA synthesis in cultured mammalian cells.

Administration of monuron to mice *in vivo* induced chromosomal aberrations and micronucleus formation in bone-marrow cells and increased the frequency of morphologically abnormal sperm.

5. Summary of Data and Evaluation

5.1 Exposure data

Monuron is a nonselective systemic herbicide which inhibits photosynthesis. It was introduced in 1952 and has been used for the control of grasses and weeds in non-cropland areas, such as rights-of-way, industrial sites and drainage ditch banks. It has been used at lower application rates in agricultural areas in some countries as a pre- or post-emergence herbicide.

Monuron has been formulated for use as wettable powder and granules.

Exposure may occur during its production and use and, at much lower levels, from consumption of foods containing residues.

5.2 Carcinogenicity in humans

No data were available to the Working Group.

5.3 Carcinogenicity in experimental animals

Monuron was tested adequately for carcinogenicity in one study in mice and in one study in rats by oral administration. No increase in tumour incidence was found in mice. In rats, dose-related increased incidences of renal and liver-cell tumours were observed in males.

5.4 Other relevant data

Monuron forms chloroaniline–haemoglobin adducts in rats. In one study, it increased the number and volume fraction of enzyme-positive foci in rat liver.

No data were available on the genetic and related effects of monuron in humans.

Table 3. Genetic and related effects of monuron

Test system	Result[a]		Dose[b] LED/HID	Reference
	Without exogenous metabolic system	With exogenous metabolic system		
SA0, Salmonella typhimurium TA100, reverse mutation	–	–	500.0000	US National Technical Information Service, Environmental Protection Agency (1977)
SA0, Salmonella typhimurium TA100, reverse mutation	–	–	2500.0000	US National Toxicology Program (1988)
SA5, Salmonella typhimurium TA1535, reverse mutation	–	–	500.0000	US National Technical Information Service, Environmental Protection Agency (1977)
SA5, Salmonella typhimurium TA1535, reverse mutation	0	+	1.5000	Seiler (1978)
SA5, Salmonella typhimurium TA1535, reverse mutation	–	–	2500.0000	US National Toxicology Program (1988)
SA7, Salmonella typhimurium TA1537, reverse mutation	–	–	500.0000	US National Technical Information Service, Environmental Protection Agency (1977)
SA7, Salmonella typhimurium TA1537, reverse mutation	–	–	2500.0000	US National Toxicology Program (1988)
SA8, Salmonella typhimurium TA1538, reverse mutation	–	–	500.0000	US National Technical Information Service, Environmental Protection Agency (1977)
SA9, Salmonella typhimurium TA98, reverse mutation	–	–	2500.0000	US National Toxicology Program (1988)
SAS, Salmonella typhimurium, reverse mutation	–	0	0.0000	Andersen et al. (1972)
ECW, Escherichia coli WP2 uvrA, reverse mutation	–	–	500.0000	US National Technical Information Service, Environmental Protection Agency (1977)
SCG, Saccharomyces cerevisiae D7, gene conversion	–	–	40000.0000	US National Technical Information Service, Environmental Protection Agency (1984)

Table 3 (contd)

Test system	Result[a] Without exogenous metabolic system	Result[a] With exogenous metabolic system	Dose[b] LED/HID	Reference
SCH, *Saccharomyces cerevisiae* D3, homozygosis by mitotic recombination	−	−	50000.0000	US National Technical Information Service, Environmental Protection Agency (1977)
SCH, *Saccharomyces cerevisiae* D7, homozygosis by mitotic recombination	−	−	40000.0000	US National Technical Information Service, Environmental Protection Agency (1984)
SCR, *Saccharomyces cerevisiae* D7, reverse mutation	−	−	40000.0000	US National Technical Information Service, Environmental Protection Agency (1984)
HSM, *Hordeum vulgare*, mutation	+	0	1000.0000	Wuu & Grant (1966)
HSC, *Hordeum vulgare*, chromosomal aberrations	+	0	500.0000	Wuu & Grant (1966)
HSC, *Hordeum vulgare*, chromosomal aberrations	+	0	500.0000	Wuu & Grant (1967)
* *Anopheles stephensi*, chromosomal aberrations	+	0	10.0000	Sharma et al. (1987)
GST, Gene mutation, mouse lymphoma L5178Y cells *in vitro*, *tk* locus	(+)	+	20.0000	US National Technical Information Service, Environmental Protection Agency (1984)
GST, Gene mutation, mouse lymphoma L5178Y cells *in vitro*, *tk* locus	−	−	1100.0000	McGregor *et al.* (1988)
SIC, Sister chromatid exchange, Chinese hamster ovary cells *in vitro*	−	+	250.0000	US National Technical Information Service, Environmental Protection Agency (1984)
SIC, Sister chromatid exchange, Chinese hamster ovary cells *in vitro*	+	+	100.0000	US National Toxicology Program (1988)
CIC, Chromosomal aberrations, Chinese hamster ovary cells *in vitro*	−	+	1300.0000	US National Toxicology Program (1988)
TCS, Cell transformation, Syrian hamster cells *in vitro*	+	0	5.0000	Amacher & Zelljadt (1983)
UHF, Unscheduled DNA synthesis, human lung fibroblasts WI38 *in vitro*	−	−	200.0000	US National Technical Information Service, Environmental Protection Agency (1984)

Table 3 (contd)

Test system	Result[a]		Dose[b] LED/HID	Reference
	Without exogenous metabolic system	With exogenous metabolic system		
CBA, Chromosomal aberrations, mouse bone marrow *in vivo*	+	0	14.4000 × 3 i.p.	Sharma *et al.* (1987)
MVM, Micronucleus test, mouse bone marrow *in vivo*	–	0	2000.0000 × 2 p.o.	Seiler (1978)
MVM, Micronucleus test, mouse bone marrow *in vivo*	+	0	2000.0000 × 2, oral	US National Technical Information Service, Environmental Protection Agency (1984)
MVM, Micronucleus test, mouse bone marrow *in vivo*	+	0	14.4000 × 3 i.p.	Sharma *et al.* (1987)
SPM, Sperm morphology, mouse *in vivo*	+	0	14.4000 × 3 i.p.	Sharma *et al.* (1987)

*Not displayed on profile

[a]+, positive; (+), weakly positive; –, negative; 0, not tested; ?, inconclusive (variable response in several experiments within an adequate study)

[b]In-vitro tests, μg/ml; in-vivo tests mg/kg bw

Monuron induced micronucleus formation, chromosomal aberrations and abnormal sperm in mice *in vivo*. It induced chromosomal aberrations in cultured mammalian cells, insects and plants, sister chromatid exchange and cell transformation in cultured mammalian cells and mutation in plants.

5.5 Evaluation[1]

No data were available from studies in humans.

There is *limited evidence* in experimental animals for the carcinogenicity of monuron.

Overall evaluation

Monuron *is not classifiable as to its carcinogenicity to humans (Group 3)*.

6. References

Amacher, D.E. & Zelljadt, I. (1983) The morphological transformation of Syrian hamster embryo cells by chemicals reportedly nonmutagenic to *Salmonella typhimurium*. *Carcinogenesis, 4,* 291-295

Andersen, K.J., Leighty, E.G. & Takahashi, M.K. (1972) Evaluation of herbicides for possible mutagenic properties. *J. agric. Food Chem., 25,* 649-656

Ben-Dyke, R., Sanderson, D.M. & Noakes, D.N. (1970) Acute toxicity data for pesticides (1970). *World Rev. Pest Control, 9,* 119-127

Budavari, S., ed. (1989) *The Merck Index,* 11th ed., Rahway, NJ, Merck & Co., p. 985

Ernst, W. (1969) Metabolism of substituted dinitrophenols and ureas in mammals and methods for the isolation and identification of metabolites. *J. S. Afr. Chem. Inst., 22,* S79-S88

Ernst, W. & Bohme, C. (1965) The metabolism of urea herbicides in the rat. Part 1. Monuron and aresin (monolinuron) (Ger.) *Food Cosmet. Toxicol., 3,* 789-796

Health and Welfare Canada (1990) *National Pesticide Residue Limits in Food,* Ottawa, Bureau of Chemical Safety, Food Directorate, Health Protection Branch

Hodge, H.C., Maynard, E.A., Downs, W.L. & Coye, R.D. (1958) Chronic toxicity of 3-(*p*-chlorophenyl)-1,1-dimethylurea (monuron). *Arch. ind. Health, 17,* 45-47

IARC (1976) *IARC Monographs on the Evaluation of Carcinogenic Risk of Chemicals to Man,* Vol. 12, *Some Carbamates, Thiocarbamates and Carbazides,* Lyon, pp. 167-176

IARC (1987) *IARC Monographs on the Evaluation of Carcinogenic Risks to Humans,* Suppl. 7, *Overall Evaluations of Carcinogenicity: An Updating of* IARC Monographs *Volumes 1 to 42,* Lyon, pp. 156-160

Innes, J.R.M., Ulland, B.M., Valerio, M.G., Petrucelli, L., Fishbein, L., Hart, E.R., Pallotta, A.J., Bates, R.R., Falk, H.L., Gart, J.J., Klein, M., Mitchell, I. & Peters, J. (1969) Bioassay of pesticides and industrial chemicals for tumorigenicity in mice: a preliminary note. *J. natl Cancer Inst., 42,* 1101-1114

Izmerov, N.F., ed. (1984) *International Register of Potentially Toxic Chemicals. Scientific Reviews of Soviet Literature on Toxicity and Hazards of Chemicals: Monuron* (Issue 77), Moscow, Centre of International Projects, United Nations Environment Programme

---

[1]For definition of the italicized terms, see Preamble, pp. 26-28.

Maronpot, R.R., Pitot, H.C. & Peraino, C. (1989) Use of rat liver altered focus models for testing chemicals that have completed two-year carcinogenicity studies. *Toxicol. Pathol.*, *17*, 651-662

McGregor, D.B., Brown, A., Cattanach, P., Edwards, I., McBride, D., Riach, C. & Caspary, W.J. (1988) Responses of the L5178Y tk$^+$/tk$^-$ mouse lymphoma cell forward mutation assay: III. 72 coded chemicals. *Environ. mol. Mutagenesis*, *12*, 85-154

Meister, R.T., ed. (1990) *Farm Chemicals Handbook '90*, Willoughby, OH, pp. C201, C301

Ross, D., Farmer, P.B., Gescher, A., Hickman, J.A. & Threadgill, M.D. (1981) The formation and metabolism of *N*-hydroxymethyl compounds. I. The oxidative *N*-demethylation of *N*-dimethyl derivatives of arylamines, aryltriazenes, arylformamidines and arylureas including the herbicide monuron. *Biochem. Pharmacol.*, *31*, 3621-3627

Royal Society of Chemistry (1986) *European Directory of Agrochemical Products*, Vol. 2, *Herbicides*, Cambridge, pp. 481-482

Royal Society of Chemistry (1989) *The Agrochemicals Handbook*, [Dialog Information Services (File 306)], Cambridge

Rubenchik, B.L., Petrun, A.S., Pliss, M.B. & Shipko, G.P. (1969) Monuron action on the liver when this herbicide is introduced together with food (Russ.). *Vopr. Pitan.*, *28*, 13-18

Rubenchik, B.L., Botsman, N.E. & Gorbanj, G.P. (1970) On carcinogenic effect of herbicide monuron (Russ.). *Vopr. Onkol.*, *16*, 51-53

Sabbioni, G. & Neumann, H.-G. (1990) Biomonitoring of arylamines: hemoglobin adducts of urea and carbamate pesticides. *Carcinogenesis*, *11*, 111-115

Sadtler Research Laboratories (1980) *The Standard Spectra, 1980, Cumulative Index*, Philadelphia, PA

Seiler, J.P. (1978) Herbicidal phenylalkylureas as possible mutagens. I. Mutagenicity tests with some urea herbicides. *Mutat. Res.*, *58*, 353-359

Sharma, G.P., Sobti, R.C., Chaudhry, A., Gill, R.K. & Ahluwalia, K.K. (1987) Mutagenic potential of a substituted urea herbicide, monuron. *Cytologia*, *52*, 841-846

Sidwell, J.A. & Ruzicka, J.H.A. (1976) The determination of substituted phenylurea herbicides and their impurities in technical and formulated products by use of liquid chromatography. *Analyst*, *101*, 111-121

US Environmental Protection Agency (1975) *Initial Scientific and Mini-economic Review of Monuron. Substitute Chemical Program* (EPA-540/1-75-028), Washington DC, US Department of Commerce, pp. 2, 5, 21, 92-93, 98-101

US Environmental Protection Agency (1983) *Registration Standard for Pesticide Products Containing Monuron as the Active Ingredient* (540/RS-83-013), Washington DC, Office of Pesticide Programs

US Food and Drug Administration (1989) Diuron. In: *Pesticide Analytical Manual*, Vol. II, *Methods Which Detect Multiple Residues*, Washington DC, US Department of Health and Human Services, p. 1

US National Technical Information Service (1968) *Evaluation of Carcinogenic, Teratogenic and Mutagenic Activities of Selected Pesticides and Industrial Chemicals*, Vol. 1, *Carcinogenic Study*, Washington DC, US Department of Commerce

US National Technical Information Service, Environmental Protection Agency (1977) *Evaluation of Selected Pesticides as Chemical Mutagens:* in vitro *and* in vivo *Studies* (EPA-600/1-77-028), Washington DC

US National Technical Information Service, Environmental Protection Agency (1984) In Vitro *and* In Vivo *Mutagenicity Studies of Environmental Chemicals* (EPA-600/1-84-008), Washington DC

US National Toxicology Program (1988) *Toxicology and Carcinogenesis Studies of Monuron (CAS No. 150-68-5) in F344/N Rats and B6C3F$_1$ Mice (Feed Studies)* (Technical Report Series No. 266), Research Triangle Park, NC

Worthing, C.R. & Walker, S.B., eds (1987) *The Pesticide Manual: A World Compendium*, 8th ed., Thornton Heath, British Crop Protection Council, pp. 584-585

Wuu, K.D. & Grant, W.F. (1966) Morphological and somatic chromosomal aberrations induced by pesticides in barley (*Hordeum vulgare*). *Can. J. Genet. Cytol.*, 8, 481-501

Wuu, K.D. & Grant, W.F. (1967) Chromosomal aberrations induced by pesticides in meiotic cells of barley. *Cytologia*, 32, 31-41

Zweig, G., ed. (1964) *Analytical Methods for Pesticides, Plant Growth Regulators, and Food Additives*, Vol. IV, *Herbicides*, New York, Academic Press, pp. 157-170

PICLORAM

1. Exposure Data

1.1 Chemical and physical data

1.1.1 *Synonyms, structural and molecular data*

Chem. Abstr. Serv. Reg. No.: 1918-02-1
Chem. Abstr. Name: 2-Pyridinecarboxylic acid, 4-amino-3,5,6-trichloro-
IUPAC Systematic Name: 4-Amino-3,5,6-trichloropyridine-2-carboxylic acid
Synonyms: 4-Aminotrichloropicolinic acid; 4-amino-3,5,6-trichloropicolinic acid; ATCP; picolinic acid, 4-amino-3,5,6-trichloro; 3,5,6-trichloro-4-aminopicolinic acid

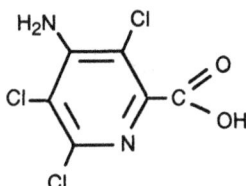

$C_6H_3Cl_3N_2O_2$ Mol. wt: 241.46

1.1.2 *Chemical and physical properties*

(a) *Description*: Colourless crystals with a chlorine-like odour (Royal Society of Chemistry, 1989)

(b) *Melting-point*: Decomposes at 215°C (Royal Society of Chemistry, 1989; Meister, 1990)

(c) *Solubility*: Slightly soluble (at 25°C) in water (0.43 g/l), dichloromethane (0.6 g/l), acetonitrile (1.6 g/l), diethyl ether (1.2 g/l) and benzene (0.2 g/l); moderately soluble (at 25°C) in acetone (19.8 g/l), isopropanol (5.5 g/l), ethanol (10.5 g/l) and methanol (18.5 g/l); very slightly soluble (at 25°C) in carbon disulfide (< 0.05 g/l) and kerosene (0.01 g/l) (US Environmental Protection Agency, 1988a; Royal Society of Chemistry, 1989)

(d) *Vapour pressure*: 6.16×10^{-7} mm Hg [0.82×10^{-7} kPa] at 35°C (Budavari, 1989)

(e) *Stability*: In aqueous solutions, decomposed by ultraviolet irradiation (Royal Society of Chemistry, 1989) but stable to hydrolysis (US Environmental Protection Agency, 1988b); very stable to acidic and basic media, but decomposed by hot concentrated alkalis; readily forms water-soluble alkali-metal and amine salts (Royal Society of Chemistry, 1989).

(f) *Conversion factor for airborne concentrations*[1]: $mg/m^3 = 9.88 \times ppm$

1.1.3 *Trade names, technical products and impurities*

The trade name is Tordon.

Picloram is available as granules and as soluble concentrates (Worthing & Walker, 1987; Royal Society of Chemistry, 1989). In the USA, it is formulated as the potassium, triisopropanolamine and triethylamine salts and as the isooctyl ester, either as pellets or as soluble concentrates in water (US Environmental Protection Agency, 1988b).

Picloram is compatible with many other herbicides and with fertilizers (Royal Society of Chemistry, 1989). It is formulated in combination with 2,4-D (see IARC, 1987a), 2,4,5-T (see IARC, 1987a), triclopyr(2-butoxyethyl), amitrole (see IARC, 1987b), atrazine (see monograph, p. 441), simazine (see monograph, p. 495), bromacil, dalapon, diuron, tebuthiuron, MCPA (see IARC, 1987a) and mecoprop (see IARC, 1986) (Royal Society of Chemistry, 1986; Worthing & Walker, 1987; Anon., 1989a).

The US Environmental Protection Agency (1988b) has limited the level of hexachlorobenzene (see IARC, 1987c) contamination in technical-grade picloram to a maximum of 200 ppm (mg/kg) and the level of nitrosamines, a potential contaminant of the triethylamine and triisopropanolamine forms of picloram, to a maximum of 1 ppm (mg/kg).

1.1.4 *Analysis*

Selected methods for the analysis of picloram in various matrices are given in Table 1.

Table 1. Methods for the analysis of picloram

Sample matrix	Sample preparation	Assay procedure[a]	Limit of detection	Reference
Water	Adjust to pH 12; wash with dichloromethane; acidify; extract with ethyl ether; derivatize with diazomethane	GC/ECD	0.14 µg/l	US Environmental Protection Agency (1989)
Soil	Extract with potassium chloride/potassium hydroxide solution; acidify; saturate with sodium chloride and equilibrate with ethyl ether; clean-up on an alumina column	GC/ECD	5 ppb (µg/ kg)	US Food and Drug Administration (1989a)
Milk	Extract with ethyl ether; clean-up on basic alumina column; partition residues from aqueous bicarbonate into ethyl ether; methylate residue; analyse	GC/ECD	0.05 ppm (mg/l)	US Food and Drug Administration (1989b)
Formulations	Acidify in acetone; exchange solvent to dimethylformamide	IR	Not reported	Ramsey (1967)

---

[1]Calculated from: $mg/m^3 = $ (molecular weight/24.45) $\times$ ppm, assuming standard temperature (25°C) and pressure (760 mm Hg [101.3 kPa])

Table 1 (contd)

Sample matrix	Sample preparation	Assay procedure[a]	Limit of detection	Reference
Crop samples	Extract with sodium hydroxide; acidify; treat with potassium permanganate; extract with ethyl ether; clean-up on a buffered celite column; methylate with diazomethane	GC/ECD	0.05 ppm (mg/kg)	US Food and Drug Administration (1989c)
Animal tissues	Extract with methanol/sodium carbonate; acidify; extract with ethyl ether; clean-up on an alumina column; treat further with potassium permanganate (liver); methylate with diazomethane	GC/ECD	0.005 ppm (mg/kg)	US Food and Drug Administration (1989d)

[a]Abbreviations: GC/ECD, gas chromatograph/electron capture detector; IR, infra-red spectrometry

1.2 Production and use

1.2.1 Production

Picloram was first introduced into commercial production in 1963. It is synthesized from α-picoline by successive chlorination, amination and hydrolysis (Ramsey, 1967).

The annual worldwide production of picloram from 1969 to the present has been 400-1600 tonnes per year. In 1981, it was estimated that 1000-1300 tonnes were produced in the USA, of which 630-850 tonnes were exported (Schutte, 1982). It is currently produced in the USA (Meister, 1990).

1.2.2 Use

Picloram is a systemic herbicide that is absorbed rapidly by roots and leaves and accumulates in new growth. It is used for the control of most annual and perennial broad-leaved weeds (except crucifers), including woody weeds, bracken, ferns and docks on grassland and non-crop areas. Most grasses are resistant to picloram, but seedling grasses may be susceptible (Worthing & Walker, 1987; Royal Society of Chemistry, 1989). Picloram is used alone or in combination with 2,4-D against deep-rooted perennials on non-crop land and in combination with 2,4-D or 2,4,5-T for brush control (Worthing & Walker, 1987).

Picloram may also be used for annual broadleaf weed control in spring and winter wheat, oats and barley; for perennial broadleaf weed control in fallow grainland; and for broadleaf annual and perennial weed control in rangeland and permanent grass pasture (Anon., 1989b).

In the USA, the potassium and triisopropanolamine salts of picloram are approved for food crop use on small grains, pastures and rangeland grasses; for use on noncrop areas and rights-of-way; and for forestry use. The triethylamine salt is approved for crop use on pastures and rangelands, and the isooctyl ester is approved for noncrop use on industrial sites and rights-of-way and for forestry use (US Environmental Protection Agency, 1988b).

A product available in the USA containing picloram and 2,4-D is applied to cut tree surfaces to kill unwanted growth (Anon., 1989b).

In the USA in 1981, it was estimated that yearly usage of picloram (active ingredient) was as follows (tonnes): utility rights-of-way, 130-160; rangeland, 100-120; forest site preparation, 70-90; pastures, 65-80; wheat, 4-5 (Schutte, 1982). By 1987, the amount used on pasture and rangeland had approximately doubled (270-410 tonnes) (Eckerman, 1987).

1.3 Occurrence

1.3.1 *Water*

Picloram was found in 420 of 744 surface water samples collected from 135 locations and in three of 64 groundwater samples collected from 30 locations. It was found in seven states of the USA. Levels (85th percentile) of 0.13 µg/l in surface water and 0.02 µg/l in groundwater were found in all positive samples; the maximal concentration found in surface water was 4.6 µg/l and that in groundwater, 0.02 µg/l (US Environmental Protection Agency, 1988c).

1.3.2 *Soil*

The main degradation pathways of picloram in the environment are photolysis and microbial degradation in aerobic soil. Field tests in Texas (USA) using a liquid formulation of picloram indicated that approximately 74% of the picloram in the test ecosystem, which contained soil, water and vegetation, was dissipated 28 days after application (Scifres *et al.*, 1977). In New Zealand, within 12 months after aerial application of 1.1 kg/ha picloram, residues in soil had fallen to 'safe levels' in 65% of locations sampled; the figure rose to 75% after 14 months (MacDiarmid, 1975).

Laboratory studies indicate that, under aerobic soil conditions, the half-time of picloram is dependent on the concentration applied and the temperature and the moisture of the soil. The major metabolite is carbon dioxide, other metabolites being present in insignificant amounts (Meikle *et al.*, 1974). Under anaerobic conditions in soil and aquatic media, picloram degrades extremely slowly in the absence of light (US Environmental Protection Agency, 1988c).

Picloram does not usually persist in soil after normal agricultural, forestry and industrial applications. In the field, picloram dissipates at a faster rate in hot, wet areas than in cool, dry locations. The half-time of picloram under most field conditions is a few months (US Environmental Protection Agency, 1988c). There is little potential for picloram to move from treated areas into runoff water (Fryer *et al.*, 1979). Although this chemical is considered to be moderately mobile, leaching is generally limited to the upper parts of most soil profiles (Grover, 1977). Instances in which picloram has entered groundwater are largely limited to misapplication or unusual soil conditions (Frank *et al.*, 1979).

1.4 Regulations and guidelines

The US Environmental Protection Agency has proposed to establish a 'maximum contaminant level' (feasible and enforceable limits to public health) in drinking-water and a 'maximum contaminant level goal' (desirable but non-enforceable) for picloram at 0.5 mg/l (Anon., 1990).

National pesticide residue limits for picloram in foods are presented in Table 2.

Table 2. National pesticide residue limits for picloram in foods[a]

Country	Residue limit (mg/kg)	Commodities
Argentina	0.5	Sorghum, maize, wheat, barley, canary grass
Australia	5	Edible offal
	0.2	Cereal grains
	0.05[b]	Meat, milk, milk products
Brazil	50[c]	Grasses
	1.0[c]	Forage
	0.2	Meat and meat products
	0.1[c]	Rice, wheat, barley, grains
	0.05	Milk, sugar-cane[c]
Canada	Negligible	Barley
Italy	0.5	Forage
USA[d]	80	Grasses, forage
	5	Kidney (cattle, goats, hogs, horses and sheep)
	3	Milled fractions (except flour) of wheat, barley and oats when used in feed
	1.0	Green forage and straw (barley, oats and wheat)
	0.5	Barley grain, flax seed and straw, liver (cattle, goats, hogs, horses and sheep), oats grain, wheat grain
	0.2	Fat, meat by-products, meat (cattle, goats, hogs, horses and sheep, excluding kidney and liver)
	0.05	Eggs, milk, poultry (fat, meat by-products, meat)

[a]From Health and Welfare Canada (1990)
[b]Set at or about the limit of detection
[c]Provisional
[d]From its application in the acid form or in the form of its potassium, triethylamine or triisopropanolamine salts, expressed as picloram

The time-weighted average occupational exposure limit for picloram in air is 10 mg/m^3 in Belgium, Finland, the Netherlands, Switzerland, the United Kingdom, the USA and Venezuela. The short-term exposure limit is 20 mg/m^3 in Finland and the United Kingdom, and the ceiling is 20 mg/m^3 in Venezuela (Cook, 1987; American Conference of Governmental Industrial Hygienists, 1989; US Occupational Safety and Health Administration, 1989).

2. Studies of Cancer in Humans

No data were available to the Working Group.

3. Studies of Cancer in Experimental Animals

Oral administration

Mouse: Groups of 50 male and 50 female B6C3F$_1$ mice, five weeks old, were fed diets containing picloram (technical-grade; at least 90% pure with 130 ppm [mg/kg] hexachlorobenzene [US Environmental Protection Agency, 1988]. The time at which chemical analysis of the technical product was carried out is not reported.) Since the maximum tolerated dose was not established beforehand, the concentration of picloram in the feed was changed during the course of the study. Low-dose groups were fed 5000 mg/kg of diet for one week and 2500 mg/kg diet for the subsequent 79 weeks; high-dose groups were fed dietary concentrations of 10 000 mg/kg of diet for one week and 5000 mg/kg of diet for the following 79 weeks. During the remaining 10 weeks of the study, the animals were fed basal diet. Groups of 40 control animals of each sex (10 matched and 30 concurrent) received the basal diet during the entire study period of 90 weeks. There was no significant difference in survival between test and control groups. The body weights of the mice were unaffected by the administration of picloram. No significant difference in tumour incidence was found between treated and control animals (US National Cancer Institute, 1978). [The Working Group noted the short duration of treatment.]

Rat: Groups of 50 male and 50 female Osborne-Mendel rats, five weeks old, were fed diets containing picloram (technical grade; at least 90% pure with 130 ppm [mg/kg] hexachlorobenzene [US Environmental Protection Agency, 1988]. The time at which chemical analysis of the technical product was carried out is not reported.) The concentrations of picloram in the feed were changed during the study: low-dose groups were fed 10 000 mg/kg of diet for 39 weeks and 5000 mg/kg diet for the subsequent 41 weeks; high-dose groups were fed dietary concentrations of 20 000 mg/kg of diet for 39 weeks and 10 000 for the following 41 weeks. During the remaining 33 weeks of the study, the animals were fed basal diet. Groups of 50 control animals of each sex (10 matched and 40 concurrent) received the basal diet during the entire study period of 113 weeks. There was no significant difference in survival between control and test groups. Mean body weights of treated rats were higher than those of the matched controls during the second year of the study. In female rats, C-cell adenomas of the thyroid occurred in 1/38 pooled controls, 3/46 low-dose and 7/46 high-dose rats ($p = 0.029$ test for trend). An increased incidence of neoplastic nodules of the liver was observed in treated females: in 0/39 pooled controls, 5/50 low-dose and 7/49 high-dose animals ($p = 0.014$; $p = 0.016$, test for trend); in males, this lesion appeared only in three animals of the low-dose group. Hepatocellular carcinomas occurred in one low-dose male rat and one high-dose female rat. A dose-related increase in the incidence of foci of cellular alteration was observed in the liver in animals of each sex (US National Cancer Institute, 1978). [The Working Group noted the short duration of treatment and the changes in dietary concentration during the study.]

Groups of 50 male and 50 female Fischer 344 rats, five weeks of age, were fed diets providing 0, 20, 60 and 200 mg/kg bw technical-grade picloram (93-94% pure; 6-7% tri- and tetrachlorinated pyridine compounds) for 24 months. Survival was similar in treated and control groups (> 68%). A dose-related increase in the combined incidence of benign and malignant liver-cell tumours was observed in males: two adenomas occurred in controls, two adenomas and two carcinomas in animals given 20 mg/kg bw, eight adenomas and two carcinomas at 60 mg/kg bw and four adenomas and two carcinomas at 200 mg/kg bw [$p = 0.04$, test for trend] (Stott *et al.*, 1990).

4. Other Relevant Data

4.1 Absorption, distribution, metabolism and excretion

4.1.1 Humans

Six male volunteers aged 40-51 years received single oral doses of 0.5 and 5 mg/kg bw picloram (99.6% pure, sodium salt) or a dermal application of 2 mg/kg bw picloram acid in an ethanolic vehicle on the back. Picloram was well absorbed when administered orally (> 90% of the dose) but was poorly absorbed through the skin (0.2% of the dose). High renal clearance (670 ml/min) of unchanged picloram (> 90% of the dose) suggests that active renal tubular secretion is most important for picloram excretion. Plasma disappearance was biphasic, with a rapid phase (half-time, approximately 1 h) and a highly variable terminal phase (half-time, 4-57 h) (Nolan *et al.*, 1984).

4.1.2 Experimental systems

Comparatively few data have been published on the disposition and metabolic fate of picloram in animals. Studies in rats and dogs, published as abstracts (Redemann, 1965a,b), suggest that picloram is excreted rapidly in the urine as unchanged material. Disposition studies (Kutschinski & Van Riley, 1969) in young cattle confirm that tissue retention is minimal with dietary intakes of 2.6-23 mg/kg per day. At the highest dietary intake level studied (1600 ppm [mg/kg]), tissue concentrations were recorded as (ppm [mg/kg]): kidney, 15-18; blood, 1.4-2; liver, 1.1-1.6; and muscle and fat, 0.3-0.5. Clearance was rapid after cessation of intake.

Treatment of rats with picloram (1-200 mg/kg bw intraperitoneally) induced a dose-dependent increase in ethoxyresorufin and ethoxycoumarin O-deethylation in rat liver. Picloram also binds to rat-liver microsomes from animals pretreated with phenobarbital and 3-methylcholanthrene, causing a typical type-I binding spectrum (Reidy *et al.*, 1987).

4.2 Toxic effects

4.2.1 Humans

No data were available to the Working Group.

4.2.2 Experimental systems

Picloram has low toxicity in experimental animals, according to the available published data. The acute oral LD_{50} in rats is approximately 8200 mg/kg bw, and the dermal LD_{50} in rabbits is > 4000 mg/kg bw (Ben-Dyke *et al.*, 1970). Bioavailability and toxicity appear to depend on the salts or formulation tested. For example, the oral LD_{50} values cited by Hayes *et al.* (1986) for the soluble potassium salt are 954 mg/kg bw in male rats and 686 mg/kg bw in female rats. No LD_{50} has been published for other salts used in commercial formulations.

The liver is the primary target organ for picloram toxicity during chronic administration. In Fischer 344 rats, centrilobular hepatocyte hypertrophy appeared as early as two weeks at the highest dose rates (500-2000 mg/kg per day) and at lower rates over longer intervals (150-500 mg/kg per day over 13 weeks; 60-200 mg/kg per day over 6-12 months). A subsequent two-year feeding study in Fischer 344 rats (Stott *et al.*, 1990) using picloram

(93-94% pure; main impurities, tri- and tetrachlorinated pyridines) at 20, 60, 200 mg/kg per day confirmed that there was dose-related enlargement of eosinophilic centrilobular hepatocytes and mild hepatomegaly, the effect being greater in males than in females.

Administration of the more soluble potassium salt in drinking-water for 90 days at 190-600 mg/kg (bw?) per day to Sprague-Dawley rats also caused liver lesions, described as an increased incidence and/or severity of hepatocyte mononuclear foci, as well as causing mild renal damage, described as multi-focal renal tubular epithelial degeneration (Hayes *et al.*, 1986). The doses used in this study, 600-1070 mg/kg per day, were clearly in the lethal range, producing significant mortality (males, 20-90%; females, 10-70%). Comparable doses given to pregnant rats by gavage over shorter periods of administration also produced mortality: 750 mg/kg per day caused 14% mortality and 1000 mg/kg per day, 26% (Thompson *et al.*, 1972).

4.3 Reproductive and developmental effects

4.3.1 *Humans*

No data were available to the Working Group.

4.3.2 *Experimental systems*

Following application of picloram to fertile mallard eggs by immersing them for 30 sec in an aqueous solution, the LC_{50} for embryonic death was equivalent to application of 100 lb/acre (112 kg/ha), an exposure level calculated to be 12 times that expected after usual application in the field, i.e., 100 gal/acre (935 litres/ha). Exposure at this level caused stunted embryos (Hoffman & Albers, 1984).

When hens' eggs were sprayed with picloram at 10 times the normal field level of application (11.2 kg/ha) before incubation and on days 4 or 18 of incubation, no effect was observed on hatching success, early performance of chicks (Somers *et al.*, 1978a) or their reproductive performance in adulthood (Somers *et al.*, 1978b).

A classical teratology study with Sprague-Dawley rats given 500, 750 or 1000 mg/kg bw picloram per day by gavage on days 6-15 of gestation provided evidence of retarded fetal growth but no teratogenic effect and no effect on postnatal survival or development (Thompson *et al.*, 1972). Similarly, administration of 40, 200 or 400 mg/kg bw per day picloram acid equivalent (given as the potassium salt) on days 6-18 of gestation to New Zealand rabbits had no embryotoxic or teratological effect (John-Greene *et al.*, 1985). In both these studies, the higher doses caused some toxicity to the mothers.

4.4 Genetic and related effects (see also Table 3 and Appendices 1 and 2)

4.4.1 *Humans*

No data were available to the Working Group.

4.4.2 *Experimental systems*

Picloram did not induce mutation in bacteriophage, *Salmonella typhimurium* or *Drosophila melanogaster*, but there is one report of induction of forward mutation in *Streptomyces coelicolor*. Mitotic recombination was induced in *Saccharomyces cerevisiae* but

Table 3. Genetic and related effects of picloram

Test system	Result[a] Without exogenous metabolic system	With exogenous metabolic system	Dose[b] LED/HID	Reference
BPF, Bacteriophage, forward mutation	–	0	500.0000	Andersen et al. (1972)
BPR, Bacteriophage T4, reverse mutation	–	0	6000.0000	Andersen et al. (1972)
SA0, Salmonella typhimurium TA100, reverse mutation	–	–	1667.0000	Mortelmans et al. (1986)
SA5, Salmonella typhimurium TA1535, reverse mutation	–	–	200.0000	Carere et al. (1978)
SA5, Salmonella typhimurium TA1535, reverse mutation	–	–	1667.0000	Mortelmans et al. (1986)
SA7, Salmonella typhimurium TA1537, reverse mutation	–	–	200.0000	Carere et al. (1978)
SA7, Salmonella typhimurium TA1537, reverse mutation	–	–	1667.0000	Mortelmans et al. (1986)
SA8, Salmonella typhimurium TA1538, reverse mutation	–	–	200.0000	Carere et al. (1978)
SA9, Salmonella typhimurium TA98, reverse mutation	–	–	1667.0000	Mortelmans et al. (1986)
SAS, Salmonella typhimurium, reverse mutation	–	–	0.0000	Andersen et al. (1972)
SAS, Salmonella typhimurium TA1536, reverse mutation	–	–	200.0000	Carere et al. (1978)
SCF, Streptomyces coelicolor, streptomycin resistance	+	0	200.0000	Carere et al. (1978)
SCH, Saccharomyces cerevisiae, mitotic recombination	+	0	5.0000	L'vova (1984)
SCH, Saccharomyces cerevisiae, mitotic recombination	+	–	5.0000	L'vova (1989)
ANG, Aspergillus nidulans, mitotic recombination	–	0	800.0000	Bignami et al. (1977)
DMX, Drosophila melanogaster, sex-linked recessive lethal mutation	–	0	1000.0000 injection	Woodruff et al. (1985)
DMX, Drosophila melanogaster, sex-linked recessive lethal mutation	–	0	5000.0000 feeding	Woodruff et al. (1985)
DMN, Drosophila melanogaster, aneuploidy	–	0	650.0000	Woodruff et al. (1983)
CHL, Chromosomal aberrations, human lymphocytes in vitro	–	0	50.0000	L'vova (1984)
CBA, Chromosomal aberrations, mouse bone marrow in vivo	–	0	10.0000	L'vova (1984)

[a] +, positive; –, negative; 0, not tested
[b] In-vitro tests, μg/ml; in-vivo tests, mg/kg bw

not in *Aspergillus nidulans*. In single studies, picloram did not induce aneuploidy in *D. melanogaster* or chromosomal aberrations in either cultured human lymphocytes or mouse bone-marrow cells *in vivo*.

5. Summary of Data Reported and Evaluation

5.1 Exposure data

Picloram is a systemic herbicide used to control broad-leaved weeds on pasture, rangeland, rights-of-way, forestland and some grains. It was first registered for use in 1963.

Picloram has been formulated as granules and soluble concentrates in the form of amine and potassium salts and esters.

Exposure to picloram may occur during its production and application and, at much lower levels, from consumption of foods containing residues.

5.2 Carcinogenicity in humans

No data were available to the Working Group.

5.3 Carcinogenicity in experimental animals

Technical-grade picloram was tested for carcinogenicity in one experiment in mice and in two experiments in rats by administration in the diet. No increase in tumour incidence was observed in mice. In rats, it increased the incidence of liver-cell tumours (mainly benign) in males in one study and in males and females in another, and of C-cell adenomas of the thyroid in female rats in one study.

5.4 Other relevant data

The liver is the primary organ for picloram toxicity following chronic administration to rats.

No data were available on the genetic and related effects of picloram in humans.

Picloram did not induce chromosomal aberrations in mouse bone-marrow cells *in vivo* nor in cultured human cells. With the exception of a single report in which forward mutation was induced in *Streptomyces coelicolor*, picloram gave negative results in all short-term tests for mutation. It induced mitotic recombination in yeast but not in fungi.

5.5 Evaluation[1]

No data were available from studies in humans.

There is *limited evidence* for the carcinogenicity of picloram of technical grades in experimental animals.

---

[1]For definition of the italicized terms, see Preamble, pp. 26-28.

Overall evaluation

Picloram *is not classifiable as to its carcinogenicity to humans (Group 3).*

6. References

American Conference of Governmental Industrial Hygienists (1989) *Threshold Limit Values and Biological Exposure Indices for 1988-1989*, Cincinnati, OH, p. 31

Andersen, K.J., Leighty, E.G. & Takahashi, M.K. (1972) Evaluation of herbicides for possible mutagenic properties. *J. agric. Food Chem.*, *20*, 649-656

Anon. (1989a) *MSDS Reference for Crop Protection 1988/1989*, New York, Chemical and Pharmaceutical Press, pp. 294-297

Anon. (1989b) *Crop Protection Chemicals Reference*, 5th ed., New York, Chemical and Pharmaceutical Press, pp. 691-712

Anon. (1990) Drinking-water regulations. *BIBRA Bull.*, *29*, 229

Ben-Dyke, R., Sanderson, D.M. & Noakes, D.N. (1970) Acute toxicity data for pesticides (1970). *World Rev. Pest Control*, *9*, 119-127

Bignami, M., Aulicino, F., Velcich, A., Carere, A. & Morpurgo, G. (1977) Mutagenic and recombinogenic action of pesticides in *Aspergillus nidulans*. *Mutat. Res.*, *46*, 395-402

Budavari, S., ed. (1989) *The Merck Index*, 11th ed., Rahway, NJ, Merck & Co., p. 1174

Carere, A., Ortali, V.A., Cardamone, G., Torracca, A.M. & Raschetti, R. (1978) Microbiological mutagenicity studies of pesticides *in vitro*. *Mutat. Res.*, *57*, 277-286

Cook, W.A., ed. (1987) *Occupational Exposure Limits—Worldwide*, Washington DC, American Industrial Hygiene Association, pp. 33, 64, 208-209

Eckerman, D.E. (1987) *Preliminary Quantitative Usage Analysis of Picloram*, Washington DC, US Environmental Protection Agency

Frank, R., Sirons, G.J. & Ripley, B.D. (1979) Herbicide contamination and decontamination of well waters in Ontario, Canada, 1968-1978. *Pestic. Monit. J.*, *13*, 120-127

Fryer, J.D., Smith, P.D. & Ludwig, J.W. (1979) Long-term persistence of picloram in a sandy loam soil. *J. environ. Qual.*, *8*, 83-86

Gorzinski, S.J., Johnson, K.A., Campbell, R.A. & Landry, T.D. (1987) Dietary toxicity of picloram herbicide in rats. *J. Toxicol. environ. Health*, *20*, 367-377

Grover, R. (1977) Mobility of dicamba, picloram and 2,4-D in soil columns. *Weed Sci.*, *25*, 159-162

Hayes, J.R., Condie, L.W. & Borzelleca, J.F. (1986) Acute, 14-day repeated dosing, and 90-day subchronic toxicity studies of potassium picloram. *Fundam. appl. Toxicol.*, *7*, 464-470

Health and Welfare Canada (1990) *National Pesticide Residue Limits in Food*, Ottawa, Bureau of Chemical Safety, Food Directorate, Health Protection Branch

Hoffman, D.J. & Albers, P.H. (1984) Evaluation of potential embryotoxicity and teratogenicity of 42 herbicides, insecticides, and petroleum contaminants to mallard eggs. *Arch. environ. Contam. Toxicol.*, *13*, 15-27

IARC (1986) *IARC Monographs on the Evaluation of the Carcinogenic Risk of Chemicals to Humans*, Vol. 41, *Some Halogenated Hydrocarbons and Pesticide Exposures*, Lyon, p. 363

IARC (1987a) *IARC Monographs on the Evaluation of Carcinogenic Risks to Humans*, Suppl. 7, *Overall Evaluations of Carcinogenicity: An Updating of* IARC Monographs *Volumes 1 to 42*, Lyon, pp. 156-160

IARC (1987b) *IARC Monographs on the Evaluation of Carcinogenic Risks to Humans*, Suppl. 7, *Overall Evaluations of Carcinogenicity: An Updating of* IARC Monographs *Volumes 1 to 42*, Lyon, pp. 92-93

IARC (1987c) *IARC Monographs on the Evaluation of Carcinogenic Risks to Humans*, Suppl. 7, *Overall Evaluations of Carcinogenicity: An Updating of* IARC Monographs *Volumes 1 to 42*, Lyon, pp. 219-220

John-Greene, J.A., Ouellette, J.H., Jeffries, T.K., Johnson, K.A. & Rao, K.S. (1985) Teratological evaluation of picloram potassium salt in rabbits. *Food chem. Toxicol.*, *23*, 753-756

Kutschinski, A.H. & Van Riley (1969) Residue in various tissues of steers fed 4-amino-3,5,6-trichloropicolinic acid. *J. agric. Food Chem.*, *17*, 283-287

L'vova, T.S. (1984) Study of mutagenic action of five worthwhile pesticides on murine marrow, cultures of human lymphocytes and on a yeast (Russ.). *Tsitol. Genet.*, *18*, 455-457

L'vova, T.S. (1989) Comparative study of the effect of a group of pesticides on recombination of yeast with and without the presence of metabolic activators (Russ.). *Tsitol. Genet.*, *24*, 68-70

MacDiarmid, B.N. (1975) Soil residues of picloram applied aerially to New Zealand brushweed. Effect of soil on pesticides. In: *Proceedings of the 28th New Zealand Weed and Pest Control Conference*, pp. 109-114

Meikle, R.W., Youngson, C.R., Hedlund, R.T., Goring, C.A.I. & Addington, W.W. (1974) Decomposition of picloram by soil microorganisms: a proposed reaction sequence. *Weed Sci.*, *22*, 263-268

Meister, R.T., ed. (1990) *Farm Chemicals Handbook '90*, Willoughby, OH, Meister Publishing Company, pp. C228-C229

Mortelmans, K., Haworth, S., Lawlor, T., Speck, W., Tainer, B. & Zeiger, E. (1986) *Salmonella* mutagenicity tests: II. Results from the testing of 270 chemicals. *Environ. Mutagenesis*, *8* (Suppl. 7), 1-119

Nolan, R.J., Freshour, N.L., Kastl, P.E. & Saunders, J.H. (1984) Pharmacokinetics of picloram in male volunteers. *Toxicol. appl. Pharmacol.*, *76*, 264-269

Ramsey, J.C. (1967) Tordon. In: Zewig, G., ed., *Analytical Methods for Pesticides, Plant Growth Regulators, and Food Additives*, Vol. 5, *Additional Principles and Methods of Analysis*, New York, Academic Press, pp. 507-525

Redemann, C.T. (1965a) The fate of 4-amino-3,5,6-trichloropicolinic acid in the dog (Abstract No. 40). In: *Proceedings of the 150th Meeting of the American Chemical Society, Atlantic City, NJ*, Washington DC, American Chemical Society, pp. 16a-17a

Redemann, C.T. (1965b) The fate of 4-amino-3,5,6-trichloropicolinic acid in the rat (Abstract No. 41). In: *Proceedings of the 150th Meeting of the American Chemical Society, Atlantic City, NJ*, Washington DC, American Chemical Society, p. 17a

Reidy, G.F., Rose, H.A. & Stacey, N.H. (1987) Effects of picloram on xenobiotic biotransformation in rat liver. *Xenobiotica*, *17*, 1057-1066

Royal Society of Chemistry (1986) *European Directory of Agrochemical Products*, Vol. 2, *Herbicides*, Cambridge, pp. 512-514

Royal Society of Chemistry (1989) *The Agrochemicals Handbook* [Dialog Information Services (File 306)], Cambridge

Schutte, W.D. (1982) *Preliminary Quantitative Usage Analysis of Picloram*, Washington DC, US Environmental Protection Agency

Scifres, C.J., McCall, H.G., Maxey, R. & Tai, R. (1977) Residual properties of 2,4,5-T and picloram in sandy rangeland soils. *J. environ. Qual.*, *6*, 36-42

Somers, J.D., Moran, E.T., Jr & Reinhart, B.S. (1978a) Hatching success and early performance of chicks from eggs sprayed with 2,4-D, 2,4,5-T and picloram at various stages of embryonic development. *Bull. environ. Contam. Toxicol.*, 20, 289-293

Somers, J.E., Moran, E.T., Jr & Reinhart, B.S. (1978b) Reproductive success of hens and cockerels originating from eggs sprayed with 2,4-D, 2,4,5-T and picloram followed by early performance of their progeny after a comparable *in ovo* exposure. *Bull. environ. Contam. Toxicol.*, 20, 111-119

Stott, W.T., Johnson, K.A., Landry, T.D., Gorzinski, S.J. & Cieszlak, F.S. (1990) Chronic toxicity and oncogenicity of picloram in Fischer 344 rats. *J. Toxicol. environ. Health*, 30, 91-104

Thompson, D.J., Emerson, J.L., Strebing, R.J., Gerbig, C.G. & Robinson, V.B. (1972) Teratology and postnatal studies on 4-amino-3,5,6-trichloropicolinic acid (picloram) in the rat. *Food Cosmet. Toxicol.*, 10, 797-803

US Environmental Protection Agency (1988a) *Pesticide Fact Sheet: Picloram*, Washington DC, Office of Pesticide Programs

US Environmental Protection Agency (1988b) *Guidance for the Reregistration of Pesticide Products Containing Picloram as the Active Ingredient* (PB89-159834, 540/RS-88-132), Washington DC

US Environmental Protection Agency (1988c) *Picloram*, Washington DC, Office of Drinking Water

US Environmental Protection Agency (1989) Method 515.1. Revision 4.0. Determination of chlorinated acids in water by gas chromatography with an electron capture detector. In: *Methods for the Determination of Organic Compounds in Drinking Water* (EPA Report No. EPA-600/4-88/039; US NTIS PB89-22046), Cincinnati, OH, Environmental Monitoring Systems Laboratory, pp. 221-253

US Food and Drug Administration (1989a) Picloram method IV. In: *Pesticide Analytical Manual*, Vol. II, *Methods Which Detect Multiple Residues*, Washington DC, US Department of Health and Human Services, pp. 19-22

US Food and Drug Administration (1989b) Picloram. In: *Pesticide Analytical Manual*, Vol. II, *Methods Which Detect Multiple Residues*, Washington DC, US Department of Health and Human Services, pp. 1-8

US Food and Drug Administration (1989c) Picloram method III. In: *Pesticide Analytical Manual*, Vol. II, *Methods Which Detect Multiple Residues*, Washington DC, US Department of Health and Human Services, pp. 13-17

US Food and Drug Administration (1989d) Picloram. In: *Pesticide Analytical Manual*, Vol. II, *Methods Which Detect Multiple Residues*, US Department of Health and Human Services, pp. 9-11

US National Cancer Institute (1978) *Bioassay of Picloram for Possible Carcinogenicity* (Technical Report Series No. 23; DHEW Publ. No. (NIH) 78-823), Washington DC

US Occupational Safety and Health Administration (1989) Air contaminants—permissible exposure limits. *US Code fed. Regul., Title 29*, Part 1910.1000

Woodruff, R.C., Phillips, J.P. & Irwin, D. (1983) Pesticide-induced complete and partial chromosome loss in screens with repair-defective females of Drosophila melanogaster. *Environ. Mutagenesis*, 5, 835-846

Woodruff, R.C., Mason, J.M., Valencia, R. & Zimmering, S. (1985) Chemical mutagenesis testing in *Drosophila*. V. Results of 53 coded compounds tested for the National Toxicology Program. *Environ. Mutagenesis*, 7, 677-702

Worthing, C.R. & Walker, S.B., eds (1987) *The Pesticide Manual: A World Compendium*, 8th ed., Thornton Heath, British Crop Protection Council, pp. 672-673

SIMAZINE

1. Exposure Data

1.1 Chemical and physical data

1.1.1 *Synonyms, structural and molecular data*

Chem. Abstr. Serv. Reg. No.: 122-34-9
Replaced CAS Reg. Nos: 11141-20-1; 12764-71-5; 39291-64-0; 119603-94-0 *Chem. Abstr.*
Name: 6-Chloro-*N,N'*-diethyl-1,3,5-triazine-2,4-diamine
IUPAC Systematic Name: 6-Chloro-N^2,N^4-diethyl-1,3,5-triazine-2,4-diamine
Synonyms: 4,6-Bis(ethylamino)-2-chlorotriazine; 2,4-bis(ethylamino)-6-chloro-*s*-triazine; 2-chloro-4,6-bis(ethylamino)-*s*-triazine

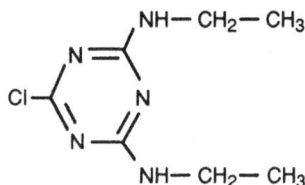

$C_7H_{12}ClN_5$ Mol. wt: 201.66

1.1.2 *Chemical and physical properties*

(a) *Description*: Colourless-to-white, odourless crystals (US Environmental Protection Agency, 1984a; Royal Society of Chemistry, 1989)
(b) *Melting-point*: 225-227°C (Royal Society of Chemistry, 1989)
(c) *Spectroscopy data*: Infrared (prism [35711]; grating [13705]) and ultraviolet [16140] spectral data have been reported (Sadtler Research Laboratories, 1980).
(d) *Solubility*: Practically insoluble in water (3.5 mg/l at 20°C), petroleum ether (2 mg/l at 20°C) and *n*-pentane (3 mg/l at 25°C); slightly soluble in dioxane and ethyl Cellosolve; soluble in chloroform (900 mg/l at 20°C), methanol (400 mg/l at 20°C) and diethyl ether (300 mg/l at 25°C) (Budavari, 1989; Royal Society of Chemistry, 1989; Meister, 1990)
(e) *Vapour pressure*: 6.1×10^{-9} mm Hg [0.8×10^{-9} kPa] at 20°C (US Environmental Protection Agency, 1988a; Royal Society of Chemistry, 1989)
(f) *Stability*: Stable in neutral, weakly acidic and weakly alkaline media; hydrolysed by stronger acids and bases; decomposed by ultraviolet irradiation (Royal Society of Chemistry, 1989)

(g) Conversion factor for airborne concentrations[1]: mg/m^3 = 8.25 × ppm

1.1.3 *Trade names, technical products and impurities*

Some examples of trade names are: Aktinit S; Aquazine; Azotop; Bitemol S 50; CAT; CDT; CET; Geigy 27,692; Gesatop; H 1803; Herbazin; Herbex; Herbatoxol S; Herboxy; Hungazin DT; Premazine; Princep; Radocon; Radokor; Simanex; Simatsin-neste; Simazin; Symazine; Tafazine; Taphazine; Triazine A 384; W 6658; Yrodazin

Simazine is registered in the USA as a technical material with 95-99.9% active ingredient (US Environmental Protection Agency, 1984b). It is available there in wettable powder, granular, liquid, flowable concentrate, soluble concentrate and dry flowable forms. The usual carrier is water, oil or clay (US Environmental Protection Agency, 1984a). In Europe, it is available as dustable powders, emulsifiable concentrates, liquid creams, granules, microgranules, suspension concentrates, soluble concentrates, ultra-low volume suspensions, water-dispersible granules and wettable powders (Royal Society of Chemistry, 1986). In the USSR, simazine is manufactured as a wettable powder or dust (Izmerov, 1983).

Simazine can be formulated with most other herbicides and fertilizers (Royal Society of Chemistry, 1986, 1989). It is formulated in the USA in combination with amitrole (see IARC, 1987a), atrazine (see monograph, p. 441), prometon, trietazine, sodium chlorate and sodium metaborate (Anon., 1989; Meister, 1990). It has also been formulated in various countries in combination with metoxuron, diquat, sodium trichloroacetate, secbumeton, MCPA (see IARC, 1987b), ametryne, paraquat dichloride, diquat dichloride, paraquat dibromide, sodium 2-(2,4-dichlorophenoxy)ethyl sulfate, 2,4-D (see IARC, 1987b), diuron, propyzamide, nonflurazon, dalapon sodium and picloram (Worthing & Walker, 1987).

1.1.4 *Analysis*

Selected methods for the analysis of simazine in various matrices are given in Table 1.

Table 1. Methods for the analysis of simazine

Sample matrix	Sample preparation	Assay procedure[a]	Limit of detection	Reference
Formulation (80% wettable powder)	Dissolve in chloroform; centrifuge	GC/FID	Not reported	Williams (1984)
Formulation (wettable powder)	Add morpholine; boil; add 50% sulfuric acid; titrate with silver nitrate	Potentiometry	Not reported	Knüsli *et al.* (1964)
Drinking-water	Extract by passing sample through liquid-solid extractor; elute with dichloromethane; concentrate by evaporation	GC/MS	0.2 μg/l	US Environmental Protection Agency (1988b)

[1]Calculated from: mg/m^3 = (molecular weight/24.45) × ppm, assuming standard temperature (25°C) and pressure (760 mm Hg [101.3 kPa])

Table 1 (contd)

Sample matrix	Sample preparation	Assay procedure[a]	Limit of detection	Reference
Drinking-water (contd)	Extract with dichloromethane; isolate extract; dry; concentrate with methyl *tert*-butyl ether	GC/NPD	0.075 μg/l	US Environmental Protection Agency (1989a)
	Extract with hexane; inject extract	GC/ECD	6.8 μg/l	US Environmental Protection Agency (1989b)
Crop samples, animal tissues	Extract with chloroform; evaporate to dryness; redissolve in carbon tetrachloride; clean-up on alumina column; convert to hydroxytriazine by treatment with acid	UV	0.05-0.1 ppm (mg/kg)	US Food and Drug Administration (1989a)
Crop samples	Extract with acetonitrile: water (70:30); clean-up on alumina column; elute with benzene: hexane (1:1); analyse benzene solution	GC/MCD	0.05 ppm (mg/kg)	US Food and Drug Administration (1989a,b)
Milk	Add methanol and sodium oxalate; extract with ethyl ether: petroleum ether (1:1); wash with water; dry with sodium sulfate and evaporate to dryness; dissolve in petroleum ether; extract with acetonitrile; backwash combined extracts with petroleum ether and evaporate to dryness	GC/MCD	0.05 ppm (mg/l)	US Food and Drug Administration (1989c)
Fish	Extract with dichloromethane-methanol; clean-up with acetonitrile/hexane partition and alumina column chromatography	GC/MCD	0.01 ppm (mg/kg)	US Food and Drug Administration (1989a,d)

[a]Abbreviations: GC/ECD, gas chromatography/electron capture detection; GC/FID, gas chromatography/flame ionization detection; GC/MCD, gas chromatography/microcoulometric detection; GC/MS, gas chromatography/mass spectrometry; GC/NPD, gas chromatography/nitrogen-phosphorous detection; UV, ultraviolet spectrophotometry

1.2 Production and use

1.2.1 *Production*

Simazine was first introduced in 1957 (US Environmental Protection Agency, 1984a). It is produced by the reaction of cyanuric chloride and monomethylamine in water or aqueous acetone (Izmerov, 1983).

It is produced currently by four companies in Israel, Switzerland and the USA (Meister, 1990). Estimated production in 1978-80 in the USA was approximately 5000 tonnes per annum, of which about 1000 tonnes were exported (Vlier Zygadlo, 1982). A major US producer reported producing an average of 4000 tonnes per annum in 1981-84 and an average of 8000 tonnes per annum in 1985-89.

1.2.2 *Use*

Simazine is a pre-emergent systemic herbicide that inhibits photosynthesis. It has been used for the control of germinating annual grasses and broad-leaved weeds in a variety of vegetables and fruit, turf and ornamental plants, and in forestry (Meister, 1990); its major use is on maize (US Environmental Protection Agency, 1984b). It is also used for total weed control on non-crop land and as an aquatic herbicide and algicide for control of algae and submerged weeds in ponds (Royal Society of Chemistry, 1989).

Methods of application include broadcast, band, soil incorporated and soil surface using ground or aerial equipment (US Environmental Protection Agency, 1984a). It is also registered for use in the USA in swimming pools, ponds and cooling towers (US Environmental Protection Agency, 1984b).

It was estimated that in the USA during the period 1978-80, yearly usage of simazine (active ingredient) was as follows: maize, 1000-1300 tonnes; aquatic uses, 700-900 tonnes; industrial sites, 600-800 tonnes; grapes, 220-290 tonnes; oranges, 220-290 tonnes; apples, 100-120 tonnes; and various other fruits, 300 tonnes (Vlier Zygadlo, 1982).

In the USSR, simazine is used on vineyards, strawberries and winter wheat sowings; it is also used to suppress couchgrass, Bermuda grass and some other perennial weeds (Izmerov, 1983).

1.3 Occurrence

1.3.1 *Water*

Simazine has been found in groundwater in California, Pennsylvania and Maryland, USA, at levels in the range of 0.2 to 3.0 µg/l. It was found in 922 of 5873 surface water samples and 202 of 2654 groundwater samples in the USA. The 85th percentile was 2.18 µg/l in surface water and 1.60 µg/l in groundwater; the maximal concentration in surface water was 1.3 mg/l and that in groundwater, 0.8 mg/l. Simazine was found in surface water in 16 states and in groundwater in eight states (US Environmental Protection Agency, 1988a).

Simazine did not hydrolyse in sterile aqueous solutions buffered at pH 5, 7 or 9 at 20°C, over a 28-day test period. Dissipation studies in pond and lake water with simazine gave variable results, with half-times ranging from 50 to 700 days. 2-Chloro-4-ethylamino-6-amino-*s*-triazine was identified in lake water but was no more persistent than simazine (US Environmental Protection Agency, 1988a).

1.3.2 *Soil*

The half-time of simazine varies depending on the soil microbial population, moisture, temperature and farming practice. Under aerobic conditions, the degradation of simazine in soil depends largely on the soil moisture and temperature (Walker, 1976). In a sandy loam soil, half-times ranged from 36 to 234 days. When applied to a loamy sand and silt loam soils and incubated (25-30°C) for 48 weeks, simazine dissipated with half-times of 16.3 and 25.5 weeks, respectively. Under anaerobic conditions, ^{14}C-simazine had a half-time of 8-12 weeks in a loamy sand soil. Degradation products included 2-chloro-4-ethylamino-6-amino-*s*-

triazine, 2-chloro-4,6-bis(amino)-*s*-triazine, 2-hydroxy-4,6-bis(ethylamino)-*s*-triazine and 2-hydroxy-4-ethylamino-6-amino-*s*-triazine (US Environmental Protection Agency, 1988a).

Studies of column leaching and adsorption/desorption indicated that simazine would be expected to be slightly to very mobile in soils ranging in texture from clay to sandy loam. Its adsorption was correlated with the content of organic matter in the soil and to a lesser degree with the cation exchange capacity and clay content (US Environmental Protection Agency, 1988a).

In field studies, simazine had a half-time of about 30-139 days in sandy loam and silt loam soils (US Environmental Protection Agency, 1988a). In a study with four New Zealand soils, with acid pH (5.4-5.5) and organic carbon levels of 4.6 and 9.4%, the half-times were 25 and 32 days, respectively (Rahman & Holland, 1985).

Field studies with simazine on Taichung (Taiwan) clay loam in different seasons and Taipei loam soils showed a significant effect of climate on degradation rate. Simazine had a half-time of 18 days in summer and 24 days in winter at Taichung; the more moderate temperature and precipitation of the autumn in Taipei resulted in a half-time of 14 days (Chen *et al.*, 1983).

1.3.3 *Food*

In the national surveillence programme in Canada, 1664 samples were analysed for simazine during the period 1984/85 to 1988/89. No residue was detected in fruit, meat, vegetables or wine (Government of Canada, 1990). No simazine residue (< 0.05 ppm [mg/kg]) was reported in a survey of 19 851 samples of various foods and feeds in the USA over 1982-86 (Luke *et al.*, 1988).

1.4 Regulations and guidelines

WHO (1987) recommended a drinking-water guideline of 17 µg/l for simazine. The maximal allowable concentration of simazine in drinking-water in Canada is 10 µg/l (Ritter & Wood, 1989). The US Environmental Protection Agency proposed to establish the 'maximal contaminant level' (feasible and enforceable limits to protect public health) and 'maximal contaminant level goal' (desirable but not enforceable) for simazine at 1 µg/l (Anon., 1990).

In the USSR, the maximal allowable concentration of simazine in workplace air is 2 mg/m^3. The single and mean daily maximal allowable concentration in the atmosphere of residential areas is 0.02 mg/m^3 (Izmerov, 1983).

National pesticide residue limits for simazine in food are presented in Table 2.

Tolerances are established for residues of simazine in sugar-cane byproducts (molasses and syrup and molasses intended for animal feed), resulting from application of the herbicide to growing sugar-cane, at 1 ppm (mg/kg); that for combined residues of simazine and its metabolites (2-amino-4-chloro-6-ethylamino-*s*-triazine and 2,4-diamino-6-chloro-*s*-triazine) in potable water when present therein as a result of application of the herbicide to growing aquatic weeds is 0.01 ppm (mg/kg) (US Environmental Protection Agency, 1989d,e).

Table 2. National pesticide residue limits for simazine in foods[a]

Country	Residue limit (mg/kg)	Commodities
Australia[b]	0.1	Asparagus, fruit, nuts
	0.05	Lupins
	0.01	Eggs, meat, milk, milk products, poultry, meat
Austria	1.0	Asparagus
	0.5	Maize
	0.1	Fish
	0.05	Other
Belgium	1.0	Asparagus
	0.1	Fruit, other vegetables, grains
	0.05	Potatoes
	0[c] (0.05)	Other foodstuffs of vegetable origin
Brazil[d]	10	Asparagus
	1.0	Conifers, rubber plants, sisal
	0.2	Maize, apples, citrus fruits, grapes, pears, sugar-cane, sorghum, pine-apples, bananas, black pepper, cocoa, coffee
	0.02	Babassu palm
Canada	Negligible	Apples, alfalfa (meat, milk and eggs), asparagus, blackberries, blueber-ries, maize, filberts/hazelnuts, fruit tree orchards (fruit), grapes, logan-berries, raspberries, strawberries, trefoil (meat, milk and eggs)
France	1.0	Asparagus
	0.1	Blackcurrants, pome fruit, raspberries, sweet maize
Germany	1.0	Asparagus
	0.1	Hops, other vegetable foodstuffs, fish, seafood and their products
Hungary	0.1	Crops and food
Italy	0.1	Citrus fruit, drupes, pomes, strawberries, grapes, olives, minor fruit, hazelnuts, artichokes, asparagus, maize, sorghum
Kenya	10	Asparagus
	0.5	Artichokes
	0.25	Almonds, apples, avocados, cherries, fresh maize including sweet (kernels plus cobs with husks removed), maize grain, cranberries, currants, dewberries, filberts, grapefruit, grapes, lemons, loganberries, macadamia nuts, olives, oranges, peaches, pears, plums, raspberries, strawberries, walnuts
	0.02	Eggs, milk, meat, fat and meat products of cattle, goats, hogs, horses, poultry and sheep
Netherlands	0.1	Cereals, fruit, vegetables
	0.05	Potatoes
	0[c] (0.05)	Other
Spain	1.0	Asparagus
	0.1	Fruit, maize grain, beans and alfalfa
	0.02	Other plant products
Switzerland	0.1	Maize, cereals, asparagus
	0.05	Berries, pome fruit

Table 2 (contd)

Country	Residue limit (mg/kg)	Commodities
USA[e]	15	Alfalfa, alfalfa forage and hay; Bermuda grass, Bermuda grass forage and hay, grass, grass forage and hay
	10	Asparagus
	0.5	Artichokes, sugar-cane
	0.25	Almonds, almonds (hulls), apples, avocados, blackberries, blueberries, boysenberries, cherries, maize (fodder, forage, fresh, grain), cranberries, currants, dewberries, filberts, grapefruit, grapes, lemons, loganberries, macadamia nuts, olives, oranges, peaches, pears, plums, raspberries, strawberries, sugar-cane
	0.2	Walnuts
	0.1	Pecans
	0.02	Fat, meat by-products, and meat of cattle, goats, hogs, horses, poultry and sheep, eggs, milk
	12[f]	Fish
	0.2[f]	Bananas
USSR[g]	1.0	Cereals
	0.2	Fruit, potatoes
	0.05	Grapes
Yugoslavia	0.5	Maize

[a]From Health and Welfare Canada (1990)
[b]Set at or about the limit of analytical determination
[c]The figure in parentheses is the lower limit for determining residues in the corresponding product according to the standard method of analysis.
[d]Provisional
[e]From US Environmental Protection Agency (1989c)
[f]Simazine and its metabolites
[g]From Izmerov (1983)

2. Studies of Cancer in Humans

One case-control study that suggested an association between ovarian cancer and exposure to herbicides in Italy mentioned simazine among the triazine herbicides to which subjects were exposed (Donna *et al.*, 1989) (see monograph on atrazine, p. 449).

3. Studies of Cancer in Experimental Animals[1]

The Working Group was aware of studies by the US National Technical Information Service (1968), Innes *et al.* (1969) and Pliss and Zabezhinsky (1970), in which simazine was tested in mice or rats by oral or subcutaneous administration and in mice by skin application. These studies were considered to be uninformative for an evaluation of carcinogenicity.

---

[1]The Working Group was aware of a study in progress in rats in which simazine was administered by oral administration (IARC, 1990).

4. Other Relevant Data

4.1 Absorption, distribution, metabolism and excretion

4.1.1 *Humans*

No data were available to the Working Group.

4.1.2 *Experimental systems*

The primary route of metabolism of simazine in rats, rabbits and other species *in vivo* and *in vitro* is *N*-dealkylation (Böhme & Bär, 1967; Adams *et al.*, 1990). [The Working Group noted that, while minor metabolites (other than some oxidation products of the alkyl side-chains) have not been identified, it is probable that the aromatic chlorine group is a site for glutathione conjugation, as occurs with atrazine (Timchalk *et al.*, 1990).]

Simazine is readily nitrosated by nitrogen oxides at an air:solid interface (Janzowski *et al.*, 1980).

4.2 Toxic effects

4.2.1 *Humans*

Simazine has been implicated as a cause of occupational contact dermatitis (Elizarov, 1972).

4.2.2 *Experimental systems*

The oral LD_{50} was reported to be > 5000 mg/kg bw in rats (Ben-Dyke *et al.*, 1970) and 973, 971 and 2367 mg/kg bw in adult female, male and weanling male rats, respectively. The dermal LD_{50} was > 2500 mg/kg bw in rats of each sex (Gaines & Linder, 1986). The lethal single dose of simazine in sheep has been estimated at 500 mg/kg bw (Hapke, 1968).

The liver and biliary system were identified as the targets for toxicity in rats given simazine by gavage at 15 mg/kg bw per day for three or 28 days (Olędzka-Słotwinska, 1974). Hypothyroidism was the most sensitive indicator of simazine toxicity in sheep at daily dose rates of 1.4-6 mg/kg bw; higher doses produced frank goitres and diffuse hepatic and cerebral damage. Necrotic and dystrophic changes of the testicular germinal epithelium were noted in rams given 6-25 mg/kg bw per day (Dshurov, 1979).

4.3 Reproductive and prenatal effects

4.3.1 *Humans*

No data were available to the Working Group.

4.3.2 *Experimental systems*

Simazine perturbed development of gonads *in ovo* and *in vitro* and reduced fertility in chicks and quail (Didier & Lutz-Ostertag, 1972). [The Working Group noted that doses and concentrations were not clearly defined.] It was reported in an abstract that simazine administered at 2.0 and 20 ppm (mg/kg) in the diet to laying mallard ducks throughout the egg production cycle caused no reproductive impairment (Fink, 1975).

Inhalation by rats of simazine at concentrations of up to 317 mg/m^3 on days 7-14 of gestation resulted in no developmental toxicity (Dilley *et al.*, 1977, abstract; Newell & Dilley, 1978). In contrast, a Bulgarian triazine herbicide (Polyzin 50) [impurities unspecified] was embryotoxic when pregnant rats were exposed by inhalation to 2 mg/m^3 in air; it was teratogenic following exposure to 0.2 and 2 mg/m^3 throughout pregnancy and to 2 mg/m^3 during the first trimester of pregnancy. Postnatal liver insufficiency occurred in the offspring (Mirkova & Ivanov, 1981). [The Working Group noted that the apparent discrepancy in effects between these studies might be due to unspecified impurities in the latter study.]

Administration of simazine to rats during the organogenetic period (gestational days 6-15) caused embryolethality at > 312 mg/kg bw, decreased fetal body weight at 2500 mg/kg bw and retarded ossification at ≥ 78 mg/kg bw. No teratogenic effect was observed (Chen *et al.*, 1981).

4.4 Genetic and related effects (see also Table 3 and Appendices 1 and 2)

4.4.1 *Humans*

No data were available to the Working Group.

4.4.2 *Experimental systems*

Simazine did not induce gene mutation in bacteria or in *Saccharomyces cerevisiae*, whereas there were mixed responses in mutation assays with plants. Simazine induced sex-linked recessive lethal mutation in *Drosophila melanogaster*.

Mutations were induced at the *tk* locus in mouse lymphoma L5178Y cells, but DNA damage, as indicated by unscheduled DNA synthesis, was not induced in cultured human fibroblasts.

Neither gene conversion nor mitotic recombination was induced in *S. cerevisiae* or aneuploidy in *Neurospora crassa*. Chromosomal aberrations were induced consistently in plants.

Dominant lethal effects, but not aneuploidy, were induced in *D. melanogaster* in a single study.

In a single study with cultured human lymphocytes, simazine induced a small increase in the frequency of sister chromatid exchange, but it had no such effect in cultured Chinese hamster cells, even at very high concentrations.

It did not induce micronucleus formation in bone-marrow cells of mice *in vivo*.

5. Summary of Data Reported and Evaluation

5.1 Exposure data

Simazine was introduced in 1957 as a systemic herbicide for use on grasses and weeds in food crops, especially maize, and for general weed control. It is available in many types of formulation, including wettable powders, granules, concentrates, suspensions and liquids. Exposure can occur during its production and application and *via* contamination of ground- and surface water.

Table 3. Genetic and related effects of simazine

Test system	Result[a] Without exogenous metabolic system	Result[a] With exogenous metabolic system	Dose[b] LED/HID	Reference
ECB, *Escherichia coli* PQ37, SOS chromotest	0	–	0.0000	Mersch–Sundermann et al. (1989)
SAD, *Salmonella typhimurium* TA1978/TA1538 differential toxicity	–	0	2000.0000	US National Technical Information Service, Environmental Protection Agency (1984)
SAD, *Salmonella typhimurium* SL525/SL4700	–	0	2000.0000	US National Technical Information Service, Environmental Protection Agency (1984)
SA0, *Salmonella typhimurium* TA100, reverse mutation	0		2500.0000	Simmon et al. (1977)
SA0, *Salmonella typhimurium* TA100, reverse mutation	0	+[c]	0.0000	Means et al. (1988)
SA0, *Salmonella typhimurium* TA100, reverse mutation	–	–	500.0000	Mersch–Sundermann et al. (1988)
SA0, *Salmonella typhimurium* TA100, reverse mutation	–	–	2500.0000	US National Technical Information Service, Environmental Protection Agency (1984)
SA2, *Salmonella typhimurium* TA102, reverse mutation	–	–	500.0000	Mersch–Sundermann et al. (1988)
SA3, *Salmonella typhimurium* TA1530, reverse mutation (spot test)	–	0	0.0000	Seiler (1973)
SA5, *Salmonella typhimurium* TA1535, reverse mutation	–	–	500.0000	US National Technical Information Service, Environmental Protection Agency (1977)
SA5, *Salmonella typhimurium* TA1535, reverse mutation	0	–	2500.0000	Simmon et al. (1977)
SA7, *Salmonella typhimurium* TA1537, reverse mutation	–	–	500.0000	US National Technical Information Service, Environmental Protection Agency (1977)
SA8, *Salmonella typhimurium* TA98, reverse mutation	–	–	500.0000	US National Technical Information Service, Environmental Protection Agency (1977)
SA8, *Salmonella typhimurium* TA1538, reverse mutation	0	–	2500.0000	Simmon et al. (1977)

Table 3 (contd)

Test system	Result[a]		Dose[b] LED/HID	Reference
	Without exogenous metabolic system	With exogenous metabolic system		
SA9, *Salmonella typhimurium* TA98, reverse mutation	0	–	2500.0000	Simmon *et al.* (1977)
SA9, *Salmonella typhimurium* TA98, reverse mutation	–	–	2500.0000	US National Technical Information Service, Environmental Protection Agency (1984)
SA9, *Salmonella typhimurium* TA98, reverse mutation	–	–	1000.0000	Mersch–Sundermann *et al.* (1988)
SAS, *Salmonella typhimurium*, reverse mutation	–	0	0.0000	Andersen *et al.* (1972)
SAS, *Salmonella typhimurium his* G46, reverse mutation (spot test)	–	0	0.0000	Seiler (1973)
SAS, *Salmonella typhimurium* TA1531, reverse mutation (spot test)	–	0	0.0000	Seiler (1973)
SAS, *Salmonella typhimurium* TA1532, reverse mutation (spot test)	–	0	0.0000	Seiler (1973)
SAS, *Salmonella typhimurium*, TA1534 reverse mutation (spot test)	–	0	0.0000	Seiler (1973)
SAS, *Salmonella typhimurium* TA97, reverse mutation	–	–	500.0000	Mersch–Sundermann *et al.* (1988)
ECF, *Escherichia coli*, forward mutation	–	0	0.0000	Fahrig (1974)
ECW, *Escherichia coli* WP2 *uvr*, reverse mutation	–	–	500.0000	US National Technical Information Service, Environmental Protection Agency (1984)
Serratia marcescens, reverse mutation	–	0	0.0000	Fahrig (1974)
SCG, *Saccharomyces cerevisiae*, gene conversion	–	0	0.0000	Fahrig (1974)
SCG, *Saccharomyces cerevisiae*, gene conversion	–	0	1000.0000[d]	Siebert & Lemperle (1974)
SCH, *Saccharomyces cerevisiae* D3, homozygosis by recombination	–	–	50000.0000	US National Technical Information Service, Environmental Protection Agency (1977)
SCR, *Saccharomyces cerevisiae* D7, reverse mutation	–	–	25000.0000	US National Technical Information Service, Environmental Protection Agency (1984)
SCG, *Saccharomyces cerevisiae* D7, gene conversion	–	–	25000.0000	US National Technical Information Service, Environmental Protection Agency (1984)

Table 3 (contd)

Test system	Result[a] Without exogenous metabolic system	With exogenous metabolic system	Dose[b] LED/HID	Reference
Saccharomyces cerevisiae D7, mitotic recombination	-	-	25000.0000	US National Technical Information Service, Environmental Protection Agency (1984)
SCR, *Saccharomyces cerevisiae*, reverse mutation	-	0	5.0000	Emnova et al. (1987)
NCN, *Neurospora crassa*, aneuploidy	-	0	0.0000	Griffiths (1979)
HSM, *Hordeum vulgare*, mutation	+	0	1000.0000	Wuu & Grant (1966)
HSM, *Hordeum vulgare*, mutation	-	0	200.0000	Stroyev (1968a)
PLM, *Rizobium meliloti*, mutation	-	0	5000.0000	Kaszubiak (1968)
PLM, *Zea mays*, chlorophyll mutation	+	0	200.0000	Morgun et al. (1982)
PLM, *Zea mays*, mutation	+	0	0.0000	Plewa et al. (1984)
PLM, *Fragaria ananassa*, mutation	+	0	0.0200	Malone and Dix (1990)
TSI, *Tradescantia paludosa*, micronuclei	-	0	200.0000	Ma et al. (1984)
HSC, *Hordeum vulgare*, chromosomal aberrations	+	0	500.0000	Wuu & Grant (1966)
HSC, *Hordeum vulgare*, chromosomal aberrations	+	0	500.0000 spray	Wuu & Grant (1967a)
HSC, *Hordeum vulgare*, chromosomal aberrations	(+)	0	500.0000	Stroyev (1968b)
HSC, *Hordeum vulgare*, chromosomal aberrations	(+)	0	500.0000[d]	Kahlon (1980)
VFC, *Vicia faba*, chromosomal aberrations	+	0	200.0000[d]	Wuu & Grant (1967b)
VFC, *Vicia faba*, chromosomal aberrations	+	0	5.0000	Hakeem & Shehab (1974)
VFC, *Vicia faba*, chromosomal aberrations	(+)	0	1000.0000	de Kergommeaux et al. (1983)
PLC, *Allium cepa*, chromosomal aberrations	+	0	20.0000	Chubutia & Ugulava (1973)
PLC, *Crepis capillaris*, chromosomal aberrations	+	0	1000.0000	Voskanyan & Avakyan (1984)
DMX, *Drosophila melanogaster*, sex-linked recessive lethal mutation	-	0	50.0000	Benes & Sram (1969)
DMX, *Drosophila melanogaster*, sex-linked recessive lethal mutation	+	0	80.0000	Murnik & Nash (1977)
DMX, *Drosophila melanogaster*, sex-linked recessive lethal mutation	+	0	200.0000	US National Technical Information Service, Environmental Protection Agency (1984)
DML, *Drosophila melanogaster*, dominant lethal test	+	0	6000.0000	Murnik & Nash (1977)
DMN, *Drosophila melanogaster*, aneuploidy	-	0	6000.0000	Murnik & Nash (1977)

Table 3 (contd)

Test system	Result[a] Without exogenous metabolic system	Result[a] With exogenous metabolic system	Dose[b] LED/HID	
GST, Gene mutation, mouse lymphoma L5178Y cells *in vitro*, *tk* locus	−	(+)	300.0000	US National Technical Information Service, Environmental Protection Agency (1984)
SIC, Sister chromatid exchange, Chinese hamster cells *in vitro*	−	−	1700.0000	US National Technical Information Service, Environmental Protection Agency (1984)
UHF, Unscheduled DNA synthesis, human lung WI 38 fibroblasts *in vitro*	−	−	200.0000	Jones *et al.* (1984)
SHL, Sister chromatid exchange, human lymphocytes *in vitro*	(+)	0	0.0000	Ghiazza *et al.* (1984)
MVM, Micronucleus test, mouse *in vivo*	−	0	500.0000	Jones *et al.* (1984)

[a] +, positive; (+), weakly positive; −, negative; 0, not tested; ?, inconclusive (variable response in several experiments within an adequate study)
[b] In-vitro tests, μg/ml; in-vivo tests, mg/kg bw
[c] Tested with extracts of simazine-treated *Zea mays*
[d] Commercial pesticide tested

Exposure could also occur through consumption of foods containing residues. Simazine residues were not detected in large-scale surveys of food products in Canada and the USA.

5.2 Carcinogenicity in humans

No adequate data were available to the Working Group.

5.3 Experimental carcinogenicity data

No adequate data were available to the Working Group.

5.4 Other relevant data

No data on the genetic and related effects of simazine in humans were available to the Working Group.

Simazine did not induce micronucleus formation in mice. It induced a small increase in the frequency of sister chromatid exchange in human cells *in vitro* but not in rodent cells. Simazine did not induce genetic damage in any other tests, except in plants where chromosomal aberrations were induced and in *Drosophila melanogaster* where dominant lethal effects and gene mutation were induced.

5.5 Evaluation[1]

There is *inadequate evidence* in humans for the carcinogenicity of simazine.

There is *inadequate evidence* in experimental animals for the carcinogenicity of simazine.

Overall evaluation

Simazine *is not classifiable as to its carcinogenicity to humans (Group 3).*

6. References

Adams, N.H., Levi, P.E. & Hodgson, E. (1990) In vitro studies of the metabolism of atrazine, simazine and terbutryn in several vertebrate species. *J. agric. Food Chem.*, 38, 1411-1417

Andersen, K.J., Leighty, E.G. & Takahashi, M.K. (1972) Evaluation of herbicides for possible mutagenic properties. *J. agric. Food Chem.*, 20, 649-656

Anon. (1989) *Crop Protection Chemicals Reference*, 5th ed., New York, Chemical and Pharmaceutical Press, pp. 538-627

Anon. (1990) Drinking-water regulations. *BIBRA Bull.*, 29, 229

Ben-Dyke, R., Sanderson, D.M. & Noakes, D.N. (1970) Acute toxicity data for pesticides (1970). *World Rev. Pest Control*, 9, 119-127

---

[1]For definition of the italicized terms, see Preamble, pp. 26-28.

Benes, V. & Sram, R. (1969) Mutagenic activity of some pesticides in *Drosophila melanogaster*. *Ind. Med.*, *38*, 442-444

Böhme, C. & Bär, F. (1967) The transformation of triazine herbicides in the animal organism (Ger.). *Food Cosmet. Toxicol.*, *5*, 23-28

Budavari, S., ed. (1989) *The Merck Index*, 11th ed., Rahway, NJ, Merck & Co., p. 1351

Chen, P.C., Chi, H.F. & Kan, S.Y. (1981) Experimental studies on the toxicity and teratogenicity of simazine (Chin.). *Chin. J. prev. Med.*, *15*, 83-85

Chen, Y.-L., Duh, J.-R. & Wang, Y.-S. (1983) The influence of climate and soil properties on the degradation of simazine in soils in Taiwan. *Proc. natl Sci. Counc. ROC(A)*, *7*, 36-41

Chubutia, R.A. & Ugulava, N.A. (1973) Cytogenetic effect of herbicides (Georgian). *Tr. Nauchno.-Issled. Inst. Zashch. Rast.*, *25*, 97-99

Didier, R. & Lutz-Ostertag, Y. (1972) Action of simazine on the genital tract of chick and quail embryos *in vivo* and *in vitro* (Fr.). *C.R. Soc. Biol.*, *166*, 1691-1693

Dilley, J.V., Chernoff, N., Kay, D., Winslow, N. & Newell, G.W. (1977) Inhalation teratology studies of five chemicals in rats (Abstract) *Toxicol. appl. Pharmacol.*, *41*, 196

Donna, A., Crosignani, P., Robutti, F., Betta, P.G., Bocca, R., Mariani, N., Ferrario, F., Fissi, R. & Berrino, F. (1989) Triazine herbicides and ovarian epithelial neoplasms. *Scand. J. Work Environ. Health*, *15*, 47-53

Dshurov, A. (1979) Histological changes in organs of sheep in chronic simazine poisoning (Ger.). *Zbl. Vet. Med. A.*, *26*, 44-54

Elizarov, G.P. (1972) Occupational skin diseases caused by simazine and propazine (Russ.). *Vestn. Derm. Venerol.*, *46*, 27-29

Emnova, E.E., Mereniouk, G.V. & Tsurkan, L.G. (1987) Genetic study of simazine-trizine herbicides on *Saccharomyces cerevisiae* (Russ.). *Tsitol. Genet.*, *21*, 127-130

Fahrig, R. (1974) Comparative mutagenicity studies with pesticides. In: Rosenfeld, C. & Davis, W., eds, *Environmental Pollution and Carcinogenic Risks* (IARC Scientific Publications No. 10), Lyon, IARC, pp. 161-181

Fink, R.J. (1975) The effect of simazine on the reproductive capability of mallard ducks (Abstract No. 168). *Toxicol. appl. Pharmacol.*, *33*, 188-189

Gaines, T.B. & Linder, R.E. (1986) Acute toxicity of pesticides in adult and weanling rats. *Fundam. appl. Toxicol.*, *7*, 299-308

Ghiazza, G., Zavarise, G., Lanero, M. & Ferraro, G. (1984) SCE (sister chromatid exchanges) induced in chromosomes of human lymphocytes by trifluralin, atrazine and simazine (Ital.). *Boll. Soc. It. Biol. sper.*, *60*, 2149-2153

Government of Canada (1990) *Report on National Surveillance Data from 1984/85 to 1988/89*, Ottawa

Griffiths, A.J.F. (1979) Neurospora prototroph selection system for studying aneuploid production. *Environ. Health Perspect.*, *31*, 75-80

Hakeem, H. & Shehab, A. (1974) Cytological effects of simazine on *Vicia faba*. *Proc. Egypt. Acad. Sci.*, *25*, 61-66

Hapke, H.J. (1968) Research into the toxicology of the weed killer simazine (Ger.). *Berl. Münch. Tierärztl. Wochenschr.*, *81*, 301-303

Health and Welfare Canada (1990) *National Pesticide Residue Limits in Food*, Ottawa, Bureau of Chemical Safety, Food Directorate, Health Protection Branch

IARC (1987a) *IARC Monographs on the Evaluation of Carcinogenic Risks to Humans*, Suppl. 7, *Overall Evaluations of Carcinogenicity: An Updating of* IARC Monographs *Volumes 1 to 42*, Lyon, pp. 92-93

IARC (1987b) *IARC Monographs on the Evaluation of Carcinogenic Risks to Humans*, Suppl. 7, *Overall Evaluations of Carcinogenicity: An Updating of* IARC Monographs *Volumes 1 to 42*, Lyon, pp. 157-160

IARC (1990) *Directory of Agents Being Tested for Carcinogenicity*, No. 14, Lyon, p. 62

Innes, J.R.M., Ulland, B.M., Valerio, M.G., Petrucelli, L., Fishbein, L., Hart, E.R., Pallotta, A.J., Bates, R.R., Falk, H.L., Gart, J.J., Klein, M., Mitchell, I. & Peters, J. (1969) Bioassay of pesticides and industrial chemicals for tumorigenicity in mice: a preliminary note. *J. natl Cancer Inst.*, *42*, 1101-1114

Izmerov, N.F., ed. (1983) *International Register of Potentially Toxic Chemicals. Scientific Reviews of Soviet Literature on Toxicity and Hazards of Chemicals: Simazine* (Issue 28), Moscow, Centre of International Projects, United Nations Environment Programme

Janzowski, C., Klein, R. & Preussmann, R. (1980) Formation of *N*-nitroso compounds of the pesticides atrazine, simazine and carbaryl with nitrogen oxides. In: Walker, E.A., Griciute, L., Castegnaro, M. & Börzsönyi, M., eds, *N-Nitroso Compounds: Analysis, Formation and Occurrence* (IARC Scientific Publications No. 31), Lyon, IARC, pp. 329-339

Kahlon, P.S. (1980) Seedling injury and chromosome aberrations induced by Bladex, Dowpon, Princep and Tenoran. *J. Tenn. Acad. Sci.*, *55*, 17-19

Kaszubiak, H. (1968) The effects of herbicides on *Rhizobium*. III. Influence of herbicides in mutation. *Acta microbiol. pol.*, *17*, 51-58

de Kergommeaux, D.J., Grant, W.F. & Sandhu, S.S. (1983) Clastogenic and physiological response of chromosomes to nine pesticides in the *Vicia faba* in vivo root tip assay system. *Mutat. Res.*, *24*, 69-84

Knüsli, E., Burchfield, H.P. & Storr, S.E.E. (1964) Simazine. In: *Analytical Methods for Pesticides, Plant Growth Regulators and Food Additives*, Vol. IV, *Herbicides*, New York, Academic Press, pp. 213-219

Luke, M.A., Masumoto, M.T., Cairns, T. & Hundley, H.K. (1988) Levels and incidences of pesticide residues in various foods and animal feeds analyzed by the Luke multiresidue methodology for fiscal years 1982-1986. *J. Assoc. off. anal. Chem.*, *71*, 415-420

Ma, T.-H., Harris, M.M., Anderson, V.A., Ahmed, I., Mohammad, K., Bare, J.L. & Lin, G. (1984) Tradescantia-micronucleus (Trad-MCN) tests on 140 health-related agents. *Mutat. Res.*, *138*, 157-167

Malone, R.P. & Dix, P.J. (1990) Mutagenesis and triazine herbicide effects in strawberry shoot cultures. *J. exp. Bot.*, *41*, 463-469

Means, J.C., Plewa, M.J. & Gentile, J.M. (1988) Assessment of the mutagenicity of fractions from *s*-triazine-treated *Zea mays*. *Mutat. Res.*, *197*, 325-326

Meister, R.T., ed. (1990) *Farm Chemicals Handbook '90*, Willoughby, OH, Meister Publishing Company, pp. C261-C262

Mersch-Sundermann, V., Dickgiesser, N., Hablizel, U. & Gruber, B. (1988) Examination of the mutagenicity of organic microcontaminations of the environment. I. Mutagenicity of selected herbicides and insecticides in the *Salmonella*-microsome test (Ames test) in relation to the pathogenic potency of contaminated ground- and drinking-water (Ger.). *Zbl. Bakt. Hyg. B.*, *186*, 247-260

Mersch-Sundermann, V., Hofmeister, A., Müller, G. & Hof, H. (1989) Examination of the muta-genicity of organic microcontaminations of the environment. III. The mutagenicity of selected herbicides and insecticides with the SOS-chromotest (Ger.). *Zbl. Hyg.*, *189*, 135-146

Mirkova, E. & Ivanov, I. (1981) A propos of the embryotoxic effect of triazine herbicide Polyzin 50 (Russ.). *Probl. Khig.*, 6, 36-43

Morgun, V.V., Logvinenko, V.F., Merezhinskii, Y.G., Lapina, T.V. & Frigorenko, N.V. (1982) Cytogenetic and genetic activity of the herbicides atrazine, simazine, prometrin and linuron (Russ.). *Tsitol. Genet.*, 16, 38-41

Murnik, M.R. & Nash, C.L. (1977) Mutagenicity of the triazine herbicides atrazine, cyanazine and simazine in *Drosophila melanogaster. J. Toxicol. environ. Health*, 3, 691-697

Newell, G.W. & Dilley, J.V. (1978) *Teratology and Acute Toxicology of Selected Pesticides Administered by Inhalation* (EPA-600/1-78-003), Research Triangle Park, NC, US Environmental Protection Agency

Olędzka-Słotwinska, H. (1974) The effect of simazine on the ultrastructure and activities of some hydrolases of the rat liver. *Ann. Med. Sect. Pol. Acad. Sci.*, 19, 141-142

Plewa, M.J., Wagner, E.D., Gentile, G.J. & Gentile, J.M. (1984) An evaluation of the genotoxic properties of herbicides following plant and animal activation. *Mutat. Res.*, 136, 233-245

Pliss, G.B. & Zabezhinsky, M.A. (1970) On carcinogenic properties of symmetrical triazine derivatives (Russ.). *Vopr. Oncol.*, 16, 82-85

Rahman, A. & Holland, P.T. (1985) Persistence and mobility of simazine in some New Zealand soils. *N. Z. J. exp. Agric.*, 13, 59-65

Ritter, L. & Wood, G. (1989) Evaluation and regulation of pesticides in drinking water: a Canadian approach. *Food. Addit. Contam.*, 6 (Suppl. 1), S87-S94

Royal Society of Chemistry (1986) *European Directory of Agrochemical Products*, Vol. 2, *Herbicides*, Cambridge, pp. 539-550

Royal Society of Chemistry (1989) *The Agrochemicals Handbook* [Dialog Information Services (File 306)], Cambridge

Sadtler Research Laboratories (1980) *The Standard Spectra, 1980, Cumulative Index*, Philadelphia, PA

Seiler, J.P. (1973) A survey on the mutagenicity of various pesticides. *Experientia*, 29, 622-623

Siebert, D. & Lemperle, E. (1974) Genetic effects of herbicides: induction of mitotic gene conversion in *Saccharomyces cerevisiae. Mutat. Res.*, 22, 111-120

Simmon, V.F., Kauhanen, K. & Tardiff, R.G. (1977) Mutagenic activity of chemicals identified in drinking water. In: Scott, D., Bridges, B.A. & Sobels, F.H., eds, *Progress in Genetic Toxicology*, Amsterdam, North Holland Biomedical Press, pp. 249-258

Stroyev, V.S. (1968a) The mutagenic effect by the action of herbicides on the barley (Russ.). *Genetika*, IV, 164-167

Stroyev, V.S. (1968b) Cytogenetic activity of the herbicides—simazine and maleic acid hydrazide (Russ.). *Genetika*, IV, 130-134

Timchalk, C., Dryzga, M.D., Langvardt, P.W., Kastl, P.E. & Osborne, D.W. (1990) Determination of the effect of tridiphane on the pharmacokinetics of [^{14}C]-atrazine following oral administration to male Fischer 344 rats. *Toxicology*, 61, 27-40

US Environmental Protection Agency (1984a) *Pesticide Fact Sheet No. 23: Simazine*, Washington DC, Office of Pesticide Programs

US Environmental Protection Agency (1984b) *Registration Standard for Pesticide Products Containing Simazine as the Active Ingredient* (PB84-212349), Washington DC

US Environmental Protection Agency (1988a) *Simazine*, Washington DC, Office of Drinking Water

US Environmental Protection Agency (1988b) Method 525. Determination of organic compounds in drinking water by liquid-solid extraction and capillary column gas chromatography/mass spectrometry. In: *Methods for the Determination of Organic Compounds in Drinking Water* (EPA Report No. EPA-600/4-88/039; US NTIS PB89-220461), Cincinnati, OH, Environmental Monitoring Systems Laboratory, pp. 325-356

US Environmental Protection Agency (1989a) Method 507. Revision 2.0. Determination of nitrogen- and phosphorus-containing pesticides in water by gas chromatography with a nitrogen-phosphorus detector. In: *Methods for the Determination of Organic Compounds in Drinking Water* (EPA Report No. EPA-600/4-88/039; US NTIS PB89-220461), Cincinnati, OH, Environmental Monitoring Systems Laboratory, pp. 143-170

US Environmental Protection Agency (1989b) Method 505. Revision 2.0. Analysis of organohalide pesticides and commercial polychlorinated biphenyl (PCB) products in water by microextraction and gas chromatography. In: *Methods for the Determination of Organic Compounds in Drinking Water* (EPA Report No. EPA-600/4-88/039; US NTIS PB89-220461), Cincinnati, OH, Environmental Monitoring Systems Laboratory, pp. 109-141

US Environmental Protection Agency (1989c) Simazine; tolerances for residues. Tolerances and exemptions from tolerances for pesticide chemicals in or on raw agricultural commodities. *US Code fed. Regul., Title 40*, Part 180.213

US Environmental Protection Agency (1989d) Simazine. Tolerances for pesticides in food. *US Code fed. Regul., Title 40*, Part 185.5350

US Environmental Protection Agency (1989e) Simazine. Tolerances for pesticides in animal feed. *US Code fed. Regul., Title 40*, Part 186.5350

US Food and Drug Administration (1989a) Simazine. In: *Pesticide Analytical Manual*, Vol. II, *Methods Which Detect Multiple Residues*, Washington DC, US Department of Health and Human Services, pp. 1-9

US Food and Drug Administration (1989b) Simazine method II. In: *Pesticide Analytical Manual*, Vol. II, *Methods Which Detect Multiple Residues*, Washington DC, US Department of Health and Human Services, p. 11

US Food and Drug Administration (1989c) Simazine method III. In: *Pesticide Analytical Manual*, Vol. II, *Methods Which Detect Multiple Residues*, Washington DC, US Department of Health and Human Services, pp. 13-20

US Food and Drug Administration (1989d) Simazine method IV. In: *Pesticide Analytical Manual*, Vol. II, *Methods Which Detect Multiple Residues*, Washington DC, US Department of Health and Human Services, pp. 21-27

US National Technical Information Service (1968) *Evaluation of Carcinogenic, Teratogenic and Mutagenic Activities of Selected Pesticides and Industrial Chemicals*, Vol. 1, *Carcinogenic Study*, Washington DC, US Department of Commerce

US National Technical Information Service, Environmental Protection Agency (1977) *Evaluation of Selected Pesticides as Chemical Mutagens*: in vitro *and* in vivo *Studies* (EPA-600/1-77-028), Washington DC

US National Technical Information Service, Environmental Protection Agency (1984) In Vitro *and* In Vivo *Mutagenicity Studies of Environmental Chemicals* (EPA-600/1-84-003), Washington DC

Vlier Zygadlo, L. (1982) *Preliminary Quantitative Usage Analysis of Simazine*, Washington DC, Office of Pesticide Programs, Environmental Protection Agency

Voskanyan, A.Z. & Avakyan, V.A. (1984) Cytogenetic effect of simazine and linuron herbicides on the chromosomes of *Crepis capillaris* (Russ.). *Biol. Zhuv. Armenii, 9*, 741-744

Walker, A. (1976) Simulation of herbicide persistence in soil. *Pestic. Sci.*, 7, 41-49

WHO (1987) *Drinking-water Quality: Guidelines for Selected Herbicides* (Environmental Health Criteria 27), Copenhagen, p. 8

Williams, S., ed. (1984) *Official Methods of Analysis of the Association of Official Analytical Chemists*, 14th ed., Washington DC, Association of Official Analytical Chemists, pp. 145-146

Worthing, C.R. & Walker, S.B., eds (1987) *The Pesticide Manual: A World Compendium*, 8th ed., Thornton Heath, British Crop Protection Council, pp. 746-747

Wuu, K.D. & Grant, W.F. (1966) Morphological and somatic chromosomal aberrations induced by pesticides in barley (*Hordeum vulgare*). *Can. J. Genet. Cytol.*, 8, 481-501

Wuu, K.D. & Grant, W.F. (1967a) Chromosomal aberrations induced by pesticides in meiotic cells of barley. *Cytologia*, 32, 31-41

Wuu, K.D. & Grant, W.F. (1967b) Chromosomal aberrations in somatic cells of *Vicia faba* by pesticides. *Nucleus*, 10, 37-46

TRIFLURALIN

1. Exposure Data

1.1 Chemical and physical data

1.1.1 Synonyms, structural and molecular data

Chem. Abstr. Serv. Reg. No.: 1582-09-8
Replaced CAS Reg. Nos: 39300-53-3; 52627-52-8; 61373-95-3; 75635-23-3
Chem. Abstr. Name: 2,6-Dinitro-N,N-dipropyl-4-(trifluoromethyl)benzenamine
IUPAC Systematic Name: α,α,α-Trifluoro-2,6-dinitro-N,N-dipropyl-*para*-toluidine; 2,6-dinitro-N,N-dipropyl-4-trifluoromethylaniline
Synonyms: 4-(Trifluoromethyl)-2,6-dinitro-N,N-dipropylaniline

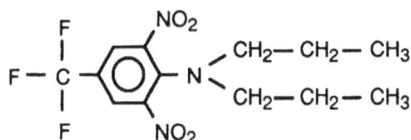

$C_{13}H_{16}F_3N_3O_4$ Mol. wt: 335.28

1.1.2 Chemical and physical properties

(a) *Description*: Yellow-orange crystals (Royal Society of Chemistry, 1989)
(b) *Boiling-point*: 139-140°C at 4.2 mm Hg [0.56 kPa] (Budavari, 1989)
(c) *Melting-point*: 48.5-49°C (technical-grade, 98% pure) (Worthing & Walker, 1987)
(d) *Spectroscopy data*: Infrared spectroscopy data have been reported (US Environmental Protection Agency, 1975).
(e) *Solubility*: Slightly soluble in water (< 1 mg/l at 27°C); freely soluble in common organic solvents, such as acetone (400 g/l), Stoddard solvent, xylene (580 g/l) and aromatic naphthas (Worthing & Walker, 1987; Budavari, 1989; Royal Society of Chemistry, 1989; Meister, 1990)
(f) *Vapour pressure*: 1.02×10^{-4} mm Hg [0.14×10^{-4} kPa] at 25°C (Royal Society of Chemistry, 1989)
(g) *Stability*: Stable to hydrolysis (US Environmental Protection Agency, 1987); decomposed by ultraviolet irradiation under acidic conditions, mainly to 2-amino-6-nitro-α,α,α-trifluoro-*para*-toluidine; at alkaline pH mainly to 2-ethyl-7-nitro-5-fluoromethylbenzimidazole (Leitis & Crosby, 1974)

(h) *Conversion factor for airborne concentrations*[1]: $mg/m^3 = 13.71 \times ppm$

1.1.3 *Trade names, technical products and impurities*

Some examples of trade names are: Agreflan; Agriflan 24; Elancolan; L 36352; Lilly 36,352; Nitran; Nitran K; Olitref; Super-Treflan; Synfloran; Trefanocide; Treflan; Trifloran; Trifluraline; Trikepin; Tristar.

In the USA, trifluralin is available as 94.5-98% active ingredient technical product (US Environmental Protection Agency, 1987). It is available as emulsifiable concentrates, granules and liquid formulations (Anon., 1989; Meister, 1990). In Europe, a soluble concentrate is also available (Royal Society of Chemistry, 1986). In the USSR, trifluralin is available as emulsifiable concentrates and in granules (Izmerov, 1985).

Trifluralin is compatible with most other pesticides and may be combined with both dry and liquid fertilizers (Royal Society of Chemistry, 1989). It is formulated in combination with isoproturon, linuron, napropamide, terbutryne, benefin (benfluralin), metribuzin, bromoxynil octanoate, ioxynil octanoate, trietazine, neburon and alachlor with petroleum distillates (Worthing & Walker, 1987; Anon., 1989).

Technical-grade trifluralin may be contaminated with N-nitrosodi-n-propylamine (Kello, 1989; see IARC, 1978). This compound is present as a result of a side-reaction between nitrosating agents and di-n-propylamine during an amination step in the manufacturing process (West & Day, 1979). In the USA, trifluralin may contain no more than 0.5 ppm (mg/kg) total N-nitrosamine (US Environmental Protection Agency, 1987) and in Italy, no more than 0.4 ppm (mg/kg) nitrosamines (Anon., 1990). In the specification of FAO (1988), trifluralin may contain no more than 1 mg/kg.

1.1.4 *Analysis*

Selected methods for the analysis of trifluralin in various matrices are given in Table 1.

Table 1. Methods for the analysis of trifluralin[a]

Sample	Sample preparation	Assay procedure	Limit of detection	Reference
Water	Extract with dichloromethane; isolate extract; dry; concentrate with solvent exchange to methyl *tert*-butyl ether	GC/ECD	0.025 μg/l	US Environmental Protection Agency (1989a)
Crops	Extract with methanol; re-extract into dichloromethane; evaporate; dissolve in hexane; clean-up on Florisil column; evaporate to dryness; dissolve in benzene	GC/ECD	0.005-0.01 ppm (mg/kg)	US Food and Drug Administration (1989)

[1]Calculated from: $mg/m^3 = (molecular\ weight/24.45) \times ppm$, assuming standard temperature (25°C) and pressure (760 mm Hg [101.3 kPa])

Table 1 (contd)

Sample	Sample preparation	Assay procedure	Limit of detection	Reference
Specified vegetables (carrots, green beans, *Brassica* vegetables)	Crops containing BHC, ethion and/or zineb require an extra TLC clean-up procedure. Develop TLC plate; scrap trifluralin region; transfer to a micro column; elute with acetone; evaporate eluate to dryness; dissolve residue in benzene	GC/ECD	< 0.01 ppm (mg/kg)	US Food and Drug Administration (1989)
Dry formulation	Extract with acetone in Soxhlet; evaporate; dilute to volume with acetone	GC/FID	Not reported	Williams (1984)
Liquid formulation	Extract with acetone	GC/FID	Not reported	Association of Official Analytical Chemists (1984)

[a]Abbreviations: BHC, benzene hexachloride; GC/ECD, gas chromatograph/electron capture detector; GC/FID, gas chromatograph/flame ionization detector; TLC, thin-layer chromatography

1.2 Production and use

1.2.1 *Production*

Trifluralin was first registered in 1963 (US Environmental Protection Agency, 1987). It is prepared by reacting di-*n*-propylamine with 2,6-dinitro-4-trifluoromethylchlorobenzene (Izmerov, 1985).

Trifluralin is produced currently in Argentina, Brazil, Guatemala, Hungary, Israel, Italy, Mexico, Spain and the USA (Meister, 1990). According to information supplied by current manufacturers, annual worldwide production is approximately 20 000-25 000 tonnes. Production by two companies (in tonnes) was: 1985, ~19 000; 1980, ~28 000; 1975, ~17 600; 1970, ~4100; 1965, ~1500. A third company produced 11 900 tonnes in 1986-89, 9400 tonnes in 1981-85 and 3200 tonnes in 1978-80.

1.2.2 *Use*

Trifluralin is a selective soil herbicide which acts by entering the seedling in the hypocotyl region and disrupting cell division. It also inhibits root development (Royal Society of Chemistry, 1989).

Trifluralin is used for pre-emergence control of many annual grasses and broad-leaved weeds in *Brassicas*, beans, peas, carrots, parsnips, lettuce, capsicums, tomatoes, artichokes, onions, garlic, vines, strawberries, raspberries, citrus fruit, oilseed rape, groundnuts, soya beans, sunflowers, safflowers, ornamental plants, cotton, sugar beets, sugar-cane and in forestry. It is also used with linuron or isoproturon for control of annual grasses and broad-leaved weeds in winter cereals. Trifluralin is normally applied to soil before planting, but it may be applied after planting of some crops (Royal Society of Chemistry, 1989). Trifluralin plus 2,4-D is used as a post-planting herbicide for transplanted rice (Worthing & Walker, 1987).

In the USA in 1980, 90% of yearly usage of trifluralin (active ingredient) was accounted for by three crops: soya beans, 9700 tonnes; cotton, 2900 tonnes; and sunflowers, 1200 tonnes (Weiler, 1980). Approximately 14-16 thousand tonnes of trifluralin (active ingredient) were used in the USA in 1987 (US Environmental Protection Agency, 1990).

1.3 Occurrence

1.3.1 *Water*

Trifluralin was found in 172 of 2047 surface water samples and in one of 507 groundwater samples in the USA. Residues were found in surface water in seven states in the USA at a concentration (85th percentile) of 0.54 µg/litre. Trifluralin has also been detected in finished drinking-water (US Environmental Protection Agency, 1988).

N-Nitroso-di-*n*-propylamine was not detected in water samples from ponds or wells located in or near fields that had been treated with trifluralin at various rates (limit of detection, 0.01 µg/litre) (West & Day, 1979).

1.3.2 *Soil*

In studies carried out anaerobically in the dark at 25°C, trifluralin at 5 ppm (mg/kg) degraded rapidly in a non-sterile silt loam soil, and < 1% of the applied material was detected after 20 days. Autoclaving and flooding of the soil decreased the rate of degradation. Under aerobic conditions, degradation was slower, with 15% of the trifluralin lost after 20 days (Parr & Smith, 1973).

^{14}C-Trifluralin applied at 1.1 kg/ha was relatively immobile in sand, sandy loam, silt, loam and clay loam columns (30 cm) eluted with 60 cm of water. More than 90% of the applied radiolabel remained in the top 0-10 cm segment (US Environmental Protection Agency, 1988).

In the field, ^{14}C-trifluralin (99% pure) applied at a rate of 0.84-6.72 kg/ha dissipated in the top 0-0.5-cm layer of a silt loam soil, with 14, 4 and 1.5% of the amount applied remaining after 1, 2 and 3 years, respectively. Some 30 minor degradation products were identified; none represented more than 2.8% of the amount applied. In a medium loam soil, trifluralin (4 lb/gal [7 kg/litre] emulsifiable concentrate) applied at 0.75 and 1.5 lb/acre [0.85 and 1.7 kg/ha] degraded, with 20 and 32%, respectively, remaining after 120 days. Trifluralin (7 kg/litre emulsifiable concentrate) applied to a sandy loam soil at 1.0 lb active ingredient/acre [1.1 kg/ha] had a half-time of 2-4 months (US Environmental Protection Agency, 1988).

Trifluralin was detected in 12% of soil samples taken from 15 states in the USA at levels ranging from 0.08 to 0.24 ppm (mg/kg). The areas from which the samples were taken were considered to use pesticides regularly according to available records (Stevens *et al.*, 1970). Trifluralin residues were also detected in 3.5% of 1729 agricultural soil samples tested in 1969 in the USA (Wiersma *et al.*, 1972). α,α,α-Trifluorotoluene-3,4,5-triamine, a degradation product of trifluralin, appeared to be a key compound in the formation of soil-bound residues (Golab *et al.*, 1979).

Maximal seasonal losses of trifluralin applied for three consecutive years at 1.4 kg/ha were less than 0.05% in the run-off (water/sediment suspensions) from silty clay loam field plots planted with cotton or soya beans under a wide range of rainfall (0.3-13 cm) (Willis et al., 1975).

1.3.3 Food

As part of the national surveillence programme in Canada, 1344 food samples were analysed for trifluralin in the period 1984-89. Residues were detected in carrots at 0.05-0.3 mg/kg in seven of 138 samples. No residue was detected in fruit, other vegetables or maize (Government of Canada, 1990).

Residues of volatile nitrosamines (N-nitrosodimethylamine, N-nitrosodi-n-propylamine or N-butyl-N-ethyl-N-nitrosamine) were not detected in crops and plants from fields treated with trifluralin at 0.56-2.2 kg/ha (limit of detection 0.2 ppb [μg/kg]) (West & Day, 1979).

1.3.4 Occupational exposure

Application of trifluralin containing 3.5-6.4 ppm (mg/kg) N-nitroso-di-n-propylamine at a rate of 0.69-2 lb/acre [0.78-2.27 kg/ha] resulted in average air concentrations of < 0.001-0.015 μg/m^3 of the nitrosamine and 0.12-37.3 μg/m^3 trifluralin (Day et al., 1982).

1.4 Regulations and guidelines

WHO (1987) recommended a drinking-water guideline level of 170 μg/litre for trifluralin. In the USSR, the maximal allowable concentration in water of open basins is 860 μg/litre and that in basins used for fish-breeding purposes, 0.3 μg/litre (Izmerov, 1985).

The tolerance established in the USA for residues of trifluralin in peppermint oil and spearmint oil is 2 ppm (mg/litre) (US Environmental Protection Agency, 1989c). National pesticide residue limits for trifluralin in foods are presented in Table 2.

Table 2. National pesticide residue limits for trifluralin in foods[a]

Country	Residue limit (mg/kg)	Commodities
Australia	0.5	Carrots
	0.05[b]	Adzuki beans, all other vegetables, cereal grains, chickpeas, cowpeas, eggs, faba beans, fruit, lablab, lupins, meat, milk, milk products, mung beans, oilseeds, peanuts, poultry meat, sugar-cane
Austria	3.0	Cauliflower
	1.0	Carrots
	0.1	Cabbage, oilseeds, sweet red/green peppers, tomatoes
	0.05	Other
Belgium	0.05	Carrots, tomatoes, onions, artichokes, cabbages and related vegetables
	0.01	Grains
	0 (0.01)[c]	Other
Brazil	0.05[d]	Carrots, garlic, onions, citrus fruit, Brassicas, eggplant, okra, peppers, tomatoes, field beans, string beans, manioc, oilseeds, coffee beans
Canada	0.5	Carrots
	Negligible	Asparagus, barley, cole crops, crambe, beans, flax, herbs, kale, lentils, mustard seed, peas, peppers, rapeseed (canola oil), rye, safflower (oil), sainfoin forage (meat, milk and eggs), Saskatoon berries, strawberries, soya beans, sunflower, tomatoes, triticale, turnips (rutabagas), wheat

Table 2 (contd)

Country	Residue limit (mg/kg)	Commodities
France	0.05	Carrots, tomatoes, onions, artichokes, cabbage
Germany	3	Cauliflower
	1.0	Carrots
	0.5	Turnips, rutabagas
	0.1	Other vegetable foodstuffs
Hungary	0.1	Crops and food
Italy	0.15	Carrots, oilseeds
	0.05	Citrus fruit, drupes, apples, pears, strawberries, grapes, garden vegetables (except carrots), potatoes, sugar beets, mint
	0.01	Wheat, barley, rye, rice
Japan	0.2	Carrots
	0.01	Rice, oats and other minor cereals, fruit, vegetables (except carrots), potatoes, etc., pulses, tea
Kenya	1.0	Carrots
	0.5	Citrus fruit, cottonseed, cucurbits, fruiting vegetables, grapes, hops, leafy vegetables, nuts, peanuts, root crop vegetables (except carrots), safflower seed, seed and pod vegetables, stone fruits, sugar-cane, sunflower seed, wheat grain
Mexico	1.0	Carrots
	0.2[e]	Alfalfa (hay)
	0.05[e]	Cotton (seed), peanuts, sugar cane, citrus fruit, celery, eggplant, broccoli, wheat, grapes, nuts, squash, safflower seed, chili peppers, cabbage, asparagus, spinach, lettuce, tomato, maize (forage), cucumber, watermelon
Netherlands	0.01[f]	All cereals
	0 (0.01)[g]	Other
Spain	1.0	Carrots
	0.05	Other plant products
Switzerland	0.05	Cereals, rapeseed, tomatoes, cabbages, peas
USA[h]	2	Mung bean sprouts
	1.0	Carrots
	0.2[e]	Alfalfa, hay
	0.1	Peanut (hulls)
	0.05[e]	Asparagus, barley (fodder, forage, hay and straw), citrus fruit, maize grain (excluding popcorn); maize (grain forage and fodder, excluding popcorn), cottonseed, cucurbits, flax seed and straw, grain crops (excluding fresh maize and rice grain), grapes, hops, legume forage, nuts, peanuts, peppermint hay, rape (seed and straw), safflower seed, sorghum (fodder and forage), spearmint hay, stone fruit, sugar-cane, sunflower seeds, upland cress, vegetables (fruiting, leafy, root excluding carrots, seed and pod), wheat (grain and straw)

Table 2 (contd)

Country	Residue limit (mg/kg)	Commodities
USSR[i]	0.05	Vegetables

[a]From Health and Welfare Canada (1990)

[b]At or about the limit of analytical determination

[c]The figure in parentheses is the lower limit for determining residues in the corresponding product according to the standard method of analysis.

[d]Provisional

[e]Tolerance for negligible residues

[f]A pesticide may be used on an eating or drinking ware or raw material without a demonstrable residue remaining. The value listed is considered to be the highest concentration at which this requirement is deemed to have been met.

[g]Residues shall be absent; the value in parentheses is the highest concentration at which this requirement is still deemed to have been met.

[h]From US Environmental Protection Agency (1989b)

[i]From Izmerov (1985)

The USSR has established a maximum allowable concentration in workplace air of 3 mg/m^3 (Cook, 1987).

2. Studies of Cancer in Humans

2.1 Case-control studies of lymphatic and haematopoietic neoplasms

In the population-based case-control study of soft-tissue sarcoma, Hodgkin's disease and non-Hodgkin's lymphoma in Kansas, USA (described in detail in the monograph on occupational exposures in spraying and application of insecticides, p. 66), three cases of non-Hodgkin's lymphoma and two controls reported use of trifluralin (odds ratio, 12.5; 95% confidence interval [CI], 1.6-116.1) (Hoar et al., 1986).

In the population-based case-control study of leukaemia among white male farmers in Iowa and Minnesota, USA (Brown et al., 1990; described in detail in the monograph on occupational exposure in spraying and application of insecticides, p. 68), 32 cases and 87 controls reported use of trifluralin (odds ratio, 1.0; 95% CI, 0.7-1.6).

[Exposure to other pesticides could not be excluded in these studies.]

2.2 Case-control study of cancer of the ovary

In the population-based case-control study of ovarian epithelial cancer in northern Italy (described in detail in the monograph on atrazine, p. 449), one case and three controls were farmers and were judged to have been exposed to trifluralin (alone or with linuron) [crude odds ratio, 0.64; 95% CI, 0.1-6.5]. These subjects were also exposed to triazine herbicides (Donna et al., 1989).

3. Studies of Cancer in Experimental Animals

3.1 Oral administration[1]

3.1.1 *Mouse*

Groups of 50 male and 50 female B6C3F$_1$ mice, six weeks old, were fed diets containing various levels of technical-grade trifluralin (purity, > 90%; analysis of the compound three years after completion of the bioassay established the presence of 84-88 ppm (mg/kg) N-nitrosodi-n-propylamine). Initially, males were fed 2000 or 4000 mg/kg of diet; due to toxicity, administration of the high dose was stopped in week 57 of the study for one week, followed by dietary administration for four weeks at the previous concentration. This cyclic administration was continued for 22 weeks. In females, the initial concentrations were 4500 and 9000 mg/kg of diet for 17 weeks; at week 18, the low and high doses were decreased to 2250 mg/kg and 4500 mg/kg, respectively. In week 57, animals in the high-dose group were administered the compound intermittently for 22 weeks (one week on trifluralin-free diet followed by four weeks on trifluralin-treated diet). From week 79, all treated animals were given control diet for a further 12 weeks. The experiment was terminated at week 90. Twenty mice of each sex were used as matched controls, and a pooled control group (60 females and 60 males) was also available. Survival of high-dose males was lower that than in the other groups: 52% of the low-dose and 55% of the control males survived at least 86 weeks compared to only 34% of the high-dose males. In female mice, survival was 95% controls, 92% low-dose and 62% high-dose mice. In females, an increased incidence of hepatocellular carcinomas was noted: control, 0/20; low-dose, 12/47; and high-dose, 21/44 (Fisher exact test, $p < 0.01$; test for trend, $p < 0.001$); in males the incidence was 4/19 controls, 12/47 low-dose and 9/49 high-dose. Hepatocellular adenomas were observed in 3/47 low-dose females and in 2/47 low-dose males. Alveolar/bronchiolar adenomas or carcinomas of the lung were observed predominantly in female treated mice: 0/19 controls, 7/43 low-dose (Fisher exact test, $p = 0.005$ when compared with pooled controls) and 3/30 high-dose (test for trend; $p < 0.026$ when compared with pooled controls). In females, squamous-cell carcinomas of the forestomach occurred in 4/45 low-dose and in 1/44 high-dose animals; no such tumour was observed in controls or treated male mice; however, a squamous-cell papilloma occurred in 1/47 low-dose males (US National Cancer Institute, 1978). [The Working Group noted that contamination of the trifluralin with N-nitrosodi-n-propylamine was observed three years after the experiment was performed and that no account was made for differential survival.]

Groups of 80 male and 80 female B6C3F$_1$ mice [age unspecified] received trifluralin (technical-grade, containing less than 0.01 µg/g N-nitrosodi-n-propylamine) in the diet at levels of 563, 2250 or 4500 mg/kg for 24 months. Groups of 120 mice of each sex received a control diet. Survival at the end of the study ranged from 67 to 80% in the various groups. Body weight gains of high-dose mice were reduced by as much as 30% compared to those of

---

[1]The Working Group was aware of a completed but as yet unpublished study in rats by oral administration (US Environmental Protection Agency, 1988).

controls during the study. There was no increased incidence of neoplasms at any site in treated mice (Francis *et al.*, 1991).

3.1.2 *Rat*

Groups of 50 male and 50 female Osborne-Mendel rats, six weeks old, were initially given 6500 or 13 000 mg/kg of diet technical-grade trifluralin (purity > 90%; analysis of the compound three years after completion of the bioassay established the presence of 84-88 ppm [mg/kg] of *N*-nitrosodi-*n*-propylamine). In week 22 of the study, the low and high concentrations were decreased to 3250 and 6500 mg/kg of diet, respectively. In week 63, administration of trifluralin to the high-dose female rats was stopped for one week and then resumed for four weeks; high-dose males received the same cyclic pattern beginning in week 69. This intermittent feeding pattern was maintained until week 78. All animals were then given control diet until week 111, when the study was terminated. Fifty rats of each sex were used as matched controls. No difference in survival was observed between treated and control groups. The combined incidence of follicular-cell adenomas and carcinomas of the thyroid in female mice was: control, 1/50; low-dose, 7/50 ($p = 0.028$ Fisher exact test); and high-dose, 0/49. Two haemangiosarcomas of the spleen were observed in the 12 low-dose females in which this organ was examined histologically (US National Cancer Institute, 1978). [The Working Group noted the incomplete histological examination of many organs in the treated groups and that contamination of the trifluralin with *N*-nitrosodi-*n*-propylamine was observed three years after the experiment was performed.]

3.2 Administration by injection

Mouse: Groups of 25 female Swiss mice, seven weeks of age, were given 13 intraperitoneal or subcutaneous injections at three-day intervals of 0.25 ml of Treflan® (44.5% trifluralin, 55.5% unspecified), for a total dose of 0.0065 mg trifluralin. Groups of 50 mice received either intraperitoneal or subcutaneous injections of saline. The animals were kept under observation for seven months from the start of treatment; one animal from each group was killed at each 15-day interval beginning one month after the end of treatment. Lymphomas (one was questionable) were reported in 5/25 mice receiving Treflan by subcutaneous injection and in 3/21 mice receiving Treflan by intraperitoneal injection. A mesothelioma was reported in one treated mouse given a subcutaneous injection and in three mice given intraperitoneal injections. No tumour was observed in control mice (Donna *et al.*, 1981). [The Working Group noted the presence of unspecified material in the Treflan mixture and the very early appearence of lymphomas.]

4. Other Relevant Data

4.1 Absorption, distribution, metabolism and excretion

4.1.1 *Humans*

No data were available to the Working Group.

4.1.2 *Experimental systems*

Few published data are available on the metabolism and disposition of trifluralin. Rats dosed orally with radiolabelled trifluralin ($^{14}CF_3$ or ^{14}C-*N*-propyl-; 100 mg/kg bw) excreted

80% of the dose in the faeces; only 8% was unchanged trifluralin (Emmerson & Anderson, 1966). Incomplete absorption was indicated by the finding that only 11-14% of the radioactivity was recovered from bile. Extensive nitro-reduction to the corresponding amines occurred, probably as a result of metabolism by the gut microflora. Absorbed trifluralin was extensively metabolized, primarily by N-dealkylation and nitro-reduction, and then excreted in the urine. The extent of N-dealkylation was indicated by the fact that approximately 20% of the dose was recovered from expired air after administration of the ^{14}C-propyl compound. [The Working Group noted that the analytical methods used in this study would have been inadequate to determine the presence of side-chain hydroxylated or benzimidazole metabolites, which have been formed by rat liver microsomes *in vitro* (Nelson *et al.*, 1977).]

4.2 Toxic effects

4.2.1 *Humans*

No data were available to the Working Group.

4.2.2 *Experimental systems*

Trifluralin has a relatively low acute toxicity in experimental animals (Worth, 1970; Ben-Dyke *et al.*, 1970; Ladonin *et al.*, 1980; Gaines & Linder, 1986). Acute oral LD_{50} values were 3700-10 000 mg/kg bw in rodents and 2000 mg/kg bw in rabbits, dogs and hens. Trifluralin did not appreciably irritate skin.

In a carcinogenesis bioassay (see section 3), no remarkable non-neoplastic toxicity was reported in rats or mice, other than reduced growth and a low incidence of forestomach acanthosis and hyperkeratosis in mice (US National Cancer Institute, 1978). [The Working Group noted that the technical-grade trifluralin used was later found to be contaminated with N-nitrosodi-n-propylamine at 84-88 ppm [mg/kg].] The report of Francis *et al.* (1991) of a study in mice using technical-grade trifluralin that was not contaminated with N-nitrosodi-n-propylamine confirmed the effects on growth and also revealed progressive glomerulonephritis in female mice. Increases in the blood level of urea nitrogen and the serum level of alkaline phosphatase and decreased erythrocyte and leukocyte counts were reported to be related to treatment in animals of each sex.

4.3 Reproductive and developmental effects

4.3.1 *Humans*

No data were available to the Working Group.

4.3.2 *Experimental systems*

Administration of 1 g/kg bw trifluralin per day by gavage to pregnant CD-1 mice on days 6-15 of gestation resulted in a significant reduction in the number of live litters and an increased rate of stillborns and of pups with pathological conditions (runts, haemorrhages on the snout, tail or feet, paralysed hind limbs, defective righting reflex and narrow pelvises). Pups were allowed to be delivered, and 88 different skeletal variants were assessed upon sacrifice at two months of age. In the trifluralin-treated group, 12/88 of these skeletal variants increased in frequency. The most obvious was the occurrence of 14 ribs, parted frontals, an undoubled foramen ovale and accessory foramina in the cervical vertebrae. These animals appeared normal in physical conformation. Three of the 25 treated mothers died (Beck, 1981).

Application of trifluralin to fertile mallard eggs, by immersing them for 30 sec in an aqueous solution, resulted in embryonic death at exposure levels calculated to be 0.8 times that expected after usual application in the field, i.e., 1.6 lb/acre (1.8 kg/ha). Exposure at this level also reduced growth and increased the rate of bill malformation and of stuntedness in the embryos (Hoffman & Albers, 1984).

4.4 Genetic and related effects (see also Table 3 and Appendices 1 and 2)

4.4.1 *Humans*

No data were available to the Working Group.

4.4.2 *Experimental systems*

Trifluralin did not induce mutation in bacteria, in *Drosophila melanogaster* or in cultured mouse lymphoma cells at the *tk* locus. In a single report, chlorophyll mutation was induced in *Zea mays*. Recombination was not induced in *Aspergillus nidulans* or *Saccharomyces cerevisiae*. Aneuploidy was induced in *Neurospora crassa* and *Hordeum vulgare*, but evidence was equivocal in *Sordaria brevicollis* and conflicting in *D. melanogaster*.

DNA repair was not induced in cultured human cells. In a single study, sister chromatid exchange was weakly induced in cultured human lymphocytes.

Chromosomal aberrations were induced by trifluralin in various plant species but not in cultured hamster CHO cells. Equivocal results were obtained in cultured human lymphocytes. In the study in which aberrations were seen, the damage may have been secondary to interference with the mitotic spindle (Donna *et al.*, 1981).

In a single study, sister chromatid exchange was not induced in Chinese hamster bone-marrow cells *in vivo*.

Conflicting evidence was obtained for the induction of aberrations in mouse bone marrow, but consistent reports are available of chromosomal aberration in mouse embryos and male germ-line cells. Dominant lethal mutations were observed in mice. [The Working Group noted that the studies in which effects were seen originated from one laboratory and were performed with a commercial formulation containing 26% trifluralin; other components or impurities were not mentioned.]

Trifluralin metabolites induced chromosomal aberrations in cultured human lymphocytes and in mouse bone-marrow cells *in vivo* (Pilinskaya, 1987).

5. Summary of Data Reported and Evaluation

5.1 Exposure data

Trifluralin is a selective pre-emergence herbicide used for the control of annual grasses and certain broadleaf weeds. It was first registered for use in 1963.

Table 3. Genetic and related effects of trifluralin

Test system	Result[a] Without exogenous metabolic system	With exogenous metabolic system	Dose[b] LED/HID	Reference
BPF, Bacteriophage, forward mutation	-	0	25.0000	Andersen et al. (1972)
BPR, Bacteriophage, reverse mutation	-	0	20.0000	Andersen et al. (1972)
SA0, Salmonella typhimurium TA100, reverse mutation	-	-	500.0000	US National Technical Information Service, Environmental Protection Agency (1977)
SA0, Salmonella typhimurium TA100, reverse mutation	-	-	250.0000	Benigni et al. (1982)
SA0, Salmonella typhimurium TA100, reverse mutation	-	-	2500.0000	Moriya et al. (1983)
SA0, Salmonella typhimurium TA100, reverse mutation	-	-	167.0000	Mortelmans et al. (1986)
SA0, Salmonella typhimurium TA100, reverse mutation	-	-	400.0000	Garriott et al. (1991)
SA5, Salmonella typhimurium TA1535, reverse mutation	-	-	500.0000	US National Technical Information Service, Environmental Protection Agency (1977)
SA5, Salmonella typhimurium TA1535, reverse mutation	-	-	250.0000	Benigni et al. (1982)
SA5, Salmonella typhimurium TA1535, reverse mutation	-	-	2500.0000	Moriya et al. (1983)
SA5, Salmonella typhimurium TA1535, reverse mutation	-	-	167.0000	Mortelmans et al. (1986)
SA5, Salmonella typhimurium TA1535, reverse mutation	-	-	400.0000	Garriott et al. (1991)
SA7, Salmonella typhimurium TA1537, reverse mutation	-	-	500.0000	US National Technical Information Service, Environmental Protection Agency (1977)
SA7, Salmonella typhimurium TA1537, reverse mutation	-	-	250.0000	Benigni et al. (1982)
SA7, Salmonella typhimurium TA1537, reverse mutation	-	-	2500.0000	Moriya et al. (1983)
SA7, Salmonella typhimurium TA1537, reverse mutation	-	-	167.0000	Mortelmans et al. (1986)
SA7, Salmonella typhimurium TA1537, reverse mutation	-	-	400.0000	Garriott et al. (1991)
SA8, Salmonella typhimurium TA1538, reverse mutation	-	-	500.0000	US National Technical Information Service, Environmental Protection Agency (1977)
SA8, Salmonella typhimurium TA1538, reverse mutation	-	-	2500.0000	Moriya et al. (1983)
SA8, Salmonella typhimurium TA1538, reverse mutation	-	-	400.0000	Garriott et al. (1990)

Table 3 (contd)

Test system	Result[a] Without exogenous metabolic system	With exogenous metabolic system	Dose[b] LED/HID	Reference
SA9, *Salmonella typhimurium* TA 98, reverse mutation	–	–	250.0000	Benigni et al. (1982)
SA9, *Salmonella typhimurium* TA 98, reverse mutation	–	–	167.0000	Mortelmans et al. (1986)
SA9, *Salmonella typhimurium* TA 98, reverse mutation	–	–	400.0000	Garriott et al. (1990)
ECW, *Escherichia coli* WP2 *uvrA*, reverse mutation	–	–	500.0000	US National Technical Information Service, Environmental Protection Agency (1977)
ECW, *Escherichia coli* WP2 *uvrA*, reverse mutation	–	–	2500.0000	Moriya et al. (1983)
SCH, *Saccharomyces cerevisiae*, D3 homozygosis by recombination	–	–	50000.0000	US National Technical Information Service, Environmental Protection Agency (1977)
ANG, *Aspergillus nidulans*, mitotic recombination	(+)	0	100.0000	Carere & Morpurgo (1981)
ANG, *Aspergillus nidulans*, mitotic recombination	+[c]	0	100.0000	Benigni et al. (1982)
ANN, *Aspergillus nidulans*, nondisjunction	–	0	10000.0000	Carere & Morpurgo (1981)
NCN, *Neurospora crassa*, aneuploidy	+	0	1.0000	Griffiths (1979)
SCN, *Saccharomyces cerevisiae*, chromosome loss (aneuploidy)	–	0	250.0000	Whittakeer et al. (1990)
*, *Sordaria brevicollis*, aneuploidy	(+)	0	50.0000	Bond & McMillan (1979)
TSL, *Tradescantia paludosa*, micronuclei	?	0	178.0000[d]	Ma et al. (1984)
ACC, *Allium cepa*, chromosomal aberrations	+	0	5.0000[d]	Kabarity & Nahas (1979)
HSC, *Hordeum vulgare*, chromosomal aberrations	+	0	40.0000	Oku (1976)
PLC, *Gossypium hirsutum*, chromosomal aberrations	+	0	1.0000	Hess & Bayer
PLC, *Zea meys*, chlorophyll mutations	+	0	0.0000[d]	Lapina et al. (1984)
PLC, *Zea meys*, chromosomal aberrations	+	0	0.0000[d]	Grigorenko et al. (1986)
VFC, *Vicia faba*, chromosomal aberrations	+	0	90.0000[d]	Wu (1972)
DMX, *Drosophila melanogaster*, sex-linked recessive lethal mutation	–	0	100.0000	Murnik (1978) (Abstract)

Table 3 (contd)

Test system	Result[a] Without exogenous metabolic system	Result[a] With exogenous metabolic system	Dose[b] LED/HID	Reference
DMX, *Drosophila melanogaster*, sex-linked recessive lethal mutation	–[e]	0	30.0000 feeding	Yoon et al. (1985)
DMX, *Drosophila melanogaster*, sex-linked recessive lethal mutation	–	0	400.0000 injection	Yoon et al. (1985)
DMN, *Drosophila melanogaster*, aneuploidy	+	0	100.0000	Murnik (1978) (abstract)
DMN, *Drosophila melanogaster*, aneuploidy	–	0	400.0000	Foureman (1988)
G51, Gene mutation mouse lymphoma, L5178Y	–	–	20.0000	Garriott et al. (1990)
CIC, Chromosomal aberrations, Chinese hamster CHO cells *in vitro*	–	–	50.0000	Garriott et al. (1990)
UHF, Unscheduled DNA synthesis, human lung fibroblasts WI38 *in vitro*	–	–	335.0000	US National Technical Information Service, Environmental Protection Agency (1977)
UHF, Unscheduled DNA synthesis, EUE cells *in vitro*	–	0	0.0000	Carere & Morpurgo (1981)
UHF, Unscheduled DNA synthesis, EUE cells *in vitro*	–	0	100.0000	Benigni et al. (1984)
SHL, Sister chromatid exchange, human lymphocytes *in vitro*	(+)	0	0.0000	Ghiazza et al. (1984)
CHL, Chromosomal aberrations, human lymphocytes *in vitro*	(+)	0	0.0000[d]	Donna et al. (1981)
CHL, Chromosomal aberrations, human lymphocytes *in vitro*	–[e]	0	40.0000	Pilinskaya (1987)
SVA, Sister chromatid exchange, Chinese hamster cells *in vivo*	–	0	500.0000	Garriott et al. (1987)
CBA, Chromosomal aberrations, mouse bone marrow *in vivo*	+	0	52.0000 × 1 i.p.[f]	Nehez et al. (1979)
CBA, Chromosomal aberrations, mouse bone marrow *in vivo*	–[e]	0	1000.0000	Pilinskaya (1987)
CGC, Chromosomal aberrations, mouse spermatogonia/spermatocytes	+	0	52.0000 × 1 i.p.[f]	Nehez et al. (1980)

Table 3 (contd)

Test system	Result[a]		Dose[b] LED/HID	Reference
	Without exogenous metabolic system	With exogenous metabolic system		
CGC, Chromosomal aberrations, mouse spermatogonia/ spermatocytes	+	0	1.6000 × 10 i.p.[f]	Nehez et al. (1982)
*Chromosomal aberrations, mouse embryos (males treated in vivo)	+	0	52.0000 × 1 i.p.[f]	Nehez et al. (1980)
DLM, Dominant lethal test, mouse	+	0	52.0000 × 1 i.p.[f]	Nehez et al. (1980)

*Not displayed on profile

[a] +, positive; (+), weakly positive; −, negative; 0, not tested; ?, inconclusive (variable response in several experiments within an adequate study)

[b] In-vitro tests, μg/ml; in-vivo tests, mg/kg bw

[c] Technical grade, +; pure, sample, −

[d] Treflan (44.5% trifluralin) tested; dose represents concentration of trifluralin

[e] The metabolites 2,6-dinitro-4-(trifluoro)aniline and 2,6-diamino-4-(trifluoro)aniline gave positive results

[f] Olitref (26% trifluralin) tested; dose represents concentration of trifluralin

Trifluralin has been formulated as emulsifiable concentrates, granules and liquids.

Exposure to trifluralin may occur during its production and application and, at much lower levels, from consumption of residues in food and water.

N-Nitrosodi-n-propylamine has been detected in technical trifluralin, and levels of nitrosamines in trifluralin have been restricted in some countries.

5.2 Carcinogenicity in humans

Use of trifluralin was associated with an increased risk for non-Hodgkin's lymphoma in a study in the USA. A study of ovarian cancer in Italy did not suggest an association with exposure to trifluralin. Both results were based on small numbers of exposed subjects. A larger US study showed no association with the occurrence of leukaemia.

5.3 Carcinogenicity in experimental animals

One technical grade of trifluralin (possibly contaminated with N-nitrosodi-n-propyl-amine) was tested for carcinogenicity in mice and rats by administration in the diet. In female mice, it induced an increased incidence of hepatocellular carcinomas; in the same study, an increase in the incidence of lung adenomas or carcinomas was observed in females. An increased incidence of squamous-cell carcinomas of the forestomach was noted in female mice at the lower but not at the higher dose. In rats, an increase in the combined incidence of follicular-cell adenomas and carcinomas of the thyroid was noted at the lower but not at the higher dose in females.

Another preparation of trifluralin was tested for carcinogenicity in mice by adminis-tration in the diet. No increase in tumour incidence was observed.

5.4 Other relevant data

In a single study, trifluralin was embryolethal and increased the incidence of skeletal variants in mice at doses that caused some maternal toxicity.

No data were available on the genetic and related effects of trifluralin in humans.

A commercial trifluralin formulation induced chromosomal aberrations in bone-marrow, embryonal cells and the male germ line in mice. Chromosomal aberrations were also induced in plants. Aneuploidy was induced in several lower eukaryotes. There was little evidence for the induction of gene mutation in any test system.

5.5. Evaluation[1]

There is *inadequate evidence* in humans for the carcinogenicity of trifluralin.

There is *limited evidence* in experimental animals for the carcinogenicity of technical-grade trifluralin.

Overall evaluation

Trifluralin *is not classifiable as to its carcinogenicity to humans (Group 3).*

---

[1]For definition of the italicized terms, see Preamble, pp. 26-28.

6. References

Andersen, K.J., Leighty, E.G. & Takahashi, M.K. (1972) Evaluation of herbicides for possible mutagenic properties. *J. agric. Food Chem.*, 20, 649-656

Anon. (1989) *Crop Protection Chemicals Reference*, 5th ed., New York, Chemical and Pharmaceutical Press, pp. 1081-1130, 1617-1632

Anon. (1990) Trifluralin. *Gazzetta Ufficiale della Republica Italiana*, Serie Generale no. 78, *24 March*, Art. 4

Beck, S.L. (1981) Assessment of adult skeletons to detect prenatal exposure to 2,4,5-T or trifluralin in mice. *Teratology*, 23, 33-55

Ben-Dyke, R., Sanderson, D.M. & Noakes, D.N. (1970) Acute toxicity data for pesticides (1970) *World Rev. Pest Control*, 9, 119-127

Benigni, R., Bignami, M., Conti, L., Crebelli, R., Dogliotti, E., Falcone, E. & Carere, A. (1982) In vitro mutational studies with trifluralin and trifluorotoluene derivatives. *Ann. Ist. super. Sanità*, 18, 123-126

Bond, D.J. & McMillan, L. (1979) Meiotic aneuploidy: its origins and induction following chemical treatment in *Sordaria brevicollis*. *Environ. Health Perspect.*, 31, 67-74

Brown, L.M., Blair, A., Gibson, R., Everett, G.D., Cantor, K.P., Schuman, L.M., Burmeister, L.F., Van Lier, S.F. & Dick, F. (1990) Pesticide exposures and other agricultural risk factors for leukemia among men in Iowa and Minnesota. *Cancer Res.*, 50, 6585-6591

Budavari, S., ed. (1989) *The Merck Index*, 11th ed., Rahway, NJ, Merck & Co., p. 1523

Carere, A. & Morpurgo, G. (1981) Comparison of the mutagenic activity of pesticides *in vitro* in various short-term assays. *Progr. Mutat. Res.*, 2, 87-104

Cook, W.A., ed. (1987) *Occupational Exposure Limits—Worldwide*, Washington DC, American Industrial Hygiene Association, p. 222

Day, E.W., Jr, Saunders, D.G., Mosier, J.W., McKinney, E.M., Powers, F.L., Griggs, R.D. & Frank, R. (1982) Estimation of inhalation exposure to *N*-nitrosodipropylamine during the application and incorporation of the herbicide trifluralin. *Environ. Sci. Technol.*, 16, 131-136

Donna, A., Betta, P.G., Gagliardi, F., Ghiazza, G.F., Gallareto, M. & Gabutto, V. (1981) Preliminary experimental contribution to the study of possible carcinogenic activity of two herbicides containing atrazine-simazine and trifluralin as active principles. *Pathologica*, 73, 707-721

Donna, A., Crosignani, P., Robutti, F., Betta, P.G., Bocca, R., Mariani, N., Ferrario, F., Fissi, R. & Berrino, F. (1989) Triazine herbicides and ovarian epithelial neoplasms. *Scand. J. Work Environ. Health*, 15, 47-53

Emmerson, J.L. & Anderson, R.C. (1966) Metabolism of trifluralin in the rat and dog. *Toxicol. appl. Pharmacol.*, 9, 84-97

FAO (1988) *FAO Specifications for Plant Protection Products, Trifluralin*, (AGP-CP/235), Rome

Foureman, P.A. (1988) The TX;Y test for the detection of nondisjunction and chromosome breakage in *Drosophila melanogaster*. II. Results of female exposures. *Mutat. Res.*, 203, 309-316

Francis, P.C., Emmerson, J.L., Adams, E.R. & Owen, N.V. (1991) Oncogenicity study of trifluralin in B6C3F$_1$ mice. *Food chem. Toxicol.*, 29, 549-555

Gaines, T.B. & Linder, R.E. (1986) Acute toxicity of pesticides in adult and weanling rats. *Fundam. appl. Toxicol.*, 7, 299-308

Garriott, M.L., Adams, E.R., Probst, G.S., Emmerson, J.L., Oberly, T.J., Kindig, D.E.F., Neal, S.B., Bewsey, B.J. & Rexroat, M.A. (1991) Genotoxicity studies on the preemergence herbicide trifluralin. *Mutat. Res.*, 260, 187-193

Ghiazza, G., Zavarise, G., Lanero, M. & Ferraro, G. (1984) SCE (sister chromatid exchange) induced in chromosomes of human lymphocytes by trifluralin, atrazine and simazine (Ital.). *Boll. Soc. It. Biol. sper.*, *60*, 2149-2153

Golab, T., Althaus, W.A. & Wooten, H.L. (1979) Fate of [^{14}C] trifluralin in soil. *Agric. Food Chem.*, *27*, 163-179

Government of Canada (1990) *Report on National Surveillance Data from 1984/85 to 1988/89*, Ottawa

Griffiths, A.J.F. (1979) Neurospora prototroph selection system for studying aneuploid production. *Environ. Health Perspect.*, *31*, 75-80

Grigorenko, N.V., Fasilchenko, V.F., Merezhinski, Y.G., Morgun, V.V., Logvinenko, V.F. & Sharmankin, S.V. (1986) Cytogenetic activity of a herbicide treflan, and its metabolites as applied to maize (Russ.). *Tsitol. Genet.*, *20*, 294-298

Health and Welfare Canada (1990) *National Pesticide Residue Limits in Food*, Ottawa, Bureau of Chemical Safety, Food Directorate, Health Protection Branch

Hess, D. & Bayer, D. (1974) The effect of trifluralin on the ultrastructure of dividing cells of the root meristem of cotton (*Gossypium hirsutum* L. 'Acala 4-42'). *J. Cell Sci.*, *15*, 429-441

Hoar, S.K., Blair, A., Holmes, F.F., Boysen, C.D., Robel, R.J., Hoover, R. & Fraumeni, J.F., Jr (1986) Agricultural herbicide use and risk of lymphoma and soft-tissue sarcoma. *J. Am. med. Assoc.*, *256*, 1141-1147

Hoffman, D.J. & Albers, P.H. (1984) Evaluation of potential embryotoxicity and teratogenicity of 42 herbicides, insecticides, and petroleum contaminants to mallard eggs. *Arch. environ. Contam. Toxicol.*, *13*, 15-27

IARC (1978) *IARC Monographs on the Evaluation of the Carcinogenic Risk of Chemicals to Humans*, Vol. 17, *Some N-Nitroso Compounds*, Lyon, pp. 177-189

Izmerov, N.F., ed. (1985) *International Register of Potentially Toxic Chemicals. Scientific Reviews of Soviet Literature on Toxicity and Hazards of Chemicals: Trifluralin* (Issue 80), Moscow, Centre of International Projects, United Nations Environment Programme

Kabarity, A. & Nahas, A. (1979) Induction of polyploidy and C-tumours after treating *Allium cepa* root tips with the herbicide 'Treflan'. *Biol. plant.*, *21*, 253-258

Kello, D. (1989) WHO drinking water quality guidelines for selected herbicides. *Food Addit. Contam.*, *6 (Suppl. 1)*, S79-S85

Ladonin, V.F., Hassan, A. & Winteringham, F.P.W. (1980) Dinitroaniline herbicides. *Chemosphere*, *9*, 67-69

Lapina, T.V., Grigorenko, N.V., Morgun, V.V., Logvinenko, V.F. & Merezhinski, M.G. (1984) Study of mutagenic effect of herbicides Treflan, Ramrod and Banvell-D on a maize (Russ.). *Tsitol. Genet.*, *18*, 119-122

Leitis, E. & Crosby, D.G. (1974) Photodecomposition of trifluralin. *J. agric. Food Chem.*, *22*, 842-848

Ma, T.-H., Harris, M.M., Anderson, V.A., Ahmed, I., Mohammad, K., Bare, J.L. & Lin, G. (1984) Tradescantia-micronucleus (Trad-MCN) tests on 140 health-related agents. *Mutat. Res.*, *138*, 157-167

Meister, R.T., ed. (1990) *Farm Chemicals Handbook '90*, Willoughby, OH, Meister Publishing Company, p. C294

Moriya, M., Ohta, T., Watanabe, K., Miyazawa, T., Kato, K. & Shirazu, Y. (1983) Further mutagenicity studies on pesticides in bacterial reversion assay systems. *Mutat. Res.*, *116*, 185-216

Mortelmans, K., Haworth, S., Lawlor, T., Speck, W., Tainer, B. & Zeiger, E. (1986) *Salmonella* mutagenicity tests: II. Results from the testing of 270 chemicals. *Environ. Mutagenesis*, *8* (Suppl. 7), 1-119

Murnik, M.R. (1978) Mutagenicity of the herbicide trifluralin in *Drosophila melanogaster* (Abstract no. 149). *Mutat. Res.*, *53*, 235-236

Nehéz, M., Páldy, A., Selypes, A., Körösfalvi, M., Lörinczi, I. & Berensci, G. (1979) The mutagenic effect of trifluralin-containing herbicide on mouse bone marrow *in vivo*. *Ecotoxicol. environ. Saf.*, *3*, 454-457

Nehéz, M., Páldy, A., Selypes, A., Körösfalvi, M., Lörinczi, I. & Berensci, G. (1980) The mutagenic effect of trifluralin-containing herbicide on mouse germ cells *in vivo*. *Ecotoxicol. environ. Saf.*, *4*, 263-266

Nehéz, M., Selypes, A., Páldy, A., Mazzag, E., Berensci, G. & Jármay, K. (1982) The effects of five weeks treatment with dinitro-o-cresol or trifluralin-containing pesticides in the germ cells of male mice. *J. appl. Toxicol.*, *2*, 179-180

Nelson, J.O., Kearney, P.C., Plimmer, J.R. & Menzer, R.E. (1977) Metabolism of trifluralin, profluralin and fluchloralin by rat liver microsomes. *Pestic. Biochem. Physiol.*, *7*, 73-82

Oku, K. (1976) Effect of some herbicides on somatic division in barley (Jpn.). *Kromosomo*, *II*, 63-68

Parr, J.F. & Smith, S. (1973) Degradation of trifluralin under laboratory conditions and soil anaerobiosis. *Soil Sci.*, *115*, 55-63

Pilinskaya, M.S.A. (1987) Evaluation of the cytogenetic effect of the herbicide treflan and of a number of its metabolites on mammalian somatic cells (Russ.). *Tsitol. Genet.*, *21*, 131-135

Royal Society of Chemistry (1986) *European Directory of Agrochemical Products*, Vol. 2, *Herbicides*, Cambridge, pp. 580-586

Royal Society of Chemistry (1989) *The Agrochemicals Handbook* [Dialog Information Services (File 306)], Cambridge

Stevens, L., Collier, C.W. & Woodham, D.W. (1970) Monitoring pesticides in soils from areas of regular, limited and no pesticide use. *Pestic. Monit. J.*, *4*, 145-166

US Environmental Protection Agency (1975) Infrared spectra of pesticides. In: *Manual of Chemical Methods for Pesticides and Devices*, Arlington, VA, Association of Official Analytical Chemists

US Environmental Protection Agency (1987) *Guidance for the Reregistration of Pesticide Products Containing Trifluralin as the Active Ingredient*, Washington DC

US Environmental Protection Agency (1988) *Trifluralin*, Washington DC, Office of Drinking Water

US Environmental Protection Agency (1989a) Method 508. Revision 3.0. Determination of chlorinated pesticides in water by gas chromatography with an electron capture detector. In: *Methods for the Determination of Organic Compounds in Drinking Water* (EPA Report No. EPA-600/4-88/039; US NTIS PB89-220461), Cincinnati, OH, Environmental Monitoring Systems Laboratory, pp. 171-198

US Environmental Protection Agency (1989b) Trifluralin; tolerances for residues. Tolerances and exemptions from tolerances for pesticide chemicals in or on raw agricultural commodities. *US Code fed. Regul.*, *Title 40*, Part 180.207

US Environmental Protection Agency (1989c) Trifluralin. Tolerances for pesticides in food. *US Code fed. Regul.*, *Title 40*, Part 185.5900

US Environmental Protection Agency (1990) *Pesticides Industry Sales and Usage: 1988 Market Estimates*, Washington DC, Office of Pesticide Programs

US Food and Drug Administration (1989) Trifluralin. In: *Pesticide Analytical Manual*, Vol. II, *Methods Which Detect Multiple Residues*, Washington DC, US Department of Health and Human Services, pp. 1-15

US National Cancer Institute (1978) *Bioassay of Trifluralin for Possible Carcinogenicity* (Technical Report Series No. 34; DHEW Publ. No. (NIH) 78-834), Bethesda, MD

US National Technical Information Service, Environmental Protection Agency (1977) *Evaluation of Selected Pesticides as Chemical Mutagens:* in vitro *and* in vivo *Studies* (EPA-600/1-77-028), Washington DC

US National Technical Information Service, Environmental Protection Agency (1984) In Vitro *and* In Vivo *Mutagenicity Studies of Environmental Chemicals* (EPA-600/1-84-003), Washington DC

Weiler, E. (1980) *Preliminary Quantitative Usage Analysis of Trifluralin*, Washington DC, US Environmental Protection Agency

West, S.D. & Day, E.W., Jr (1979) Determination of volatile nitrosamines in crops and soils treated with dinitroaniline herbicides. *Agric. Food Chem.*, 27, 1075-1080

Whittaker, S.G., Zimmermann, F.K., Dicus, B., Piegorsch, W.W., Resnick, M.A. & Fogel, S. (1990) Detection of induced mitotic chromosome loss in *Saccharomyces cerevisiae*—an interlaboratory assessment of 12 chemicals. *Mutat. Res.*, 241, 225-242

WHO (1987) *Drinking-water Quality: Guidelines for Selected Herbicides* (Environmental Health Criteria 27), Copenhagen, p. 8

Wiersma, G.B., Tai, H. & Sand, P.F. (1972) Pesticide residue levels in soils FY 1969—National Soils Monitoring Program. *Pestic. Monit. J.*, 6, 194-201

Williams, S., ed. (1984) *Official Methods of Analysis of the Association of Official Analytical Chemists*, 14th ed., Washington DC, Association of Official Analytical Chemists, pp. 108-109,

Willis, G.H., Rogers, R.L. & Southwick, L.M. (1975) Losses of diuron, linuron, fenac and trifluralin in surface drainage water. *J. environ. Qual.*, 4, 399-402

Worth, H.M. (1970) The toxicological evaluation of benefin and trifluralin. In: Deichmann, W.B., Peñalver, R.A. & Radomski, J.L., eds, *Pesticides Symposia. Inter-American Conferences on Toxicology and Occupational Medicine*, Miami, FL, Halos and Associates, Inc., pp. 263-267

Worthing, C.R. & Walker, S.B., eds (1987) *The Pesticide Manual: A World Compendium*, 8th ed., Thornton Heath, British Crop Protection Council, pp. 832-833

Wu, T.-P. (1972) Some cytological effects of treflan and mitomycin C on root tips of *Vicia faba* L. *Taiwania*, 17, 248-254

Yoon, J.S., Mason, J.M., Valencia, R., Woodruff, R.C. & Zimmering, S. (1985) Chemical mutagenesis testing in *Drosophila*. IV. Results of 45 coded compounds tested for the National Toxicology Program. *Environ. Mutagenesis*, 7, 349-367

SUMMARY OF FINAL EVALUATIONS

Agent	Degree of evidence of carcinogenicity[a,b]		Overall evaluation of carcinogenicity to humans[a]
	Humans	Animals	
Aldicarb	ND	I	3
Atrazine	I	L	2B[c]
Captafol	ND	S	2A[c]
Chlordane	I	S	2B
DDT	I	S	2B
Deltamethrin	ND	I	3
Dichlorvos	I	S	2B
Fenvalerate	ND	I	3
Heptachlor	I	S	2B
Monuron	ND	L	3
Occupational exposures in spraying and application of nonarsenical insecticides	L		2A
Pentachlorophenol	I	S	2B
Permethrin	ND	I	3
Picloram	ND	L (tech.-grade)	3
Simazine	I	I	3
Thiram	I	I	3
Trifluralin	I	L (tech.-grade)	3
Ziram	ND	L	3

[a]I, inadequate evidence; S, sufficient evidence; L, limited evidence; ND, no data
[b]For definitions of degrees of evidence and groupings of evaluations, see Preamble, pp. 26-28.
[c]Other relevant data influenced the making of the overall evaluation.

APPENDIX 1

SUMMARY TABLES OF
GENETIC AND RELATED EFFECTS

Summary table of genetic and related effects of aldicarb

Nonmammalian systems													Mammalian systems																										
Proka-ryotes		Lower eukaryotes		Plants				Insects					*In vitro*															*In vivo*												
													Animal cells								Human cells								Animals								Humans				
D	G	D	R	G	A	D	G	C	R	G	C	A	D	G	S	M	C	A	T	I	D	G	S	M	C	A	T	I	D	G	S	M	C	DL	A	D	S	M	C	A
?	−													+							−¹	+¹	+			+¹							+¹							

A, aneuploidy; C, chromosomal aberrations; D, DNA damage; DL, dominant lethal mutation; G, gene mutation; I, inhibition of intercellular communication; M, micronuclei; R, mitotic recombination and gene conversion; S, sister chromatid exchange; T, cell transformation

In completing the tables, the following symbols indicate the consensus of the Working Group with regard to the results for each endpoint:

+   considered to be positive for the specific endpoint and level of biological complexity

+¹   considered to be positive, but only one valid study was available to the Working Group

−   considered to be negative

−¹   considered to be negative, but only one valid study was available to the Working Group

?   considered to be equivocal or inconclusive (e.g., there were contradictory results from different laboratories; there were confounding exposures; the results were equivocal)

Summary table of genetic and related effects of chlordane

Nonmammalian systems[a]											Mammalian systems																											
Proka-ryotes		Lower eukaryotes		Plants			Insects				In vitro																	In vivo												
											Animal cells							Human cells									Animals							Humans					
D	G	D	R	A	D	G	C	R	G	C	D	G	S	M	C	A	T	I	D	G	S	M	C	A	T	I	D	G	S	M	C	DL	A	D	S	M	C	A
-	-		+¹		+¹						-	+							+	?		-¹			+¹								-						

A, aneuploidy; C, chromosomal aberrations; D, DNA damage; DL, dominant lethal mutation; G, gene mutation; I, inhibition of intercellular communication; M, micronuclei; R, mitotic recombination and gene conversion; S, sister chromatid exchange; T, cell transformation

In completing the tables, the following symbols indicate the consensus of the Working Group with regard to the results for each endpoint:

+ considered to be positive for the specific endpoint and level of biological complexity

+¹ considered to be positive, but only one valid study was available to the Working Group

- considered to be negative

-¹ considered to be negative, but only one valid study was available to the Working Group

? considered to be equivocal or inconclusive (e.g. there were contradictory results from different laboratories; there were confounding exposures; the results were equivocal)

[a]Sister chromatid exchange in fish *in vivo*: +¹

Summary table of genetic and related effects of heptachlor

Nonmammalian systems											Mammalian systems																												
Prokaryotes	Lower eukaryotes			Plants			Insects				In vitro																		In vivo											
											Animal cells								Human cells									Animals							Humans				
D	G	D	R	G	A	D	G	M	C	R	D	G	S	M	C	A	T	I	D	G	S	M	C	A	T	I	D	G	S	M	C	DL	A	D	S	M	C	A
–		$-^1$		$+^1$	$+^1$	+				$-^1$	–							$+^1$	+							$+^1$						–						–

A, aneuploidy; C, chromosomal aberrations; D, DNA damage; DL, dominant lethal mutation; G, gene mutation; I, inhibition of intercellular communication; M, micronuclei; R, mitotic recombination and gene conversion; S, sister chromatid exchange; T, cell transformation

In completing the table, the following symbols indicate the consensus of the Working Group with regard to the results for each endpoint:

+   considered to be positive for the specific endpoint and level of biological complexity

$+^1$ considered to be positive, but only one valid study was available to the Working Group

–   considered to be negative

$-^1$ considered to be negative, but only one valid study was available to the Working Group

?   considered to be equivocal or inconclusive (e.g., there were contradictory results from different laboratories; there were confounding exposures; the results were equivocal)

Summary table of genetic and related effects of DDT

Nonmammalian systems												Mammalian systems																					
Proka-ryotes	Lower eukaryotes			Plants			Insects					In vitro														In vivo							
												Animal cells								Human cells						Animals[a]							Humans	
D	D	G	R	A	D	G	C	R	G	C	A	D	G	S	M	C	A	T	I	D	G	S	M	C	A	T	I	D	G	S	M	C	DL	A	D	S	M	C	A
-			-¹		-¹		-	+¹	?			?			-¹		+	?		-			-¹		+	-		-¹		?	-		-	?				?¹	

A, aneuploidy; C, chromosomal aberrations; D, DNA damage; DL, dominant lethal mutation; G, gene mutation; I, inhibition of intercellular communication; M, micronuclei; R, mitotic recombination and gene conversion; S, sister chromatid exchange; T, cell transformation

In completing the tables, the following symbols indicate the consensus of the Working Group with regard to the results for each endpoint:

+   considered to be positive for the specific endpoint and level of biological complexity

+¹   considered to be positive, but only one valid study was available to the Working Group

–   considered to be negative

–¹   considered to be negative, but only one valid study was available to the Working Group

?   considered to be equivocal or inconclusive (e.g. there were contradictory results from different laboratories; there were confounding exposures; the results were equivocal)

[a]Sperm morphology, ?; Gap junctional area reduction, +¹; Mouse host-mediated assay, –

Summary table of genetic and related effects of *para,para'*-TDE

Nonmammalian systems													Mammalian systems																											
Proka-ryotes		Lower eukaryotes				Plants			Insects						In vitro																		In vivo								
															Animal cells									Human cells								Animals[b]								Humans		
D	G	D	R	G	A	D	G	A	D	G	C	R	C	A	D	G	S	M	C	A	T	I	D	G	S	M	C	A	T	I	D	G	S	M	C	DL	A	D	S	M	C	A
−															−[a]			?			−¹	+¹																				

A, aneuploidy; C, chromosomal aberrations; D, DNA damage; DL, dominant lethal mutation; G, gene mutation; I, inhibition of intercellular communication; M, micronuclei; R, mitotic recombination and gene conversion; S, sister chromatid exchange; T, cell transformation

In completing the table, the following symbols indicate the consensus of the Working Group with regard to the results for each endpoint:

+ considered to be positive for the specific endpoint and level of biological complexity

+¹ considered to be positive, but only one valid study was available to the Working Group

− considered to be negative

−¹ considered to be negative, but only one valid study was available to the Working Group

? considered to be equivocal or inconclusive (e.g., there were contradictory results from different laboratories; there were confounding exposures; the results were equivocal)

[a]Isomers not specified

[b]Mouse host-mediated assay, −¹

Summary table of genetic and related effects of *ortho,para'*-TDE

Nonmammalian systems											Mammalian systems																						
Proka-ryotes		Lower eukaryotes			Plants		Insects			In vitro																In vivo								
									Animal cells									Human cells							Animals[b]							Humans		
D	G	D	R	G	A	D	G	C	R	C	A	D	G	S	M	C	A	T	I	D	G	S	M	C	A	T	DL	A	D	G	S	M	C	A	D	S	M	C	A
–[1]														–[1]	–	–[1]		?				–[1]																	

A, aneuploidy; C, chromosomal aberrations; D, DNA damage; DL, dominant lethal mutation; G, gene mutation; I, inhibition of intercellular communication; M, micronuclei; R, mitotic recombination and gene conversion; S, sister chromatid exchange; T, cell transformation

In completing the tables, the following symbols indicate the consensus of the Working Group with regard to the results for each endpoint:

+   considered to be positive for the specific endpoint and level of biological complexity

+[1] considered to be positive, but only one valid study was available to the Working Group

–   considered to be negative

–[1] considered to be negative, but only one valid study was available to the Working Group

?   considered to be equivocal or inconclusive (e.g., there were contradictory results from different laboratories; there were confounding exposures; the results were equivocal)

[a]Isomers not specified

[b]Mouse host-mediated assay, –[1]

Summary table of genetic and related effects of para,para'-DDE

Nonmammalian systems												Mammalian systems																											
Prokaryotes		Lower eukaryotes				Plants				Insects		*In vitro*																*In vivo*											
												Animal cells								Human cells								Animals[b]							Humans				
D	G	D	R	G	A	D	G	C	R	G	C	A	D	G	S	M	C	A	T	D	G	S	M	C	A	T	I	D	G	S	M	C	DL	A	D	S	M	C	A
–[1][b]	–		+[a]							+[1]	–[1]		–	+	?	+										–[1]	+[1]												

A, aneuploidy; C, chromosomal aberrations; D, DNA damage; DL, dominant lethal mutation; G, gene mutation; I, inhibition of intercellular communication; M, micronuclei; R, mitotic recombination and gene conversion; S, sister chromatid exchange; T, cell transformation

In completing the tables, the following symbols indicate the consensus of the Working Group with regard to the results for each endpoint:

+   considered to be positive for the specific endpoint and level of biological complexity

+[1]   considered to be positive, but only one valid study was available to the Working Group

–   considered to be negative

–[1]   considered to be negative, but only one valid study was available to the Working Group

?   considered to be equivocal or inconclusive (e.g., there were contradictory results from different laboratories; there were confounding exposures; the results were equivocal)

[a]DNA rearrangement in recombinant plasmid in *Saccharomyces cerevisiae*, +

[b]Mouse host-mediated assay, –[1]

Summary table of genetic and related effects of deltamethrin

Nonmammalian systems				Mammalian systems		
Proka-ryotes	Lower eukaryotes	Plants	Insects	In vitro		In vivo
				Animal cells	Human cells	Animals[a] / Humans

D	G	D	R	G	A	D	G	C	R	D	G	S	M	C	A	D	G	S	M	C	A	T	I	D	G	S	M	C	DL	A	D	S	M	C	A
$-^1$								+^{1}							$-^1$							$-^1$			+^{1}					+^{1}					

A, aneuploidy; C, chromosomal aberrations; D, DNA damage; DL, dominant lethal mutation; G, gene mutation; I, inhibition of intercellular communication; M, micronuclei; R, mitotic recombination and gene conversion; S, sister chromatid exchange; T, cell transformation

In completing the tables, the following symbols indicate the consensus of the Working Group with regard to the results for each endpoint:

+   considered to be positive for the specific endpoint and level of biological complexity

+^{1} considered to be positive, but only one valid study was available to the Working Group

–   considered to be negative

–^{1} considered to be negative, but only one valid study was available to the Working Group

?   considered to be equivocal or inconclusive (e.g., there were contradictory results from different laboratories; there were confounding exposures; the results were equivocal)

[a]Sperm abnormalities, +^{1}

Summary table of genetic and related effects of dichlorvos

Nonmammalian systems														Mammalian systems																				
Proka-ryotes[a]		Lower eukaryotes			Plants				Insects					*In vitro*															*In vivo*						
														Animal cells								Human cells							Animals[b]						Humans
D	G	D	R	G	A	D	G	M	C	R	G	C	A	D	G	S	M	C	A	T	I	D	G	S	M	C	A	T	I	D	G	S	M	C	DL	A	D	S	M	C	A
+	+	+	+	+[1]	+[1]	+	+[1]	+	+	−	+[1]	+[1]		?[1]	+[1]	+	+	+			−[1]	+	+						−[1]	−[1]		−[1]	−[1]	−							

A, aneuploidy; C, chromosomal aberrations; D, DNA damage; DL, dominant lethal mutation; G, gene mutation; I, inhibition of intercellular communication; M, micronuclei; R, mitotic recombination and gene conversion; S, sister chromatid exchange; T, cell transformation

In completing the table, the following symbols indicate the consensus of the Working Group with regard to the results for each endpoint:

+   considered to be positive for the specific endpoint and level of biological complexity

+[1]   considered to be positive, but only one valid study was available to the Working Group

−   considered to be negative

−[1]   considered to be negative, but only one valid study was available to the Working Group

?   considered to be equivocal or inconclusive (e.g. there were contradictory results from different laboratories; there were confounding exposures; the results were equivocal)

[a] DNA binding, +

[b] Sperm morphology, ?[1]; DNA binding *in vivo*, −

Summary table of genetic and related effects of fenvalerate

Nonmammalian systems													Mammalian systems																										
Proka-ryotes		Lower eukaryotes				Plants		Insects					In vitro																In vivo											
													Animal cells								Human cells								Animals*							Humans				
D	G	D	R	G	A	D	G	C	R	G	C	A	D	G	S	M	C	A	T	I	D	G	S	M	C	A	T	I	D	G	S	M	C	DL	A	D	S	M	C	A
-										-¹	-¹	+¹							+¹			+¹						+¹				+¹	+¹							

A, aneuploidy; C, chromosomal aberrations; D, DNA damage; DL, dominant lethal mutation; G, gene mutation; I, inhibition of intercellular communication; M, micronuclei; R, mitotic recombination and gene conversion; S, sister chromatid exchange; T, cell transformation

In completing the tables, the following symbols indicate the consensus of the Working Group with regard to the results for each endpoint:

+   considered to be positive for the specific endpoint and level of biological complexity

+¹   considered to be positive, but only one valid study was available to the Working Group

−   considered to be negative

−¹   considered to be negative, but only one valid study was available to the Working Group

?   considered to be equivocal or inconclusive (e.g., there were contradictory results from different laboratories; there were confounding exposures; the results were equivocal)

*Sperm morphology, +¹

Summary table of genetic and related effects of permethrin

Nonmammalian systems												Mammalian systems																											
												In vitro																In vivo											
Proka-ryotes		Lower eukaryotes			Plants			Insects				Animal cells								Human cells								Animals							Humans				
D	G	R	G	A	D	G	C	R	G	C	A	D	G	S	M	C	A	T	I	D	G	S	M	C	A	T	I	D	G	S	M	C	DL	A	D	S	M	C	A
–										–[1]			–[1]													–[1]													

A, aneuploidy; C, chromosomal aberrations; D, DNA damage; DL, dominant lethal mutation; G, gene mutation; I, inhibition of intercellular communication; M, micronuclei; R, mitotic recombination and gene conversion; S, sister chromatid exchange; T, cell transformation

In completing the tables, the following symbols indicate the consensus of the Working Group with regard to the results for each endpoint:

+   considered to be positive for the specific endpoint and level of biological complexity

+[1]   considered to be positive, but only one valid study was available to the Working Group

–   considered to be negative

–[1]   considered to be negative, but only one valid study was available to the Working Group

?   considered to be equivocal or inconclusive (e.g. there were contradictory results from different laboratories; there were confounding exposures; the results were equivocal)

Summary table of genetic and related effects of captafol

Nonmammalian systems															Mammalian systems																				
Proka-ryotes		Lower eukaryotes				Plants		Insects							In vitro																In vivo				
															Animal cells								Human cells								Animals						Humans				
D	G	D	R	G	A	D	G	C	R	G	C	A			D	G	S	M	C	A	T	I	D	G	S	M	C	A	T	I	D	G	S	M	C	DL	A	D	S	M	C	A
+1	+	+1		+1	−1												+	+1	+							+1	+1	+1									+					

A, aneuploidy; C, chromosomal aberrations; D, DNA damage; DL, dominant lethal mutation; G, gene mutation; I, inhibition of intercellular communication; M, micronuclei; R, mitotic recombination and gene conversion; S, sister chromatid exchange; T, cell transformation

In completing the tables, the following symbols indicate the consensus of the Working Group with regard to the results for each endpoint:

+   considered to be positive for the specific endpoint and level of biological complexity

+1   considered to be positive, but only one valid study was available to the Working Group

−   considered to be negative

−1   considered to be negative, but only one valid study was available to the Working Group

?   considered to be equivocal or inconclusive (e.g., there were contradictory results from different laboratories; there were confounding exposures; the results were equivocal)

Summary table of genetic and related effects of pentachlorophenol

Nonmammalian systems												Mammalian systems																										
Proka-ryotes		Lower eukaryotes				Plants				Insects			*In vitro*																*In vivo**										
													Animal cells								Human cells								Animals							Humans				
D	G	D	R	G	A	D	G	C	R	G	C	A	D	G	S	M	C	A	T	I	D	G	S	M	C	A	T	I	D	G	S	M	C	DL	A	D	S	M	C	A
?		+		+1						-1			-	?		+	+	-1					-1		-1						+1						-1			+1

A, aneuploidy; C, chromosomal aberrations; D, DNA damage; DL, dominant lethal mutation; G, gene mutation; I, inhibition of intercellular communication; M, micronuclei; R, mitotic recombination and gene conversion; S, sister chromatid exchange; T, cell transformation

In completing the tables, the following symbols indicate the consensus of the Working Group with regard to the results for each endpoint:

+ considered to be positive for the specific endpoint and level of biological complexity

+1 considered to be positive, but only one valid study was available to the Working Group

– considered to be negative

–1 considered to be negative, but only one valid study was available to the Working Group

? considered to be equivocal or inconclusive (e.g., there were contradictory results from different laboratories; there were confounding exposures; the results were equivocal)

*Sperm morphology test, –1

Summary table of genetic and related effects of thiram

Nonmammalian systems										Mammalian systems																										
Proka-ryotes		Lower eukaryotes		Plants			Insects			In vitro															In vivo											
										Animal cells								Human cells							Animals[a]							Humans				
D	G	R	A	D	G	C	R	G	C	D	G	S	M	C	A	T	I	D	G	S	M	C	A	T	D	G	S	M	C	DL	A	D	S	M	C	A
?	+		+[1]	+[1]	+[1]			+[1]		?	-[1]	?[1]						+[1]	+[1]										+	+[1]						

A, aneuploidy; C, chromosomal aberrations; D, DNA damage; DL, dominant lethal mutation; G, gene mutation; I, inhibition of intercellular communication; M, micronuclei; R, mitotic recombination and gene conversion; S, sister chromatid exchange; T, cell transformation

In completing the tables, the following symbols indicate the consensus of the Working Group with regard to the results for each endpoint:

+   considered to be positive for the specific endpoint and level of biological complexity

+[1]   considered to be positive, but only one valid study was available to the Working Group

−   considered to be negative

−[1]   considered to be negative, but only one valid study was available to the Working Group

?   considered to be equivocal or inconclusive (e.g., there were contradictory results from different laboratories; there were confounding exposures; the results were equivocal)

[a] Sperm morphology test, +

Summary table of genetic and related effects of ziram

Nonmammalian systems															Mammalian systems																				
Proka-ryotes		Lower eukaryotes				Plants			Insects					In vitro														In vivo								
														Animal cells							Human cells							Animals							Humans				
D	G	D	R	G	A	D	G	A	D	R	G	C	A	D	G	S	M	C	A	T	D	G	S	M	C	A	T	D	G	S	M	C	DL	A	D	G	S	M	C	A
+¹	+		-¹				-¹				+	-¹		+¹		+¹	-¹			+¹				+¹							+¹	+¹	?							+¹

A, aneuploidy; C, chromosomal aberrations; D, DNA damage; DL, dominant lethal mutation; G, gene mutation; I, inhibition of intercellular communication; M, micronuclei; R, mitotic recombination and gene conversion; S, sister chromatid exchange; T, cell transformation

In completing the tables, the following symbols indicate the consensus of the Working Group with regard to the results for each endpoint:

+   considered to be positive for the specific endpoint and level of biological complexity

+¹   considered to be positive, but only one valid study was available to the Working Group

–   considered to be negative

–¹   considered to be negative, but only one valid study was available to the Working Group

?   considered to be equivocal or inconclusive (e.g., there were contradictory results from different laboratories; there were confounding exposures; the results were equivocal)

Summary table of genetic and related effects of atrazine

Nonmammalian systems											Mammalian systems																											
											In vitro																In vivo											
Prokaryotes		Lower eukaryotes			Plants			Insects			Animal cells								Human cells								Animals							Humans				
D	G	D	R	G	A	D	G	C	R	G	D	G	S	M	C	A	T	I	D	G	S	M	C	A	T	I	D	G	S	M	C	DL	A	D	S	M	C	A
–		–	+	+	+	+	+	?	+[1]	+[1]		–[1]	–[1]		–				–[1]		–[1]							+[1][a]		–[1][b]		?[1]						

A, aneuploidy; C, chromosomal aberrations; D, DNA damage; DL, dominant lethal mutation; G, gene mutation; I, inhibition of intercellular communication; M, micronuclei; R, mitotic recombination and gene conversion; S, sister chromatid exchange; T, cell transformation

In completing the tables, the following symbols indicate the consensus of the Working Group with regard to the results for each endpoint:

+   considered to be positive for the specific endpoint and level of biological complexity

+[1]   considered to be positive, but only one valid study was available to the Working Group

–   considered to be negative

–[1]   considered to be negative, but only one valid study was available to the Working Group

?   considered to be equivocal or inconclusive (e.g., there were contradictory results from different laboratories; there were confounding exposures; the results were equivocal)

[a] Mouse, host-mediated assay, +[1]

[b] Sperm head morphological abnormality test, –[1]

Summary table of genetic and related effects of monuron

Nonmammalian systems												Mammalian systems																									
Proka-ryotes	Lower eukaryotes			Plants			Insects					In vitro														In vivo[a]											
												Animal cells							Human cells							Animals							Humans				
D	D	G	R	D	G	A	D	R	G	C	A	D	G	S	M	C	A	T	D	G	S	M	C	A	T	D	G	S	M	C	DL	A	D	S	M	C	A
–	–			+1	+		–1			+1[b]		?	+		+1			+1	–1										+		+1						

A, aneuploidy; C, chromosomal aberrations; D, DNA damage; DL, dominant lethal mutation; G, gene mutation; I, inhibition of intercellular communication; M, micronuclei; R, mitotic recombination and gene conversion; S, sister chromatid exchange; T, cell transformation

In completing the tables, the following symbols indicate the consensus of the Working Group with regard to the results for each endpoint:

+   considered to be positive for the specific endpoint and level of biological complexity

+1   considered to be positive, but only one valid study was available to the Working Group

–   considered to be negative

–1   considered to be negative, but only one valid study was available to the Working Group

?   considered to be equivocal or inconclusive (e.g., there were contradictory results from different laboratories; there were confounding exposures; the results were equivocal)

[a]Sperm-head morphological abnormality test, +1

[b]Polytene chromosomal damage

Summary table of genetic and related effects of picloram

Nonmammalian systems											Mammalian systems																								
Proka-ryotes		Lower eukaryotes				Plants		Insects			In vitro																	In vivo									
											Animal cells								Human cells								Animals								Humans				
D	G	D	R	G	A	D	G	C	R	G	A	C	T	I	D	G	S	M	C	A	T	I	D	G	S	M	C	A	T	I	D	G	S	M	C	DL	A	D	S	M	C	A
-			+	+¹					-		-¹																	-¹										-¹				

A, aneuploidy; C, chromosomal aberrations; D, DNA damage; DL, dominant lethal mutation; G, gene mutation; I, inhibition of intercellular communication; M, micronuclei; R, mitotic recombination and gene conversion; S, sister chromatid exchange; T, cell transformation

In completing the tables, the following symbols indicate the consensus of the Working Group with regard to the results for each endpoint:

+ considered to be positive for the specific endpoint and level of biological complexity
+¹ considered to be positive, but only one valid study was available to the Working Group
− considered to be negative
−¹ considered to be negative, but only one valid study was available to the Working Group
? considered to be equivocal or inconclusive (e.g., there were contradictory results from different laboratories; there were confounding exposures; the results were equivocal)

Summary table of genetic and related effects of simazine

Nonmammalian systems											Mammalian systems																											
											In vitro																In vivo											
Proka-ryotes		Lower eukaryotes		Plants		Insects					Animal cells								Human cells								Animals							Humans				
D	G	R	A	D	G	C	R	G	C	A	D	G	S	M	C	A	T	I	D	G	S	M	C	A	T	I	D	G	S	M	C	DL	A	D	S	M	C	A
-	-	-	-¹	?		+		+		+¹	?¹		-¹						-¹	?¹										-¹								

A, aneuploidy; C, chromosomal aberrations; D, DNA damage; DL, dominant lethal mutation; G, gene mutation; I, inhibition of intercellular communication; M, micronuclei; R, mitotic recombination and gene conversion; S, sister chromatid exchange; T, cell transformation

In completing the tables, the following symbols indicate the consensus of the Working Group with regard to the results for each endpoint:

+   considered to be positive for the specific endpoint and level of biological complexity

+¹   considered to be positive, but only one valid study was available to the Working Group

−   considered to be negative

−¹   considered to be negative, but only one valid study was available to the Working Group

?   considered to be equivocal or inconclusive (e.g. there were contradictory results from different laboratories; there were confounding exposures; the results were equivocal)

Summary table of genetic and related effects of trifluralin

Nonmammalian systems												Mammalian systems																											
												In vitro															In vivo													
Prokaryotes		Lower eukaryotes			Plants			Insects				Animal cells								Human cells								Animals							Humans					
D	G	D	R	G	A	D	G	E	R	G	C	A	D	G	S	M	C	A	T	I	D	G	S	M	C	A	T	I	D	G	S	M	C	DL	A	D	S	M	C	A
-		-		+		+[1]	+		-			?			-[1]	-[1]	-[1]				-		?[1]					?			-[1]		+	+[1]						+[1]

A, aneuploidy; C, chromosomal aberrations; D, DNA damage; DL, dominant lethal mutation; G, gene mutation; I, inhibition of intercellular communication; M, micronuclei; R, mitotic recombination and gene conversion; S, sister chromatid exchange; T, cell transformation

In completing the tables, the following symbols indicate the consensus of the Working Group with regard to the results for each endpoint:

+   considered to be positive for the specific endpoint and level of biological complexity

+[1]   considered to be positive, but only one valid study was available to the Working Group

-   considered to be negative

-[1]   considered to be negative, but only one valid study was available to the Working Group

?   considered to be equivocal or inconclusive (e.g., there were contradictory results from different laboratories; there were confounding exposures; the results were equivocal)

APPENDIX 2

ACTIVITY PROFILES FOR
GENETIC AND RELATED EFFECTS

APPENDIX 2

ACTIVITY PROFILES FOR
GENETIC AND RELATED EFFECTS

Methods

The x–axis of the activity profile (Waters *et al.*, 1987, 1988) represents the bioassays in phylogenetic sequence by endpoint, and the values on the y-axis represent the logarithmically transformed lowest effective doses (LED) and highest ineffective doses (HID) tested. The term 'dose', as used in this report, does not take into consideration length of treatment or exposure and may therefore be considered synonymous with concentration. In practice, the concentrations used in all the in-vitro tests were converted to µg/ml, and those for in-vivo tests were expressed as mg/kg bw. Because dose units are plotted on a log scale, differences in molecular weights of compounds do not, in most cases, greatly influence comparisons of their activity profiles. Conventions for dose conversions are given below.

Profile–line height (the magnitude of each bar) is a function of the LED or HID, which is associated with the characteristics of each individual test system—such as population size, cell–cycle kinetics and metabolic competence. Thus, the detection limit of each test system is different, and, across a given activity profile, responses will vary substantially. No attempt is made to adjust or relate responses in one test system to those of another.

Line heights are derived as follows: for negative test results, the highest dose tested without appreciable toxicity is defined as the HID. If there was evidence of extreme toxicity, the next highest dose is used. A single dose tested with a negative result is considered to be equivalent to the HID. Similarly, for positive results, the LED is recorded. If the original data were analysed statistically by the author, the dose recorded is that at which the response was significant ($p < 0.05$). If the available data were not analysed statistically, the dose required to produce an effect is estimated as follows: when a dose-related positive response is observed with two or more doses, the lower of the doses is taken as the LED; a single dose resulting in a positive response is considered to be equivalent to the LED.

In order to accommodate both the wide range of doses encountered and positive and negative responses on a continuous scale, doses are transformed logarithmically, so that effective (LED) and ineffective (HID) doses are represented by positive and negative numbers, respectively. The response, or logarithmic dose unit (LDU_{ij}), for a given test system i and chemical j is represented by the expressions

LDU_{ij} = $-\log_{10}$ (dose), for HID values; LDU ≤ 0

and   (1)

LDU_{ij} = $-\log_{10}$ (dose $\times$ 10^{-5}), for LED values; LDU ≥ 0.

These simple relationships define a dose range of 0 to -5 logarithmic units for ineffective doses (1-100 000 µg/ml or mg/kg bw) and 0 to +8 logarithmic units for effective doses (100 000-0.001 µg/ml or mg/kg bw). A scale illustrating the LDU values is shown in Figure 1. Negative responses at doses less than 1 µg/ml (mg/kg bw) are set equal to 1. Effectively, an LED value $\geq$100 000 or an HID value $\leq$1 produces an LDU = 0; no quantitative information is gained from such extreme values. The dotted lines at the levels of log dose units 1 and -1 define a 'zone of uncertainty' in which positive results are reported at such high doses (between 10 000 and 100 000 µg/ml or mg/kg bw) or negative results are reported at such low dose levels (1 to 10 µg/ml or mg/kg bw) as to call into question the adequacy of the test.

Fig. 1. Scale of log dose units used on the y–axis of activity profiles

Positive (µg/ml or mg/kg bw)		Log dose units	
0.001	....	8	————
0.01	....	7	—
0.1	....	6	—
1.0	....	5	—
10	....	4	—
100	....	3	—
1000	....	2	—
10 000	....	1	—
100 000	.... 1	0	————
	.... 10	-1	—
	.... 100	-2	—
	.... 1000	-3	—
	.... 10 000	-4	—
	.... 100 000	-5	————

Negative
(µg/ml or mg/kg bw)

LED and HID are expressed as µg/ml or mg/kg bw.

In practice, an activity profile is computer generated. A data entry programme is used to store abstracted data from published reports. A sequential file (in ASCII) is created for each compound, and a record within that file consists of the name and Chemical Abstracts Service number of the compound, a three–letter code for the test system (see below), the qualitative test result (with and without an exogenous metabolic system), dose (LED or HID), citation number and additional source information. An abbreviated citation for each publication is stored in a segment of a record accessing both the test data file and the citation file. During processing of the data file, an average of the logarithmic values of the data subset is calculated, and the length of the profile line represents this average value. All dose values are plotted for each profile line, regardless of whether results are positive or negative. Results obtained in the absence of an exogenous metabolic system are indicated by a bar (–), and results obtained in the presence of an exogenous metabolic system are indicated by an upward–directed arrow (↑). When all results for a given assay are either positive or negative, the mean of the LDU values is plotted as a solid line; when conflicting data are reported for the same assay (i.e., both positive and negative results), the majority data are shown by a solid line and the minority data by a dashed line (drawn to the extreme conflicting response). In the few cases in which the numbers of positive and negative results are equal, the solid line is drawn in the positive direction and the maximal negative response is indicated with a dashed line.

Profile lines are identified by three–letter code words representing the commonly used tests. Code words for most of the test systems in current use in genetic toxicology were defined for the US Environmental Protection Agency's GENE–TOX Program (Waters, 1979; Waters & Auletta, 1981). For *IARC Monographs* Supplement 6, Volume 44 and subsequent volumes, including this publication, codes were redefined in a manner that should facilitate inclusion of additional tests. Naming conventions are described below.

Data listings are presented in the text and include endpoint and test codes, a short test code definition, results [either with (M) or without (NM) an exogenous activation system], the associated LED or HID value and a short citation. Test codes are organized phylogenetically and by endpoint from left to right across each activity profile and from top to bottom of the corresponding data listing. Endpoints are defined as follows: A, aneuploidy; C, chromosomal aberrations; D, DNA damage; F, assays of body fluids; G, gene mutation; H, host–mediated assays; I, inhibition of intercellular communication; M, micronuclei; P, sperm morphology; R, mitotic recombination or gene conversion; S, sister chromatid exchange; and T, cell transformation.

Dose conversions for activity profiles

Doses are converted to μg/ml for in-vitro tests and to mg/kg bw per day for in-vivo experiments.

1. In–vitro test systems

    (a) Weight/volume converts directly to μg/ml.

    (b) Molar (M) concentration × molecular weight = mg/ml = 10^3 μg/ml; mM concentration × molecular weight = μg/ml.

    (c) Soluble solids expressed as % concentration are assumed to be in units of mass per volume (i.e., 1% = 0.01 g/ml = 10 000 μg/ml; also, 1 ppm = 1 μg/ml).

    (d) Liquids and gases expressed as % concentration are assumed to be given in units of volume per volume. Liquids are converted to weight per volume using the density (D) of the solution (D = g/ml). Gases are converted from volume to mass using the ideal gas law, PV = nRT. For exposure at 20–37°C at standard atmospheric pressure, 1% (v/v) = 0.4 μg/ml × molecular weight of the gas. Also, 1 ppm (v/v) = 4×10^{-5} μg/ml × molecular weight.

(e) In microbial plate tests, it is usual for the doses to be reported as weight/plate, whereas concentrations are required to enter data on the activity profile chart. While remaining cognisant of the errors involved in the process, it is assumed that a 2-ml volume of top agar is delivered to each plate and that the test substance remains in solution within it; concentrations are derived from the reported weight/plate values by dividing by this arbitrary volume. For spot tests, a 1-ml volume is used in the calculation.

(f) Conversion of particulate concentrations given in $\mu g/cm^2$ are based on the area (A) of the dish and the volume of medium per dish; i.e., for a 100–mm dish: $A = \pi R^2 = \pi \times (5\ cm)^2 = 78.5\ cm^2$. If the volume of medium is 10 ml, then $78.5\ cm^2 = 10$ ml and $1\ cm^2 = 0.13$ ml.

2. In–vitro systems using in–vivo activation

For the body fluid–urine (BF–) test, the concentration used is the dose (in mg/kg bw) of the compound administered to test animals or patients.

3. In–vivo test systems

(a) Doses are converted to mg/kg bw per day of exposure, assuming 100% absorption. Standard values are used for each sex and species of rodent, including body weight and average intake per day, as reported by Gold et al. (1984). For example, in a test using male mice fed 50 ppm of the agent in the diet, the standard food intake per day is 12% of body weight, and the conversion is dose = 50 ppm $\times$ 12% = 6 mg/kg bw per day.

Standard values used for humans are: weight – males, 70 kg; females, 55 kg; surface area, 1.7 m^2; inhalation rate, 20 l/min for light work, 30 l/min for mild exercise.

(b) When reported, the dose at the target site is used. For example, doses given in studies of lymphocytes of humans exposed in vivo are the measured blood concentrations in $\mu g/ml$.

Codes for test systems

For specific nonmammalian test systems, the first two letters of the three–symbol code word define the test organism (e.g., SA– for *Salmonella typhimurium*, EC– for *Escherichia coli*). If the species is not known, the convention used is –S–. The third symbol may be used to define the tester strain (e.g., SA8 for *S. typhimurium* TA1538, ECW for *E. coli* WP2*uvrA*). When strain designation is not indicated, the third letter is used to define the specific genetic endpoint under investigation (e.g., ––D for differential toxicity, ––F for forward mutation, ––G for gene conversion or genetic crossing-over, ––N for aneuploidy, ––R for reverse mutation, ––U for unscheduled DNA synthesis). The third letter may also be used to define the general endpoint under investigation when a more complete definition is not possible or relevant (e.g., ––M for mutation, ––C for chromosomal aberration).

For mammalian test systems, the first letter of the three–letter code word defines the genetic endpoint under investigation: A–– for aneuploidy, B–– for binding, C–– for chromosomal aberration, D–– for DNA strand breaks, G–– for gene mutation, I–– for inhibition of intercellular communication, M–– for micronucleus formation, R–– for DNA repair, S–– for sister chromatid exchange, T–– for cell transformation and U–– for unscheduled DNA synthesis.

For animal (i.e., non–human) test systems *in vitro*, when the cell type is not specified, the code letters –IA are used. For such assays *in vivo*, when the animal species is not specified, the code letters –VA are used. Commonly used animal species are identified by the third letter (e.g., ––C for Chinese hamster, ––M for mouse, ––R for rat, ––S for Syrian hamster).

For test systems using human cells *in vitro*, when the cell type is not specified, the code letters –IH are used. For assays on humans *in vivo*, when the cell type is not specified, the code letters –VH are used. Otherwise, the second letter specifies the cell type under investigation (e.g., –BH for bone marrow, –LH for lymphocytes).

Some other specific coding conventions used for mammalian systems are as follows: BF– for body fluids, HM– for host–mediated, ––L for leukocytes or lymphocytes *in vitro* (–AL, animals; –HL, humans), –L– for leukocytes *in vivo* (–LA, animals; –LH, humans), ––T for transformed cells.

Note that these are examples of major conventions used to define the assay code words. The alphabetized listing of codes must be examined to confirm a specific code word. As might be expected from the limitation to three symbols, some codes do not fit the naming conventions precisely. In a few cases, test systems are defined by first-letter code words, for example: MST, mouse spot test; SLP, mouse specific locus test, postspermatogonia; SLO, mouse specific locus test, other stages; DLM, dominant lethal test in mice; DLR, dominant lethal test in rats; MHT, mouse heritable translocation test.

The genetic activity profiles and listings were prepared in collaboration with Environmental Health Research and Testing Inc. (EHRT) under contract to the US Environmental Protection Agency; EHRT also determined the doses used. The references cited in each genetic activity profile listing can be found in the list of references in the appropriate monograph.

References

Garrett, N.E., Stack, H.F., Gross, M.R. & Waters, M.D. (1984) An analysis of the spectra of genetic activity produced by known or suspected human carcinogens. *Mutat. Res., 134,* 89–111

Gold, L.S., Sawyer, C.B., Magaw, R., Backman, G.M., de Veciana, M., Levinson, R., Hooper, N.K., Havender, W.R., Bernstein, L., Peto, R., Pike, M.C. & Ames, B.N. (1984) A carcinogenic potency database of the standardized results of animal bioassays. *Environ. Health Perspect., 58,* 9–319

Waters, M.D. (1979) *The GENE–TOX program.* In: Hsie, A.W., O'Neill, J.P. & McElheny, V.K., eds, *Mammalian Cell Mutagenesis: The Maturation of Test Systems* (Banbury Report 2), Cold Spring Harbor, NY, CSH Press, pp. 449–467

Waters, M.D. & Auletta, A. (1981) The GENE–TOX program: genetic activity evaluation. *J. chem. Inf. comput. Sci., 21,* 35–38

Waters, M.D., Stack, H.F., Brady, A.L., Lohman, P.H.M., Haroun, L. & Vainio, H. (1987) Appendix 1: Activity profiles for genetic and related tests. In: *IARC Monographs on the Evaluation of the Carcinogenic Risk of Chemicals to Humans,* Suppl. 6, *Genetic and Related Effects: An Updating of Selected* IARC Monographs *from Volumes 1 to 42,* Lyon, IARC, pp. 687–696

Waters, M.D., Stack, H.F., Brady, A.L., Lohman, P.H.M., Haroun, L. & Vainio, H. (1988) Use of computerized data listings and activity profiles of genetic and related effects in the review of 195 compounds. *Mutat. Res.*, *205*, 295–312

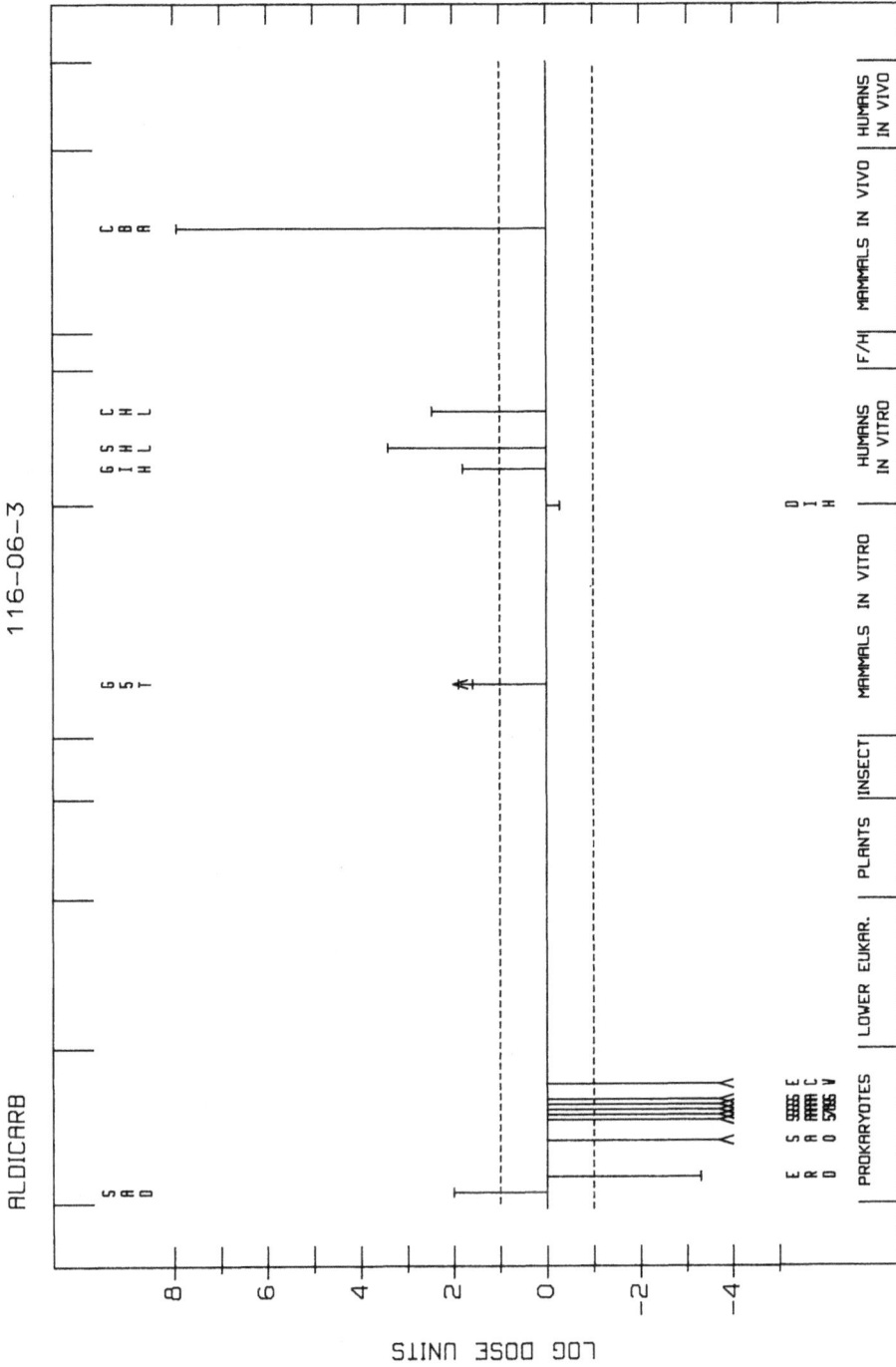

ALDICARB

116-06-3

LOG DOSE UNITS

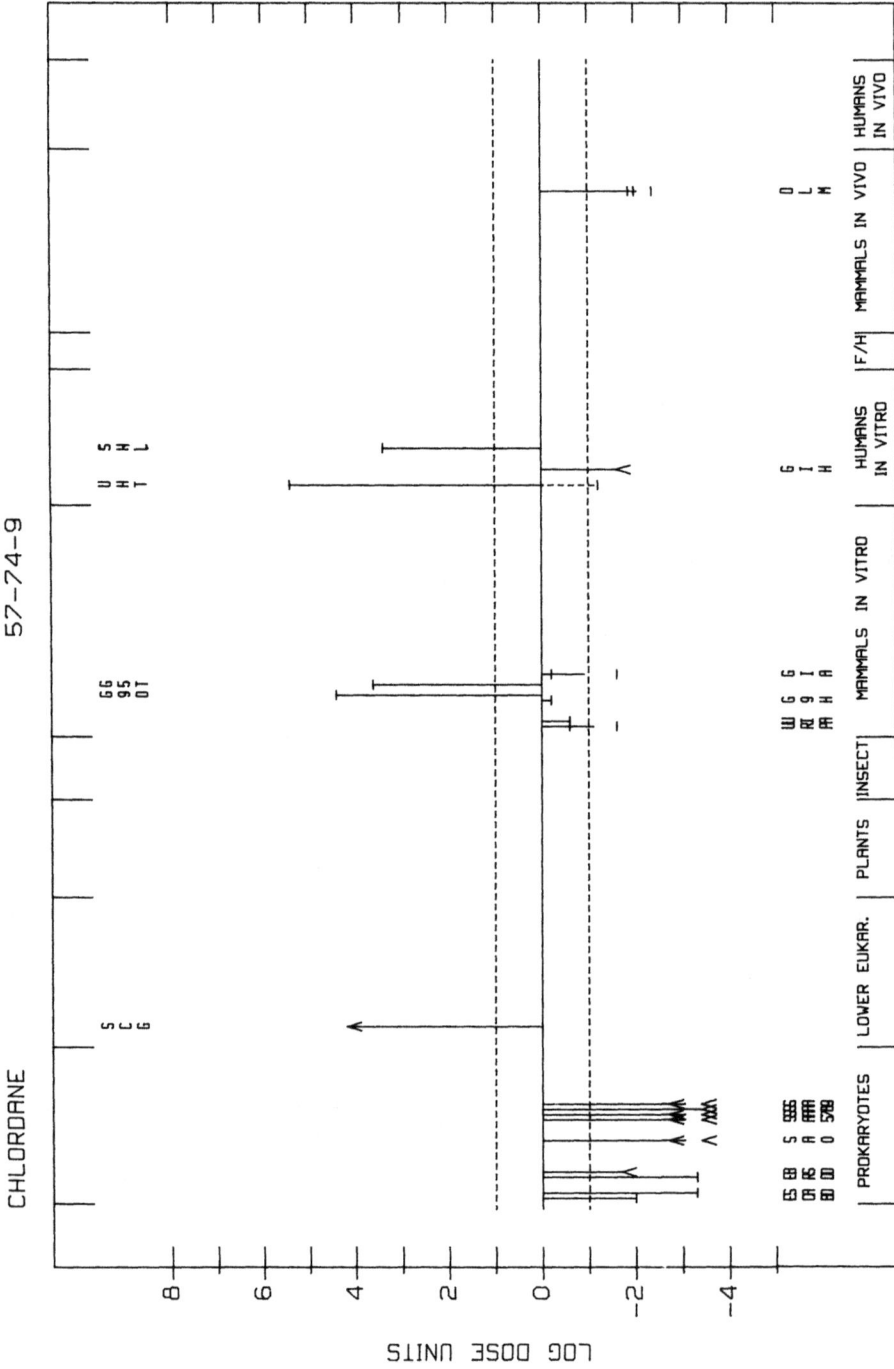

CHLORDANE

57-74-9

LOG DOSE UNITS

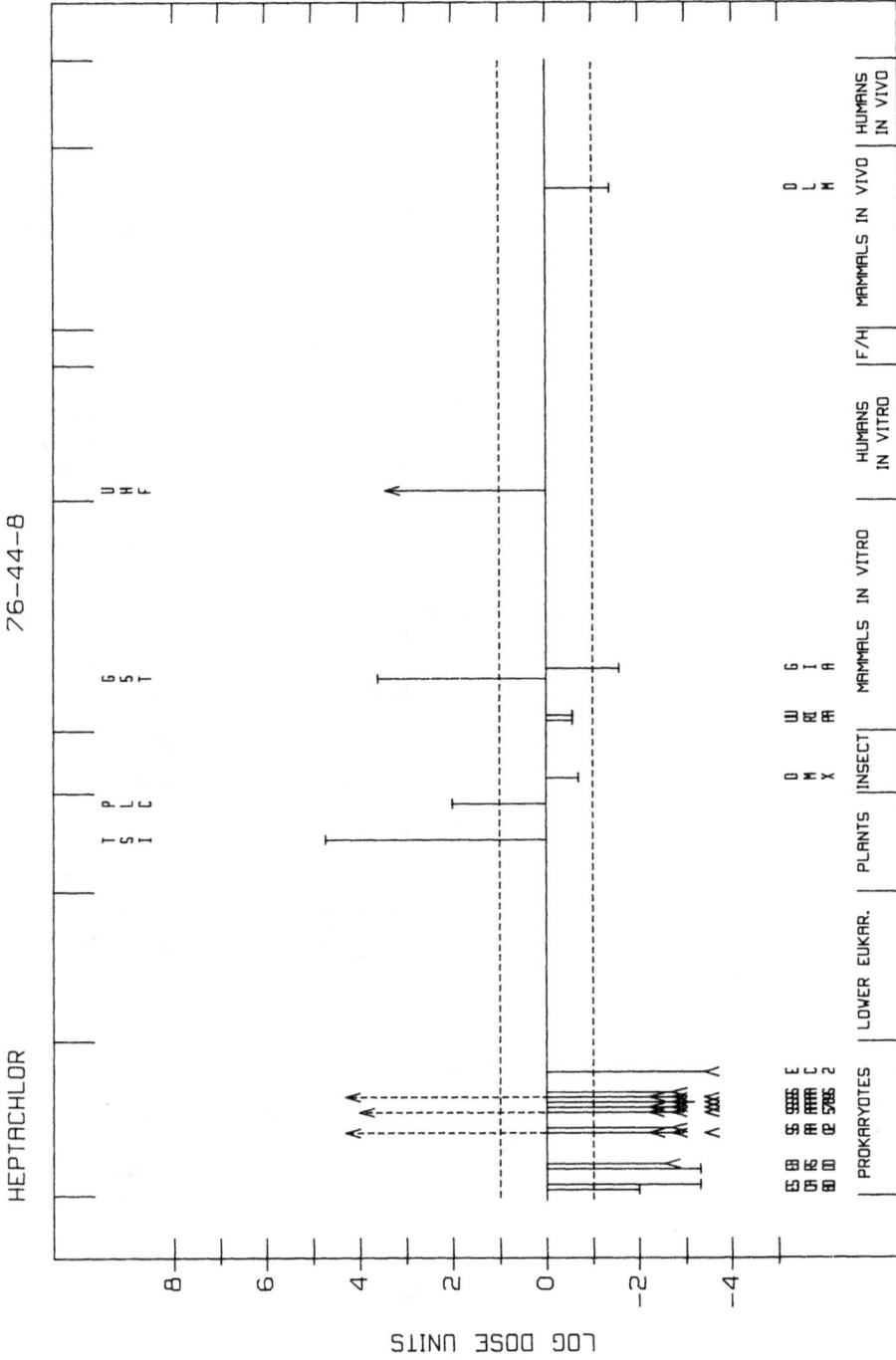

HEPTACHLOR

76-44-8

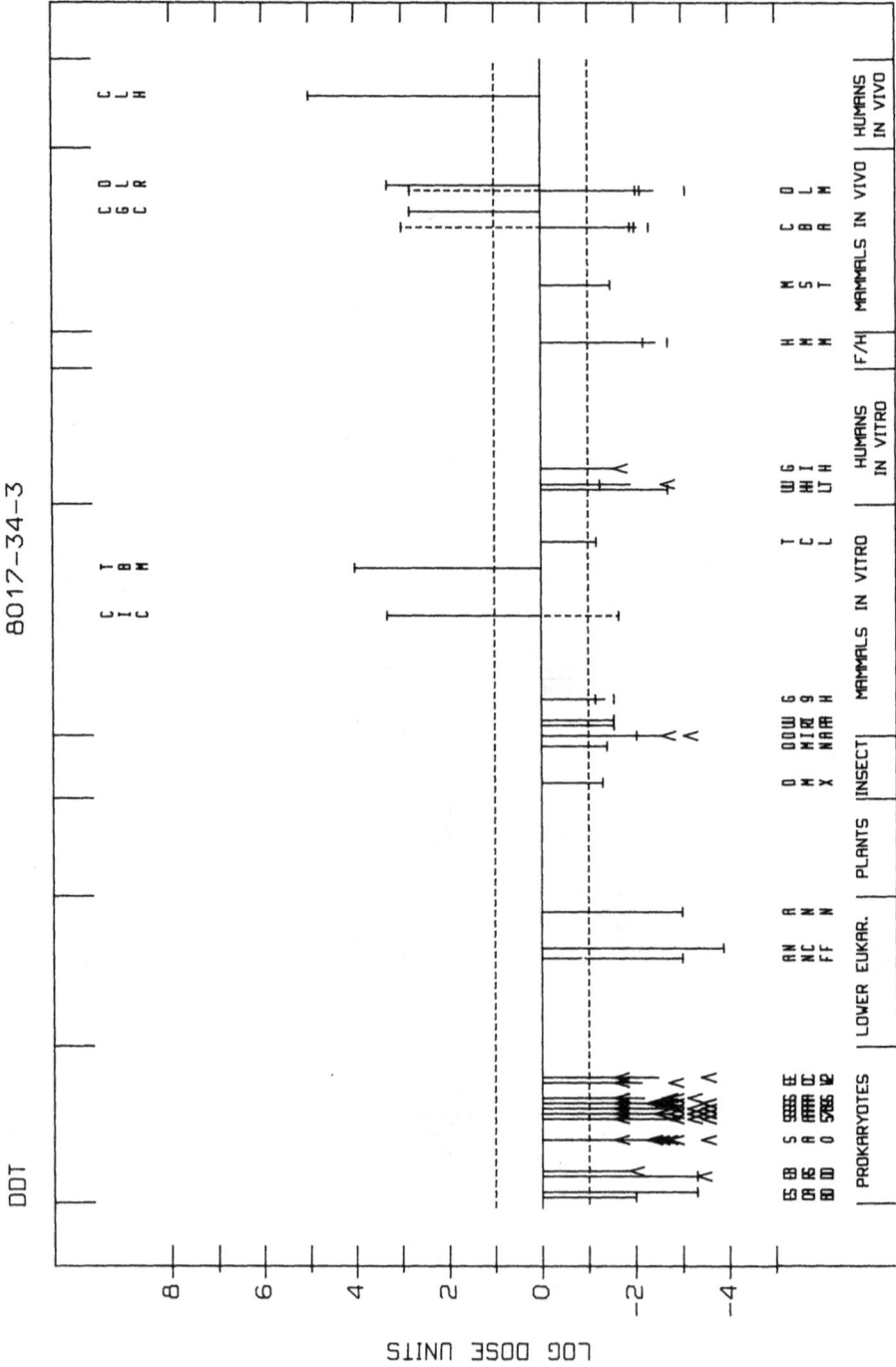

DDT

8017-34-3

LOG DOSE UNITS

8 6 4 2 0 -2 -4

PROKARYOTES | LOWER EUKAR. | PLANTS | INSECT | MAMMALS IN VITRO | HUMANS IN VITRO | F/H | MAMMALS IN VIVO | HUMANS IN VIVO

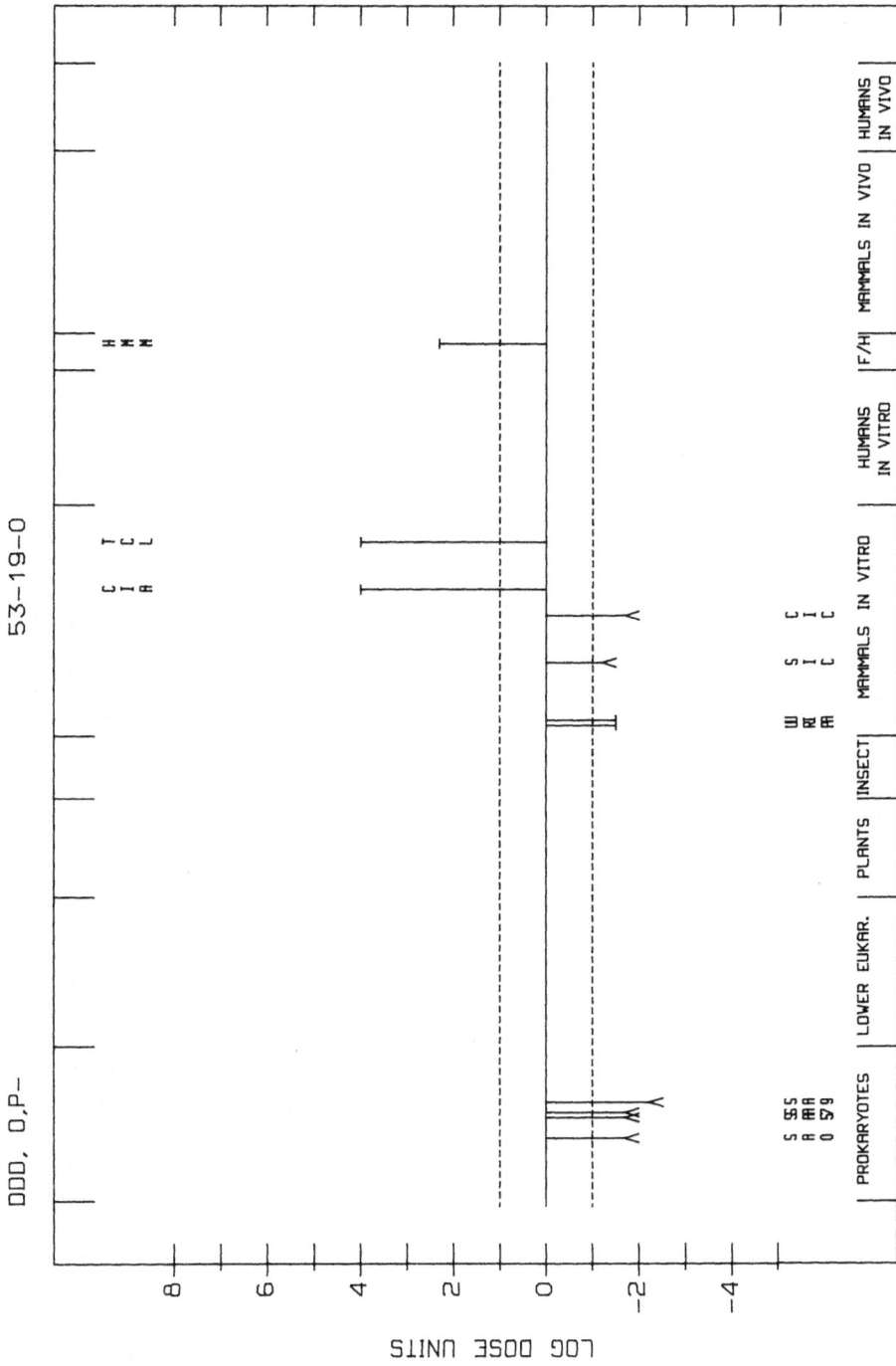

DDD, O,P-   53-19-0

LOG DOSE UNITS

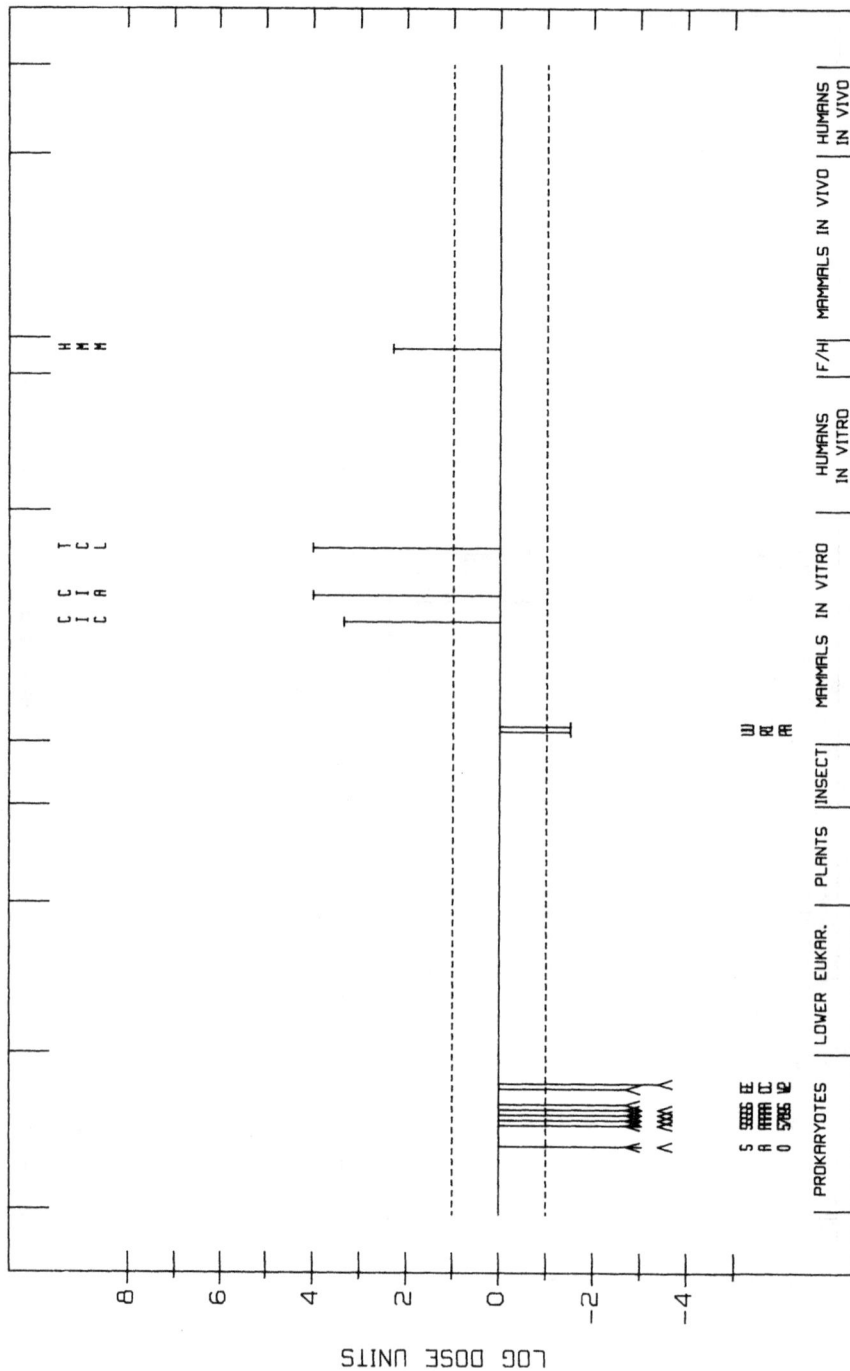

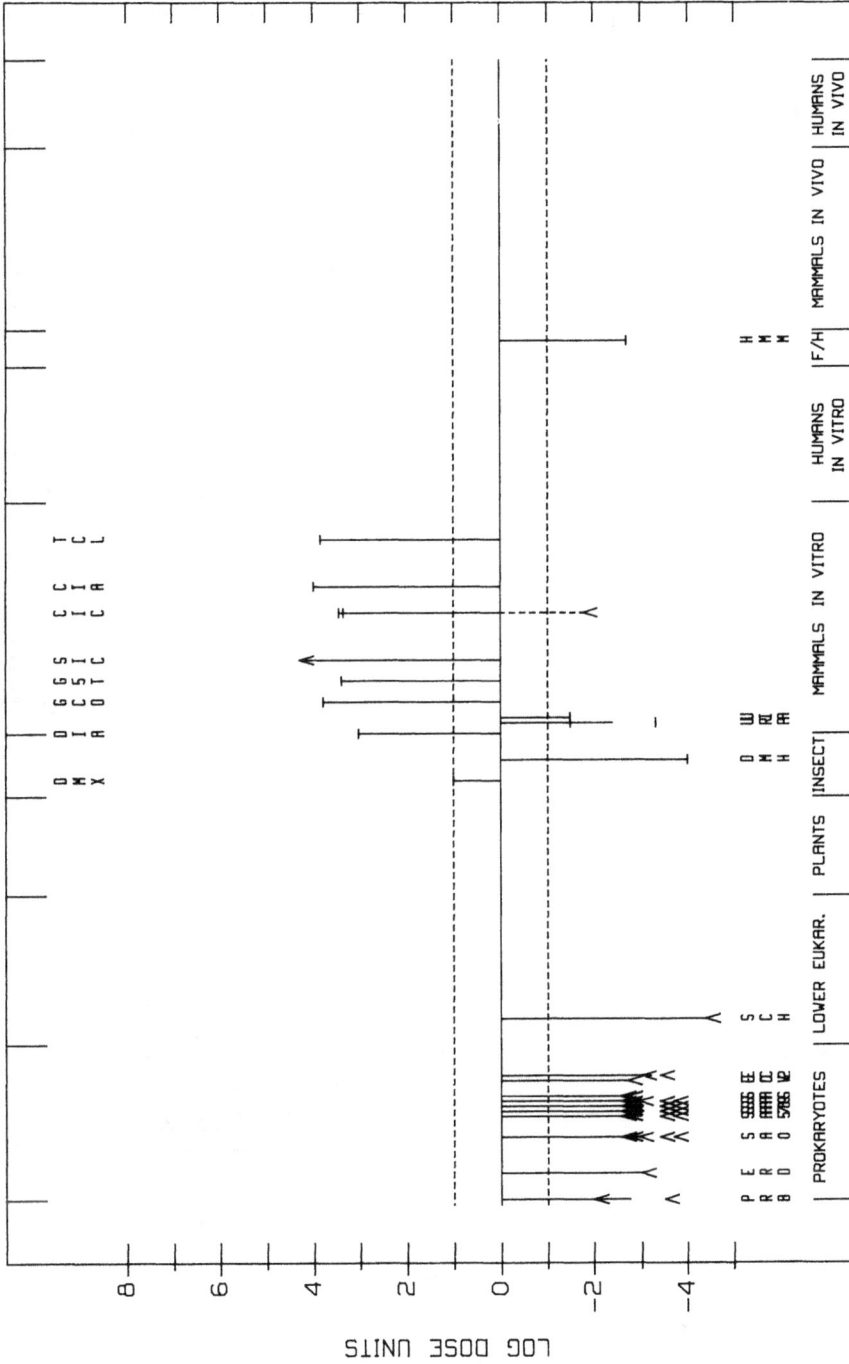

DDE, P,P-

72-55-9

DELTAMETHRIN

52918-63-5

LOG DOSE UNITS

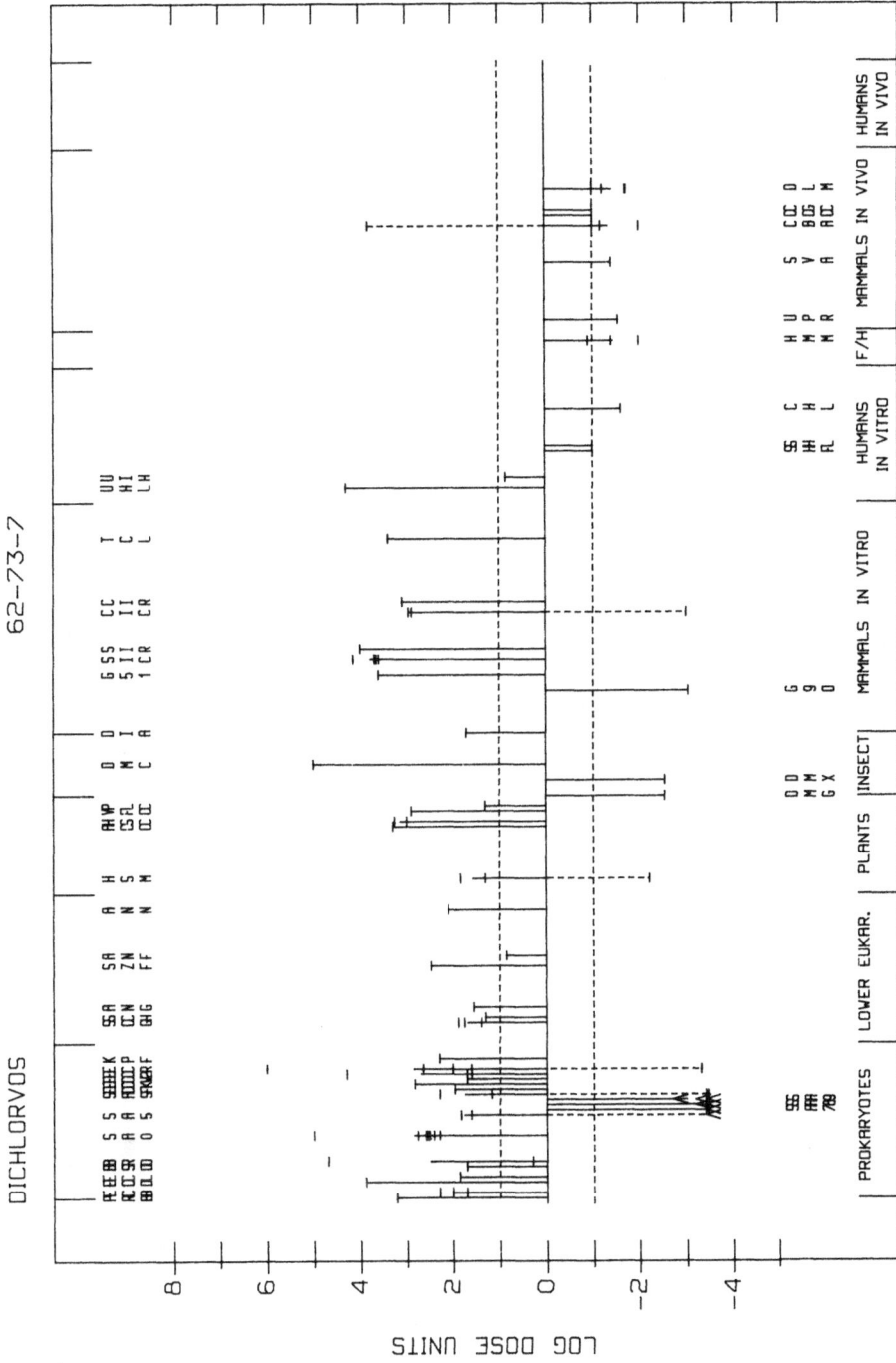

DICHLORVOS

62-73-7

LOG DOSE UNITS

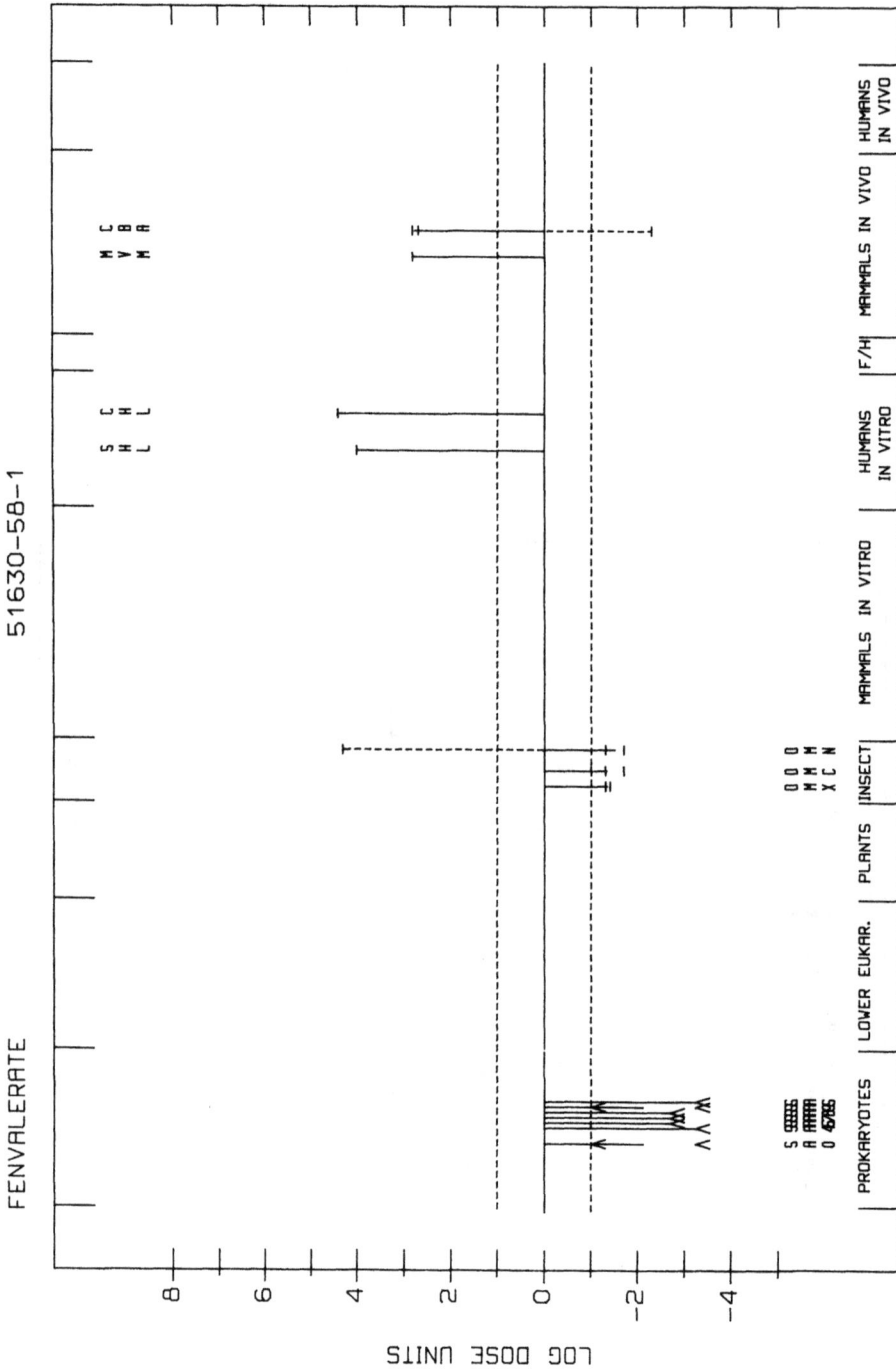

FENVALERATE

51630-58-1

LOG DOSE UNITS

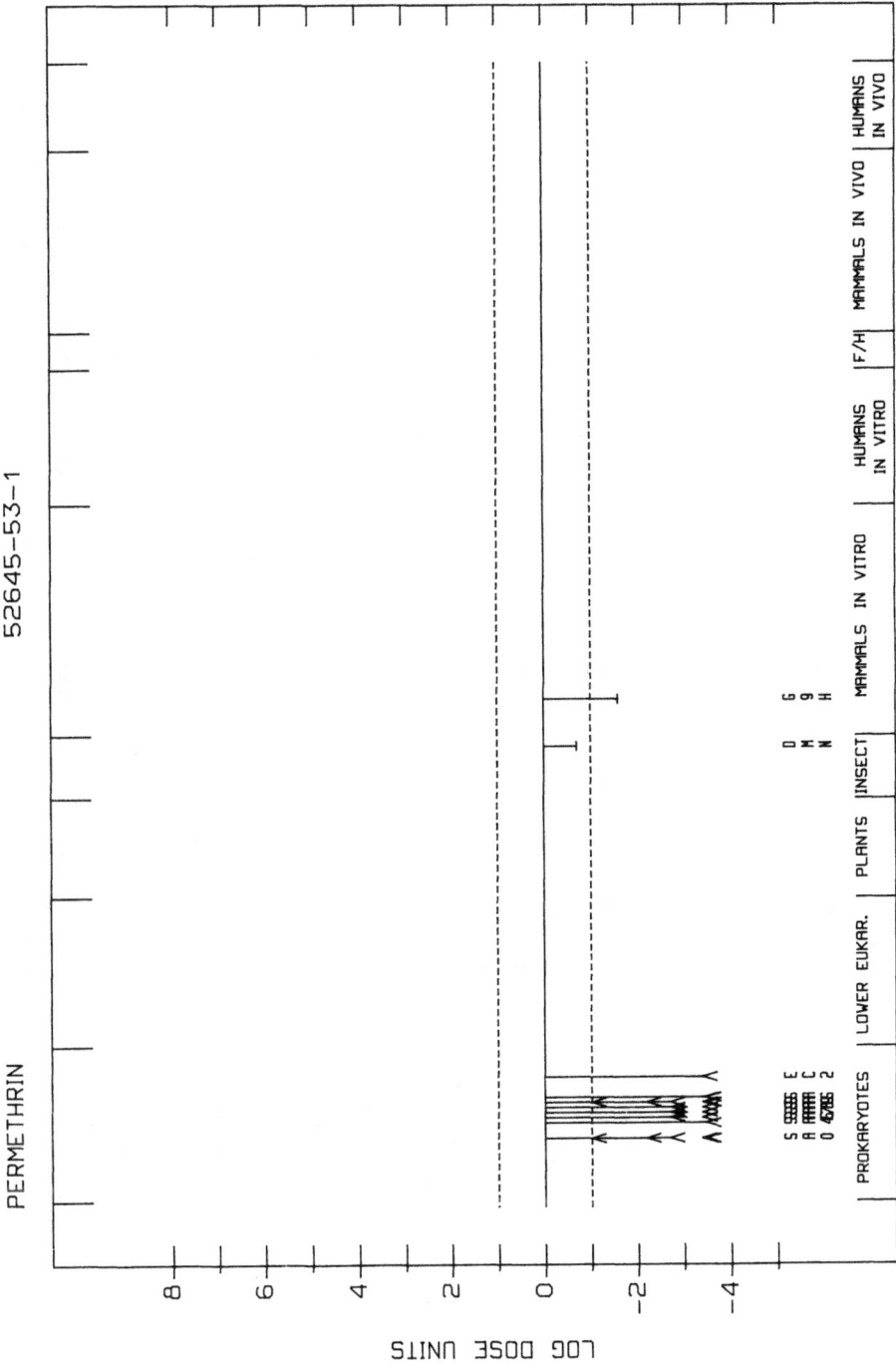

PERMETHRIN

52645-53-1

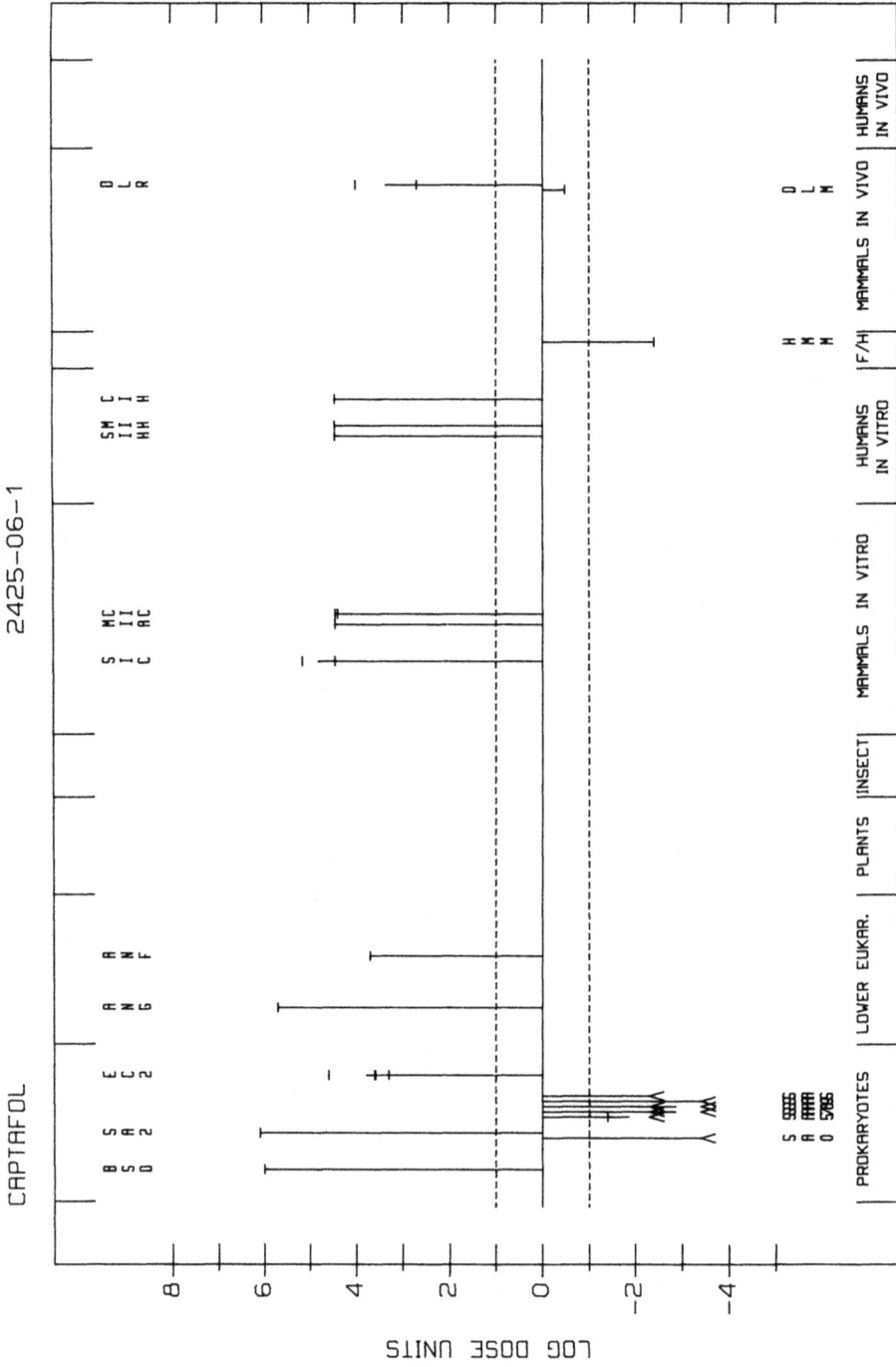

PENTACHLOROPHENOL   87-86-5

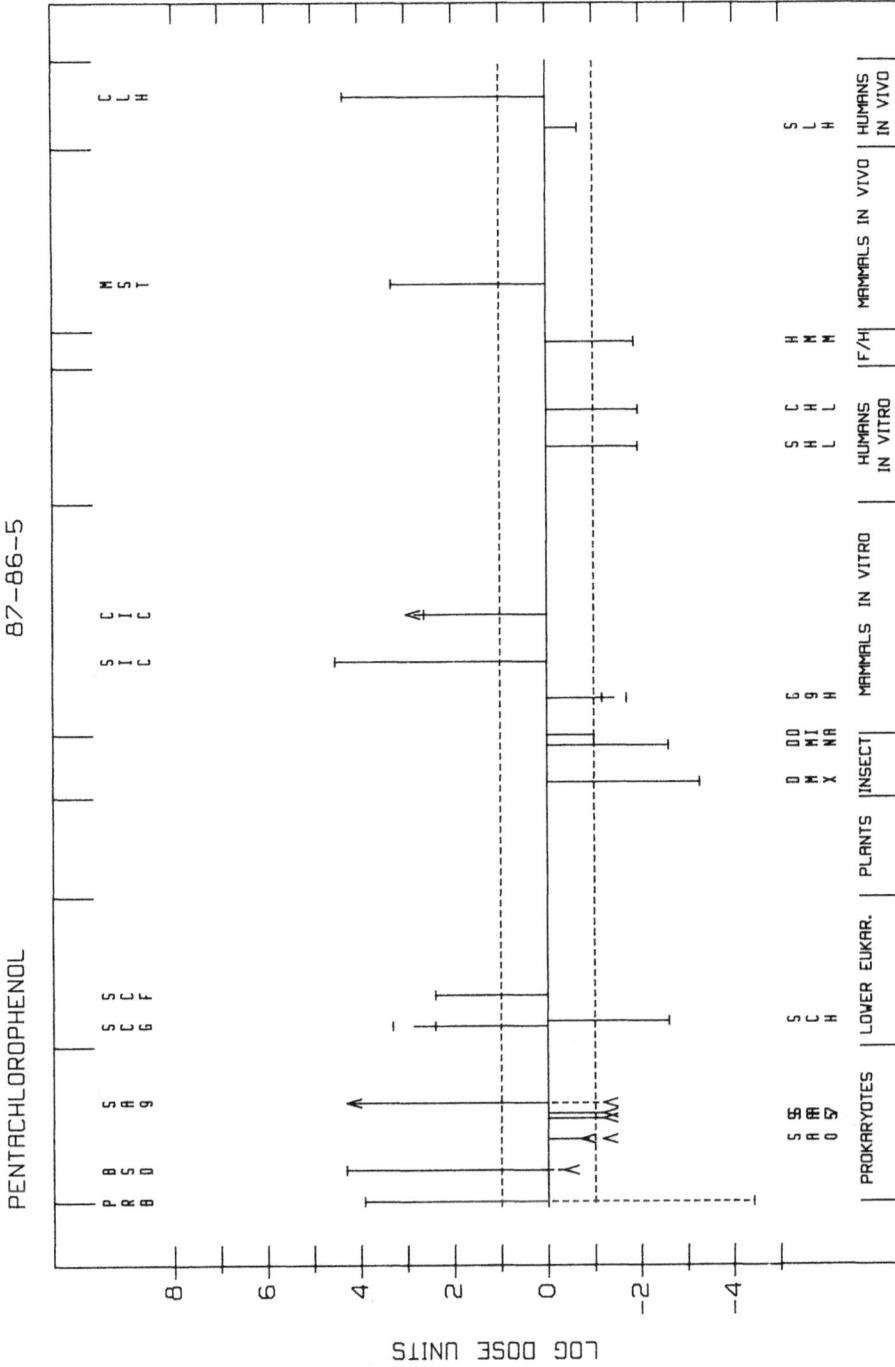

THIRAM   137-26-8

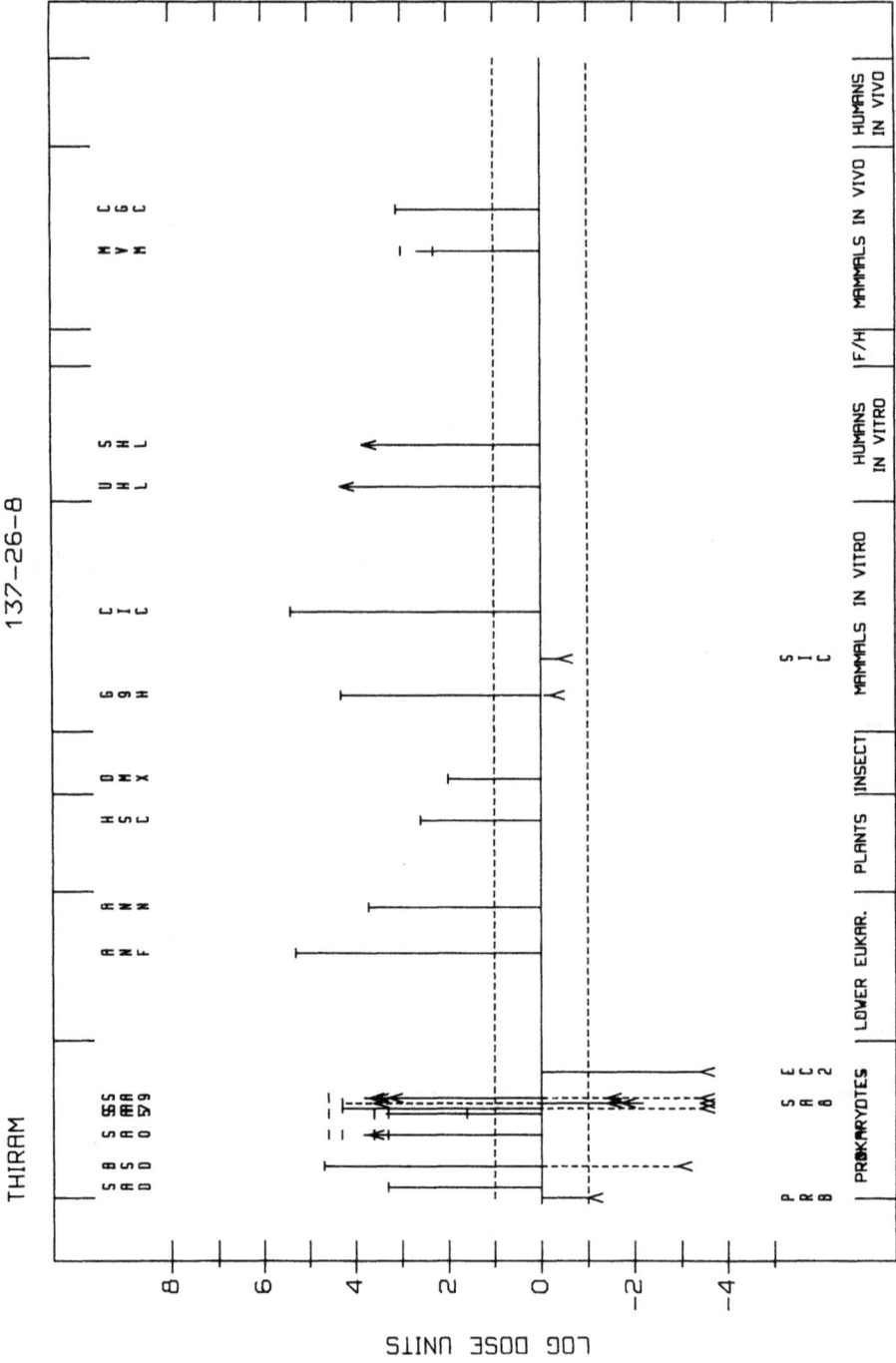

LOG DOSE UNITS

ZIRAM

137-30-4

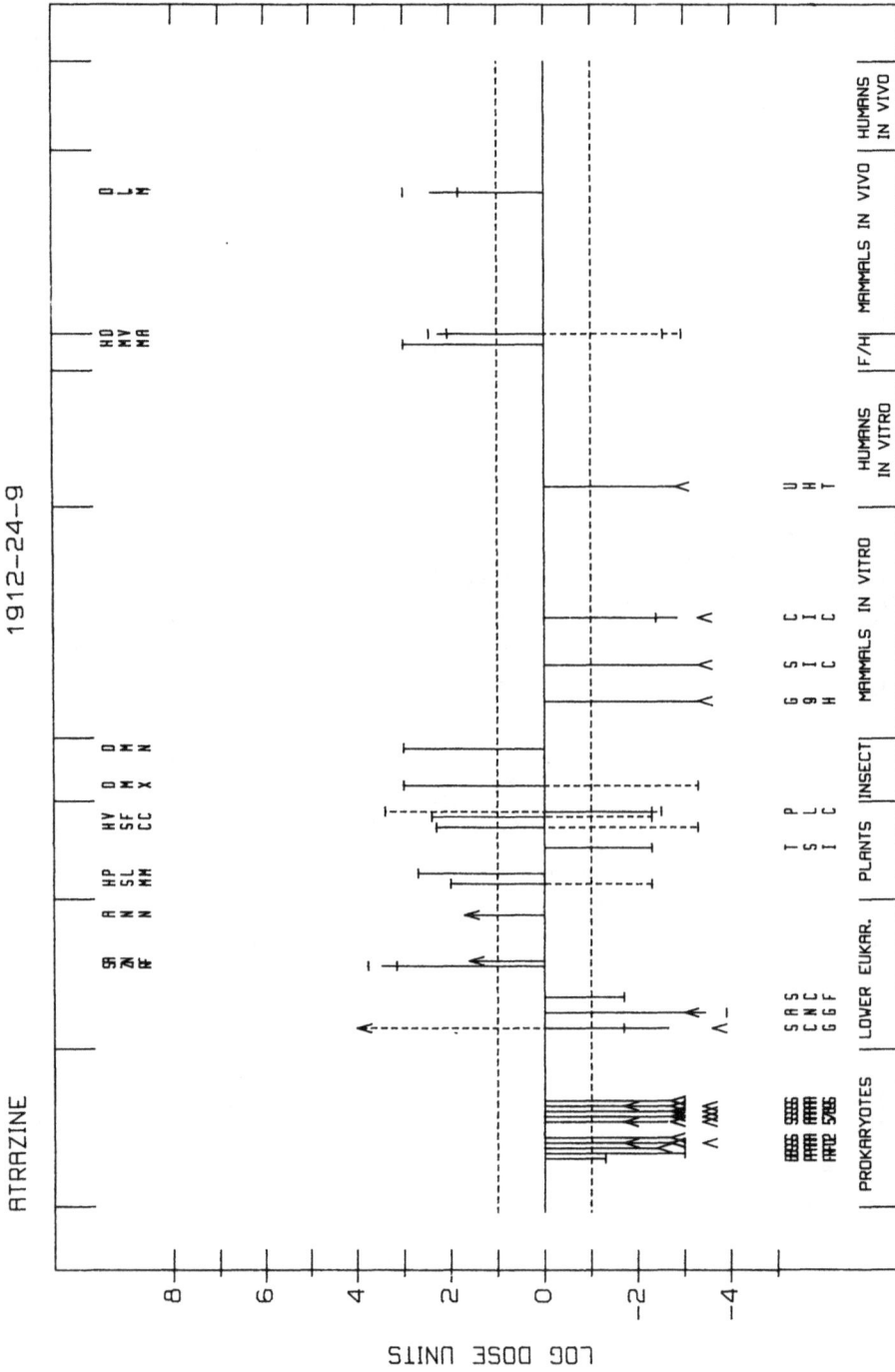

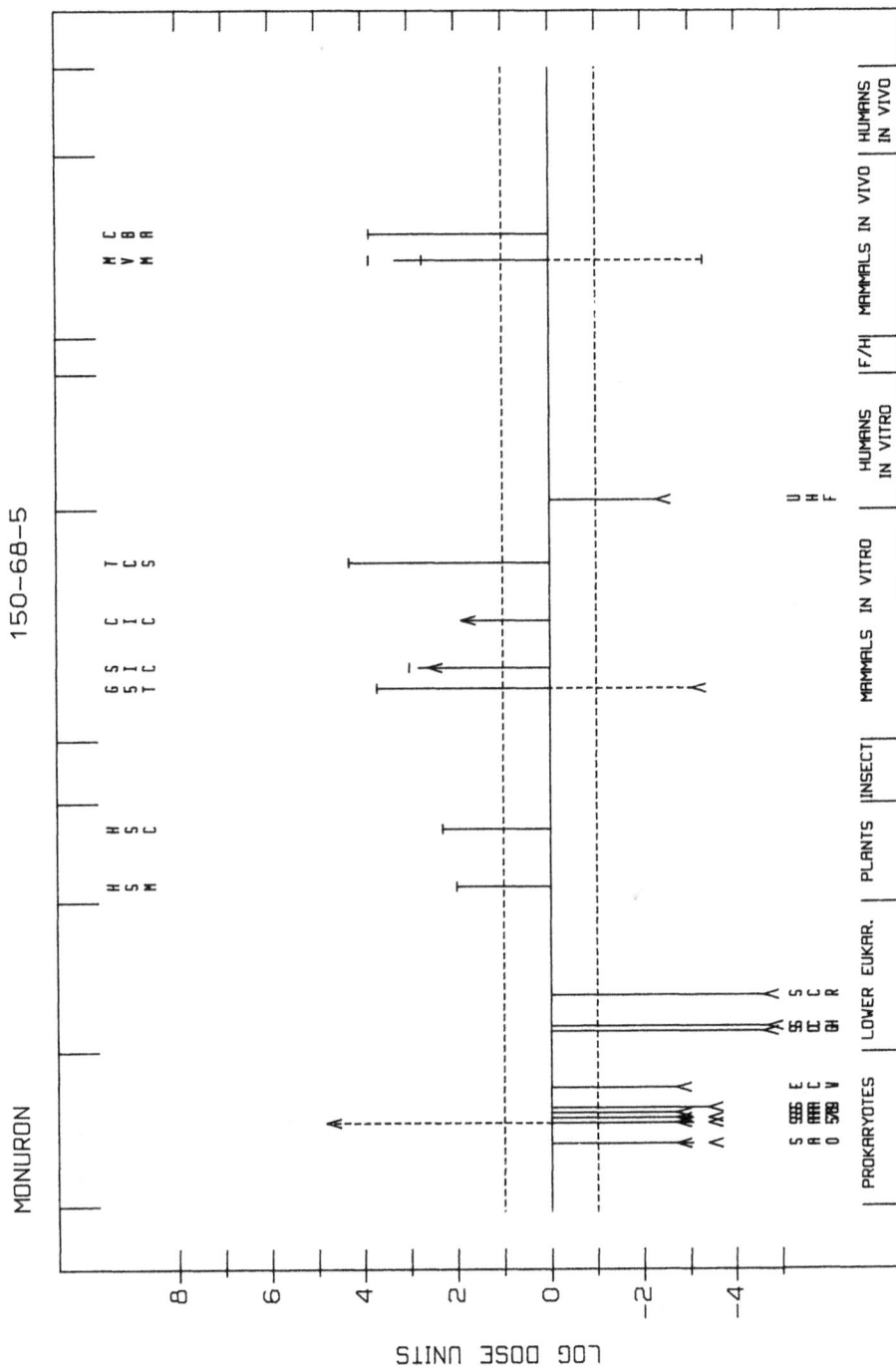

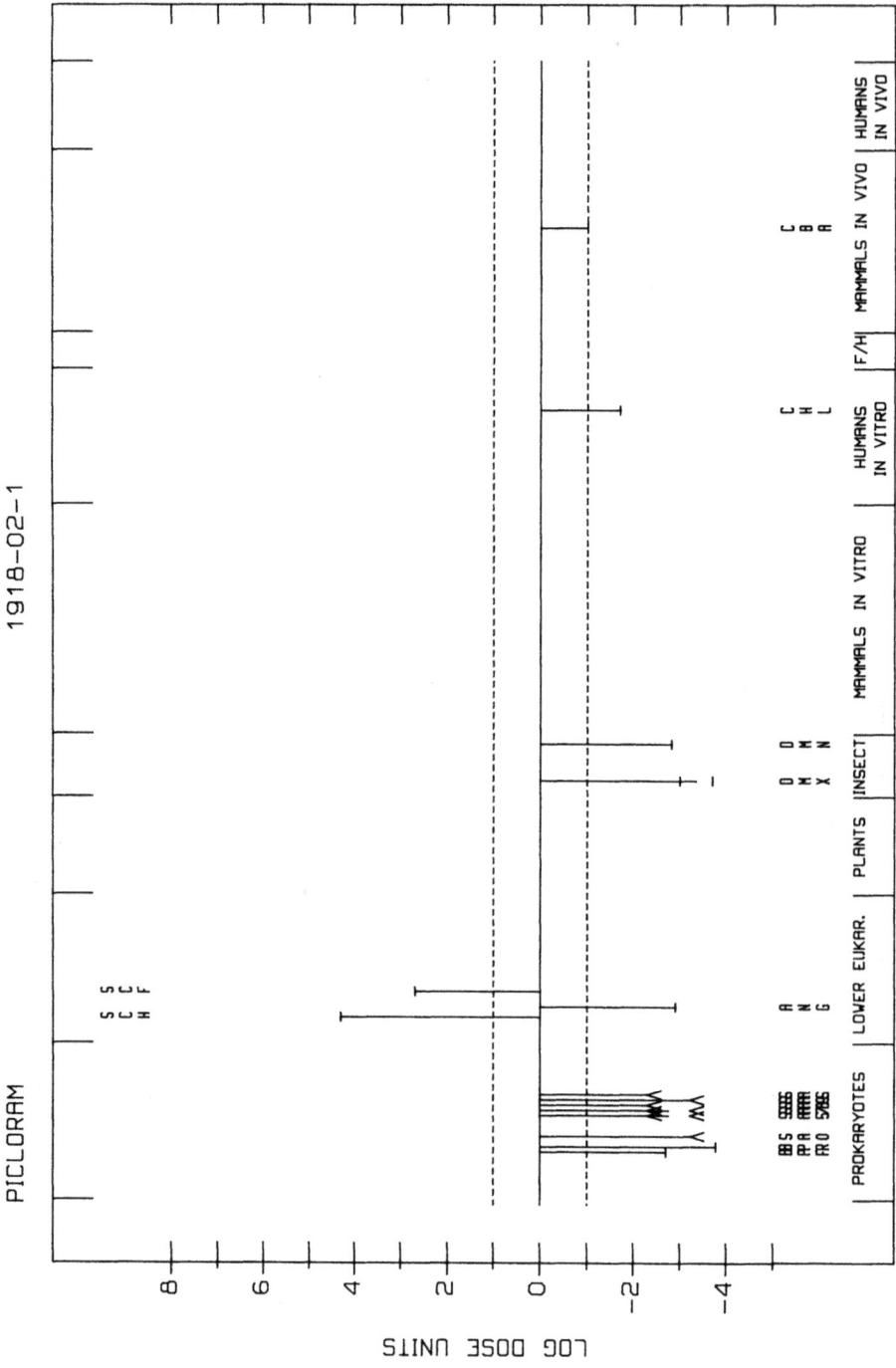

PICLORAM   1918-02-1

SIMAZINE   122-34-9

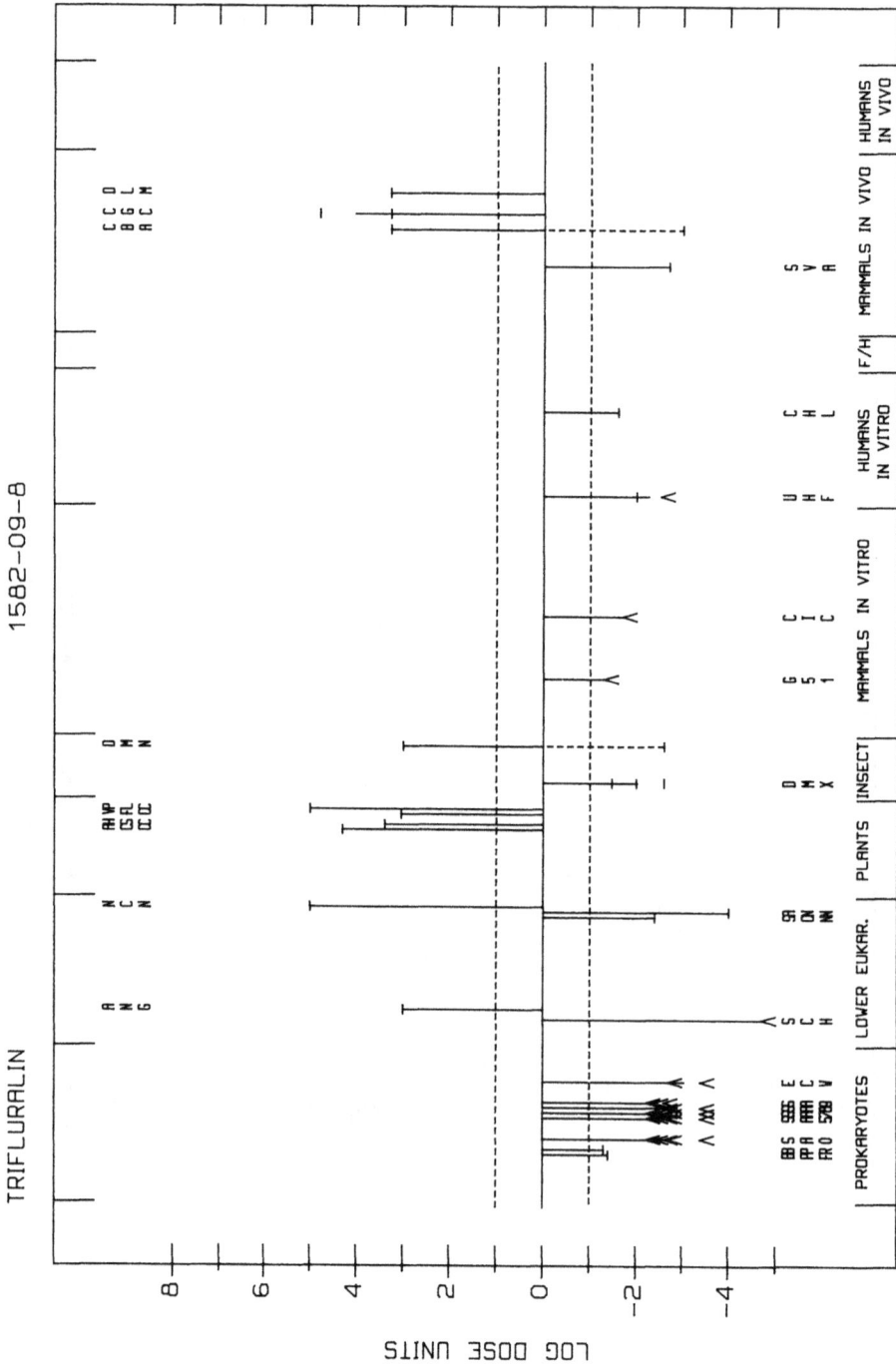

CUMULATIVE CROSS INDEX TO *IARC MONOGRAPHS ON THE EVALUATION OF CARCINOGENIC RISKS TO HUMANS*

The volume, page and year are given. References to corrigenda are given in parentheses.

A

A-α-C	*40*, 245 (1986); *Suppl. 7*, 56 (1987)
Acetaldehyde	*36*, 101 (1985) (*corr. 42*, 263); *Suppl. 7*, 77 (1987)
Acetaldehyde formylmethylhydrazone (*see* Gyromitrin)	
Acetamide	*7*, 197 (1974); *Suppl. 7*, 389 (1987)
Acetaminophen (*see* Paracetamol)	
Acridine orange	*16*, 145 (1978); *Suppl. 7*, 56 (1987)
Acriflavinium chloride	*13*, 31 (1977); *Suppl. 7*, 56 (1987)
Acrolein	*19*, 479 (1979); *36*,133 (1985); *Suppl. 7*, 78 (1987);
Acrylamide	*39*, 41 (1986); *Suppl. 7*, 56 (1987)
Acrylic acid	*19*, 47 (1979); *Suppl. 7*, 56 (1987)
Acrylic fibres	*19*, 86 (1979); *Suppl. 7*, 56 (1987)
Acrylonitrile	*19*, 73 (1979); *Suppl. 7*, 79 (1987)
Acrylonitrile–butadiene–styrene copolymers	*19*, 91 (1979); *Suppl. 7*, 56 (1987)
Actinolite (*see* Asbestos)	
Actinomycins	*10*, 29 (1976) (*corr. 42*, 255); *Suppl. 7*, 80 (1987)
Adriamycin	*10*, 43 (1976); *Suppl. 7*, 82 (1987)
AF-2	*31*, 47 (1983); *Suppl. 7*, 56 (1987)
Aflatoxins	*1*, 145 (1972) (*corr. 42*, 251); *10*, 51 (1976); *Suppl. 7*, 83 (1987)
Aflatoxin B_1 (*see* Aflatoxins)	
Aflatoxin B_2 (*see* Aflatoxins)	
Aflatoxin G_1 (*see* Aflatoxins)	
Aflatoxin G_2 (*see* Aflatoxins)	
Aflatoxin M_1 (*see* Aflatoxins)	
Agaritine	*31*, 63 (1983); *Suppl. 7*, 56 (1987)
Alcohol drinking	*44*
Aldicarb	*53*, 93
Aldrin	*5*, 25 (1974); *Suppl. 7*, 88 (1987)
Allyl chloride	*36*, 39 (1985); *Suppl. 7*, 56 (1987)
Allyl isothiocyanate	*36*, 55 (1985); *Suppl. 7*, 56 (1987)
Allyl isovalerate	*36*, 69 (1985); *Suppl. 7*, 56 (1987)
Aluminium production	*34*, 37 (1984); *Suppl. 7*, 89 (1987)
Amaranth	*8*, 41 (1975); *Suppl. 7*, 56 (1987)
5-Aminoacenaphthene	*16*, 243 (1978); *Suppl. 7*, 56 (1987)

2-Aminoanthraquinone	27, 191 (1982); *Suppl.* 7, 56 (1987)
para-Aminoazobenzene	8, 53 (1975); *Suppl.* 7, 390 (1987)
ortho-Aminoazotoluene	8, 61 (1975) (*corr.* 42, 254);.
	Suppl. 7, 56 (1987)
para-Aminobenzoic acid	16, 249 (1978); *Suppl.* 7, 56 (1987)
4-Aminobiphenyl	1, 74 (1972) (*corr.* 42, 251);
	Suppl. 7, 91 (1987)
2-Amino-3,4-dimethylimidazo[4,5-*f*]quinoline (*see* MeIQ)	
2-Amino-3,8-dimethylimidazo[4,5-*f*]quinoxaline (*see* MeIQx)	
3-Amino-1,4-dimethyl-5*H*-pyrido[4,3-*b*]indole (*see* Trp-P-1)	
2-Aminodipyrido[1,2-*a*:3′,2′-*d*]imidazole (*see* Glu-P-2)	
1-Amino-2-methylanthraquinone	27, 199 (1982); *Suppl.* 7, 57 (1987)
2-Amino-3-methylimidazo[4,5-*f*]quinoline (*see* IQ)	
2-Amino-6-methyldipyrido[1,2-*a*:3′,2′-*d*]-imidazole (*see* Glu-P-1)	
2-Amino-3-methyl-9*H*-pyrido[2,3-*b*]indole (*see* MeA-α-C)	
3-Amino-1-methyl-5*H*-pyrido[4,3-*b*]indole (*see* Trp-P-2)	
2-Amino-5-(5-nitro-2-furyl)-1,3,4-thiadiazole	7, 143 (1974); *Suppl.* 7, 57 (1987)
4-Amino-2-nitrophenol	16, 43 (1978); *Suppl.* 7, 57 (1987)
2-Amino-5-nitrothiazole	31, 71 (1983); *Suppl.* 7, 57 (1987)
2-Amino-9*H*-pyrido[2,3-*b*]indole [*see* A-α-C)	
11-Aminoundecanoic acid	39, 239 (1986); *Suppl.* 7, 57 (1987)
Amitrole	7, 31 (1974); 41, 293 (1986) (*corr.*
	52, 513; *Suppl.* 7, 92 (1987)
Ammonium potassium selenide (*see* Selenium and selenium compounds)	
Amorphous silica (*see also* Silica)	*Suppl.* 7, 341 (1987)
Amosite (*see* Asbestos)	
Ampicillin	50, 153 (1990)
Anabolic steroids (*see* Androgenic (anabolic) steroids)	
Anaesthetics, volatile	11, 285 (1976); *Suppl.* 7, 93 (1987)
Analgesic mixtures containing phenacetin (*see also* Phenacetin)	*Suppl.* 7, 310 (1987)
Androgenic (anabolic) steroids	*Suppl.* 7, 96 (1987)
Angelicin and some synthetic derivatives (*see also* Angelicins)	40, 291 (1986)
Angelicin plus ultraviolet radiation (*see also* Angelicin and some synthetic derivatives)	*Suppl.* 7, 57 (1987)
Angelicins	*Suppl.* 7, 57 (1987)
Aniline	4, 27 (1974) (*corr.* 42, 252);
	27, 39 (1982); *Suppl.* 7, 99 (1987)
ortho-Anisidine	27, 63 (1982); *Suppl.* 7, 57 (1987)
para-Anisidine	27, 65 (1982); *Suppl.* 7, 57 (1987)
Anthanthrene	32, 95 (1983); *Suppl.* 7, 57 (1987)
Anthophyllite (*see* Asbestos)	
Anthracene	32, 105 (1983); *Suppl.* 7, 57 (1987)
Anthranilic acid	16, 265 (1978); *Suppl.* 7, 57 (1987)
Antimony trioxide	47, 291 (1989)
Antimony trisulfide	47, 291 (1989)
ANTU (*see* 1-Naphthylthiourea)	
Apholate	9, 31 (1975); *Suppl.* 7, 57 (1987)
Aramite®	5, 39 (1974); *Suppl.* 7, 57 (1987)
Areca nut (*see* Betel quid)	
Arsanilic acid (*see* Arsenic and arsenic compounds)	
Arsenic and arsenic compounds	1, 41 (1972); 2, 48 (1973);
	23, 39 (1980); *Suppl.* 7, 100 (1987)

Arsenic pentoxide (*see* Arsenic and arsenic compounds)
Arsenic sulphide (*see* Arsenic and arsenic compounds)
Arsenic trioxide (*see* Arsenic and arsenic compounds)
Arsine (*see* Arsenic and arsenic compounds)
Asbestos   *2*, 17 (1973) (*corr. 42*, 252);
                                                                       14 (1977) (*corr. 42*, 256); Suppl. 7,
                                                                       106 (1987) (*corr. 45*, 283)
Atrazine   *53*, 441
Attapulgite   *42*, 159 (1987); *Suppl. 7*, 117 (1987)
Auramine (technical-grade)   *1*, 69 (1972) (*corr. 42*, 251); *Suppl.
                                                                       7*, 118 (1987)
Auramine, manufacture of (*see also* Auramine, technical-grade)   *Suppl. 7*, 118 (1987)
Aurothioglucose   *13*, 39 (1977); *Suppl. 7*, 57 (1987)
Azacitidine   *26*, 37 (1981); *Suppl. 7*, 57 (1987);
                                                                       50, 47 (1990)
5-Azacytidine (*see* Azacitidine)
Azaserine   *10*, 73 (1976) (*corr. 42*, 255);
                                                                       Suppl. 7, 57 (1987)
Azathioprine   *26*, 47 (1981); *Suppl. 7*, 119 (1987)
Aziridine   *9*, 37 (1975); *Suppl. 7*, 58 (1987)
2-(1-Aziridinyl)ethanol   *9*, 47 (1975); *Suppl. 7*, 58 (1987)
Aziridyl benzoquinone   *9*, 51 (1975); *Suppl. 7*, 58 (1987)
Azobenzene   *8*, 75 (1975); *Suppl. 7*, 58 (1987)

B

Barium chromate (*see* Chromium and chromium compounds)
Basic chromic sulphate (*see* Chromium and chromium compounds)
BCNU (*see* Bischloroethyl nitrosourea)
Benz[*a*]acridine   *32*, 123 (1983); *Suppl. 7*, 58 (1987)
Benz[*c*]acridine   *3*, 241 (1973); *32*, 129 (1983);
                                                                       Suppl. 7, 58 (1987)
Benzal chloride (*see also* α-Chlorinated toluenes)   *29*, 65 (1982); *Suppl. 7*, 148 (1987)
Benz[*a*]anthracene   *3*, 45 (1973); *32*, 135 (1983);
                                                                       Suppl. 7, 58 (1987)
Benzene   *7*, 203 (1974) (*corr. 42*, 254); *29*, 93,
                                                                       391 (1982); *Suppl. 7*, 120 (1987)
Benzidine   *1*, 80 (1972); *29*, 149, 391 (1982);
                                                                       Suppl. 7, 123 (1987)
Benzidine-based dyes   *Suppl. 7*, 125 (1987)
Benzo[*b*]fluoranthene   *3*, 69 (1973); *32*, 147 (1983);
                                                                       Suppl. 7, 58 (1987)
Benzo[*j*]fluoranthene   *3*, 82 (1973); *32*, 155 (1983); *Suppl.
                                                                       7*, 58 (1987)
Benzo[*k*]fluoranthene   *32*, 163 (1983); *Suppl. 7*, 58 (1987)
Benzo[*ghi*]fluoranthene   *32*, 171 (1983); *Suppl. 7*, 58 (1987)
Benzo[*a*]fluorene   *32*, 177 (1983); *Suppl. 7*, 58 (1987)
Benzo[*b*]fluorene   *32*, 183 (1983); *Suppl. 7*, 58 (1987)
Benzo[*c*]fluorene   *32*, 189 (1983); *Suppl. 7*, 58 (1987)
Benzo[*ghi*]perylene   *32*, 195 (1983); *Suppl. 7*, 58 (1987)
Benzo[*c*]phenanthrene   *32*, 205 (1983); *Suppl. 7*, 58 (1987)

Benzo[a]pyrene	3, 91 (1973); 32, 211 (1983); Suppl. 7, 58 (1987)
Benzo[e]pyrene	3, 137 (1973); 32, 225 (1983); Suppl. 7, 58 (1987)
para-Benzoquinone dioxime	29, 185 (1982); Suppl. 7, 58 (1987)
Benzotrichloride (see also α-Chlorinated toluenes)	29, 73 (1982); Suppl. 7, 148 (1987)
Benzoyl chloride	29, 83 (1982) (corr. 42, 261); Suppl. 7, 126 (1987)
Benzoyl peroxide	36, 267 (1985); Suppl. 7, 58 (1987)
Benzyl acetate	40, 109 (1986); Suppl. 7, 58 (1987)
Benzyl chloride (see also α-Chlorinated toluenes)	11, 217 (1976) (corr. 42, 256); 29, 49 (1982); Suppl. 7, 148 (1987)
Benzyl violet 4B	16, 153 (1978); Suppl. 7, 58 (1987)
Bertrandite (see Beryllium and beryllium compounds)	
Beryllium and beryllium compounds	1, 17 (1972); 23, 143 (1980) (corr. 42, 260); Suppl. 7, 127 (1987)
Beryllium acetate (see Beryllium and beryllium compounds)	
Beryllium acetate, basic (see Beryllium and beryllium compounds)	
Beryllium–aluminium alloy (see Beryllium and beryllium compounds)	
Beryllium carbonate (see Beryllium and beryllium compounds)	
Beryllium chloride (see Beryllium and beryllium compounds)	
Beryllium–copper alloy (see Beryllium and beryllium compounds)	
Beryllium–copper–cobalt alloy (see Beryllium and beryllium compounds)	
Beryllium fluoride (see Beryllium and beryllium compounds)	
Beryllium hydroxide (see Beryllium and beryllium compounds)	
Beryllium–nickel alloy (see Beryllium and beryllium compounds)	
Beryllium oxide (see Beryllium and beryllium compounds)	
Beryllium phosphate (see Beryllium and beryllium compounds)	
Beryllium silicate (see Beryllium and beryllium compounds)	
Beryllium sulphate (see Beryllium and beryllium compounds)	
Beryl ore (see Beryllium and beryllium compounds)	
Betel quid	37, 141 (1985); Suppl. 7, 128 (1987)
Betel-quid chewing (see Betel quid)	
BHA (see Butylated hydroxyanisole)	
BHT (see Butylated hydroxytoluene)	
Bis(1–aziridinyl)morpholinophosphine sulphide	9, 55 (1975); Suppl. 7, 58 (1987)
Bis(2–chloroethyl)ether	9, 117 (1975); Suppl. 7, 58 (1987)
N,N–Bis(2–chloroethyl)–2–naphthylamine	4, 119 (1974) (corr. 42, 253); Suppl. 7, 130 (1987)
Bischloroethyl nitrosourea (see also Chloroethyl nitrosoureas)	26, 79 (1981); Suppl. 7, 150 (1987)
1,2–Bis(chloromethoxy)ethane	15, 31 (1977); Suppl. 7, 58 (1987)
1,4–Bis(chloromethoxymethyl)benzene	15, 37 (1977); Suppl. 7, 58 (1987)
Bis(chloromethyl)ether	4, 231 (1974) (corr. 42, 253); Suppl. 7, 131 (1987)
Bis(2–chloro–1–methylethyl)ether	41, 149 (1986); Suppl. 7, 59 (1987)
Bis(2,3–epoxycyclopentyl)ether	47, 231 (1989)
Bisphenol A diglycidyl ether (see Glycidyl ethers)	
Bitumens	35, 39 (1985); Suppl. 7, 133 (1987)
Bleomycins	26, 97 (1981); Suppl. 7, 134 (1987)
Blue VRS	16, 163 (1978); Suppl. 7, 59 (1987)
Boot and shoe manufacture and repair	25, 249 (1981); Suppl. 7, 232 (1987)
Bracken fern	40, 47 (1986); Suppl. 7, 135 (1987)

Brilliant Blue FCF — *16*, 171 (1978) *(corr. 42*, 257); *Suppl. 7*, 59 (1987)

Bromochloroacetonitrile *(see* Halogenated acetonitriles)
Bromodichloromethane — *52*, 179 (1991)
Bromoethane — *52*, 299 (1991)
Bromoform — *52*, 213 (1991)
1,3-Butadiene — *39*, 155 (1986) *(corr. 42*, 264); *Suppl. 7*, 136 (1987)

1,4-Butanediol dimethanesulphonate — *4*, 247 (1974); *Suppl. 7*, 137 (1987)
n-Butyl acrylate — *39*, 67 (1986); *Suppl. 7*, 59 (1987)
Butylated hydroxyanisole — *40*, 123 (1986); *Suppl. 7*, 59 (1987)
Butylated hydroxytoluene — *40*, 161 (1986); *Suppl. 7*, 59 (1987)
Butyl benzyl phthalate — *29*, 193 (1982) *(corr. 42*, 261); *Suppl. 7*, 59 (1987)

β-Butyrolactone — *11*, 225 (1976); *Suppl. 7*, 59 (1987)
γ-Butyrolactone — *11*, 231 (1976); *Suppl. 7*, 59 (1987)

C

Cabinet-making *(see* Furniture and cabinet-making)
Cadmium acetate *(see* Cadmium and cadmium compounds)
Cadmium and cadmium compounds — 2, 74 (1973); *11*, 39 (1976) *(corr. 42*, 255); *Suppl. 7*, 139 (1987)

Cadmium chloride *(see* Cadmium and cadmium compounds)
Cadmium oxide *(see* Cadmium and cadmium compounds)
Cadmium sulphate *(see* Cadmium and cadmium compounds)
Cadmium sulphide *(see* Cadmium and cadmium compounds)
Caffeine — *51*, 291 (1991)
Calcium arsenate *(see* Arsenic and arsenic compounds)
Calcium chromate *(see* Chromium and chromium compounds)
Calcium cyclamate *(see* Cyclamates)
Calcium saccharin *(see* Saccharin)
Cantharidin — *10*, 79 (1976); *Suppl. 7*, 59 (1987)
Caprolactam — *19*, 115 (1979) *(corr. 42*, 258); *39*, 247 (1986) *(corr. 42*, 264); *Suppl. 7*, 390 (1987)

Captafol — *53*, 353
Captan — *30*, 295 (1983); *Suppl. 7*, 59 (1987)
Carbaryl — *12*, 37 (1976); *Suppl. 7*, 59 (1987)
Carbazole — *32*, 239 (1983); *Suppl. 7*, 59 (1987)
3-Carbethoxypsoralen — *40*, 317 (1986); *Suppl. 7*, 59 (1987)
Carbon blacks — *3*, 22 (1973); *33*, 35 (1984); *Suppl. 7*, 142 (1987)

Carbon tetrachloride — *1*, 53 (1972); *20*, 371 (1979); *Suppl. 7*, 143 (1987)

Carmoisine — *8*, 83 (1975); *Suppl. 7*, 59 (1987)
Carpentry and joinery — *25*, 139 (1981); *Suppl. 7*, 378 (1987)
Carrageenan — *10*, 181 (1976) *(corr. 42*, 255); *31*, 79 (1983); *Suppl. 7*, 59 (1987)
Catechol — *15*, 155 (1977); *Suppl. 7*, 59 (1987)
CCNU *(see* 1-(2-Chloroethyl)-3-cyclohexyl-1-nitrosourea)

Ceramic fibres (*see* Man–made mineral fibres)
Chemotherapy, combined, including alkylating agents (*see* MOPP and
  other combined chemotherapy including alkylating agents)
Chlorambucil   *9*, 125 (1975); *26*, 115 (1981);
                                                                     Suppl. 7, 144 (1987)
Chloramphenicol   *10*, 85 (1976); *Suppl. 7*, 145 (1987);
                                                                     50, 169 (1990)
Chlorendic acid   *48*, 45 (1990)
Chlordane (*see also* Chlordane/Heptachlor)   *20*, 45 (1979) (*corr. 42*, 258)
Chlordane/Heptachlor   *Suppl. 7*, 146 (1987); *53*, 115
Chlordecone   *20*, 67 (1979); *Suppl. 7*, 59 (1987)
Chlordimeform   *30*, 61 (1983); *Suppl. 7*, 59 (1987)
Chlorinated dibenzodioxins (other than TCDD)   *15*, 41 (1977); *Suppl. 7*, 59 (1987)
Chlorinated drinking-water   *52*, 45 (1991)
Chlorinated paraffins   *48*, 55 (1990)
α–Chlorinated toluenes   *Suppl. 7*, 148 (1987)
Chlormadinone acetate (*see also* Progestins; Combined oral   *6*, 149 (1974); *21*, 365 (1979)
  contraceptives)
Chlornaphazine (*see N,N*–Bis(2–chloroethyl)–2–naphthylamine)
Chloroacetonitrile (*see* Halogenated acetonitriles)
Chlorobenzilate   *5*, 75 (1974); *30*, 73 (1983);
                                                                     Suppl. 7, 60 (1987)
Chlorodibromomethane   *52*, 243 (1991)
Chlorodifluoromethane   *41*, 237 (1986) (*corr. 51*, 483);
                                                                     Suppl. 7, 149 (1987)
Chloroethane   *52*, 315 (1991)
1–(2–Chloroethyl)–3–cyclohexyl–1–nitrosourea   (*see also*   *26*, 137 (1981) (*corr. 42*, 260);
  Chloroethyl nitrosoureas)   *Suppl. 7*, 150 (1987)
1–(2–Chloroethyl)–3–(4–methylcyclohexyl)–1–nitrosourea (*see also*   *Suppl. 7*, 150 (1987)
  Chloroethyl nitrosoureas)
Chloroethyl nitrosoureas   *Suppl. 7*, 150 (1987)
Chlorofluoromethane   *41*, 229 (1986); *Suppl. 7*, 60 (1987)
Chloroform   *1*, 61 (1972); *20*, 401 (1979);
                                                                     Suppl. 7, 152 (1987)
Chloromethyl methyl ether (technical–grade) (*see also*
  Bis(chloromethyl)ether)   *4*, 239 (1974)
(4–Chloro–2–methylphenoxy)acetic acid (*see* MCPA)
Chlorophenols   *Suppl. 7*, 154 (1987)
Chlorophenols (occupational exposures to)   *41*, 319 (1986)
Chlorophenoxy herbicides   *Suppl. 7*, 156 (1987)
Chlorophenoxy herbicides (occupational exposures to)   *41*, 357 (1986)
4–Chloro–*ortho*–phenylenediamine   *27*, 81 (1982); *Suppl. 7*, 60 (1987)
4–Chloro–*meta*–phenylenediamine   *27*, 82 (1982); *Suppl. 7*, 60 (1987)
Chloroprene   *19*, 131 (1979); *Suppl. 7*, 160 (1987)
Chloropropham   *12*, 55 (1976); *Suppl. 7*, 60 (1987)
Chloroquine   *13*, 47 (1977); *Suppl. 7*, 60 (1987)
Chlorothalonil   *30*, 319 (1983); *Suppl. 7*, 60 (1987)
para–Chloro–*ortho*–toluidine and its strong acid salts   *16*, 277 (1978); *30*, 65 (1983);
  (*see also* Chlordimeform)   *Suppl. 7*, 60 (1987); *48*, 123 (1990)
Chlorotrianisene (*see also* Nonsteroidal oestrogens)   *21*, 139 (1979)
2–Chloro–1,1,1–trifluoroethane   *41*, 253 (1986); *Suppl. 7*, 60 (1987)
Chlorozotocin   *50*, 65 (1990)

Contraceptives, oral (*see* Combined oral contraceptives; Sequential oral contraceptives)

Copper 8–hydroxyquinoline	*15*, 103 (1977); *Suppl. 7*, 61 (1987)
Coronene	*32*, 263 (1983); *Suppl. 7*, 61 (1987)
Coumarin	*10*, 113 (1976); *Suppl. 7*, 61 (1987)
Creosotes (*see also* Coal-tars)	*Suppl. 7*, 177 (1987)
meta-Cresidine	*27*, 91 (1982); *Suppl. 7*, 61 (1987)
para-Cresidine	*27*, 92 (1982); *Suppl. 7*, 61 (1987)
Crocidolite (*see* Asbestos)	
Crude oil	*45*, 119 (1989)
Crystalline silica (*see also* Silica)	*Suppl. 7*, 341 (1987)
Cycasin	*1*, 157 (1972) (*corr. 42*, 251); *10*, 121 (1976); *Suppl. 7*, 61 (1987)
Cyclamates	*22*, 55 (1980); *Suppl. 7*, 178 (1987)
Cyclamic acid (*see* Cyclamates)	
Cyclochlorotine	*10*, 139 (1976); *Suppl. 7*, 61 (1987)
Cyclohexanone	*47*, 157 (1989)
Cyclohexylamine (*see* Cyclamates)	
Cyclopenta[*cd*]pyrene	*32*, 269 (1983); *Suppl. 7*, 61 (1987)
Cyclopropane (*see* Anaesthetics, volatile)	
Cyclophosphamide	*9*, 135 (1975); *26*, 165 (1981); *Suppl. 7*, 182 (1987)

D

2,4–D (*see also* Chlorophenoxy herbicides; Chlorophenoxy herbicides, occupational exposures to)	*15*, 111 (1977)
Dacarbazine	*26*, 203 (1981); *Suppl. 7*, 184 (1987)
Dantron	*50*, 265 (1990)
D & C Red No. 9	*8*, 107 (1975); *Suppl. 7*, 61 (1987)
Dapsone	*24*, 59 (1980); *Suppl. 7*, 185 (1987)
Daunomycin	*10*, 145 (1976); *Suppl. 7*, 61 (1987)
DDD (*see* DDT)	
DDE (*see* DDT)	
DDT	*5*, 83 (1974) (*corr. 42*, 253); *Suppl. 7*, 186 (1987); *53*, 179
Decabromodiphenyl oxide	*48*, 73 (1990)
Deltamethrin	*53*, 251
Diacetylaminoazotoluene	*8*, 113 (1975); *Suppl. 7*, 61 (1987)
N,N'-Diacetylbenzidine	*16*, 293 (1978); *Suppl. 7*, 61 (1987)
Dichlorvos	*53*, 267
Diallate	*12*, 69 (1976); *30*, 235 (1983); *Suppl. 7*, 61 (1987)
2,4–Diaminoanisole	*16*, 51 (1978); *27*, 103 (1982); *Suppl. 7*, 61 (1987)
4,4'–Diaminodiphenyl ether	*16*, 301 (1978); *29*, 203 (1982); *Suppl. 7*, 61 (1987)
1,2–Diamino–4–nitrobenzene	*16*, 63 (1978); *Suppl. 7*, 61 (1987)
1,4–Diamino–2–nitrobenzene	*16*, 73 (1978); *Suppl. 7*, 61 (1987)
2,6–Diamino–3–(phenylazo)pyridine (*see* Phenazopyridine hydrochloride)	
2,4–Diaminotoluene (*see also* Toluene diisocyanates)	*16*, 83 (1978); *Suppl. 7*, 61 (1987)

2,5-Diaminotoluene (*see also* Toluene diisocyanates)	*16*, 97 (1978); *Suppl. 7*, 61 (1987)
ortho-Dianisidine (*see* 3,3′-Dimethoxybenzidine)	
Diazepam	*13*, 57 (1977); *Suppl. 7*, 189 (1987)
Diazomethane	*7*, 223 (1974); *Suppl. 7*, 61 (1987)
Dibenz[*a,h*]acridine	*3*, 247 (1973); *32*, 277 (1983); *Suppl. 7*, 61 (1987)
Dibenz[*a,j*]acridine	*3*, 254 (1973); *32*, 283 (1983); *Suppl. 7*, 61 (1987)
Dibenz[*a,c*]anthracene	*32*, 289 (1983) (*corr. 42*, 262); *Suppl. 7*, 61 (1987)
Dibenz[*a,h*]anthracene	*3*, 178 (1973) (*corr. 43*, 261); *32*, 299 (1983); *Suppl. 7*, 61 (1987)
Dibenz[*a,j*]anthracene	*32*, 309 (1983); *Suppl. 7*, 61 (1987)
7*H*-Dibenzo[*c,g*]carbazole	*3*, 260 (1973); *32*, 315 (1983); *Suppl. 7*, 61 (1987)
Dibenzodioxins, chlorinated (other than TCDD) (*see* Chlorinated dibenzodioxins (other than TCDD))	
Dibenzo[*a,e*]fluoranthene	*32*, 321 (1983); *Suppl. 7*, 61 (1987)
Dibenzo[*h,rst*]pentaphene	*3*, 197 (1973); *Suppl. 7*, 62 (1987)
Dibenzo[*a,e*]pyrene	*3*, 201 (1973); *32*, 327 (1983); *Suppl. 7*, 62 (1987)
Dibenzo[*a,h*]pyrene	*3*, 207 (1973); *32*, 331 (1983); *Suppl. 7*, 62 (1987)
Dibenzo[*a,i*]pyrene	*3*, 215 (1973); *32*, 337 (1983); *Suppl. 7*, 62 (1987)
Dibenzo[*a,l*]pyrene	*3*, 224 (1973); *32*, 343 (1983); *Suppl. 7*, 62 (1987)
Dibromoacetonitrile (*see* Halogenated acetonitriles)	
1,2-Dibromo-3-chloropropane	*15*, 139 (1977); *20*, 83 (1979); *Suppl. 7*, 191 (1987)
Dichloroacetonitrile (*see* Halogenated acetonitriles)	
Dichloroacetylene	*39*, 369 (1986); *Suppl. 7*, 62 (1987)
ortho-Dichlorobenzene	*7*, 231 (1974); *29*, 213 (1982); *Suppl. 7*, 192 (1987)
para-Dichlorobenzene	*7*, 231 (1974); *29*, 215 (1982); *Suppl. 7*, 192 (1987)
3,3′-Dichlorobenzidine	*4*, 49 (1974); *29*, 239 (1982); *Suppl. 7*, 193 (1987)
trans-1,4-Dichlorobutene	*15*, 149 (1977); *Suppl. 7*, 62 (1987)
3,3′-Dichloro-4,4′-diaminodiphenyl ether	*16*, 309 (1978); *Suppl. 7*, 62 (1987)
1,2-Dichloroethane	*20*, 429 (1979); *Suppl. 7*, 62 (1987)
Dichloromethane	*20*, 449 (1979); *41*, 43 (1986); *Suppl. 7*, 194 (1987)
2,4-Dichlorophenol (*see* Chlorophenols; Chlorophenols, occupational exposures to)	
(2,4-Dichlorophenoxy)acetic acid (*see* 2,4-D)	
2,6-Dichloro-*para*-phenylenediamine	*39*, 325 (1986); *Suppl. 7*, 62 (1987)
1,2-Dichloropropane	*41*, 131 (1986); *Suppl. 7*, 62 (1987)
1,3-Dichloropropene (technical-grade)	*41*, 113 (1986); *Suppl. 7*, 195 (1987)
Dichlorvos	*20*, 97 (1979); *Suppl. 7*, 62 (1987); *53*, 267
Dicofol	*30*, 87 (1983); *Suppl. 7*, 62 (1987)

Dicyclohexylamine (*see* Cyclamates)
Dieldrin   *5*, 125 (1974); *Suppl. 7*, 196 (1987)
Dienoestrol (*see also* Nonsteroidal oestrogens)   *21*, 161 (1979)
Diepoxybutane   *11*, 115 (1976) (*corr. 42*, 255); *Suppl. 7*, 62 (1987)

Diesel and gasoline engine exhausts   *46*, 41 (1989)
Diesel fuels   *45*, 219 (1989) (*corr. 47*, 505)
Diethyl ether (*see* Anaesthetics, volatile)
Di(2-ethylhexyl)adipate   *29*, 257 (1982); *Suppl. 7*, 62 (1987)
Di(2-ethylhexyl)phthalate   *29*, 269 (1982) (*corr. 42*, 261); *Suppl. 7*, 62 (1987)

1,2-Diethylhydrazine   *4*, 153 (1974); *Suppl. 7*, 62 (1987)
Diethylstilboestrol   *6*, 55 (1974); *21*, 173 (1979) (*corr. 42*, 259); *Suppl. 7*, 273 (1987)

Diethylstilboestrol dipropionate (*see* Diethylstilboestrol)
Diethyl sulphate   *4*, 277 (1974); *Suppl. 7*, 198 (1987)
Diglycidyl resorcinol ether   *11*, 125 (1976); *36*, 181 (1985); *Suppl. 7*, 62 (1987)

Dihydrosafrole   *1*, 170 (1972); *10*, 233 (1976); *Suppl. 7*, 62 (1987)

1,8-Dihydroxyanthraquinone (*see* Dantron)
Dihydroxybenzenes (*see* Catechol; Hydroquinone; Resorcinol)
Dihydroxymethylfuratrizine   *24*, 77 (1980); *Suppl. 7*, 62 (1987)
Dimethisterone (*see also* Progestins; Sequential oral   *6*, 167 (1974); *21*, 377 (1979)
   contraceptives)
Dimethoxane   *15*, 177 (1977); *Suppl. 7*, 62 (1987)
3,3'-Dimethoxybenzidine   *4*, 41 (1974); *Suppl. 7*, 198 (1987)
3,3'-Dimethoxybenzidine-4,4'-diisocyanate   *39*, 279 (1986); *Suppl. 7*, 62 (1987)
para-Dimethylaminoazobenzene   *8*, 125 (1975); *Suppl. 7*, 62 (1987)
para-Dimethylaminoazobenzenediazo sodium sulphonate   *8*, 147 (1975); *Suppl. 7*, 62 (1987)
trans-2-[(Dimethylamino)methylimino]-5-[2-(5-nitro-2-furyl)-   *7*, 147 (1974) (*corr. 42*, 253); *Suppl. 7*, 62 (1987)
   vinyl]-1,3,4-oxadiazole
4,4'-Dimethylangelicin plus ultraviolet radiation (*see also*   *Suppl. 7*, 57 (1987)
   Angelicin and some synthetic derivatives)
4,5'-Dimethylangelicin plus ultraviolet radiation (*see also*   *Suppl. 7*, 57 (1987)
   Angelicin and some synthetic derivatives)
Dimethylarsinic acid (*see* Arsenic and arsenic compounds)
3,3'-Dimethylbenzidine   *1*, 87 (1972); *Suppl. 7*, 62 (1987)
Dimethylcarbamoyl chloride   *12*, 77 (1976); *Suppl. 7*, 199 (1987)
Dimethylformamide   *47*, 171 (1989)
1,1-Dimethylhydrazine   *4*, 137 (1974); *Suppl.7*, 62 (1987)
1,2-Dimethylhydrazine   *4*, 145 (1974) (*corr. 42*, 253); *Suppl. 7*, 62 (1987)

Dimethyl hydrogen phosphite   *48*, 85 (1990)
1,4-Dimethylphenanthrene   *32*, 349 (1983); *Suppl. 7*, 62 (1987)
Dimethyl sulphate   *4*, 271 (1974); *Suppl. 7*, 200 (1987)
3,7-Dinitrofluoranthene   *46*, 189 (1989)
3,9-Dinitrofluoranthene   *46*, 195 (1989)
1,3-Dinitropyrene   *46*, 201 (1989)
1,6-Dinitropyrene   *46*, 215 (1989)
1,8-Dinitropyrene   *33*, 171 (1984); *Suppl. 7*, 63 (1987); *46*, 231 (1989)

Ferric oxide	*1*, 29 (1972); *Suppl. 7*, 216 (1987)
Ferrochromium (*see* Chromium and chromium compounds)	
Fluometuron	*30*, 245 (1983); *Suppl. 7*, 63 (1987)
Fluoranthene	*32*, 355 (1983); *Suppl. 7*, 63 (1987)
Fluorene	*32*, 365 (1983); *Suppl. 7*, 63 (1987)
Fluorides (inorganic, used in drinking–water)	*27*, 237 (1982); *Suppl. 7*, 208 (1987)
5–Fluorouracil	*26*, 217 (1981); *Suppl. 7*, 210 (1987)
Fluorspar (*see* Fluorides)	
Fluosilicic acid (*see* Fluorides)	
Fluroxene (*see* Anaesthetics, volatile)	
Formaldehyde	*29*, 345 (1982); *Suppl. 7*, 211 (1987)
2–(2–Formylhydrazino)–4–(5–nitro–2–furyl)thiazole	*7*, 151 (1974) (*corr. 42*, 253); *Suppl. 7*, 63 (1987)
Frusemide (*see* Furosemide)	
Fuel oils (heating oils)	*45*, 239 (1989) (*corr. 47*, 505)
Furazolidone	*31*, 141 (1983); *Suppl. 7*, 63 (1987)
Furniture and cabinet–making	*25*, 99 (1981); *Suppl. 7*, 380 (1987)
Furosemide	*50*, 277 (1990)
2–(2–Furyl)–3–(5–nitro–2–furyl)acrylamide (*see* AF–2)	
Fusarenon–X	*11*, 169 (1976); *31*, 153 (1983); *Suppl. 7*, 64 (1987)

G

Gasoline	*45*, 159 (1989) (*corr. 47*, 505)
Gasoline engine exhaust (*see* Diesel and gasoline engine exhausts)	
Glass fibres (*see* Man-made mineral fibres)	
Glasswool (*see* Man-made mineral fibres)	
Glass filaments (*see* Man-made mineral fibres)	
Glu–P–1	*40*, 223 (1986); *Suppl. 7*, 64 (1987)
Glu–P–2	*40*, 235 (1986); *Suppl. 7*, 64 (1987)
L–Glutamic acid, 5–[2–(4–hydroxymethyl)phenylhydrazide] (*see* Agaratine)	
Glycidaldehyde	*11*, 175 (1976); *Suppl. 7*, 64 (1987)
Glycidyl ethers	*47*, 237 (1989)
Glycidyl oleate	11, 183 (1976); *Suppl. 7*, 64 (1987)
Glycidyl stearate	*11*, 187 (1976); *Suppl. 7*, 64 (1987)
Griseofulvin	*10*, 153 (1976); *Suppl. 7*, 391 (1987)
Guinea Green B	*16*, 199 (1978); *Suppl. 7*, 64 (1987)
Gyromitrin	*31*, 163 (1983); *Suppl. 7*, 391 (1987)

H

Haematite	*1*, 29 (1972); *Suppl. 7*, 216 (1987)
Haematite and ferric oxide	*Suppl. 7*, 216 (1987)
Haematite mining, underground, with exposure to radon	*1*, 29 (1972); *Suppl. 7*, 216 (1987)
Hair dyes, epidemiology of	*16*, 29 (1978); *27*, 307 (1982)
Halogenated acetonitriles	*52*, 269 (1991)
Halothane (*see* Anaesthetics, volatile)	
α–HCH (*see* Hexachlorocyclohexanes)	
β–HCH (*see* Hexachlorocyclohexanes)	
γ–HCH (*see* Hexachlorocyclohexanes)	

Heating oils (*see* Fuel oils)
Heptachlor (*see also* Chlordane/Heptachlor)   *5*, 173 (1974); *20*, 129 (1979)
Hexachlorobenzene   *20*, 155 (1979); *Suppl. 7*, 219 (1987)
Hexachlorobutadiene   *20*, 179 (1979); *Suppl. 7*, 64 (1987)
Hexachlorocyclohexanes   *5*, 47 (1974); *20*, 195 (1979)
                                                    (*corr. 42*, 258); *Suppl. 7*, 220 (1987)

Hexachlorocyclohexane, technical-grade (*see* Hexachloro-
    cyclohexanes)
Hexachloroethane   *20*, 467 (1979); *Suppl. 7*, 64 (1987)
Hexachlorophene   *20*, 241 (1979); *Suppl. 7*, 64 (1987)
Hexamethylphosphoramide   *15*, 211 (1977); *Suppl. 7*, 64 (1987)
Hexoestrol (*see* Nonsteroidal oestrogens)
Hycanthone mesylate   *13*, 91 (1977); *Suppl. 7*, 64 (1987)
Hydralazine   *24*, 85 (1980); *Suppl. 7*, 222 (1987)
Hydrazine   *4*, 127 (1974); *Suppl. 7*, 223 (1987)
Hydrochlorothiazide   *50*, 293 (1990)
Hydrogen peroxide   *36*, 285 (1985); *Suppl. 7*, 64 (1987)
Hydroquinone   *15*, 155 (1977); *Suppl. 7*, 64 (1987)
4-Hydroxyazobenzene   *8*, 157 (1975); *Suppl. 7*, 64 (1987)
17α-Hydroxyprogesterone caproate (*see also* Progestins)   *21*, 399 (1979) (*corr. 42*, 259)
8-Hydroxyquinoline   *13*, 101 (1977); *Suppl. 7*, 64 (1987)
8-Hydroxysenkirkine   *10*, 265 (1976); *Suppl. 7*, 64 (1987)
Hypochlorite salts   *52*, 159 (1991)

I

Indeno[1,2,3-*cd*]pyrene   *3*, 229 (1973); *32*, 373 (1983);
                                                    Suppl. 7, 64 (1987)

Insecticides, occupational exposures in spraying and application of   *53*, 45
IQ   *40*, 261 (1986); *Suppl. 7*, 64 (1987)
Iron and steel founding   *34*, 133 (1984); *Suppl. 7*, 224 (1987)
Iron–dextran complex   *2*, 161 (1973); *Suppl. 7*, 226 (1987)
Iron–dextrin complex   *2*, 161 (1973) (*corr. 42*, 252);
                                                    Suppl. 7, 64 (1987)

Iron oxide (*see* Ferric oxide)
Iron oxide, saccharated (*see* Saccharated iron oxide)
Iron sorbitol–citric acid complex   *2*, 161 (1973); *Suppl. 7*, 64 (1987)
Isatidine   *10*, 269 (1976); *Suppl. 7*, 65 (1987)
Isoflurane (*see* Anaesthetics, volatile)
Isoniazid (*see* Isonicotinic acid hydrazide)
Isonicotinic acid hydrazide   *4*, 159 (1974); *Suppl. 7*, 227 (1987)
Isophosphamide   *26*, 237 (1981); *Suppl. 7*, 65 (1987)
Isopropyl alcohol   *15*, 223 (1977); *Suppl. 7*, 229 (1987)
Isopropyl alcohol manufacture (strong-acid process) *Suppl. 7*, 229 (1987)
    (*see also* Isopropyl alcohol)
Isopropyl oils   *15*, 223 (1977); *Suppl. 7*, 229 (1987)
Isosafrole   *1*, 169 (1972); *10*, 232 (1976);
                                                    Suppl. 7, 65 (1987)

J

Jacobine   *10*, 275 (1976); *Suppl. 7*, 65 (1987)

Jet fuel	*45*, 203 (1989)
Joinery (*see* Carpentry and joinery)	

K

Kaempferol	31, 171 (1983); *Suppl.* 7, 65 (1987)
Kepone (*see* Chlordecone)	

L

Lasiocarpine	*10*, 281 (1976); *Suppl.* 7, 65 (1987)
Lauroyl peroxide	*36*, 315 (1985); Suppl. 7, 65 (1987)
Lead acetate (*see* Lead and lead compounds)	
Lead and lead compounds	*1*, 40 (1972) (*corr. 42*, 251); *2*, 52, 150 (1973); *12*, 131 (1976); *23*, 40, 208, 209, 325 (1980); *Suppl.* 7, 230 (1987)
Lead arsenate (*see* Arsenic and arsenic compounds)	
Lead carbonate (*see* Lead and lead compounds)	
Lead chloride (*see* Lead and lead compounds)	
Lead chromate (*see* Chromium and chromium compounds)	
Lead chromate oxide (*see* Chromium and chromium compounds)	
Lead naphthenate (*see* Lead and lead compounds)	
Lead nitrate (*see* Lead and lead compounds)	
Lead oxide (*see* Lead and lead compounds)	
Lead phosphate (*see* Lead and lead compounds)	
Lead subacetate (*see* Lead and lead compounds)	
Lead tetroxide (*see* Lead and lead compounds)	
Leather goods manufacture	*25*, 279 (1981); *Suppl.* 7, 235 (1987)
Leather industries	*25*, 199 (1981); *Suppl.* 7, 232 (1987)
Leather tanning and processing	*25*, 201 (1981); *Suppl.* 7, 236 (1987)
Ledate (*see also* Lead and lead compounds)	*12*, 131 (1976)
Light Green SF	*16*, 209 (1978); *Suppl.* 7, 65 (1987)
Lindane (*see* Hexachlorocyclohexanes)	
The lumber and sawmill industries (including logging)	*25*, 49 (1981); *Suppl.* 7, 383 (1987)
Luteoskyrin	*10*, 163 (1976); *Suppl.* 7, 65 (1987)
Lynoestrenol (*see also* Progestins; Combined oral contraceptives)	*21*, 407 (1979)

M

Magenta	*4*, 57 (1974) (*corr. 42*, 252); *Suppl.* 7, 238 (1987)
Magenta, manufacture of (*see also* Magenta)	*Suppl.* 7, 238 (1987)
Malathion	*30*, 103 (1983); *Suppl.* 7, 65 (1987)
Maleic hydrazide	*4*, 173 (1974) (*corr. 42*, 253); *Suppl.* 7, 65 (1987)
Malonaldehyde	*36*, 163 (1985); *Suppl.* 7, 65 (1987)
Maneb	*12*, 137 (1976); *Suppl.* 7, 65 (1987)
Man–made mineral fibres	*43*, 39 (1988)
Mannomustine	*9*, 157 (1975); *Suppl.* 7, 65 (1987)
Mate	*51*, 273 (1991)
MCPA (*see also* Chlorophenoxy herbicides; Chlorophenoxy herbicides, occupational exposures to)	*30*, 255 (1983)

MeA–α–C	*40*, 253 (1986); *Suppl. 7*, 65 (1987)
Medphalan	*9*, 168 (1975); *Suppl. 7*, 65 (1987)
Medroxyprogesterone acetate	*6*, 157 (1974); *21*, 417 (1979)
	(*corr. 42*, 259); *Suppl. 7*, 289 (1987)
Megestrol acetate (*see* also Progestins; Combined oral contraceptives)	
MeIQ	*40*, 275 (1986); *Suppl. 7*, 65 (1987)
MeIQx	*40*, 283 (1986); *Suppl. 7*, 65 (1987)
Melamine	*39*, 333 (1986); *Suppl. 7*, 65 (1987)
Melphalan	*9*, 167 (1975); *Suppl. 7*, 239 (1987)
6–Mercaptopurine	*26*, 249 (1981); *Suppl. 7*, 240 (1987)
Merphalan	*9*, 169 (1975); *Suppl. 7*, 65 (1987)
Mestranol (*see also* Steroidal oestrogens)	*6*, 87 (1974); *21*, 257 (1979)
	(*corr. 42*, 259)
Methanearsonic acid, disodium salt (*see* Arsenic and arsenic compounds)	
Methanearsonic acid, monosodium salt (*see* Arsenic and arsenic compounds	
Methotrexate	*26*, 267 (1981); *Suppl. 7*, 241 (1987)
Methoxsalen (*see* 8–Methoxypsoralen)	
Methoxychlor	*5*, 193 (1974); *20*, 259 (1979);
	Suppl. 7, 66 (1987)
Methoxyflurane (*see* Anaesthetics, volatile)	
5–Methoxypsoralen	*40*, 327 (1986); *Suppl. 7*, 242 (1987)
8–Methoxypsoralen (*see also* 8–Methoxypsoralen plus ultraviolet radiation)	*24*, 101 (1980)
8–Methoxypsoralen plus ultraviolet radiation	*Suppl. 7*, 243 (1987)
Methyl acrylate	*19*, 52 (1979); *39, 99* (1986);
	Suppl. 7, 66 (1987)
5–Methylangelicin plus ultraviolet radiation (*see also* Angelicin and some synthetic derivatives)	*Suppl. 7*, 57 (1987)
2–Methylaziridine	*9*, 61 (1975); *Suppl. 7*, 66 (1987)
Methylazoxymethanol acetate	*1*, 164 (1972); *10*, 131 (1976);
	Suppl. 7, 66 (1987)
Methyl bromide	*41*, 187 (1986) (*corr. 45*, 283);
	Suppl. 7, 245 (1987)
Methyl carbamate	*12*, 151 (1976); *Suppl. 7*, 66 (1987)
Methyl–CCNU [*see* 1–(2–Chloroethyl)–3–(4–methylcyclohexyl)–1–nitrosourea]	
Methyl chloride	*41*, 161 (1986); *Suppl. 7*, 246 (1987)
1–, 2–, 3–, 4–, 5– and 6–Methylchrysenes	*32*, 379 (1983); *Suppl. 7*, 66 (1987)
N–Methyl–N,4–dinitrosoaniline	*1*, 141 (1972); *Suppl. 7*, 66 (1987)
4,4'–Methylene bis(2–chloroaniline)	*4*, 65 (1974) (*corr. 42*, 252);
	Suppl. 7, 246 (1987)
4,4'–Methylene bis(N,N–dimethyl)benzenamine	*27*, 119 (1982); *Suppl. 7*, 66 (1987)
4,4'–Methylene bis(2–methylaniline)	*4*, 73 (1974); *Suppl. 7*, 248 (1987)
4,4'–Methylenedianiline	*4*, 79 (1974) (*corr. 42, 252*);
	39, 347 (1986); *Suppl. 7*, 66 (1987)
4,4'–Methylenediphenyl diisocyanate	*19*, 314 (1979); *Suppl. 7*, 66 (1987)
2–Methylfluoranthene	*32*, 399 (1983); *Suppl. 7*, 66 (1987)
3–Methylfluoranthene	*32*, 399 (1983); *Suppl. 7*, 66 (1987)
Methylglyoxal	*51*, 443 (1991)

1-Naphthylthiourea — *30*, 347 (1983); *Suppl. 7*, 263 (1987)
Nickel acetate (*see* Nickel and nickel compounds)
Nickel ammonium sulphate (*see* Nickel and nickel compounds)
Nickel and nickel compounds — *2*, 126 (1973) (*corr. 42*, 252); *11*, 75 (1976); *Suppl. 7*, 264 (1987) (*corr. 45, 283*); *49*, 257 (1990)

Nickel carbonate (*see* Nickel and nickel compounds)
Nickel carbonyl (*see* Nickel and nickel compounds)
Nickel chloride (*see* Nickel and nickel compounds)
Nickel-gallium alloy (*see* Nickel and nickel compounds)
Nickel hydroxide (*see* Nickel and nickel compounds)
Nickelocene (*see* Nickel and nickel compounds)
Nickel oxide (*see* Nickel and nickel compounds)
Nickel subsulphide (*see* Nickel and nickel compounds)
Nickel sulphate (*see* Nickel and nickel compounds)
Niridazole — *13*, 123 (1977); *Suppl. 7*, 67 (1987)
Nithiazide — *31*, 179 (1983); *Suppl. 7*, 67 (1987)
Nitrilotriacetic acid and its salts — *48*, 181 (1990)
5-Nitroacenaphthene — *16*, 319 (1978); *Suppl. 7*, 67 (1987)
5-Nitro-*ortho*-anisidine — *27*, 133 (1982); *Suppl. 7*, 67 (1987)
9-Nitroanthracene — *33*, 179 (1984); *Suppl. 7*, 67 (1987)
7-Nitrobenz[*a*]anthracene — *46*, 247 (1989)
6-Nitrobenzo[*a*]pyrene — *33*, 187 (1984); *Suppl. 7*, 67 (1987); *46*, 255 (1989)
4-Nitrobiphenyl — *4*, 113 (1974); *Suppl. 7*, 67 (1987)
6-Nitrochrysene — *33*, 195 (1984); *Suppl. 7*, 67 (1987); *46*, 267 (1989)
Nitrofen (technical-grade) — *30*, 271 (1983); *Suppl. 7*, 67 (1987)
3-Nitrofluoranthene — *33*, 201 (1984); *Suppl. 7*, 67 (1987)
2-Nitrofluorene — *46*, 277 (1989)
Nitrofural — *7*, 171 (1974); *Suppl. 7*, 67 (1987); *50*, 195 (1990)

5-Nitro-2-furaldehyde semicarbazone (*see* Nitrofural)
Nitrofurantoin — *50*, 211 (1990)
Nitrofurazone (*see* Nitrofural)
1-[(5-Nitrofurfurylidene)amino]-2-imidazolidinone — *7*, 181 (1974); *Suppl. 7*, 67 (1987)
N-[4-(5-Nitro-2-furyl)-2-thiazolyl]acetamide — *1*, 181 (1972); *7*, 185 (1974); *Suppl. 7*, 67 (1987)

Nitrogen mustard — *9*, 193 (1975); *Suppl. 7*, 269 (1987)
Nitrogen mustard *N*-oxide — *9*, 209 (1975); *Suppl. 7*, 67 (1987)
1-Nitronaphthalene — *46*, 291 (1989)
2-Nitronaphthalene — *46*, 303 (1989)
3-Nitroperylene — *46*, 313 (1989)
2-Nitropropane — *29*, 331 (1982); *Suppl. 7*, 67 (1987)
1-Nitropyrene — *33*, 209 (1984); *Suppl. 7*, 67 (1987); *46*, 321 (1989)
2-Nitropyrene — *46*, 359 (1989)
4-Nitropyrene — *46*, 367 (1989)
N-Nitrosatable drugs — *24*, 297 (1980) (*corr. 42*, 260)
N-Nitrosatable pesticides — *30*, 359 (1983)
N'-Nitrosoanabasine — *37*, 225 (1985); *Suppl. 7*, 67 (1987)
N'-Nitrosoanatabine — *37*, 233 (1985); *Suppl. 7*, 67 (1987)

N-Nitrosodi-n-butylamine	4, 197 (1974); 17, 51 (1978); Suppl. 7, 67 (1987)
N-Nitrosodiethanolamine	17, 77 (1978); Suppl. 7, 67 (1987)
N-Nitrosodiethylamine	1, 107 (1972) (corr. 42, 251); 17, 83 (1978) (corr. 42, 257); Suppl. 7, 67 (1987)
N-Nitrosodimethylamine	1, 95 (1972); 17, 125 (1978) (corr. 42, 257); Suppl. 7, 67 (1987)
N-Nitrosodiphenylamine	27, 213 (1982); Suppl. 7, 67 (1987)
para-Nitrosodiphenylamine	27, 227 (1982) (corr. 42, 261); Suppl. 7, 68 (1987)
N-Nitrosodi-n-propylamine	17, 177 (1978); Suppl. 7, 68 (1987)
N-Nitroso-N-ethylurea (see N-Ethyl-N-nitrosourea)	
N-Nitrosofolic acid	17, 217 (1978); Suppl. 7, 68 (1987)
N-Nitrosoguvacine	37, 263 (1985); Suppl. 7, 68 (1987)
N-Nitrosoguvacoline	37, 263 (1985); Suppl. 7, 68 (1987)
N-Nitrosohydroxyproline	17, 304 (1978); Suppl. 7, 68 (1987)
3-(N-Nitrosomethylamino)propionaldehyde	37, 263 (1985); Suppl. 7, 68 (1987)
3-(N-Nitrosomethylamino)propionitrile	37, 263 (1985); Suppl. 7, 68 (1987)
4-(N-Nitrosomethylamino)-4-(3-pyridyl)-1-butanal	37, 205 (1985); Suppl. 7, 68 (1987)
4-(N-Nitrosomethylamino)-1-(3-pyridyl)-1-butanone	37, 209 (1985); Suppl. 7, 68 (1987)
N-Nitrosomethylethylamine	17, 221 (1978); Suppl. 7, 68 (1987)
N-Nitroso-N-methylurea (see N-Methyl-N-nitrosourea)	
N-Nitroso-N-methylurethane (see N-Methyl-N-methylurethane)	
N-Nitrosomethylvinylamine	17, 257 (1978); Suppl. 7, 68 (1987)
N-Nitrosomorpholine	17, 263 (1978); Suppl. 7, 68 (1987)
N'-Nitrosonornicotine	17, 281 (1978); 37, 241 (1985); Suppl. 7, 68 (1987)
N-Nitrosopiperidine	17, 287 (1978); Suppl. 7, 68 (1987)
N-Nitrosoproline	17, 303 (1978); Suppl. 7, 68 (1987)
N-Nitrosopyrrolidine	17, 313 (1978); Suppl. 7, 68 (1987)
N-Nitrososarcosine	17, 327 (1978); Suppl. 7, 68 (1987)
Nitrosoureas, chloroethyl (see Chloroethyl nitrosoureas)	
5-Nitro-ortho-toluidine	48, 169 (1990)
Nitrous oxide (see Anaesthetics, volatile)	
Nitrovin	31, 185 (1983); Suppl. 7, 68 (1987)
NNA (see 4-(N-Nitrosomethylamino)-4-(3-pyridyl)-1-butanal)	
NNK (see 4-(N-Nitrosomethylamino)-1-(3-pyridyl)-1-butanone)	
Nonsteroidal oestrogens (see also Oestrogens, progestins and combinations)	Suppl. 7, 272 (1987)
Norethisterone (see also Progestins; Combined oral contraceptives)	6, 179 (1974); 21, 461 (1979)
Norethynodrel (see also Progestins; Combined oral contraceptives	6, 191 (1974); 21, 461 (1979) (corr. 42, 259)
Norgestrel (see also Progestins, Combined oral contraceptives)	6, 201 (1974); 21, 479 (1979)
Nylon 6	19, 120 (1979); Suppl. 7, 68 (1987)

O

Ochratoxin A	10, 191 (1976); 31, 191 (1983) (corr. 42, 262); Suppl. 7, 271 (1987)
Oestradiol-17β (see also Steroidal oestrogens)	6, 99 (1974); 21, 279 (1979)

Oestradiol 3–benzoate (*see* Oestradiol–17β)
Oestradiol dipropionate (*see* Oestradiol–17β)
Oestradiol mustard   9, 217 (1975)
Oestradiol–17β–valerate (*see* Oestradiol–17β)
Oestriol (*see also* Steroidal oestrogens)   6, 117 (1974); 21, 327 (1979)
Oestrogen–progestin combinations (*see* Oestrogens, progestins
   and combinations)
Oestrogen–progestin replacement therapy (*see also* Oestrogens,   *Suppl. 7*, 308 (1987)
   progestins and combinations)
Oestrogen replacement therapy (*see also* Oestrogens, progestins   *Suppl. 7*, 280 (1987)
   and combinations)
Oestrogens (*see* Oestrogens, progestins and combinations)
Oestrogens, conjugated (*see* Conjugated oestrogens)
Oestrogens, nonsteroidal (*see* Nonsteroidal oestrogens)
Oestrogens, progestins and combinations   6 (1974); 21 (1979);
                                                                                                              Suppl. 7, 272 (1987)
Oestrogens, steroidal (*see* Steroidal oestrogens)
Oestrone (*see also* Steroidal oestrogens)   6, 123 (1974); 21, 343 (1979)
                                                                                                              (*corr. 42*, 259)
Oestrone benzoate (*see* Oestrone)
Oil Orange SS   8, 165 (1975); *Suppl. 7*, 69 (1987)
Oral contraceptives, combined (*see* Combined oral contraceptives)
Oral contraceptives, investigational (*see* Combined oral
   contraceptives)
Oral contraceptives, sequential (*see* Sequential oral contraceptives)
Orange I   8, 173 (1975); *Suppl. 7*, 69 (1987)
Orange G   8, 181 (1975); *Suppl. 7*, 69 (1987)
Organolead compounds (*see also* Lead and lead compounds)   *Suppl. 7*, 230 (1987)
Oxazepam   13, 58 (1977); *Suppl. 7*, 69 (1987)
Oxymetholone (*see also* Androgenic (anabolic) steroids)   13, 131 (1977)
Oxyphenbutazone   13, 185 (1977); *Suppl. 7*, 69 (1987)

P

Paint manufacture and painting (occupational exposures in)   47, 329 (1989)
Panfuran S (*see also* Dihydroxymethylfuratrizine)   24, 77 (1980); *Suppl. 7*, 69 (1987)
Paper manufacture (*see* Pulp and paper manufacture)
Paracetamol   50, 307 (1990)
Parasorbic acid   10, 199 (1976) (*corr. 42*, 255);
                                                                                                              Suppl. 7, 69 (1987)
Parathion   30, 153 (1983); *Suppl. 7*, 69 (1987)
Patulin   10, 205 (1976); 40, 83 (1986);
                                                                                                              Suppl. 7, 69 (1987)
Penicillic acid   10, 211 (1976); *Suppl. 7*, 69 (1987)
Pentachloroethane   41, 99 (1986); *Suppl. 7*, 69 (1987)
Pentachloronitrobenzene (*see* Quintozene)
Pentachlorophenol (*see also* Chlorophenols; Chlorophenols,   20, 303 (1979); 53, 371
   occupational exposures to)
Permethrin   53, 329
Perylene   32, 411 (1983); *Suppl. 7*, 69 (1987)
Petasitenine   31, 207 (1983); *Suppl. 7*, 69 (1987)
Petasites japonicus (*see* Pyrrolizidine alkaloids)

Petroleum refining (occupational exposures in)   *45*, 39 (1989)
Some petroleum solvents   *47*, 43 (1989)
Phenacetin   *13*, 141 (1977); *24*, 135 (1980);
                                                   Suppl. 7, 310 (1987)
Phenanthrene   *32*, 419 (1983); *Suppl. 7*, 69 (1987)
Phenazopyridine hydrochloride   *8*, 117 (1975); *24*, 163 (1980)
                                                   (*corr. 42*, 260); *Suppl. 7*, 312 (1987)
Phenelzine sulphate   *24*, 175 (1980); *Suppl. 7*, 312 (1987)
Phenicarbazide   *12*, 177 (1976); *Suppl. 7*, 70 (1987)
Phenobarbital   *13*, 157 (1977); *Suppl. 7*, 313 (1987)
Phenol   *47*, 263 (1989) (*corr. 50*, 385)
Phenoxyacetic acid herbicides (*see* Chlorophenoxy herbicides)
Phenoxybenzamine hydrochloride   *9*, 223 (1975); *24*, 185 (1980);
                                                   Suppl. 7, 70 (1987)
Phenylbutazone   *13*, 183 (1977); *Suppl. 7*, 316 (1987)
meta-Phenylenediamine   *16*, 111 (1978); *Suppl. 7*, 70 (1987)
para-Phenylenediamine   *16*, 125 (1978); *Suppl. 7*, 70 (1987)
Phenyl glycidyl ether (*see* Glycidyl ethers)
N-Phenyl-2-naphthylamine   *16*, 325 (1978) (*corr. 42*, 257);
                                                   Suppl. 7, 318 (1987)
ortho-Phenylphenol   *30*, 329 (1983); *Suppl. 7*, 70 (1987)
Phenytoin   *13*, 201 (1977); *Suppl. 7*, 319 (1987)
Picloram   *53*, 481
Piperazine oestrone sulphate (*see* Conjugated oestrogens)
Piperonyl butoxide   *30*, 183 (1983); *Suppl. 7*, 70 (1987)
Pitches, coal-tar (*see* Coal-tar pitches)
Polyacrylic acid   *19*, 62 (1979); *Suppl. 7*, 70 (1987)
Polybrominated biphenyls   *18*, 107 (1978); *41*, 261 (1986);
                                                   Suppl. 7, 321 (1987)
Polychlorinated biphenyls   *7*, 261 (1974); *18*, 43 (1978) (*corr.*
                                                   42, 258);
                                                   Suppl. 7, 322 (1987)
Polychlorinated camphenes (*see* Toxaphene)
Polychloroprene   *19*, 141 (1979); *Suppl. 7*, 70 (1987)
Polyethylene   *19*, 164 (1979); *Suppl. 7*, 70 (1987)
Polymethylene polyphenyl isocyanate   *19*, 314 (1979); *Suppl. 7*, 70 (1987)
Polymethyl methacrylate   *19*, 195 (1979); *Suppl. 7*, 70 (1987)
Polyoestradiol phosphate (*see* Oestradiol-17β)
Polypropylene   *19*, 218 (1979); *Suppl. 7*, 70 (1987)
Polystyrene   *19*, 245 (1979); *Suppl. 7*, 70 (1987)
Polytetrafluoroethylene   *19*, 288 (1979); *Suppl. 7*, 70 (1987)
Polyurethane foams   *19*, 320 (1979); *Suppl. 7*, 70 (1987)
Polyvinyl acetate   *19*, 346 (1979); *Suppl. 7*, 70 (1987)
Polyvinyl alcohol   *19*, 351 (1979); *Suppl. 7*, 70 (1987)
Polyvinyl chloride   *7*, 306 (1974); *19*, 402 (1979);
                                                   Suppl. 7, 70 (1987)
Polyvinyl pyrrolidone   *19*, 463 (1979); *Suppl. 7*, 70 (1987)
Ponceau MX   *8*, 189 (1975); *Suppl. 7*, 70 (1987)
Ponceau 3R   *8*, 199 (1975); *Suppl. 7*, 70 (1987)
Ponceau SX   *8*, 207 (1975); *Suppl. 7*, 70 (1987)
Potassium arsenate (*see* Arsenic and arsenic compounds)
Potassium arsenite (*see* Arsenic and arsenic compounds)

Potassium bis(2–hydroxyethyl)dithiocarbamate | *12*, 183 (1976); *Suppl. 7*, 70 (1987)
Potassium bromate | *40*, 207 (1986); *Suppl. 7*, 70 (1987)
Potassium chromate (*see* Chromium and chromium compounds)
Potassium dichromate (*see* Chromium and chromium compounds)
Prednimustine | *50*, 115 (1990)
Prednisone | *26*, 293 (1981); *Suppl. 7*, 326 (1987)
Procarbazine hydrochloride | *26*, 311 (1981); *Suppl. 7*, 327 (1987)
Proflavine salts | *24*, 195 (1980); *Suppl. 7*, 70 (1987)
Progesterone (*see also* Progestins; Combined oral contraceptives) | *6*, 135 (1974); *21*, 491 (1979) (*corr. 42*, 259)

Progestins (*see also* Oestrogens, progestins and combinations) | *Suppl. 7*, 289 (1987)
Pronetalol hydrochloride | *13*, 227 (1977) (*corr. 42*, 256); *Suppl. 7*, 70 (1987)

1,3–Propane sultone | *4*, 253 (1974) (*corr. 42*, 253); *Suppl. 7*, 70 (1987)
Propham | *12*, 189 (1976); *Suppl. 7*, 70 (1987)
β–Propiolactone | *4*, 259 (1974) (*corr. 42*, 253); *Suppl. 7*, 70 (1987)
n–Propyl carbamate | *12*, 201 (1976); *Suppl. 7*, 70 (1987)
Propylene | *19*, 213 (1979); *Suppl. 7*, 71 (1987)
Propylene oxide | *11*, 191 (1976); *36*, 227 (1985) (*corr. 42*, 263); *Suppl. 7*, 328 (1987)
Propylthiouracil | *7*, 67 (1974); *Suppl. 7*, 329 (1987)
Ptaquiloside (*see also* Bracken fern) | *40*, 55 (1986); *Suppl. 7*, 71 (1987)
Pulp and paper manufacture | *25*, 157 (1981); *Suppl. 7*, 385 (1987)
Pyrene | *32*, 431 (1983); *Suppl. 7*, 71 (1987)
Pyrido[3,4–*c*]psoralen | *40*, 349 (1986); *Suppl. 7*, 71 (1987)
Pyrimethamine | *13*, 233 (1977); *Suppl. 7*, 71 (1987)
Pyrrolizidine alkaloids (*see* Hydroxysenkirkine; Isatidine; Jacobine; Lasiocarpine; Monocrotaline; Retrorsine; Riddelliine; Seneciphylline; Senkirkine)

Q

Quercetin (*see also* Bracken fern) | *31*, 213 (1983); *Suppl. 7*, 71 (1987)
para–Quinone | *15*, 255 (1977); *Suppl. 7*, 71 (1987)
Quintozene | *5*, 211 (1974); *Suppl. 7*, 71 (1987)

R

Radon | *43*, 173 (1988) (*corr. 45*, 283)
Reserpine | *10*, 217 (1976); *24*, 211 (1980) (*corr. 42*, 260); *Suppl. 7*, 330 (1987)
Resorcinol | *15*, 155 (1977); *Suppl. 7*, 71 (1987)
Retrorsine | *10*, 303 (1976); *Suppl. 7*, 71 (1987)
Rhodamine B | *16*, 221 (1978); *Suppl. 7*, 71 (1987)
Rhodamine 6G | *16*, 233 (1978); *Suppl. 7*, 71 (1987)
Riddelliine | *10*, 313 (1976); *Suppl. 7*, 71 (1987)
Rifampicin | *24*, 243 (1980); *Suppl. 7*, 71 (1987)
Rockwool (*see* Man–made mineral fibres)
The rubber industry | *28* (1982) (*corr. 42*, 261); *Suppl. 7*, 332 (1987)

Rugulosin   *40*, 99 (1986); *Suppl. 7*, 71 (1987)

S

Saccharated iron oxide   *2*, 161 (1973); *Suppl. 7*, 71 (1987)
Saccharin   *22*, 111 (1980) (*corr. 42*, 259);
                                                             Suppl. 7, 334 (1987)
Safrole   *1*, 169 (1972); *10*, 231 (1976);
                                                             Suppl. 7, 71 (1987)

The sawmill industry (including logging) (*see* The lumber and
   sawmill industry (including logging))
Scarlet Red   *8*, 217 (1975); *Suppl. 7*, 71 (1987)
Selenium and selenium compounds   *9*, 245 (1975) (*corr. 42*, 255);
                                                             Suppl. 7, 71 (1987)

Selenium dioxide (*see* Selenium and selenium compounds)
Selenium oxide (*see* Selenium and selenium compounds)
Semicarbazide hydrochloride   *12*, 209 (1976) (*corr. 42*, 256);
                                                             Suppl. 7, 71 (1987)

Senecio jacobaea L. (*see* Pyrrolizidine alkaloids)
Senecio longilobus (*see* Pyrrolizidine alkaloids)
Seneciphylline   *10*, 319, 335 (1976); *Suppl. 7*, 71
                                                             (1987)
Senkirkine   *10*, 327 (1976); *31*, 231 (1983);
                                                             Suppl. 7, 71 (1987)
Sepiolite   *42*, 175 (1987); *Suppl. 7*, 71 (1987)
Sequential oral contraceptives (*see also* Oestrogens, progestins   *Suppl. 7*, 296 (1987)
   and combinations)
Shale-oils   *35*, 161 (1985); *Suppl. 7*, 339 (1987)
Shikimic acid (*see also* Bracken fern)   *40*, 55 (1986); *Suppl. 7*, 71 (1987)
Shoe manufacture and repair (*see* Boot and shoe manufacture
   and repair)
Silica (*see also* Amorphous silica; Crystalline silica)   *42*, 39 (1987)
Simazine   *53*, 495
Slagwool (*see* Man-made mineral fibres)
Sodium arsenate (*see* Arsenic and arsenic compounds)
Sodium arsenite (*see* Arsenic and arsenic compounds)
Sodium cacodylate (*see* Arsenic and arsenic compounds)
Sodium chlorite   *52*, 145 (1991)
Sodium chromate (*see* Chromium and chromium compounds)
Sodium cyclamate (*see* Cyclamates)
Sodium dichromate (*see* Chromium and chromium compounds)
Sodium diethyldithiocarbamate   *12*, 217 (1976); *Suppl. 7*, 71 (1987)
Sodium equilin sulphate (*see* Conjugated oestrogens)
Sodium fluoride (*see* Fluorides)
Sodium monofluorophosphate (*see* Fluorides)
Sodium oestrone sulphate (*see* Conjugated oestrogens)
Sodium *ortho*-phenylphenate (*see also ortho*-Phenylphenol) *30*, 329 (1983); *Suppl. 7*, 392 (1987)
Sodium saccharin (*see* Saccharin)
Sodium selenate (*see* Selenium and selenium compounds)
Sodium selenite (*see* Selenium and selenium compounds)
Sodium silicofluoride (*see* Fluorides)

Soots — *3*, 22 (1973); *35*, 219 (1985); *Suppl. 7*, 343 (1987)

Spironolactone — *24*, 259 (1980); *Suppl. 7*, 344 (1987)
Stannous fluoride (*see* Fluorides)
Steel founding (*see* Iron and steel founding)
Sterigmatocystin — *1*, 175 (1972); *10*, 245 (1976); *Suppl. 7*, 72 (1987)

Steroidal oestrogens (*see also* Oestrogens, progestins and combinations) — *Suppl. 7*, 280 (1987)
Streptozotocin — *4*, 221 (1974); *17*, 337 (1978); *Suppl. 7*, 72 (1987)

Strobane® (*see* Terpene polychlorinates)
Strontium chromate (*see* Chromium and chromium compounds)
Styrene — *19*, 231 (1979) (*corr. 42*, 258); *Suppl. 7*, 345 (1987)

Styrene–acrylonitrile copolymers — *19*, 97 (1979); *Suppl. 7*, 72 (1987)
Styrene–butadiene copolymers — *19*, 252 (1979); *Suppl. 7*, 72 (1987)
Styrene oxide — *11*, 201 (1976); *19*, 275 (1979); *36*, 245 (1985); *Suppl. 7*, 72 (1987)

Succinic anhydride — *15*, 265 (1977); *Suppl. 7*, 72 (1987)
Sudan I — *8*, 225 (1975); *Suppl. 7*, 72 (1987)
Sudan II — *8*, 233 (1975); *Suppl. 7*, 72 (1987)
Sudan III — *8*, 241 (1975); *Suppl. 7*, 72 (1987)
Sudan Brown RR — *8*, 249 (1975); *Suppl. 7*, 72 (1987)
Sudan Red 7B — *8*, 253 (1975); *Suppl. 7*, 72 (1987)
Sulfafurazole — *24*, 275 (1980); *Suppl. 7*, 347 (1987)
Sulfallate — *30*, 283 (1983); *Suppl. 7*, 72 (1987)
Sulfamethoxazole — *24*, 285 (1980); *Suppl. 7*, 348 (1987)
Sulphisoxazole (*see* Sulfafurazole)
Sulphur mustard (*see* Mustard gas)
Sunset Yellow FCF — *8*, 257 (1975); *Suppl. 7*, 72 (1987)
Symphytine — *31*, 239 (1983); *Suppl. 7*, 72 (1987)

T

2,4,5-T (*see also* Chlorophenoxy herbicides; Chlorophenoxy herbicides, occupational exposures to) — *15*, 273 (1977)
Talc — *42*, 185 (1987); *Suppl. 7*, 349 (1987)
Tannic acid — *10*, 253 (1976) (*corr. 42*, 255); *Suppl. 7*, 72 (1987)

Tannins (*see also* Tannic acid) — *10*, 254 (1976); *Suppl. 7*, 72 (1987)
TCDD (*see* 2,3,7,8-Tetrachlorodibenzo-*para*-dioxin)
TDE (*see* DDT)
Tea — *51*, 207 (1991)
Terpene polychlorinates — *5*, 219 (1974); *Suppl. 7*, 72 (1987)
Testosterone (*see also* Androgenic (anabolic) steroids) — *6*, 209 (1974); *21*, 519 (1979)
Testosterone oenanthate (*see* Testosterone)
Testosterone propionate (*see* Testosterone)
2,2′,5,5′-Tetrachlorobenzidine — *27*, 141 (1982); *Suppl. 7*, 72 (1987)
2,3,7,8-Tetrachlorodibenzo-*para*-dioxin — *15*, 41 (1977); *Suppl. 7*, 350 (1987)
1,1,1,2-Tetrachloroethane — *41*, 87 (1986); *Suppl. 7*, 72 (1987)
1,1,2,2-Tetrachloroethane — *20*, 477 (1979); *Suppl. 7*, 354 (1987)

Tetrachloroethylene   *20*, 491 (1979); *Suppl. 7*, 355 (1987)
2,3,4,6-Tetrachlorophenol (*see* Chlorophenols; Chlorophenols,
   occupational exposures to)
Tetrachlorvinphos   *30*, 197 (1983); *Suppl. 7*, 72 (1987)
Tetraethyllead (*see* Lead and lead compounds)
Tetrafluoroethylene   *19*, 285 (1979); *Suppl. 7*, 72 (1987)
Tetrakis(hydroxymethyl) phosphonium salts   *48*, 95 (1990)
Tetramethyllead (*see* Lead and lead compounds)
Textile manufacturing industry, exposures in   *48*, 215 (1990) (*corr. 51*, 483)
Theobromine   *51*, 421 (1991)
Theophylline   *51*, 391 (1991)
Thioacetamide   *7*, 77 (1974); *Suppl. 7*, 72 (1987)
4,4'-Thiodianiline   *16*, 343 (1978); *27*, 147 (1982);
                                                               Suppl. 7, 72 (1987)
Thiotepa   *9*, 85 (1975); *Suppl. 7*, 368 (1987);
                                                               50, 123 (1990)
Thiouracil   *7*, 85 (1974); *Suppl. 7*, 72 (1987)
Thiourea   *7*, 95 (1974); *Suppl. 7*, 72 (1987)
Thiram   *12*, 225 (1976); *Suppl. 7*, 72 (1987)
                                                               53, 403
Titanium dioxide   *47*, 307 (1989)
Tobacco habits other than smoking (*see* Tobacco products,
   smokeless)
Tobacco products, smokeless   *37* (1985) (*corr. 42*, 263; *52*, 513);
                                                               Suppl. 7, 357 (1987)
Tobacco smoke   *38* (1986) (*corr. 42*, 263); *Suppl. 7*,
                                                               357 (1987)
Tobacco smoking (*see* Tobacco smoke)
ortho-Tolidine (*see* 3,3'-Dimethylbenzidine)
2,4-Toluene diisocyanate (*see also* Toluene diisocyanates)   *19*, 303 (1979); *39*, 287 (1986)
2,6-Toluene diisocyanate (*see also* Toluene diisocyanates)   *19*, 303 (1979); *39*, 289 (1986)
Toluene   *47*, 79 (1989)
Toluene diisocyanates   *39*, 287 (1986) (*corr. 42*, 264);
                                                               Suppl. 7, 72 (1987)
Toluenes, α-chlorinated (*see* α-Chlorinated toluenes)
ortho-Toluenesulphonamide (*see* Saccharin)
ortho-Toluidine   *16*, 349 (1978); *27*, 155 (1982);
                                                               Suppl. 7, 362 (1987)
Toxaphene   *20*, 327 (1979); *Suppl. 7*, 72 (1987)
Tremolite (*see* Asbestos)
Treosulphan   *26*, 341 (1981); *Suppl. 7*, 363 (1987)
Triaziquone (*see* Tris(aziridinyl)-*para*-benzoquinone)
Trichlorfon   *30*, 207 (1983); *Suppl. 7*, 73 (1987)
Trichlormethine   *9*, 229 (1975); *Suppl. 7*, 73 (1987);
                                                               50, 143 (1990)
Trichloroacetonitrile (*see* Halogenated acetonitriles)
1,1,1-Trichloroethane   *20*, 515 (1979); *Suppl. 7*, 73 (1987)
1,1,2-Trichloroethane   *20*, 533 (1979); *Suppl. 7*, 73 (1987);
                                                               52, 337 (1991)
Trichloroethylene   *11*, 263 (1976); *20*, 545 (1979);
                                                               Suppl. 7, 364 (1987)

U

V

Vinyl fluoride   *39*, 147 (1986); *Suppl. 7*, 73 (1987)
Vinylidene chloride   *19*, 439 (1979); *39*, 195 (1986);
                                                    Suppl. 7, 376 (1987)
Vinylidene chloride–vinyl chloride copolymers   *19*, 448 (1979) (*corr. 42*, 258);
                                                    Suppl. 7, 73 (1987)
Vinylidene fluoride   *39*, 227 (1986); *Suppl. 7*, 73 (1987)
N-Vinyl-2-pyrrolidone   *19*, 461 (1979); *Suppl. 7*, 73 (1987)

W

Welding   *49*, 447 (1990) (*corr. 52*, 513)
Wollastonite   *42*, 145 (1987); *Suppl. 7*, 377 (1987)
Wood industries   *25* (1981); *Suppl. 7*, 378 (1987)

X

Xylene   *47*, 125 (1989)
2,4–Xylidine   *16*, 367 (1978); *Suppl. 7*, 74 (1987)
2,5–Xylidine   *16*, 377 (1978); *Suppl. 7*, 74 (1987)

Y

Yellow AB   *8*, 279 (1975); *Suppl. 7*, 74 (1987)
Yellow OB   *8*, 287 (1975); *Suppl. 7*, 74 (1987)

Z

Zearalenone   *31*, 279 (1983); *Suppl. 7*, 74 (1987)
Zectran   *12*, 237 (1976); *Suppl. 7*, 74 (1987)
Zinc beryllium silicate (*see* Beryllium and beryllium compounds)
Zinc chromate (*see* Chromium and chromium compounds)
Zinc chromate hydroxide (*see* Chromium and chromium
    compounds)
Zinc potassium chromate (*see* Chromium and chromium
    compounds)
Zinc yellow (*see* Chromium and chromium compounds)
Zineb   *12*, 245 (1976); *Suppl. 7*, 74 (1987)
Ziram   *12*, 259 (1976); *Suppl. 7*, 74 (1987);
                                                    53, 423

PUBLICATIONS OF THE INTERNATIONAL
AGENCY FOR RESEARCH ON CANCER
Scientific Publications Series

(Available from Oxford University Press through local bookshops)

No. 1 **Liver Cancer**
1971; 176 pages (*out of print*)

No. 2 **Oncogenesis and Herpesviruses**
Edited by P.M. Biggs, G. de-Thé and L.N. Payne
1972; 515 pages (*out of print*)

No. 3 **N-Nitroso Compounds: Analysis and Formation**
Edited by P. Bogovski, R. Preussman and E.A. Walker
1972; 140 pages (*out of print*)

No. 4 **Transplacental Carcinogenesis**
Edited by L. Tomatis and U. Mohr
1973; 181 pages (*out of print*)

No. 5/6 **Pathology of Tumours in Laboratory Animals, Volume 1, Tumours of the Rat**
Edited by V.S. Turusov
1973/1976; 533 pages; £50.00

No. 7 **Host Environment Interactions in the Etiology of Cancer in Man**
Edited by R. Doll and I. Vodopija
1973; 464 pages; £32.50

No. 8 **Biological Effects of Asbestos**
Edited by P. Bogovski, J.C. Gilson, V. Timbrell and J.C. Wagner
1973; 346 pages (*out of print*)

No. 9 **N-Nitroso Compounds in the Environment**
Edited by P. Bogovski and E.A. Walker
1974; 243 pages; £21.00

No. 10 **Chemical Carcinogenesis Essays**
Edited by R. Montesano and L. Tomatis
1974; 230 pages (*out of print*)

No. 11 **Oncogenesis and Herpesviruses II**
Edited by G. de-Thé, M.A. Epstein and H. zur Hausen
1975; Part I: 511 pages
Part II: 403 pages; £65.00

No. 12 **Screening Tests in Chemical Carcinogenesis**
Edited by R. Montesano, H. Bartsch and L. Tomatis
1976; 666 pages; £45.00

No. 13 **Environmental Pollution and Carcinogenic Risks**
Edited by C. Rosenfeld and W. Davis
1975; 441 pages (*out of print*)

No. 14 **Environmental N-Nitroso Compounds. Analysis and Formation**
Edited by E.A. Walker, P. Bogovski and L. Griciute
1976; 512 pages; £37.50

No. 15 **Cancer Incidence in Five Continents, Volume III**
Edited by J.A.H. Waterhouse, C. Muir, P. Correa and J. Powell
1976; 584 pages; (*out of print*)

No. 16 **Air Pollution and Cancer in Man**
Edited by U. Mohr, D. Schmähl and L. Tomatis
1977; 328 pages (*out of print*)

No. 17 **Directory of On-going Research in Cancer Epidemiology 1977**
Edited by C.S. Muir and G. Wagner
1977; 599 pages (*out of print*)

No. 18 **Environmental Carcinogens. Selected Methods of Analysis. Volume 1: Analysis of Volatile Nitrosamines in Food**
Editor-in-Chief: H. Egan
1978; 212 pages (*out of print*)

No. 19 **Environmental Aspects of N-Nitroso Compounds**
Edited by E.A. Walker, M. Castegnaro, L. Griciute and R.E. Lyle
1978; 561 pages (*out of print*)

No. 20 **Nasopharyngeal Carcinoma: Etiology and Control**
Edited by G. de-Thé and Y. Ito
1978; 606 pages (*out of print*)

No. 21 **Cancer Registration and its Techniques**
Edited by R. MacLennan, C. Muir, R. Steinitz and A. Winkler
1978; 235 pages; £35.00

No. 22 **Environmental Carcinogens. Selected Methods of Analysis. Volume 2: Methods for the Measurement of Vinyl Chloride in Poly(vinyl chloride), Air, Water and Foodstuffs**
Editor-in-Chief: H. Egan
1978; 142 pages (*out of print*)

No. 23 **Pathology of Tumours in Laboratory Animals. Volume II: Tumours of the Mouse**
Editor-in-Chief: V.S. Turusov
1979; 669 pages (*out of print*)

No. 24 **Oncogenesis and Herpesviruses III**
Edited by G. de-Thé, W. Henle and F. Rapp
1978; Part I: 580 pages, Part II: 512 pages (*out of print*)

Prices, valid for September 1991, are subject to change without notice

List of IARC Publications

No. 25 **Carcinogenic Risk. Strategies for Intervention**
Edited by W. Davis and
C. Rosenfeld
1979; 280 pages (*out of print*)

No. 26 **Directory of On-going Research in Cancer Epidemiology 1978**
Edited by C.S. Muir and G. Wagner
1978; 550 pages (*out of print*)

No. 27 **Molecular and Cellular Aspects of Carcinogen Screening Tests**
Edited by R. Montesano,
H. Bartsch and L. Tomatis
1980; 372 pages; £29.00

No. 28 **Directory of On-going Research in Cancer Epidemiology 1979**
Edited by C.S. Muir and G. Wagner
1979; 672 pages (*out of print*)

No. 29 **Environmental Carcinogens. Selected Methods of Analysis. Volume 3: Analysis of Polycyclic Aromatic Hydrocarbons in Environmental Samples**
Editor-in-Chief: H. Egan
1979; 240 pages (*out of print*)

No. 30 **Biological Effects of Mineral Fibres**
Editor-in-Chief: J.C. Wagner
1980; Volume 1: 494 pages; Volume 2: 513 pages; £65.00

No. 31 **N-Nitroso Compounds: Analysis, Formation and Occurrence**
Edited by E.A. Walker, L. Griciute,
M. Castegnaro and M. Börzsönyi
1980; 835 pages (*out of print*)

No. 32 **Statistical Methods in Cancer Research. Volume 1. The Analysis of Case-control Studies**
By N.E. Breslow and N.E. Day
1980; 338 pages; £20.00

No. 33 **Handling Chemical Carcinogens in the Laboratory**
Edited by R. Montesano et al.
1979; 32 pages (*out of print*)

No. 34 **Pathology of Tumours in Laboratory Animals. Volume III. Tumours of the Hamster**
Editor-in-Chief: V.S. Turusov
1982; 461 pages; £39.00

No. 35 **Directory of On-going Research in Cancer Epidemiology 1980**
Edited by C.S. Muir and G. Wagner
1980; 660 pages (*out of print*)

No. 36 **Cancer Mortality by Occupation and Social Class 1851-1971**
Edited by W.P.D. Logan
1982; 253 pages; £22.50

No. 37 **Laboratory Decontamination and Destruction of Aflatoxins B_1, B_2, G_1, G_2 in Laboratory Wastes**
Edited by M. Castegnaro et al.
1980; 56 pages; £6.50

No. 38 **Directory of On-going Research in Cancer Epidemiology 1981**
Edited by C.S. Muir and G. Wagner
1981; 696 pages (*out of print*)

No. 39 **Host Factors in Human Carcinogenesis**
Edited by H. Bartsch and
B. Armstrong
1982; 583 pages; £46.00

No. 40 **Environmental Carcinogens. Selected Methods of Analysis. Volume 4: Some Aromatic Amines and Azo Dyes in the General and Industrial Environment**
Edited by L. Fishbein,
M. Castegnaro, I.K. O'Neill and
H. Bartsch
1981; 347 pages; £29.00

No. 41 **N-Nitroso Compounds: Occurrence and Biological Effects**
Edited by H. Bartsch, I.K. O'Neill,
M. Castegnaro and M. Okada
1982; 755 pages; £48.00

No. 42 **Cancer Incidence in Five Continents, Volume IV**
Edited by J. Waterhouse, C. Muir,
K. Shanmugaratnam and J. Powell
1982; 811 pages (*out of print*)

No. 43 **Laboratory Decontamination and Destruction of Carcinogens in Laboratory Wastes: Some N-Nitrosamines**
Edited by M. Castegnaro et al.
1982; 73 pages; £7.50

No. 44 **Environmental Carcinogens. Selected Methods of Analysis. Volume 5: Some Mycotoxins**
Edited by L. Stoloff, M. Castegnaro,
P. Scott, I.K. O'Neill and H. Bartsch
1983; 455 pages; £29.00

No. 45 **Environmental Carcinogens. Selected Methods of Analysis. Volume 6: N-Nitroso Compounds**
Edited by R. Preussmann, I.K.
O'Neill, G. Eisenbrand, B.
Spiegelhalder and H. Bartsch
1983; 508 pages; £29.00

No. 46 **Directory of On-going Research in Cancer Epidemiology 1982**
Edited by C.S. Muir and G. Wagner
1982; 722 pages (*out of print*)

No. 47 **Cancer Incidence in Singapore 1968–1977**
Edited by K. Shanmugaratnam,
H.P. Lee and N.E. Day
1983; 171 pages (*out of print*)

No. 48 **Cancer Incidence in the USSR (2nd Revised Edition)**
Edited by N.P. Napalkov,
G.F. Tserkovny, V.M. Merabishvili,
D.M. Parkin, M. Smans and
C.S. Muir
1983; 75 pages; £12.00

No. 49 **Laboratory Decontamination and Destruction of Carcinogens in Laboratory Wastes: Some Polycyclic Aromatic Hydrocarbons**
Edited by M. Castegnaro et al.
1983; 87 pages; £9.00

No. 50 **Directory of On-going Research in Cancer Epidemiology 1983**
Edited by C.S. Muir and G. Wagner
1983; 731 pages (*out of print*)

No. 51 **Modulators of Experimental Carcinogenesis**
Edited by V. Turusov and R.
Montesano
1983; 307 pages; £22.50

List of IARC Publications

No. 52 Second Cancers in Relation to Radiation Treatment for Cervical Cancer: Results of a Cancer Registry Collaboration
Edited by N.E. Day and J.C. Boice, Jr
1984; 207 pages; £20.00

No. 53 Nickel in the Human Environment
Editor-in-Chief: F.W. Sunderman, Jr
1984; 529 pages; £41.00

No. 54 Laboratory Decontamination and Destruction of Carcinogens in Laboratory Wastes: Some Hydrazines
Edited by M. Castegnaro et al.
1983; 87 pages; £9.00

No. 55 Laboratory Decontamination and Destruction of Carcinogens in Laboratory Wastes: Some N-Nitrosamides
Edited by M. Castegnaro et al.
1984; 66 pages; £7.50

No. 56 Models, Mechanisms and Etiology of Tumour Promotion
Edited by M. Börzsönyi, N.E. Day, K. Lapis and H. Yamasaki
1984; 532 pages; £42.00

No. 57 N-Nitroso Compounds: Occurrence, Biological Effects and Relevance to Human Cancer
Edited by I.K. O'Neill, R.C. von Borstel, C.T. Miller, J. Long and H. Bartsch
1984; 1013 pages; £80.00

No. 58 Age-related Factors in Carcinogenesis
Edited by A. Likhachev, V. Anisimov and R. Montesano
1985; 288 pages; £20.00

No. 59 Monitoring Human Exposure to Carcinogenic and Mutagenic Agents
Edited by A. Berlin, M. Draper, K. Hemminki and H. Vainio
1984; 457 pages; £27.50

No. 60 Burkitt's Lymphoma: A Human Cancer Model
Edited by G. Lenoir, G. O'Conor and C.L.M. Olweny
1985; 484 pages; £29.00

No. 61 Laboratory Decontamination and Destruction of Carcinogens in Laboratory Wastes: Some Haloethers
Edited by M. Castegnaro et al.
1985; 55 pages; £7.50

No. 62 Directory of On-going Research in Cancer Epidemiology 1984
Edited by C.S. Muir and G. Wagner
1984; 717 pages (out of print)

No. 63 Virus-associated Cancers in Africa
Edited by A.O. Williams, G.T. O'Conor, G.B. de-Thé and C.A. Johnson
1984; 773 pages; £22.00

No. 64 Laboratory Decontamination and Destruction of Carcinogens in Laboratory Wastes: Some Aromatic Amines and 4-Nitrobiphenyl
Edited by M. Castegnaro et al.
1985; 84 pages; £6.95

No. 65 Interpretation of Negative Epidemiological Evidence for Carcinogenicity
Edited by N.J. Wald and R. Doll
1985; 232 pages; £20.00

No. 66 The Role of the Registry in Cancer Control
Edited by D.M. Parkin, G. Wagner and C.S. Muir
1985; 152 pages; £10.00

No. 67 Transformation Assay of Established Cell Lines: Mechanisms and Application
Edited by T. Kakunaga and H. Yamasaki
1985; 225 pages; £20.00

No. 68 Environmental Carcinogens. Selected Methods of Analysis. Volume 7. Some Volatile Halogenated Hydrocarbons
Edited by L. Fishbein and I.K. O'Neill
1985; 479 pages; £42.00

No. 69 Directory of On-going Research in Cancer Epidemiology 1985
Edited by C.S. Muir and G. Wagner
1985; 745 pages; £22.00

No. 70 The Role of Cyclic Nucleic Acid Adducts in Carcinogenesis and Mutagenesis
Edited by B. Singer and H. Bartsch
1986; 467 pages; £40.00

No. 71 Environmental Carcinogens. Selected Methods of Analysis. Volume 8: Some Metals: As, Be, Cd, Cr, Ni, Pb, Se Zn
Edited by I.K. O'Neill, P. Schuller and L. Fishbein
1986; 485 pages; £42.00

No. 72 Atlas of Cancer in Scotland, 1975–1980. Incidence and Epidemiological Perspective
Edited by I. Kemp, P. Boyle, M. Smans and C.S. Muir
1985; 285 pages; £35.00

No. 73 Laboratory Decontamination and Destruction of Carcinogens in Laboratory Wastes: Some Antineoplastic Agents
Edited by M. Castegnaro et al.
1985; 163 pages; £10.00

No. 74 Tobacco: A Major International Health Hazard
Edited by D. Zaridze and R. Peto
1986; 324 pages; £20.00

No. 75 Cancer Occurrence in Developing Countries
Edited by D.M. Parkin
1986; 339 pages; £20.00

No. 76 Screening for Cancer of the Uterine Cervix
Edited by M. Hakama, A.B. Miller and N.E. Day
1986; 315 pages; £25.00

List of IARC Publications

No. 77 **Hexachlorobenzene:**
Proceedings of an International
Symposium
Edited by C.R. Morris and
J.R.P. Cabral
1986; 668 pages; £50.00

No. 78 **Carcinogenicity of Alkylating**
Cytostatic Drugs
Edited by D. Schmähl and
J.M. Kaldor
1986; 337 pages; £25.00

No. 79 **Statistical Methods in**
Cancer Research. Volume III: The
Design and Analysis of Long-term
Animal Experiments
By J.J. Gart, D. Krewski, P.N. Lee,
R.E. Tarone and J. Wahrendorf
1986; 213 pages; £20.00

No. 80 **Directory of On-going**
Research in Cancer Epidemiology
1986
Edited by C.S. Muir and G. Wagner
1986; 805 pages; £22.00

No. 81 **Environmental Carcinogens:**
Methods of Analysis and Exposure
Measurement. Volume 9: Passive
Smoking
Edited by I.K. O'Neill,
K.D. Brunnemann, B. Dodet and D.
Hoffmann
1987; 383 pages; £35.00

No. 82 **Statistical Methods in**
Cancer Research. Volume II: The
Design and Analysis of Cohort
Studies
By N.E. Breslow and N.E. Day
1987; 404 pages; £30.00

No. 83 **Long-term and Short-term**
Assays for Carcinogens: A Critical
Appraisal
Edited by R. Montesano,
H. Bartsch, H. Vainio, J. Wilbourn
and H. Yamasaki
1986; 575 pages; £48.00

No. 84 **The Relevance of *N*-Nitroso**
Compounds to Human Cancer:
Exposure and Mechanisms
Edited by H. Bartsch, I.K. O'Neill
and R. Schulte- Hermann
1987; 671 pages; £50.00

No. 85 **Environmental Carcinogens:**
Methods of Analysis and Exposure
Measurement. Volume 10: Benzene
and Alkylated Benzenes
Edited by L. Fishbein and
I.K. O'Neill
1988; 327 pages; £35.00

No. 86 **Directory of On-going**
Research in Cancer Epidemiology
1987
Edited by D.M. Parkin and
J. Wahrendorf
1987; 676 pages; £22.00

No. 87 **International Incidence of**
Childhood Cancer
Edited by D.M. Parkin, C.A. Stiller,
C.A. Bieber, G.J. Draper,
B. Terracini and J.L. Young
1988; 401 pages; £35.00

No. 88 **Cancer Incidence in Five**
Continents Volume V
Edited by C. Muir, J. Waterhouse, T.
Mack, J. Powell and S. Whelan
1987; 1004 pages; £50.00

No. 89 **Method for Detecting DNA**
Damaging Agents in Humans:
Applications in Cancer Epidemiology
and Prevention
Edited by H. Bartsch, K. Hemminki
and I.K. O'Neill
1988; 518 pages; £45.00

No. 90 **Non-occupational Exposure**
to Mineral Fibres
Edited by J. Bignon, J. Peto and
R. Saracci
1989; 500 pages; £45.00

No. 91 **Trends in Cancer Incidence**
in Singapore 1968–1982
Edited by H.P. Lee , N.E. Day and
K. Shanmugaratnam
1988; 160 pages; £25.00

No. 92 **Cell Differentiation, Genes**
and Cancer
Edited by T. Kakunaga,
T. Sugimura, L. Tomatis and
H. Yamasaki
1988; 204 pages; £25.00

No. 93 **Directory of On-going**
Research in Cancer Epidemiology
1988
Edited by M. Coleman and
J. Wahrendorf
1988; 662 pages (*out of print*)

No. 94 **Human Papillomavirus and**
Cervical Cancer
Edited by N. Muñoz, F.X. Bosch and
O.M. Jensen
1989; 154 pages; £19.00

No. 95 **Cancer Registration:**
Principles and Methods
Edited by O.M. Jensen,
D.M. Parkin, R. MacLennan,
C.S. Muir and R. Skeet
1991; 288 pages; £28.00

No. 96 **Perinatal and**
Multigeneration Carcinogenesis
Edited by N.P. Napalkov,
J.M. Rice, L. Tomatis and
H. Yamasaki
1989; 436 pages; £48.00

No. 97 **Occupational Exposure to**
Silica and Cancer Risk
Edited by L. Simonato,
A.C. Fletcher, R. Saracci and
T. Thomas
1990; 124 pages; £19.00

No. 98 **Cancer Incidence in Jewish**
Migrants to Israel, 1961–1981
Edited by R. Steinitz, D.M. Parkin,
J.L. Young, C.A. Bieber and
L. Katz
1989; 320 pages; £30.00

No. 99 **Pathology of Tumours in**
Laboratory Animals, Second
Edition, Volume 1, Tumours of the
Rat
Edited by V.S. Turusov and
U. Mohr
740 pages; £85.00

No. 100 **Cancer: Causes,**
Occurrence and Control
Editor-in-Chief L. Tomatis
1990; 352 pages; £24.00

List of IARC Publications

No. 101 **Directory of On-going Research in Cancer Epidemiology 1989/90**
Edited by M. Coleman and J. Wahrendorf
1989; 818 pages; £36.00

No. 102 **Patterns of Cancer in Five Continents**
Edited by S.L. Whelan and D.M. Parkin
1990; 162 pages; £25.00

No. 103 **Evaluating Effectiveness of Primary Prevention of Cancer**
Edited by M. Hakama, V. Beral, J.W. Cullen and D.M. Parkin
1990; 250 pages; £32.00

No. 104 **Complex Mixtures and Cancer Risk**
Edited by H. Vainio, M. Sorsa and A.J. McMichael
1990; 442 pages; £38.00

No. 105 **Relevance to Human Cancer of N-Nitroso Compounds, Tobacco Smoke and Mycotoxins**
Edited by I.K. O'Neill, J. Chen and H. Bartsch
1991; 614 pages; £70.00

No. 106 **Atlas of Cancer Incidence in the German Democratic Republic**
Edited by W.H. Mehnert, M. Smans and C.S. Muir
Publ. due 1992; c.328 pages; £42.00

No. 107 **Atlas of Cancer Mortality in the European Economic Community**
Edited by M. Smans, C.S. Muir and P. Boyle
Publ. due 1991; approx. 230 pages; £35.00

No. 108 **Environmental Carcinogens: Methods of Analysis and Exposure Measurement. Volume 11: Polychlorinated Dioxins and Dibenzofurans**
Edited by C. Rappe, H.R. Buser, B. Dodet and I.K. O'Neill
1991; 426 pages; £45.00

No. 109 **Environmental Carcinogens: Methods of Analysis and Exposure Measurement. Volume 12: Indoor Air Contaminants**
Edited by B. Seifert, B. Dodet and I.K. O'Neill
Publ. due 1992; approx. 400 pages

No. 110 **Directory of On-going Research in Cancer Epidemiology 1991**
Edited by M. Coleman and J. Wahrendorf
1991; 753 pages; £38.00

No. 111 **Pathology of Tumours in Laboratory Animals, Second Edition, Volume 2, Tumours of the Mouse**
Edited by V.S. Turusov and U. Mohr
Publ. due 1992; approx. 500 pages

No. 112 **Autopsy in Epidemiology and Medical Research**
Edited by E. Riboli and M. Delendi
1991; 288 pages; £25.00

No. 113 **Laboratory Decontamination and Destruction of Carcinogens in Laboratory Wastes: Some Mycotoxins**
Edited by M. Castegnaro, J. Barek, J.-M. Frémy, M. Lafontaine, M. Miraglia, E.B. Sansone and G.M. Telling
1991; 64 pages; £11.00

No. 114 **Laboratory Decontamination and Destruction of Carcinogens in Laboratory Wastes: Some Polycyclic Heterocyclic Hydrocarbons**
Edited by M. Castegnaro, J. Barek, J. Jacob, U. Kirso, M. Lafontaine, E.B. Sansone, G.M. Telling and T. Vu Duc
1991; 50 pages; £8.00

No. 115 **Mycotoxins, Endemic Nephropathy and Urinary Tract Tumours**
Edited by M. Castegnaro, R. Plestina, G. Dirheimer, I.N. Chernozemsky and H Bartsch
1991; 340 pages; £45.00

No. 117 **Directory of On-going Research in Cancer Epidemiology 1991**
Edited by M. Coleman, J. Wahrendorf & E. Démaret
1992; 773 pages; £42.00

IARC MONOGRAPHS ON THE EVALUATION OF CARCINOGENIC RISKS TO HUMANS

(Available from booksellers through the network of WHO Sales Agents)

Volume 1 Some Inorganic Substances, Chlorinated Hydrocarbons, Aromatic Amines, *N*-Nitroso Compounds, and Natural Products
1972; 184 pages (*out of print*)

Volume 2 Some Inorganic and Organometallic Compounds
1973; 181 pages (*out of print*)

Volume 3 Certain Polycyclic Aromatic Hydrocarbons and Heterocyclic Compounds
1973; 271 pages (*out of print*)

Volume 4 Some Aromatic Amines, Hydrazine and Related Substances, *N*-Nitroso Compounds and Miscellaneous Alkylating Agents
1974; 286 pages; Sw. fr. 18

Volume 5 Some Organochlorine Pesticides
1974; 241 pages (*out of print*)

Volume 6 Sex Hormones
1974; 243 pages (*out of print*)

Volume 7 Some Anti-Thyroid and Related Substances, Nitrofurans and Industrial Chemicals
1974; 326 pages (*out of print*)

Volume 8 Some Aromatic Azo Compounds
1975; 375 pages; Sw. fr. 36

Volume 9 Some Aziridines, *N*-, *S*- and *O*-Mustards and Selenium
1975; 268 pages; Sw.fr. 27

Volume 10 Some Naturally Occurring Substances
1976; 353 pages (*out of print*)

Volume 11 Cadmium, Nickel, Some Epoxides, Miscellaneous Industrial Chemicals and General Considerations on Volatile Anaesthetics
1976; 306 pages (*out of print*)

Volume 12 Some Carbamates, Thiocarbamates and Carbazides
1976; 282 pages; Sw. fr. 34

Volume 13 Some Miscellaneous Pharmaceutical Substances
1977; 255 pages; Sw. fr. 30

Volume 14 Asbestos
1977; 106 pages (*out of print*)

Volume 15 Some Fumigants, The Herbicides 2,4-D and 2,4,5-T, Chlorinated Dibenzodioxins and Miscellaneous Industrial Chemicals
1977; 354 pages; Sw. fr. 50.

Volume 16 Some Aromatic Amines and Related Nitro Compounds - Hair Dyes, Colouring Agents and Miscellaneous Industrial Chemicals
1978; 400 pages; Sw. fr. 50

Volume 17 Some *N*-Nitroso Compounds
1987; 365 pages; Sw. fr. 50

Volume 18 Polychlorinated Biphenyls and Polybrominated Biphenyls
1978; 140 pages; Sw. fr. 20

Volume 19 Some Monomers, Plastics and Synthetic Elastomers, and Acrolein
1979; 513 pages; Sw. fr. 60

Volume 20 Some Halogenated Hydrocarbons
1979; 609 pages (*out of print*)

Volume 21 Sex Hormones (II)
1979; 583 pages; Sw. fr. 60

Volume 22 Some Non-Nutritive Sweetening Agents
1980; 208 pages; Sw. fr. 25

Volume 23 Some Metals and Metallic Compounds
1980; 438 pages (*out of print*)

Volume 24 Some Pharmaceutical Drugs
1980; 337 pages; Sw. fr. 40

Volume 25 Wood, Leather and Some Associated Industries
1981; 412 pages; Sw. fr. 60

Volume 26 Some Antineoplastic and Immunosuppressive Agents
1981; 411 pages; Sw. fr. 62

Volume 27 Some Aromatic Amines, Anthraquinones and Nitroso Compounds, and Inorganic Fluorides Used in Drinking Water and Dental Preparations
1982; 341 pages; Sw. fr. 40

Volume 28 The Rubber Industry
1982; 486 pages; Sw. fr. 70

Volume 29 Some Industrial Chemicals and Dyestuffs
1982; 416 pages; Sw. fr. 60

Volume 30 Miscellaneous Pesticides
1983; 424 pages; Sw. fr. 60

Volume 31 Some Food Additives, Feed Additives and Naturally Occurring Substances
1983; 314 pages; Sw. fr. 60

Volume 32 Polynuclear Aromatic Compounds, Part 1: Chemical, Environmental and Experimental Data
1984; 477 pages; Sw. fr. 60

Volume 33 Polynuclear Aromatic Compounds, Part 2: Carbon Blacks, Mineral Oils and Some Nitroarenes
1984; 245 pages; Sw. fr. 50

Volume 34 Polynuclear Aromatic Compounds, Part 3: Industrial Exposures in Aluminium Production, Coal Gasification, Coke Production, and Iron and Steel Founding
1984; 219 pages; Sw. fr. 48

Volume 35 Polynuclear Aromatic Compounds, Part 4: Bitumens, Coal-tars and Derived Products, Shale-oils and Soots
1985; 271 pages; Sw. fr. 70

List of IARC Publications

IARC TECHNICAL REPORTS*

No. 1 Cancer in Costa Rica
Edited by R. Sierra,
R. Barrantes, G. Muñoz Leiva, D.M.
Parkin, C.A. Bieber and
N. Muñoz Calero
1988; 124 pages;
Sw. fr. 30.-

**No. 2 SEARCH: A Computer
Package to Assist the Statistical
Analysis of Case-control Studies**
Edited by G.J Macfarlane,
P. Boyle and P. Maisonneuve (in
press)

**No. 3 Cancer Registration in the
European Economic Community**
Edited by M.P. Coleman and
E. Démaret
1988; 188 pages;
Sw. fr. 30.-

**No. 4 Diet, Hormones and Cancer:
Methodological Issues for
Prospective Studies**
Edited by E. Riboli and
R. Saracci
1988; 156 pages;
Sw. fr. 30.-

No. 5 Cancer in the Philippines
Edited by A.V. Laudico,
D. Esteban and D.M. Parkin
1989; 186 pages;
Sw. fr. 30.-

**No. 6 La genèse du Centre
International de Recherche sur le
Cancer**
Par R. Sohier et A.G.B. Sutherland
1990; 104 pages
Sw. fr. 30.-

**No. 7 Epidémiologie du cancer dans
les pays de langue latine**
1990; 310 pages
Sw. fr. 30.-

**No. 8 Comparative Study of
Anti-smoking Legislation in
Countries of the European Economic
Community**
Edited by A. Sasco
1990; c. 80 pages
Sw. fr. 30.-
(English and French editions
available) (in press)

DIRECTORY OF AGENTS BEING TESTED FOR CARCINOGENICITY (Until Vol. 13 Information Bulletin on the Survey of Chemicals Being Tested for Carcinogenicity)*

No. 8 Edited by M.-J. Ghess,
H. Bartsch and L. Tomatis
1979; 604 pages; Sw. fr. 40.-

No. 9 Edited by M.-J. Ghess,
J.D. Wilbourn, H. Bartsch and
L. Tomatis
1981; 294 pages; Sw. fr. 41.-

No. 10 Edited by M.-J. Ghess,
J.D. Wilbourn and H. Bartsch
1982; 362 pages; Sw. fr. 42.-

No. 11 Edited by M.-J. Ghess,
J.D. Wilbourn, H. Vainio and
H. Bartsch
1984; 362 pages; Sw. fr. 50.-

No. 12 Edited by M.-J. Ghess,
J.D. Wilbourn, A. Tossavainen and
H. Vainio
1986; 385 pages; Sw. fr. 50.-

No. 13 Edited by M.-J. Ghess,
J.D. Wilbourn and A. Aitio 1988;
404 pages; Sw. fr. 43.-

No. 14 Edited by M.-J. Ghess,
J.D. Wilbourn and H. Vainio
1990; 370 pages; Sw. fr. 45.-

NON-SERIAL PUBLICATIONS †

Alcool et Cancer
By A. Tuyns (in French only)
1978; 42 pages; Fr. fr. 35.-

**Cancer Morbidity and Causes of
Death Among Danish Brewery
Workers**
By O.M. Jensen
1980; 143 pages; Fr. fr. 75.-

**Directory of Computer Systems Used
in Cancer Registries**
By H.R. Menck and D.M. Parkin
1986; 236 pages; Fr. fr. 50.-

---

* Available from booksellers through the network of WHO sales agents.

†Available directly from IARC